Radiotherapy Physics: in Practice

Second edition

Edited by

J.R. Williams

Consultant Medical Physicist, Western General Hospital, Edinburgh

and

D.I. Thwaites

Consultant Medical Physicist, Western General Hospital, Edinburgh

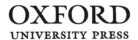

OXFORD

UNIVERSITY PRESS

This book has been printed digitally and produced in a standard specification
in order to ensure its continuing availability

OXFORD
UNIVERSITY PRESS

Great Clarendon Street, Oxford OX2 6DP

Oxford University Press is a department of the University of Oxford.
It furthers the University's objective of excellence in research, scholarship,
and education by publishing world-wide in

Oxford New York

Auckland Bangkok Buenos Aires Cape Town Chennai
Dar es Salaam Delhi Hong Kong Istanbul Karachi Kolkata
Kuala Lumpur Madrid Melbourne Mexico City Mumbai Nairobi
São Paulo Shanghai Taipei Tokyo Toronto

Oxford is a registered trade mark of Oxford University Press
in the UK and in certain other countries

Published in the United States
by Oxford University Press Inc., New York

ISBN 0-19-262878-x

Printed in Great Britain by
Antony Rowe Ltd., Eastbourne

Preface to second edition

Since the first edition of this book was published, there have been significant changes in radiotherapy equipment and techniques, which we have tried to reflect in this revision. Many improvements that have occurred can be traced to developing computer technology. Examples of developments include the routine use of MLCs, the delivery of IMRT, advances in imaging technologies for planning (e.g. MRI, CT-simulator) and for treatment verification (EPIDs). There have been significant changes in dosimetry, which have resulted in new dosimetry protocols.

The basic structure of the book has been retained, except that the longest chapter on treatment planning has been divided into three parts to cover basic and advanced photon therapy, and electron treatments. In recognition of the developing application of quality-management systems to radiotherapy, we have added an extra chapter on this subject.

Sadly, since the first edition of this book was published, Stan Klevenhagen, who was a good friend to us all, has died. We have kept his name as first author on the chapter on kilovoltage X-rays in recognition of his contribution to this work and, more generally, in the field of radiotherapy physics.

We would like to acknowledge all the contributors to this new edition and thank them for their forbearance during the editing process.

J.R. Williams and D.I. Thwaites

Preface to first edition

Radiotherapy or radiation oncology has been one of the principal modalities for the treatment of malignant disease for more than 50 years. From the outset its advancement has depended on the work of physicists and engineers, in particular for the development of high-energy accelerators for X-ray and electron beams, and in the production of radioactive sources. In addition, the clinical application of ionizing radiations for therapy is based on a foundation of dosimetric concepts and instrumentation. Many of these developments have begun with the initiative and active participation of the medical physicist, who is best placed to bring together the requirements of the clinician with the technologies available. An example is the introduction of computerized treatment-planning systems; most commercial systems are based on software written by medical physicists directly involved in the practice of radiotherapy.

The role of the physicist in future developments in radiation oncology will continue. To cite just one example, a current major area of development is concerned with conformal therapy in which the irradiated volume is shaped to fit the tumour-bearing tissue more precisely in three dimensions than could be achieved previously. This requires developments in the control of the treatment unit and in the methods of dose calculation and of treatment verification. In all of these, the contribution of medical physics is essential. The physicist is also closely involved in the routine daily practice of radiotherapy, as a member of the multidisciplinary team, which is necessary to deliver optimized treatment to each individual patient. Medical physics plays a pivotal role in many areas, including treatment equipment, dosimetry, treatment planning, and radiation protection. The physicist is essential to the continuing provision of quality and safety in radiotherapy treatment.

This book is primarily aimed at the trainee physicist and is intended as a practical guide to the subject without going into the background theory, which is adequately covered in other standard texts. Information is given on treatment equipment, particularly the criteria for selection and for the planning of new installations and their acceptance tests, commissioning, and on going quality-control programmes. The background for an understanding of dosimetry protocols is described, as well as their practical implementation. Clinical dosimetry is considered, in terms of both the collection of data and the calculation of dose and treatment planning for the individual patient. Although mainly concerned with external beam therapy, techniques for sealed and unsealed source therapies are also discussed. The importance of quality assurance and the associated quality-control procedures is stressed throughout.

In clinical practice, radiation oncology is a collaborative effort of different groups, in particular radiation oncologists, radiographers, medical physicists, and medical physics technicians. Although the book is mainly intended for physicists who are training in this area of specialization, it should also provide valuable insights for the experienced physicist, as well as for technicians and other specialist staff who need to know more about the technologies and methods underlying their work.

In bringing this book together we would like to thank our colleagues for their encouragement and assistance and in particular our families for their patience and support.

J.R. Williams and D.I. Thwaites

Contents

The colour plates can be found between pp. 142–3

Chapter 3: **Absolute dose determination for high-energy photon and electron beams**
B.J. Mijnheer, D.I. Thwaites, and J.R. Williams

Chapter 6: Kilovoltage X-rays
S.C. Klevenhagen, D.I. Thwaites, and R.J. Aukett   99

Chapter 11: **Treatment verification and *in vivo* dosimetry**

W.P.M. Mayles, S. Heisig, and H.M.O. Mayles   220

List of Contributors

Dr E.G.A. Aird
Medical Physics Department
Mount Vernon Hospital
Northwood
Middlesex HA6 2RN, UK

Dr P.R. Almond
Department of Radiation Oncology
James Graham Brown Cancer Center
University of Louisville
Louisville
Kentucky 40292, USA

Mr R.J. Aukett
Medical Physics Department
Leicester Royal Infirmary
Infirmary Square
Leicester LE1 5WW, UK

Ms S.J. Chittenden
Joint Department of Physics
Royal Marsden NHS Trust and Institute of Cancer Research
Downs Road
Sutton
Surrey SM2 5PT, UK

Dr M.A. Flower
Joint Department of Physics
Royal Marsden NHS Trust and Institute of Cancer Research
Downs Road
Sutton
Surrey SM2 5PT, UK

Mrs S. Heisig
Joint Department of Physics
Royal Marsden NHS Trust and Institute of Cancer Research
Downs Road
Sutton
Surrey SM2 5PT, UK

Dr J.L. Horton
Department of Radiation Physics
The University of Texas
M D Anderson Cancer Center
1515 Holcombe Boulevard
Houston
Texas 77030, USA

Dr K.-A. Johansson
Department of Radiation Physics
Sahlgren Hospital
University of Göteborg
S-413 45 Göteborg, Sweden

Mr T.M. Kehoe
Department of Oncology Physics
Clinical Oncology
Lothian University Hospitals NHS Trust
Western General Hospital
Edinburgh EH4 2XU, UK

Dr K. Mah
Department of Medical Physics
Toronto Sunnybrook Cancer Centre
2075 Bayview Avenue
Toronto M4N 3M5, Canada

Mrs H.M.O. Mayles
Physics Department
Clatterbridge Centre for Oncology
Bebington
Merseyside L63 4JY, UK

Dr W.P.M. Mayles
Physics Department
Clatterbridge Centre for Oncology
Bebington
Merseyside L63 4JY, UK

Dr A.L. McKenzie
Radiotherapy Physics Unit
Bristol Oncology Centre
Horfield Road
Bristol BS2 8ED, UK

Dr S.G. McNee
Department of Clinical Physics and Bioengineering
Beatson Oncology Centre
Western Infimary
Glasgow G11 6NT, UK

Dr B.J. Mijnheer
Radiotherapy Department
The Netherlands Cancer Institute
Plesmanlaan 121
1066CX Amsterdam, The Netherlands

Dr. A.T. Redpath
Department of Oncology Physics
Clinical Oncology
Lothian University Hospitals NHS Trust
Western General Hospital
Edinburgh EH4 2XU, UK

Miss A.M.E. Rembowska
Radiotherapy Physics Department
Royal South Hants Hospital
Brinton's Terrace
Southampton
Hampshire SO14 0YG, UK

Dr G. Sernbo
Department of Radiation Physics
Salgren Hospital
University of Göteborg
S-413 45 Göteborg, Sweden

Dr D.I. Thwaites
Department of Oncology Physics
Clinical Oncology
Lothian University Hospitals NHS Trust
Western General Hospital
Edinburgh EH4 2XU, UK

Dr J. Van Dam
Department of Radiotherapy
University Hospital Gasthuisberg
Herestraat 49
3000 Leuven, Belgium

Mr J. Van Dyk
Department of Clinical Physics
London Regional Cancer Centre
790 Commissioners Road East
London
Ontario N6A 4L6, Canada

Mr J.R. Williams
Department of Medical Physics and
Medical Engineering
Lothian University Hospitals NHS Trust
Western General Hospital
Edinburgh EH4 2XU, UK

Abbreviations

This is a list of common abbreviations used in several chapters in this publication. The Appendix to Chapter 3 includes further abbreviations for national bodies concerned with dosimetry protocols.

AAPM	American Association of Physicists in Medicine
AKR	Air kerma rate
ALARA	As low as reasonably achievable
BEV	Beam's eye view
BIR	British Institute of Radiology
csda	Continuous slowing down approximation
CT	Computerized tomography
CTV	Clinical Target Volume
d_{80}	Depth of 80% dose
DAH	Dose–area histogram
DICOM	Digital imaging and communications in medicine
DRR	Digitally-reconstructed radiograph
$d_{\max}$	Depth of dose maximum
DVH	Dose–volume histogram
EPID	Electronic portal imaging device
ESTRO	European Society for Therapeutic Radiology and Oncology
FWHM	Full width half maximum
GTV	Gross tumour volume
HDR	High dose rate
HVD	Half-value depth
HVL	Half-value layer
IAEA	International Atomic Energy Agency
ICRP	International Commission on Radiological Protection
ICRU	International Commission on Radiation Units and Measurements
IEC	International Electrotechnical Commission
IMRT	Intensity-modulated radiation therapy
IPEM	Institute of Physics and Engineering in Medicine
ISL	Inverse square law
ISO	International Organization for Standardization
LDR	Low dose rate
LQ	Linear–quadratic
MDR	Medium dose rate
MIRD	Medical Internal Radiation Dose
MLC	Multi-leaf collimator
MRI	Magnetic Resonance Imaging
mu	Monitor units
NPL	National Physical Laboratory
OAR	Off–axis ratio
OD	Optical density
ODI	Optical distance indicator
PACS	Picture archive and communication system

PET	Positron emission tomography
PMMA	Polymethylmethacrylate (also known as Perspex; Lucite; Plexiglas)
PSF	Peak scatter factor
PTB	Physikalisch Technische Bundesanstalt
PTV	Planning target volume
QA	Quality assurance
QC	Quality control
SAD	Source–axis distance (isocentre distance)
SAR	Scatter–air ratio
SCD	Source–chamber distance
SMR	Scatter–maximum ratio
SPECT	Single photon emission computed tomography
SSD	Source–surface distance
STT	Segmented treatment table
TAR	Tissue–air ratio
TBI	Total body irradiation
TLD	Thermoluminescent dosimetry
TMR	Tissue–maximum ratio
TPR	Tissue–phantom ratio
TPS	Treatment–planning system
WHO	World Health Organization

Chapter 1
Introduction

J.R. Williams and D.I. Thwaites

1. The development of radiotherapy

The beginnings of radiotherapy followed quickly on the discovery of ionizing radiations. X-rays were identified by Roentgen in 1895 and radioactivity by Becquerel in the following year. It was recognized at a very early stage that these radiations produced dramatic effects on normal tissues and it was a natural progression that within a few years of the discovery of radioactivity the effects of radiation should be investigated on superficial tumours. In the early days, progress in radiation therapy was largely determined by the production of satisfactory sources. The isolation of radium by the Curies was one key to this development, as was the improvement in the technology associated with X-ray production. In parallel with the developments of radiation sources, there came the recognition that it was essential to be able to define and measure the quantity of radiation being delivered. The formation of the International Committee on Radiological Units (ICRU), now called the International Commission on Radiation Units and Measurements, in 1925 was a key element in this area.

The principal advances in radiotherapy have come about since the 1940s. Two of these arose from technological developments, which were given impetus by wartime activities. The first lay in the production of new radionuclides from the reactors and particle accelerators used in high-energy physics and nuclear research. A number of these have been used for both sealed and unsealed source therapy and ^{60}Co is one of the most common sources for external beam therapy. The second major development was the linear accelerator, which was made possible by the technology developed for radar. It has become the most important radiotherapy source.

Whilst these technical developments were taking place, major advances were also proceeding in the clinical arena. Scientific methods were being applied to the analysis of clinical results and to develop a firm basis for treatment of cancer by radiation, notably in Manchester, Paris, Stockholm, and New York. In parallel with this, the science of radiobiology was developing. This began to explain clinical observations, to provide a rationale for clinical methods, and at the same time to suggest improvements in treatment techniques. All of this work was underpinned by increased understanding and formalization of dosimetric methods.

During this period, the hazards of radiation and the need for radiation protection became more clearly understood. It is axiomatic that, from the earliest times, radiotherapists should have been aware of the immediate or deterministic effects because these limit the dose that can be delivered to the tumour site. However, the stochastic effects, such as the induction of cancer, have become more clearly understood, so that treatment by radiation has been increasingly restricted to those patients with life-threatening disease for whom there is no other effective form of therapy (ICRP 1985). There are few non-malignant conditions that are still treated by ionizing radiations. In addition, developments in radiation protection have lead to much tighter controls on the radiation dose that might be received by staff. This has had consequences on the design and operation of treatment equipment and in particular has led to the development of systems for the remote handling of sealed radioactive sources used in brachytherapy.

In the last 25 years it is developments in computer hardware and methods that have had one of the most important influences on the practice of radiotherapy. Although initially they were only seen as calculating machines that could perform the task of treatment plan summation more quickly and accurately than could be achieved by hand, they were soon recognized as an essential aid to the optimization of dose delivery. The role of computers and computing techniques has now spread to all areas of the radiotherapy institute. They are incorporated into equipment control, safety systems, digital imaging systems, communications networks, and patient administration.

2. Radiotherapeutic aims

Tumour cells are those that proliferate readily outside the body's normal control mechanisms. Malignant cancers are those in which the cells are able to metastasize, i.e. to spread from their original site and to invade other tissues. There are many types of tumour cell: some grow together to form a solid mass either within or on the surface of a particular organ or tissue; others (such as leukaemias and lymphomas) are able to move freely round the body in the blood or the lymphatic system. If it is not treated, cancer will inhibit and finally destroy the function of the host tissue or organ.

Cancer therapy is concerned with the removal or killing of the cancer cells and the halting of further proliferation. The main forms of treatment are: surgery for the bulk removal of tumour; drugs both to kill and to prevent proliferation of cancer cells (chemotherapy); harnessing of the body's own defence systems (immunotherapy); and the use of ionizing radiations (radiotherapy). These modalities may be used singly or in combination.

All types of living cell can be killed by ionizing radiation but the dose required to achieve a particular level of cell killing is extremely variable, i.e. cells have different radiosensitivities. The principal problem in radiotherapy is that tumour cells are not treated in isolation. The tumour mass is sited on, or within, a tissue whose function must be conserved following treatment and it is surrounded by healthy structures through which it may be necessary to direct the radiation beam. The tumour mass may also spread and infiltrate some of these tissues. It is inevitable, therefore, that if all the cancer is to be eliminated, some healthy tissues will also receive a high dose.

Radiation killing of individual cells is stochastic, i.e. is statistical in nature, because it depends on the occurrence of individual ionizing events. However, when the effect of radiation on a large collection of cells is considered, whether it is a tumour mass or an organ, the effect is largely deterministic, i.e. there is a dose threshold below which no clinical effect will be observed and a dose above which the effect will be observed in every individual. This is illustrated in Figure 1.1, where two curves are drawn: one for tumour and the other for the limiting normal tissue. Tumours that may be successfully treated by radiotherapy are those in which the tumour curve lies to the left of the curve for the limiting normal tissues, so that the dose required to achieve a high probability of complete regression of the tumour is lower than the dose that produces a significant number of complications in normal tissue.

The figure illustrates the primary aim of radiotherapy, which is to give the highest possible dose to the cancer-bearing tissues and thus the maximum probability of

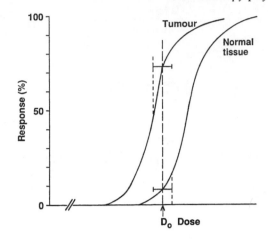

Figure 1.1 Probability of tumour control and normal tissue morbidity against dose. D_0 is the intended treatment dose and the vertical dotted lines indicate the changes in response due to small changes in dose.

complete tumour regression. The dose to the tumour is limited by the need to restrict the dose to normal tissues, so that the probability of clinically significant damage to normal tissue is kept to an acceptable level. There are certain tumours for which these aims are incompatible, e.g. in stomach cancer the radiosensitivity of the normal tissue is much greater than that of the cancer.

In some advanced cancers the aims of radiotherapy may be more limited. Radiotherapy may be used for palliation at lower doses to produce partial tumour regression for temporary symptomatic relief, rather than for radical or curative purposes.

Radiotherapeutic success is most probable when the two curves in Figure 1.1 are widely separated. Optimization of the treatment technique may allow a greater dose to be delivered to the tumour-bearing volume without an increase in dose to the limiting normal tissue. However, it is not possible to reduce the dose to normal tissue if it is infiltrated by tumour. The shape and relative positions of the dose–response curves depend on the overall treatment time and the number of fractions into which it is divided. Optimization of therapy includes the selection of the most appropriate fractionation scheme.

3. Radiotherapy methods

There are three principal routes for the administration of radiotherapy. These are:

(1) external beam therapy;

(2) sealed-source therapy (brachytherapy);

(3) unsealed-source therapy.

3.1 *External beam therapy*

External beam treatment is the most common form of radiotherapy and it will be the principal concern of this book. It is normally performed with photon beams; these are most commonly high-energy X-rays produced by a linear accelerator, but gamma-ray beams from cobalt units and lower energy X-rays in the energy range 50–300 kV may also be used. In addition, megavoltage electron beams, which can be used to treat relatively superficial tumours to a much improved geometrical precision than photons, have become an increasingly used modality. External beam therapy with other particle radiations has been proposed and, in the case of neutrons, extensively tested. Neutrons now appear to offer no therapeutic advantage. Charged particle beams, such as protons and pi-mesons, may offer some clinical benefit due to their pattern of energy deposition. However, they are associated with very expensive generating equipment and their role in radiotherapy has not been established. They will not be considered in this book.

Some of the current developments in external beam therapy arise from the increasing use of computers. They have not only enabled plans to be calculated in three dimensions but are also able to control the treatment unit, so that the high-dose region may be tailored to the target volume in three dimensions. This development is in parallel with those in imaging techniques, such as X-ray computed tomography (CT), which have depended on the revolution in digital computing.

CT allows the radiotherapist to define the target volume much more precisely in two or three dimensions, whilst magnetic resonance imaging (MRI), coupled with CT, is playing an increasingly significant role in the accurate delineation of the tumour volume in specific sites. Other imaging modalities, such as positron emission tomography (PET) are also being applied. In many centres, methods of shaping the high-dose volume (conformal therapy) are being used and developed further, based on static blocks and multi-leaf collimators. These techniques require more sophisticated treatment planning methods and, following the rapid advancement in computer hardware, Monte Carlo calculation methods are now on the brink of being feasible as the basis for routine treatment planning. This is expected to lead to considerably improved accuracy, particularly for those situations in which complex field shapes are used or when there are major inhomogeneities. At the same time, those evolving intensity modulated radiotherapy (IMRT) techniques require more sophisticated verification and quality assurance methods.

Another area of development in external beam therapy is the use of alternative fractionation schemes in which the treatment is given in a shorter time period but with more than one fraction delivered on each day; this is a good example of where better understanding of radiobiology has led to advances in clinical methods.

It is also likely that the combination of radiotherapy with other treatment modalities, such as chemotherapy, will be better optimized in the future in order to benefit from the possible synergistic effects between them.

The selection, acceptance testing, and commissioning of equipment for megavoltage (high energy) photon and electron treatment will be considered in Chapter 2. Chapters 7 to 10 describe the equipment and methods that may be used for planning this form of therapy. The differences in equipment and methods used for lower or kilovoltage energies will be described in Chapter 6.

3.2 *Brachytherapy*

Brachytherapy is treatment using sealed radioactive sources placed within the tumour volume to give a very localized dose, which serves to minimize the dose to the surrounding normal tissues. Brachytherapy is limited to small, localized tumours that are accessible for the application of the sources, and will be described in Chapter 12.

Developments in this area include the use of small, high dose-rate sources, which can be inserted through catheters to sites for which a prolonged applicator insertion would not be clinically practical, e.g. for treatment of the bronchus.

3.3 *Unsealed-source therapy*

The third treatment modality involves the use of unsealed radioactive sources which, when administered to the patient, localize in the tumour volume. This is the least common of the radiotherapy treatment modalities and is often administered outside the radiation oncology department. It is described in Chapter 13.

A potentially exciting development in this field is targeted therapy, e.g. using antibodies labelled with high activity radionuclides to treat disseminated tumours and metastatic disease.

4. Requirements for accuracy and precision

The accuracy and precision of two aspects of radiotherapy must be considered: one is the dose to the tumour and surrounding tissue: and the other is the spatial geometry of treatment delivery.

Figure 1.1 provides a diagrammatic illustration of the need for accuracy in dose delivery. Increasing the dose by even a small percentage above D_0 would cause a significant increase in normal tissue complications, whereas a reduction in dose would significantly decrease the probability of tumour control. It is the steepness of the dose–response curves that provides the guide for the specification for accuracy.

In 1976 the ICRU recommended that the dose to the target volume should be delivered to within ±5% (ICRU 1976), while more recent reviews of the clinical data have led to recommended tolerance levels of ±3%, given as one relative standard deviation (Mijnheer *et al.* 1987; Brahme *et al.* 1988). This is to be seen as an overall uncertainty on the dose received by the patient at the end of all the steps contributing to radiotherapy dosimetry. It leads in turn to tighter requirements on each step in the process. Absolute accuracy of basic dosimetry in the energy range used in radiotherapy is considered to be in the range of 2–3%. However, in itself this uncertainty is not a problem within a given modality, provided that all centres are using the same basic physical input data by following compatible dosimetry protocols. The absorbed dose required to destroy a tumour is not derived by theoretical means, it is found empirically. What is important is precision, so that the experience gained from patients treated in the past can be applied in the treatment of a patient today, or so that experience in one centre may be transferred to another with confidence. The clinical experience which provides the data for curves of the type shown in Figure 1.1 is critically dependent on the quality of the dose data. Therefore, in the communication of clinical experience, it is essential that the reported dose is consistent with protocols, not just for the estimation of dose itself, but also in the way that the dose delivered to the patient is specified, that is in the method of dose specification and the fractionation scheme employed.

Increasing attention is being paid to target volume and margin specification, along with patient immobilization and analysis of geometric accuracy and precision. This has become increasingly significant as the routine use of CT in treatment planning has grown and also as the concepts involved in conformal therapy have percolated through practice. There is a large and growing body of information on these aspects from studies using electronic portal imaging devices (EPIDs).

The methods of measuring absorbed dose at a reference point in a megavoltage photon or electron beam will be considered in Chapter 3, and doses relative to that point in Chapter 4. Dosimetry of kilovoltage X-ray beams will be considered separately in Chapter 6. Chapter 11 is concerned with treatment verification.

5. Quality assurance

Linked with accuracy of dose delivery is the need for the development of a programme of quality assurance (QA). This has been well described by the World Health Organization (1988). QA is a term that is often used loosely to describe the procedures followed to test the technical aspects of the functioning of some system or subsystem. More correctly, this activity should be described as quality control (QC) and is only one part of the overall quality system. In a treatment that has such a high potential for harm to the individual patient, the requirement for an effective QA programme cannot be overemphasized. It should be recognized that, in this context, harm is not simply overdosage but includes all forms of inaccuracy or deficiency resulting in sub-optimum treatment.

There are international standards for quality assurance and quality systems (ISO 1994), which have been applied to radiotherapy (SSCSMAC 1991; AAPM 1994; ESTRO 1995, 1998). An initial requirement is the formulation of a QA policy by the radiotherapy manager who has overall responsibility for the implementation of that policy. Included in the QA system are requirements for full periodic reviews of the system, for documentation of all activities and control of that documentation, for inspection and testing of equipment and the action to be taken in cases of non-compliance with defined action levels, for the calibration and control of test equipment, for the training of staff, and for internal quality audits. It is only by adopting an effective system of quality management that the quality of treatment can be fully assured. Some comprehensive reviews provide a guide to QA and QC procedures over the whole range of physics activities in radiotherapy (AAPM 1994; IPEM 1999). All the recent sets of recommendations (e.g. AAPM 1994; ESTRO 1995, 1998; IPEM 1999) stress the mutual interdependence of QA standards and requirements between the different areas and professional groups involved in radiation oncology, which underlines the need for an integrated, comprehensive approach. The clinical quality standards are increasingly 'evidence-based', relying on formal detailed review and analysis of the evolving information available in the literature (e.g. SBU 1996; COIN 1999).

It has been estimated that approximately 2.5 million patients around the world are treated by radiotherapy each year and it can be argued, on a cost–benefit basis and by reference to the needs for precision in treatment delivery, that effective quality assurance, even if it improves cure rates by just a few per cent, will have a more beneficial effect than many of the more expensive technical developments outlined previously. Development in quality systems should therefore be seen as of great importance in radiotherapy.

Quality assurance systems are considered in detail in Chapter 14. Throughout this book quality control procedures will be emphasized, in particular Chapter 5 describes a QC programme for external beam therapy equipment, while Chapter 11 considers methods of testing the overall accuracy and precision of radiation delivery to individual patients in both the dosimetric and geometric aspects.

6. The role of medical physics

Medical physics covers many subspecialities dealing with different branches of the physical sciences and of medicine. It was in the field of radiotherapy that the role of the physicist was first established in medicine. This is not surprising since it has been the discoveries of the science of physics that have given the clinician the tools for radiotherapy. The successful application of radiotherapy requires the active participation of the physicist in a multidisciplinary group, including radiation oncologists and radiographers. The detailed role of the physicist varies from place to place but the following core activities can be identified (see IPSM 1989; ESTRO/EFOMP 1996):

(1) as a member of the team to prepare specifications and select new equipment, to advise on equipment layout and on matters concerning radiation protection and to perform acceptance tests on the new installation;

(2) to undertake commissioning measurements including beam calibration and the measurement of all dosimetry data required for treatment;

(3) to be responsible for the maintenance of the treatment unit and other associated equipment either directly under his or her own supervision or indirectly; the physicist should monitor equipment performance and its continued suitability for the clinical purpose;

(4) to be responsible for all dosimetric measurement, calibrations, etc.;

(5) commonly to take overall responsibility for treatment planning and always to have an essential role in the development or implementation of new treatment techniques, the selection and quality control of treatment planning systems and the control of treatment planning data;

(6) to be responsible for the supply, safe keeping, preparation and dosimetry of sources used for unsealed and sealed source therapy.

This book is concerned with all these aspects of the physicist's activities in radiotherapy and is intended as a practical guide both to methods and to the selection and quality control of equipment.

7. References

American Association of Physicists in Medicine (1994). Comprehensive QA for radiation oncology. Report of Task Group 40. *Med. Phys.*, **21**, 581–618.

Brahme, A., Chavaudra, J., Landberg, T., McCullough, E.C., Nüssling F., Rawlinson, J.A., *et al.* (1988). Accuracy requirements and quality assurance of external beam therapy with photons and electrons. *Acta Oncol.*, 27 Suppl. 1., 1–26.

Clinical Oncology Information Network (1999). *Guidelines for external beam radiotherapy*. Report of the Generic Radiotherapy Working Group. Royal College of Radiologists, London.

European Society for Therapeutic Radiology and Oncology (Thwaites, D.I., Scalliet, P., Leer, J.W., and Overgaard, J.) (1995). Quality assurance in radiotherapy. (ESTRO advisory report to the Commission of the European Union for the 'Europe against Cancer' programme.) *Radioth. Oncol.*, **35**, 61–73.

European Society for Therapeutic Radiology and Oncology (1998). *Practical guidelines for the implementation of a quality system in radiotherapy*. ESTRO Booklet no. 4. ESTRO, Brussels.

European Society for Therapeutic Radiology and Oncology/European Federation of Medical Physics (1996). *Quality assurance in radiotherapy: the importance of medical physics staffing levels*. Recommendations of an ESTRO/EFOMP joint task group (Belletti, S., Dutreix, A., Garavaglia, G., Gfirtner, H., Haywood, J., Jessen, K.A.). *Radioth. Oncol.*, **41**, 89–94.

Institute of Physics and Engineering in Medicine (1999). *Physical aspects of quality control in radiotherapy* IPEM Report no. 81, IPEM, York.

Institute of Physical Sciences in Medicine (1989). *The role of the physical scientist in radiotherapy*. IPSM (IPEM), York.

International Commission on Radiation Units and Measurements (1976). D*etermination of absorbed dose in a patient irradiated by beams of X or gamma rays in radiotherapy procedures*. ICRU Report 24. ICRU, Bethesda.

International Commission on Radiological Protection (1985). Protection of the patient in radiation therapy. (ICRP publication 44.) *Ann. ICRP*, **15**, No. 2.

International Organization for Standardization (1994). *ISO 9002: 1994 Quality systems – model for quality assurance in production, installation and servicing*. ISO, Geneva.

Mijnheer, B.J., Batterman, J.J., and Wambersie, A. (1987). What degree of accuracy is required and can be achieved in photon and neutron therapy? *Radioth. Oncol.*, **8**, 237–52.

SBU (Swedish Council on Technology Assessment in Health Care) (1996). Radiotherapy for cancer. Vols 1 and 2. *Acta Oncol,*. Suppl 6.

Standing Subcommittee on Cancer of the Standing Medical Advisory Committee (1991). *Quality Assurance in Radiotherapy*. DoH, London.

World Health Organization (1988). *Quality Assurance in Radiotherapy*. WHO, Geneva.

Chapter 2

Planning and acceptance testing of megavoltage therapy installations

P.R. Almond and J.L. Horton

1. Introduction

Planning and acceptance testing of a megavoltage therapy installation is a major undertaking whatever the size of the institution or department. Because the equipment and site preparation are expensive, and most of the machines are complex and can be supplied by several different manufacturers, it is imperative that a great deal of thought and care go into the decision, with the aim being that the specification of the machine that is installed meets the need of the institution at that time and for the projected lifetime of the equipment. In this chapter, the various types of equipment that are available and their general specification are described. Criteria for machine selection are then presented, followed by a discussion of treatment-room design and protection considerations. Finally, acceptance test procedures, which ensure that the institution obtains the equipment that was planned, are presented.

2. Types of equipment

2.1 Cobalt-60 machines

The cobalt unit was the workhorse machine in radiation oncology for many years because of its reliability and acceptable per cent depth dose. Although the per cent depth dose is less than ideal for some cases, it can be used to treat most sites. Arc therapy may be required for the treatment of deeper lesions using this unit. Cobalt units still have a place in the modern clinic, particularly for head and neck lesions and palliation. Disadvantages of the cobalt unit are a wider penumbra than a linear accelerator beam, the need to correct the output monthly to allow for decay, the need to change the source at least every 5 years, and lower output. Advantages are minimal maintenance requirements and high reliability, approaching 99%.

2.2 Linear accelerators

Linear accelerators have become the treatment machines of choice in most radiation oncology departments, and they are available with a wide range of capabilities. Many small clinics choose a low-energy X-ray-only unit as their first machine. As the patient load grows they might decide to purchase a dual X-ray energy unit with electron beam capabilities. Linear accelerators may include asymmetric jaws, dynamic wedges, computer control, information management systems, multi-leaf collimators, and electronic portal imaging devices, either as standard or optional equipment. This range of options enhances the attractiveness of linear accelerators relative to cobalt units. Other reasons for their popularity are: minimal penumbra; acceptably flat and symmetric beams; and reasonable reliability. Linear accelerators, typically, have a higher dose rate and more clearance between final beam shaping devices and isocentre than cobalt units.

2.2.1 Low-energy linear accelerators with X-rays only

A low-energy linear accelerator with X-rays only is a popular unit for small clinics. Most tumour sites can be treated with 6 MV X-rays, although this treatment may not be the most elegant. Most large clinics have at least one of these machines in their armamentarium for treating head and neck, lymphoma, and breast. The reliability of these machines should be 97% or greater.

2.2.2 Low-energy linear accelerators with X-rays and electrons

Some manufacturers provide low-energy X-ray units with electron capabilities up to 13 MeV, which is a good choice for a small clinic or for the treatment of head and neck, or breast patients in a larger department. For these treatment sites it would be reasonable to purchase a machine with asymmetric jaws and electronic portal imaging. The reliability of these machines should approach that of the X-ray-only unit.

2.2.3 High-energy accelerators

Most present day high-energy accelerators have dual X-ray energies, as well as electron capability. A reasonable choice for the two X-ray energies would be the lowest and highest energies available: usually 6 MV and 18 or 20 MV. This choice gives the clinic the greatest range of capabilities. A mixture of these two energies can also yield intermediate central axis per cent depth doses when required. All sites can be treated on this type of machine. The reliability of these machines should exceed 95%.

2.3 Special machines and ancillary equipment

2.3.1 Stereotactic radiosurgery

The original specialized stereotactic radiosurgery machines were general purpose low-energy X-ray medical linacs but with gantry, collimator and table bearings with increased specifications for improved isocentric accuracy. However, more recently one manufacturer has introduced a stereotactic radiosurgery machine that is a 6 MV X-ray linac mounted on a C-arm, rather than a conventional gantry. This design eliminates the need for couch rotation during treatment.

Another new design consists of an S-band linac that produces a 6 MV X-ray beam. This accelerator is mounted on an industrial robot. The robot can position the linac at varying distances from the patient and point the beam at varying angles toward the target. The system also includes two orthogonally-mounted diagnostic X-ray fluoroscopy units, a treatment planning system with inverse planning capability, and a treatment couch. During the treatment planning process, digitally reconstructed radiographs (DRRs) are produced that present a view of the patient as would be imaged by the fluoroscopy system. The treatment plan consists of a number of different radiation points or 'nodes' (distances and angles) with associated radiation times. During a treatment session, the fluoroscopy units image the patient to assure the patient is in the position corresponding to that predicted by the DRRs before radiation is delivered at each treatment node. If the patient is within 1 cm of the expected position the system can compensate and then irradiate. If the patient is incorrectly positioned by more than 1 cm, the patient position must be corrected before irradiation.

2.3.2 Intra-operative linear accelerators

The intra-operative machine is a specialized linear accelerator for delivery of electrons to the patient in an intra-operative setting. These machines typically offer electron energies up to approximately 20 MeV and are chosen for their electron beam characteristics and reliability.

An interesting new machine is a portable self-shielded accelerator. It consists of two 6 MeV S-band linacs mounted in tandem capable of delivering electron beams of up to 12 MeV. Although lower energy than other intra-operative machines, it can treat a significant number of patients who can benefit from this modality. Its advantages include the ability to transport it between several operating suites and the self-shielding obviates the need for addition of shielding to the operating suite.

2.3.3 Microtrons

The medical microtron has yet to realize its full promise. The racetrack microtron accelerates electrons up to 50 MeV, either for electron-beam treatment or production of X-ray treatment beams. This computer-controlled unit, equipped with a multi-leaf collimator (MLC), provides a platform for intensity modulated radiation therapy (IMRT). Since the accelerator is not mounted on the gantry, it has the potential to deliver electron beams to multiple treatment rooms. Patient throughput can be increased by switching beams between different treatment rooms, treating a patient in one room while setting up patients in other rooms. Of course, beam line components and gantries are not inexpensive, resulting in little real savings over purchasing multiple accelerators. Additionally, if the microtron is down, all rooms it serves are down. The next few years should reveal if the microtron can be fully exploited clinically.

2.3.4 Intensity modulation radiation therapy devices

Although the concept of intensity modulated radiation therapy (IMRT) dates back at least 35 years, more recently, with the widespread use of computer-controlled linear accelerators, IMRT has became a topic of great interest. Active research has been pursued with linacs and microtrons fitted with MLCs and with the linac mounted on the robotic manipulator described above.

Another approach is a device that is added to a conventional medical linac. This device consists of a specialized MLC that is placed in the accelerator's blocking tray slots. There are 20 pairs of leaves each 1 cm wide and 2 cm long, resulting in irradiation of a strip of tissue up to 4 cm in the patient's superior–inferior axis and 20 cm in the orthogonal axes. The leaves are rapidly inserted in or retracted from the X-ray beam under pneumatic pressure. During treatment the linac is arced about the patient as the leaves move in and out of the beam. The extent of the arc and the amount of time each leaf intercepts the beam is determined during the inverse planning process. In most cases multiple arcs are required because of the limited range of tissue irradiated in the superior–inferior dimension. To deliver these additional arcs, the couch is precisely incremented under control of a specialized crane capable of sub-millimetre positioning accuracy.

2.3.5 Electronic portal imaging devices

An important tool in conformal radiation therapy is real-time imaging of the treated area. This imaging is accomplished with electronic portal imaging devices (EPIDs). This relatively recent innovation is receiving wide acceptance for routine treatments, in addition to its use for conformal radiation therapy. These devices have the potential to replace film for imaging treatment portals. EPIDs also have the potential for use as transit dosimeters. For IMRT this application may be as important as an imaging technology. Presently available EPIDs are of two types: either a fluoroscopic screen viewed by a television camera; or an array of liquid ionization chambers. Amorphous silicon detectors are under development.

2.3.6 Information-management systems

The increasing complexity of radiation therapy requires the development of new models in planning facilities. A radiation therapy department can no longer be thought of as simulation room, treatment-planning room, treatment room, etc. The integration and management of all the information involved in the process is becoming increasingly important, particularly with IMRT and EPIDs. Planning a radiation therapy facility for the twenty-first century requires careful attention to information management systems (IMS) and design of areas to accommodate their associated equipment. The information management system itself should network all treatment machines, MLCs, treatment-planning computers, simulators, EPIDS, and CT scanners. It should integrate:

(1) a record and verify system for patient simulation, planning and treatment;

(2) a scheduling system within the radiation therapy department and with the hospital for both the patients and the physicians;

(3) a charge-capture system for billing purposes.

Not only does the IMS require planning of the computer network with the associated cabling, routers, hubs, and servers, but probably more importantly from the physicist's view is the planning of the treatment console area. This area is becoming quite a challenge as the number of computers and monitors required to support record and verify systems, scheduling, EPIDs, MLCs, and the treatment machine, and to monitor the patient during treatment may easily exceed half-a-dozen. It is not a trivial task to design a console area to accommodate all these monitors and position them for optimum use by the technologist (radiographer). Careful attention must be paid to these details early in the planning process.

3. Equipment specification

3.1 Mechanical

Since modern megavoltage-therapy machines are complex, the equipment specifications can be quite involved. A form on which the specifications can be listed is shown in Figure 2.1. Most of this information can be obtained directly from the manufacturer. The first two major headings, i.e. 'GENERAL' and 'COUCH', have to do with the mechanical specifications of the equipment and relate to the limits and accuracy of the patient set-up. The last two major headings, i.e. 'PHOTONS' and 'ELECTRONS', are concerned with radiation-performance specifications. In addition to these specifications, power, chilled water, and air-handling requirements should also be specified.

Therapy equipment must perform with a high degree of mechanical accuracy and precision, and rigid specifications are required on both the simulator and treatment machine. Physicians are usually dissatisfied with field alignment errors of 5 mm or greater, and conformal therapy demands even tighter tolerances.

The mechanical performance of the equipment must be a fraction of the total allowable misalignment because there are a number of steps in the treatment process. The patient is simulated on a simulator before treatment and then treated on the therapy machine for up to 70 fractions. The limit of the ability of a technologist (radiographer) to position a patient reproducibly is generally accepted to be approximately 2 mm. If the mechanical tolerances for each parameter on the simulator and treatment machines is 2 mm or 2°, then the combination of the technologist's 2 mm set-up error will occasionally add to the inaccuracy of the machine to produce total errors that exceed 5 mm.

This simple analysis establishes that mechanical tolerance should be 1–2 mm or 1–2° for most therapy machine motions. These limits are readily achievable by the manufacturer and can be verified with standard test equipment in a reasonable time by the user. These parameters can be maintained on a continuing basis with a properly designed quality assurance programme (see Chapter 5). This philosophy is borne out in publications of national or international organizations, such as the International Electrotechnical Commission (IEC), which recommend similar tolerances (IEC 1989b).

3.2 Radiation performance

Even if the machine is mechanically aligned with the tumour to within 1 mm for every treatment, satisfactory

MANUFACTURER: _____   MACHINE: _____
DELIVERY TIME: _____   PRICE ESTIMATE: _____

GENERAL

Accelerator: _____
RF Power: _____
Bending Magnet: _____
Treatment Control: _____
Record & Verify: _____
Isocenter: _____
Isocenter Height: _____
Isocenter to Photon Jaws: _____
Isocenter to Electron Jaws: _____
Gantry Rotation: _____
Collimator Rotation: _____
Recommended Room Size: _____

COUCH

Vertical: _____
Lateral: _____
Longitudinal: _____
Couch Rotation: _____
Table Top Rotation: _____
Table Width: _____

PHOTONS

Energies: _____
%DD for 10 x 10 at 10 cm: _____
Wedges: _____
Field Sizes: _____
Asym Photon Jaws: _____
Dose Rate: _____
Flatness: _____
Symmetry: _____
Arc Therapy: _____

ELECTRONS

Energies: _____
X-Ray Cont: _____
Dose Rate: _____
Collimation: _____
Meth of Flatness: _____
Flatness: _____
Symmetry: _____
Arc Therapy: _____

MANUFACTURER: _____   MACHINE: _____

MISCELLANEOUS

Positive Features:

1. _____
2. _____
3. _____
4. _____

Negative Features:

1. _____
2. _____
3. _____
4. _____

Figure 2.1 Sample chart for listing the various parameter specifications for a given manufacturer's machine and for summarizing positive and negative features.

results will not be achieved unless the radiation produced also meets certain specifications. These typically address the energy, or central axis per cent depth dose, and the symmetry and flatness of the beam, the penumbra, and monitor constancy, linearity, and end effect.

Symmetry and flatness of the beam are required to be within reasonable tolerances to ensure the aim of acceptably uniform doses across the whole area of the field covering the target area. The practical problem inherent in this is that flatness varies with depth, due largely to scatter effects in electron beams and to variations in quality across the beam for photon beams. In addition, by definition, as the field edges are approached, areas of inhomogeneous dose distribution

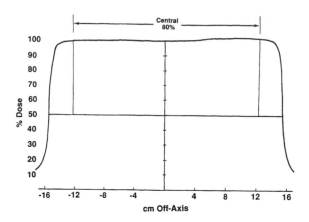

Figure 2.2 X-ray beam profile illustrating the central 80% over which beam flatness is specified.

Table 2.1 Field flatness parameters for photon beams (from IEC 1989a)

Field dimension F	d_m	d_d	max/min
5–30 cm	0.1 F	0.2 F	1.06
>30 cm	3 cm	6 cm	1.10

are encountered. Therefore, these parameters must be specified under defined measurement conditions, to include at least the depth and that part of the field that must meet the stated criteria.

Traditionally, specifications of symmetry and flatness have been in the two principal planes (planes that pass through the central axis and intersect the sides of the field at 90°) of the beam at 100 cm SSD. The specification is usually stated for the central 80% of these planes as illustrated in Figure 2.2. The transverse profile is measured and the distance between the 50% dose levels (FWHM) is determined; the area that is 80% of FWHM, and centred on the central axis, can then be considered. Of course, this area is not 80% of the treatment area, since there are two dimensions; rather, it is 64% (0.8 × 0.8) of the total area at best. If the beam has circular symmetry, then this measurement is along a radius and the area enclosed in this 'central 80%' is approximately 50% of the total area defined by the rectangular collimators.

A more meaningful definition may be the uniformity index first proposed by Svensson and Hettinger (1971). This is the ratio of the area enclosed by the 90% isodose to the area inside the 50% isodose at some reference depth. The 100% value is the value on the central axis of the beam at the depth of the reference plane. For photons the reference depth is usually taken as 10 cm; for electrons the reference depth has been variously proposed as the depth of maximum dose d_{max}, the depth of 90% dose, d_{90}, or half of the depth of the 85% or of the 80% dose [$\frac{1}{2}$]d_{85} or [$\frac{1}{2}$]d_{80}. The capabilities of present-day machines justify the use of d_{90} as the therapeutic range.

In a manner similar to Svensson and Hettinger, the International Electrotechnical Commission (IEC 1989b) specifies field uniformity in reference planes perpendicular to the central axis of the radiation beam. For photons, flatness is specified as the ratio of the maximum

dose anywhere within the radiation beam to minimum dose within the flattened area of the reference plane at a standard measurement depth of 10 cm in a water phantom, with the chamber at 100 cm from the source, i.e. SSD equal to 90 cm. Eight vertices on the major axes and diagonals of the field define the flattened area. Four vertices are located along the major axes a distance d_m inside the geometric field edge, defined as 50% of the dose on the central axis. The other four vertices are located on the diagonals inside the field a distance d_d from the corners of the field. The distances d_m and d_d and the ratio of the maximum dose to the minimum dose depend on the field dimension F (side of square field). These factors are listed in Table 2.1.

The maximum to minimum dose ratio within this area and under these measurement conditions should not exceed 1.06 for fields of 5 × 5 cm² to 30 × 30 cm² and 1.10 for larger fields. The IEC also specifies that within the flattened area, the ratio of the maximum dose to the dose on the central axis at the depth of maximum central axis dose should not exceed 1.07 for field dimensions 5–30 cm and 1.09 for field dimensions greater than 30 cm. For symmetry, the IEC specification is that the doses at any two points equidistant from the central axis and inside the flattened area at the standard measurement depth should not differ by more than 3%.

For electron beams, IEC specifies flatness and symmetry within an area 1 cm inside the 90% isodose contour at the 'standard measurement depth'. The standard measurement depth is one-half the depth of the distal 80% dose on the central axis. The symmetry is specified as the variation at any two points equidistant from the central axis within the flattened area. This symmetry ratio should not exceed 1.05.

For electrons, measurements are also required at the 'base depth', or depth of the 90% dose on the central axis, depth of maximum dose on the central axis, and 0.5 mm. At these depths IEC specifies that:

(1) the maximum distance between the 90% isodose contour and the edge of the projection of the geometric field on both major axes at the standard measurement depth should not exceed 10 mm;

(2) the maximum distance between the 90% contour and the corner of the geometric field at the standard measurement depth should not exceed 20 mm;

(3) the maximum distance between the 80% contour and the edge of the projection of the geometric field on both major axes at the base depth should not exceed 15 mm;

(4) the ratio of the highest absorbed dose anywhere in the beam at the standard measurement depth to the dose on the central axis at the depth of maximum dose should not exceed 1.03;

(5) the ratio of the highest absorbed dose anywhere in the beam at a depth of 0.5 mm to the dose on the central axis at the depth of maximum dose should not exceed 1.09.

4. Machine-selection criteria

The criteria for selecting a machine can be quite complex and time consuming. The time that elapses between deciding to acquire a piece of equipment until the first patient is treated can be of the order of 1–2 years. If changes are made during this period, then both the time and the cost are likely to increase.

The various steps taken in acquiring a megavoltage machine are shown in Figure 2.3 and are described below.

1. Equipment is purchased for a number of reasons:

    (i) to replace a machine that is worn out, outdated, or does not meet the current clinical needs;

    (ii) to add new equipment because of an increased clinical load;

    (iii) to introduce new treatment techniques;

    (iv) a move into a brand-new facility.

In the case of a replacement machine, the new equipment will generally have to fit into existing space, while if the machine is to meet a new need then the space can be designed to accommodate it.

1a. If the equipment is to be a replacement, but with the same basic characteristics as the old machine, then the task reduces to finding equipment that meets these requirements and which can be accommodated in the available space. However, in most cases new capabilities are required, and the selection process becomes similar to obtaining a piece of equipment for a new facility or to meet a new need.

2. The acquisition of a new piece of equipment should be determined by the clinical needs not only at the time that the machine will be first used but during the lifetime of the equipment, which is generally taken as 10 years. The types of patients to be treated will determine if a low- or high-energy photon machine is required and if electrons are necessary. The clinical requirements may include total body irradiation, total skin treatments, or intra-operative considerations and, if protocol patients are to be treated, the types of beams may be specified.

3. The above considerations will indicate whether a low- or high-energy photon machine is required, if electron beams at specified energies are needed, if there are special requirements on field size, etc. Other considerations may need to be taken into account, depending on the local situation.

4, 4a. At this point, additional capabilities of the machine should be considered. Are arc treatments with photons and/or electrons required? Are asymmetric jaws necessary? Is conformal or dynamic therapy desired? Are there plans for stereotactic radiosurgery? Is a multi-leaf collimator required? What about on-line megavoltage imaging? What kind of wedges are desirable, etc., etc.? If the institution is a training and/or research centre, then those programmes should be considered with respect to the capabilities of the machine.

5. By this time a fairly clear picture should have been formed as to the kind of machine required: whether it is low- or high-energy photon; if electrons are required; what kind of accessories and capabilities will be needed. At this point, discussions with the manufacturers will indicate the equipment that is available to meet these needs. It is often useful to develop a chart similar to the one shown in Figure 2.1, which summarizes the main features of each machine.

6, 7. Next, the non-technical aspects (cost, delivery time, and service) should be considered and the relative importance of each should be ranked. If there is a pressing need for a machine, then cost may be secondary to the delivery and installation time. Cost considerations should include not only the purchase price but also the operational costs, maintenance contracts, spare-part costs, and the payment schedule. Replacement costs and frequency of replacement of major components (e.g. klystron versus magnetron), as well as warranty implications, should be considered. Delivery time should also include installation time and the anticipated time to complete all the measurements necessary before treatment can commence. Service and availability of spare parts is of prime importance. How close is the nearest service office? What is their inventory list of spare parts? What is their policy of night-time and weekend work? Even the best machine is compromised if an extended period is required for servicing.

8, 8a, 9. If a competitive bidding process is required, then a specification document (Request for Proposal) based upon the above considerations should be prepared and sent to all manufacturers. When the bids are returned, they should be carefully reviewed to ensure that they meet the requirements in the specification document. The length of this document will depend on

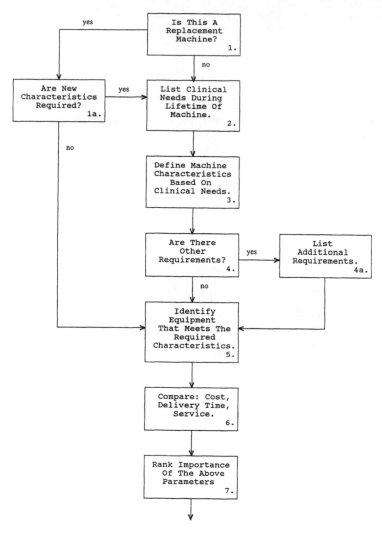

Figure 2.3 Steps required in acquiring a megavoltage therapy machine.

how such things as beam flatness, symmetry, table movement, and electrical requirements, etc. are specified. In general, the more specific this document, the more detailed should be the response from the manufacturer.

10, 10a.   Although consideration of space is included here, it may well be considered earlier in the process. Shielding should also be considered at this time. If it is a replacement machine, then the fixed space and shielding requirements could eliminate some machines. Regulations may have changed since the original machine was installed requiring additional shielding even for the same energy machine. If a specification document is sent out, then space requirements should be detailed in that document. Ideally, the environment for a new machine should be designed specifically for it with adequate space

for shielding for the machine, the control area, and any other areas that may be required. The treatment room should be large enough to accommodate all the desired procedures, including total body and total skin irradiations. Access to the treatment area must also be considered. Component parts of the accelerator are often bulky and heavy, requiring corridor, elevator, and door-opening space to accommodate the equipment when it is installed.

11, 11a.   In general, cost will be considered throughout the selection process, but the overall costs will not be determined until the above steps have been completed. If the total cost of the project (equipment, space, shielding, installation, etc.) is over budget and the budget cannot be modified, then means of reducing expenses must be

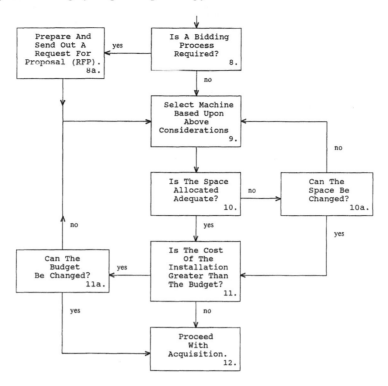

Figure 2.3 (*continued*)

found. This can be done in a number of ways, such as eliminating some of the accessories, modifying the space, changing to a less expensive machine, etc.

12. If the above steps are followed, then a machine will have been selected that meets the needs of the institution. Of course, the means of acquiring the machine depends upon the local situation. However, it is useful to establish a time line that indicates when certain tasks should be completed and when the machine is scheduled for clinical use.

Although the above 12 steps are shown in a linear fashion, some of them can be carried out in parallel or in a different order. Some may take very little time, while others can be time consuming, but it is important not to deviate too far from the scheme. The aim is to have an installation that meets the institution's clinical need. Without careful planning it is very easy to end up with an installation which, because of its limitations, dictates its clinical use rather than the other way around.

5. Treatment room and design

In the design of the treatment room and its radiation protection, several points must be considered. These include location, size and shape, shielding calculations, console area, and certain other considerations.

5.1 Location

The location of the megavoltage treatment room is generally determined by radiation safety considerations. Because of the large amount of shielding required, most megavoltage installations are placed in the basement and, if possible, in corner rooms so that two walls are backed by earthfill. If two units are being installed, then they should be adjoining so that there is the advantage of a common wall as a primary barrier. If the equipment is to go into a building that is not below ground, then a single-storey building may reduce the shielding requirements because of unoccupied areas above and below. However, if additional floors might be added later, adequate ceiling shielding should be constructed at this time. Since the placement of the room is determined by shielding needs, the rest of the department is usually designed around it. Care should be taken that patient and staff access is convenient, that patient flow is optimized, and that ancillary services, such as a mechanical room, power supplies, water, air conditioning, physics support, etc., are available. If intra-operative radiotherapy is planned, then access to elevators and closeness to the operative suite should be taken into account. Future possible expansion of the department with additional treatment machines should also be considered. If several treatment rooms are being built, then it is advisable to design the shielding and size to accommodate the highest energy machines on the market, even though the initial use of the room may be for a lower energy machine, or even left vacant. In the future, if a higher energy machine is required, the room will accommodate it without modification.

5.2 Size and shape

The size and shape of the room will depend on the equipment that is installed and the use to which it is put. In general, the manufacturers are very helpful, and will provide typical room sizes and layouts and assistance in designing the facility. Some machines are mounted on a wall, others use free-standing gantries, and some require an extra partition across the room. The internal dimensions for most rooms will be of the order of 6×6 m^2 (not including the maze). However, if special procedures are anticipated, the room size may be larger. If total body and total skin irradiations are planned, then the lateral dimension of the room may be increased to produce a large field (for a horizontal beam) at an extended distance, as shown in Figure 2.4. This particular machine was a 20 MV X-ray unit and a maze (required for neutron as well as photon protection) was incorporated into the design to obtain the extended distance. This figure also illustrates the use of outside walls, a corner room, and adjoining walls. If intra-operative radiotherapy is anticipated, then the room will need to accommodate the extra anaesthesia equipment used during these procedures and the increased number of staff required for patient set-up.

5.3 Shielding calculations

Several methods of calculating barrier thickness can be used, and the National Council on Radiation Protection and Measurements (NCRP) have described the general methods and philosophies for room design. NCRP Report 49 (1976) provides data for energies up to 10 MeV, NCRP Report 51 (1977) goes up to energies of 100 MeV, and NCRP Report 79 (1984) considers the problem of neutron contamination from medical linear accelerators when therapy equipment operates at energies above 10 MeV. Other recommendations exist, which apply to different radiation protection systems and legislation. For example, the Institute of Physics and Engineering in Medicine (IPEM formerly IPSM) has produced guidance on room design as part of wider radiotherapy protection recommendations, which incorporate consideration of United Kingdom protection legislation (IPSM 1986; IPEM 1997).

In order to calculate barrier thickness all of the following must be known for any given energy beam:

(1) workload, W;

(2) use factor, U;

(3) occupancy factor of adjoining space, T;

(4) leakage radiation.

The workload W is the output produced by the therapy unit per week at 1 m. The use factor U is the percentage of time that the therapy beam is directed at the barrier under consideration. The occupancy factor T is the proportion of time that the area beyond the barrier is occupied, although in some national regulations T must be set equal to unity under all circumstances.

The amount of radiation penetrating the barrier must be kept 'as low as reasonably achievable' (ALARA). For 'uncontrolled areas', open to the public, the permitted amount of radiation is less than that for 'controlled areas', which can only be entered by radiation workers. Most facilities are designed to the 'uncontrolled area' limits.

If the shielding transmission ratio for X-rays (B_{Xt}) is defined as the value by which the X-ray beam that is incident on the face of the shielding barrier is to be attenuated by the barrier, then for a radiotherapy installation:

$$B_{Xt} \leq 1 \times 10^{-3} \left(\frac{H_{mt}d^2}{W_{Xt}QTU} \right) \qquad (1)$$

where W_{Xt} is the workload in Gy m^2 week^{-1} for the X-rays and Q is the quality factor for the radiation (for X-rays $Q = 1$), d is the distance between the X-ray source and the reference point in metres, T is the occupancy factor (see Table 2.2), U is the use factor for the barrier of interest (see Table 2.3), and H_{mt} is the dose rate limit in mSv week^{-1}.

The barrier thickness can be obtained from published curves of transmission B_{Xt} versus barrier thickness for the appropriate X-ray energy and shielding material or from tenth-value layer data.

The number N of tenth-value layers is given by:

$$N = \log_{10} \left(\frac{1}{B_{Xt}} \right)$$

The shielding barrier thickness S can be calculated from:

$$S = T_1 + (N-1)T_e$$

where T_1 is the first tenth-value layer, facing the radiation source, and T_e represents the subsequent tenth-value layers. Values of T_1 and T_e for X-rays in concrete, steel, and lead are given in Figures 2.5, 2.6, and 2.7, as a function of the electron energy incident on a thick target.

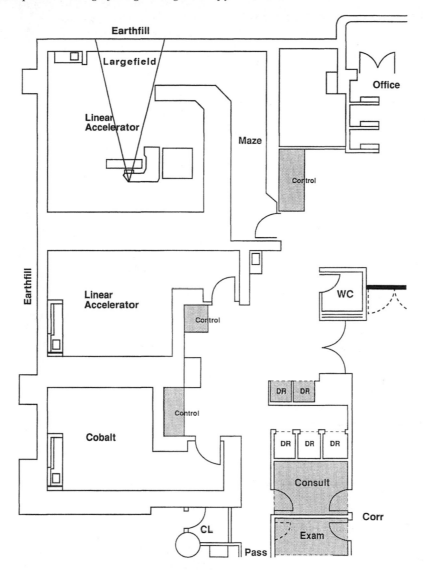

Figure 2.4 Floor plan for a three-machine installation. The installation is below ground and the outside walls are backed by earthfill. A single primary barrier between adjacent machines, an extended maze for neutron shielding, and an extended distance for larger fields are illustrated.

Table 2.2 Area occupancy factor *T* (adapted from NCRP 1976)

Non-occupationally exposed persons

T = 1	Full occupancy: work areas such as offices, laboratories, shops, wards, nurses' stations, living quarters, children's play areas, occupied space in nearby buildings.
T = 1/4	Partial occupancy: corridors, toilets, elevators using operators, unattended parking lots.
T = 1/16	Occasional occupancy: stairways, unattended elevators, janitors' closets, outside areas used only for pedestrians or vehicular traffic.

The use of occupancy factors for non-occupationally exposed persons assumes that only a small portion of the total population is exposed and hence that the genetically significant dose is small.

Occupationally exposed persons

The occupancy factor for occupationally exposed persons, in general, can be assumed to be unity.

Table 2.3 Use factors U for primary protective barriers[a]

Barrier	U
Floor	1
Walls	$\frac{1}{4}$
Ceiling	b

The above factors are to be used only if specific values for a given installation are not available.
[a]The use factor for secondary barriers is usually 1.
[b]The use factor for the ceiling of a therapy installation depends on the type of equipment and techniques used. Generally, it is not more than $\frac{1}{4}$.

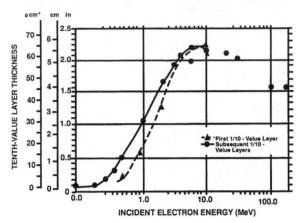

Figure 2.7 Dose-equivalent index tenth-value layers for broad-beam X-rays in lead (redrawn from NCRP 1977).

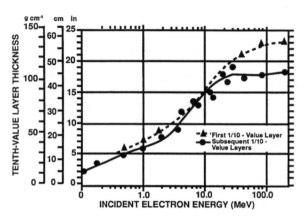

Figure 2.5 Dose-equivalent index tenth-value layers for broad-beam X-rays in concrete (redrawn from NCRP 1977).

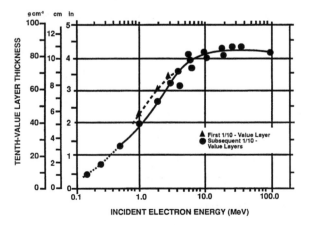

Figure 2.6 Dose-equivalent index tenth-value layers for broad-beam X-rays in steel (redrawn from NCRP 1977).

There are various classes of radiation around a megavoltage machine. The primary radiation is the radiation in the main beam: it requires the greatest shielding and barriers struck by this radiation are designated 'primary barriers'. The leakage radiation is the radiation that penetrates the shielding around the accelerator and consists of X-rays with the same energy as the primary beam. If the accelerator is operating above 10–15 MV, neutrons are also present in the leakage radiation with an average energy of approximately 1 MeV. Scatter radiation is radiation that has been scattered once by either the patient or a barrier. For high-energy X-rays, the maximum energy of Compton photons scattered to 90° is 0.511 MeV, and this value is taken as the energy for scattered X-rays. Because this energy is less than the leakage radiation energy, facilities that are designed as safe for the leakage radiation are in general safe for scattered radiation (with the exception of the room entrance if there is a short maze). Barriers against leakage and scatter radiation are referred to as secondary barriers.

The same equations can be used to determine the barrier thickness for the leakage photon radiation where $U = 1$, since leakage is assumed to be isotropic and the workload is taken as the fraction of W_X that is allowed as leakage radiation, which in most instances is 0.1% of W_X.

When medical accelerators are operated above 10–15 MV, photonuclear reactions will produce neutrons. For medical linear accelerators, the neutron production may be as high as 5 mSv per photon Gy. Examination of the concrete shielding for photons and neutrons reveals that the photons are always more penetrating than the neutrons for the energies of interest. NCRP Report 79 (1984) concludes:

Since practical therapy rooms need concrete walls at least two X-ray tenth–value layers thick, adequate concrete shielding for the photons will always be adequate for the neutrons as well.

However, great care should be taken if iron or lead is used for part of the shielding in order to reduce the overall thickness as discussed in NCRP Report 79 (1984) and by Dudziak (1969) and Shure *et al.* (1969). Not only is the attenuation of neutrons poorer but (γ,n) and (n, γ) interactions in iron or lead can create problems. In such cases, sandwich arrangements of lead, steel, and poly-ethylene or concrete are generally required to provide adequate shielding.

Figure 2.8 shows a typical room layout with an entrance maze. The layout of the maze is important; a correctly designed maze will reduce both the neutron dose and the scattered photon dose at the entrance. Depending upon the levels of these scattered radiations, a shielded door may be necessary. Kersey (1979) has described an empirical method for calculating the dose at the end of a maze and the example below is taken from his paper.

If W_X^n Gy week^{-1} is the dose at 1 m for the neutron-producing X-rays and it is assumed that the neutron dose is 0.5% of the therapy dose (Sv Gy^{-1}) measured at the same distance from the source, then the neutron dose W_n at the isocentre is:

$$W_n = W_X^n \times \left(\frac{0.5}{100}\right) \times 10^3 \text{ mSv week}^{-1}$$

and the neutron dose I_p at point P at the entrance of the maze inside the room (Figure 2.8) at a distance of d_1 m from the isocentre is:

$$I_p = \frac{W_n}{d_1^2} = \frac{W_X^n(0.5/100)}{d_1^2} \times 10^3 \text{ mSv week}^{-1} \quad (2)$$

Kersey found that the neutron dose decreases logarithmically as the distance down the maze increases. The tenth-value distance (TVD) is defined as the distance along the centre line of the maze that attenuates the equivalent dose from neutrons by a factor of 10. In most instances the TVD is 5 m. Therefore, if the total attenuating path PQ measured along the centre line of the maze is d_2 m, then the number of TVDs is $d_2/5$.

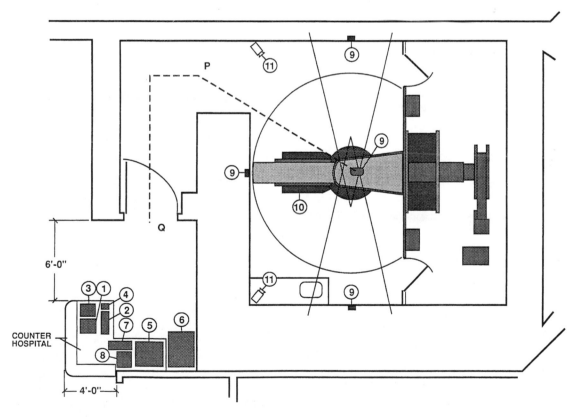

Figure 2.8 Points of calculation for neutron calculations: P, inside entrance to the maze; Q, entrance to the door. The console layout is also illustrated: 1, treatment control terminal; 2, treatment control keyboard; 3, monitor; 4, keypad; 5, printer; 6, control cabinet; 7, laser control; 8, TV monitor; 9, laser lights; 10, patient support; 11, TV cameras.

The neutron dose at Q is:

$$I_Q = \frac{I_p}{10^{d_2/5}} \text{ mSv week}^{-1}. \qquad (3)$$

If the value of I_Q is above the dose limit, either the maze must be extended or modified, or a shielding door installed. Such doors are generally made of steel-clad polyethylene or borated polyethylene, incorporating some lead downstream of the polyethylene to reduce the neutron capture gamma rays.

The scattered X-ray dose at the room entrance should be calculated but, in general, if the neutron dose is reduced to safe levels the X-ray dose will also be safe since the ratio of neutron dose to X-ray dose at the room entrance is approximately 5:1 (Kersey 1979). McCall described an alternative method for designing mazes for neutron protection, and this technique is fully described in NCRP Report 79 (1984).

5.4 Console area

Adequate space must be planned for the console area. It is not unusual to have two monitors and keyboards associated with running the machine, and two visual monitors (one stationary wide-angle, and the other pan and zoom) with camera controls and an audio system (Figure 2.8). Record-and-verify systems, multi-leaf collimators, and megavoltage imaging systems may all require console space. The institution or department may have a patient management and billing system that requires additional monitors and keyboards at the control console. If this is a new installation, then this space can be designed specifically for the equipment. Planning inputs should be obtained from radiation oncologists, physicists, radiographers (radiotherapy technologists), departmental managers, architects, etc. The position of the console area relative to the room entrance is also important. In the past the consoles were often placed next to the entrance door up against the wall (Figure 2.4). This resulted in the radiographers seated with their backs to approaching patients and with the room monitors, etc. in full view.

5.5 Other considerations

Although this section has been primarily concerned with the radiation-shielding aspects of the treatment room, there are other considerations. The electrical power supply, air conditioning, and chilled water requirements for the equipment must be taken into account. Medical physicists should work with the appropriate engineers and the manufacturers to ensure that those facilities are available. Some medical physics societies have produced comprehensive guidelines on the design of radiotherapy treatment rooms, e.g. IPEM 1997.

6. Acceptance testing

Upon delivery of the equipment, the physicist must perform a series of acceptance tests to ensure that it meets the written specifications. These tests can be classified as mechanical, radiation therapy performance, and general.

6.1 Mechanical

6.1.1 Axis of rotation of collimator

The X-ray collimator jaws are attached to the gantry by a circular bearing. This collimator unit also provides a platform for the electron collimators (cones or trimmers) and the cross-hair. The collimator bearing rotates about an axis normal to the plane of the bearing. The X-ray collimators should open symmetrically around this axis, and the X-ray electron and virtual light sources should all be aligned with it. Clearly, this axis is a key aspect of any linear accelerator and its position should be carefully defined.

Although any rigid indicator attached to the collimator housing can be used to find this rotation axis, a particularly useful device is shown in Figure 2.9. This consists of a flat tray with an adjustable rod mounted on

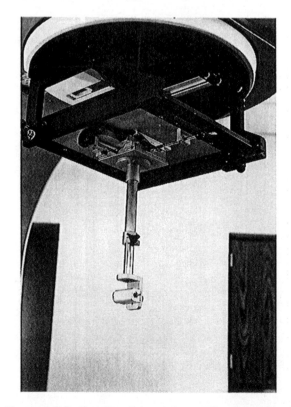

Figure 2.9 Device for determining collimator axis of rotation.

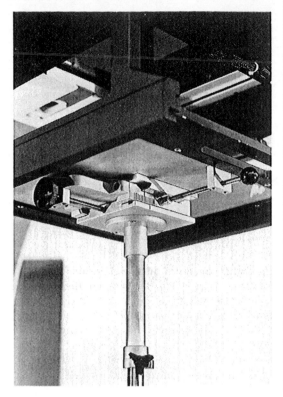

Figure 2.10 Adjustment for the device shown in Figure 2.9.

it. The tray is designed to fit in the blocking tray slot and the rod is telescopically adjustable so that its length can be changed. Its position on the plate can be changed by movement of the positioning screws shown in Figure 2.10. The distal end of the rod is terminated by a block to hold a ballpoint pen cartridge, and the block can be rotated to position the pen either parallel or perpendicular to the telescopic rod.

To find the collimator axis of rotation with this device, the tray is placed in the blocking tray slot. With the gantry at 0°, the length of the rod is adjusted to place the point of the pen at the nominal isocentre distance with the pen pointing vertically downward. The rod is adjusted on the blocking tray to place the pen near the nominal collimator axis of rotation. A piece of millimetre graph paper is attached to the treatment table and the table is raised to contact the pen. As the collimator is rotated through its entire range (either 180° or 360°) the pen traces out a semicircular or circular arc. The position of the rod on the tray can be adjusted to place it near the centre of this arc. Each subsequent tracing will produce arcs with smaller radii as the axis of rotation is approached. If the collimator bearing has no run-out, i.e. the rotation truly occurs about a single axis, the pen should trace out a point limited by the width of the

marker when the pen is positioned on the collimator axis of rotation. The bearings used by most manufacturers will produce a trace less than 1 mm in radius, and generally the trace will be a point. This point is the intersection of the collimator axis of rotation and the plane passing through the isocentre.

6.1.2 Photon jaw motion

The photon jaws should open and close symmetrically about the collimator axis of rotation. This can be verified by rigidly attaching a machinist dial indicator to a position on the gantry that does not move with collimator rotation. The feeler of the dial indicator is brought into contact with one jaw and the reading noted. After rotating the jaws through 180°, the feeler is brought into contact with the opposite jaw and this reading is recorded. The collimator symmetry is then half the difference of the readings. This value, projected to isocentre, should be less than 1 mm. The opposite set of jaws should be measured in the same manner.

The two sets of jaws should be perpendicular to each other. This can be checked by rotating the gantry to 90° and rotating the collimator to place one set of jaws horizontally. A spirit level placed on the horizontal jaws should indicate horizontal level. Likewise placing the level on the vertical jaws should indicate vertical. The collimator angle read-out can be checked at this point. The collimator angle indicator should read one of the cardinal angles 0°, 90°, 180°, or 270°, depending on the position of the jaws. Rotation of the collimator through 90° should place the jaws that were horizontal in the vertical position and the vertical jaws in the horizontal position. This can be verified with the spirit level. This test can be performed at 90° intervals and the collimator angle read-out verified at each position.

6.1.3 Congruence of light and radiation field

The light field alignment can be checked on the same piece of millimetre graph paper that was used to delineate the collimator axis of rotation. With this piece of paper at the nominal isocentre distance and the gantry at 0° (directed vertically downward), the edges of the light field produced by the X-ray jaws should be symmetric about the collimator axis. This symmetry should be checked at all the cardinal angles of the collimator. This light field symmetry should be 1 mm or better about the collimator axis. The edges of the light field should be noted on the graph paper and they should meet at right angles. After the collimator is rotated through 180°, the edges of the light field should be in the same position as before the rotation.

The cross-hair should be positioned to project its image on the collimator axis of rotation. This position should be checked as the collimator is rotated. The image of the cross-hair should not deviate from the collimator axis during rotation by more than 1 mm at the isocentre.

At this point the congruence of light and radiation fields can be checked by placing ready-pack X-ray film perpendicular to the collimator axis at the isocentre distance. The light field projection can be demarcated on the film by placing radio-opaque objects in the light field with their outside edges aligned with the light field edge, by pricking the ready-pack film with a pin in the corners, or by outlining the light field on the ready-pack film with a ballpoint pen with enough pressure to mark the emulsion. Sufficient build-up material is placed on the film to position near d_{max} and the film is then irradiated to yield an optical density of between 1 and 2. The light field edges should correspond to the 50% dose level to within 2 mm. This congruence should be verified over the range of field sizes and at two distances. The exposures of different distances will demonstrate whether the virtual light and X-ray sources are at the same distance from the isocentre.

At this point, since the light field has just been aligned to the collimator axis of rotation, a misalignment of the light and radiation field indicates that the X-ray source is not aligned with the collimator axis of rotation. If this is the case, then any adjustment should not be taken lightly. The waveguide, bending magnet, and flattening filter should be aligned with the collimator axis in the factory. This alignment procedure is complex and should only be performed by factory-trained personnel. If there is a misalignment, then its magnitude, its effect on treatment, and whether appropriately trained individuals should be called in to verify the problem must be determined.

6.1.4 Gantry angle indicators

The accuracy of the gantry angle indicators can be checked by placing a spirit level on a 'true' surface, such as the face of the collimator housing or the rails that support the blocking tray. This level should indicate horizontal with the gantry at 0° or 180°, and vertical with the gantry at 90° or 270°. Angles at 45°, 135°, 225°, and 315° can be verified with the 45° mitre indicator available on most spirit levels. If necessary, intermediate angles can be checked with an inclinometer. The indicators should be accurate to within 0.5°.

6.1.5 Mechanical axis of gantry rotation

The mechanical axis of gantry rotation can be determined with the same device that was used to find the collimator axis of rotation. Again with the gantry at 0°, the device is placed in the blocking tray slot and the marking pen is positioned at the nominal isocentre distance, but for this test the pen is horizontal rather than vertical. A piece of millimetre graph paper can be secured to a plastic block to support the paper in a vertical plane. The block is

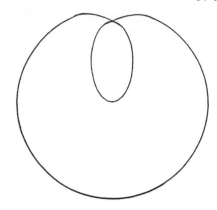

Figure 2.11 A limicon: trace produced when there is severe gantry sag.

placed on the treatment table and positioned to contact the marking pen. When the gantry is rotated through 360° the pen will trace a circle. With the telescopic feature of the rod, the pen can be moved to the centre of this circle and the gantry again rotated through 360°. A smaller circle will be traced. This iterative process can be continued until an irreducible circle is reached. This circle is a measure of the apparent run-out of the gantry bearing, the term 'apparent run-out' is used because the size of the circle is a combination of the bearing run-out and the flexing of the gantry itself. This flexing occurs because of the weight cantilevered off the gantry, which causes gravity to twist the gantry differently as it rotates. When the gantry is pointing vertically down, the axis of the collimator will tilt towards the gantry stand, whereas with the gantry pointing vertically upwards the collimator axis will tend to point away from the gantry stand. If the gantry sag is severe, a limacon, as shown in Figure 2.11, rather than a circle will be traced out by the pen. The radius of the circle enclosing the limacon is the radius of uncertainty of the mechanical axis of gantry rotation. This radius should not exceed 2 mm and preferably should be 1 mm or less.

Gantry flex obviously introduces positional uncertainty along the axis of gantry rotation and this can also be determined with the rod-and-pen device. For this test, an aluminium rod can be wrapped in millimetre graph paper and supported in a fixed position off the end of the treatment table collinear with the mechanical axis of gantry rotation. The rod and graph paper should be aligned with the cross-hairs. The pen of the rod-and-pen device is again placed vertically and contacted against the graph paper. As the gantry is rotated, the pen will trace a line along the graph paper. The run-out of the gantry in the axial direction can be measured when the paper is removed from the rod.

The ideal mechanical isocentre is the intersection of the collimator axis of rotation with the gantry axis of rotation. Because of structural flexing of the gantry, the isocentre is not a point but a 'zone of uncertainty' limited to approximately 2 mm. For most radiotherapy applications this is more than adequate, and in the rest of this chapter we shall refer to the mechanical isocentre as if it were a point. Specialized applications, such as stereotactic radiosurgery, may require modifications or ancillary devices, but this subject is beyond the scope of this chapter.

6.1.6 Radiation isocentre

The radiation isocentre can now be found. For this procedure a ready-pack film is secured to a plastic block with tape. The plane of the film is then placed in the vertical plane traced out by the collimator axis as the gantry is rotated. The film plane should be perpendicular to the gantry axis of rotation and the approximate centre of the film should be at isocentre height. A pin prick should be made in the film to denote the mechanical axis of rotation of the gantry. A second block should be placed against the film, so that the film is sandwiched between the plastic blocks. A check should then be made to ensure that the plane of the film is still in the plane traced out by the collimator axis as the gantry rotates and that the pin prick still demarcates the gantry axis. The collimator jaw should be closed down to a small field size, approximately 1×1 mm^2 if possible, and the film exposed to produce an optical density of 0.3–0.5. Without moving the film, the gantry should be rotated to another angle, perhaps 50°, and exposed again. This process should be continued until exposures have been made from all four quadrants of the gantry position. Angles that prevent the exit of one beam from overlapping the entrance of another should be chosen. When the film is processed, a pattern of a multi-arm cross will be revealed, and this pattern is referred to as 'star shot'. The point where the central axis of all the beams intersect is the radiation isocentre. Indeed, because of gantry flex, the 'point' may be a couple of millimetres wide but should not exceed 4 mm, and this point should be no more than 1 or 2 mm away from the pin prick delineating the mechanical isocentre.

6.1.7 Optical distance indicator

The accuracy of the optical distance indicator (ODI) can be checked next. A useful device is shown in Figure 2.12. It consists of a vertical rod, with detents every 5 cm, mounted on a weighted base. A white plastic plate can be moved vertically along the rod. Initially the white plate should be raised to the detent at mid-height on the rod. The device can then be positioned to place the top of the plastic plate at the isocentre. When the ODI is illuminated it should read 100 cm (or isocentre distance) on the plate. By moving the plate up and down the rod,

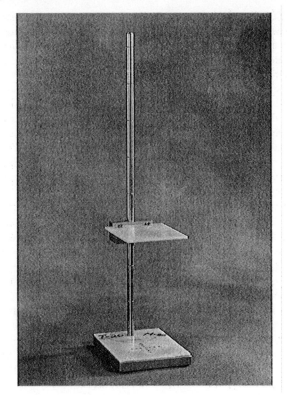

Figure 2.12 Device for checking the ODI.

the ODI can be checked over the range 80–120 cm very quickly. The ODI should be within 2 mm of the correct value of this range.

6.1.8 Field size indicators

The accuracy of the field-size indicators can be checked by taping millimetre graph paper to the table. With the gantry at 0° and the table at isocentre height, various field sizes from 2×2 cm^2 to 40×40 cm^2 can be set and the indicators compared with the light field observed on the graph paper. The asymmetric jaw indicators should also be checked by setting asymmetric fields over the range of travel for the asymmetric jaw.

For machines equipped with MLCs, similar tests should be conducted for MLC fields. The tests should be repeated at different gantry and collimator angles and on different days to check for reproducibility. Any interlocks for the MLC position relative to the jaws should also be checked at this time.

6.1.9 Treatment table rotation

Most treatment tables are mounted on a turntable that rides on a bearing. The axis of rotation of this bearing should be collinear with the axis of rotation of the collimator when the gantry points vertically downwards.

This design permits table rotation about the isocentre. The development of three-dimensional treatments and stereotactic radiosurgery with their non-coplanar beams demands very precise alignment of the collimator and table axes of rotation. The isocentre should be defined as the intersection of the gantry axes of rotation with the axis of rotation of the collimator and treatment table.

The axis of rotation of the treatment table bearing can be determined with the rod-and-pen device used to find the axis of rotation of the collimator and the gantry. For this experiment the tray is again placed in the blocking tray slot with the gantry positioned at 0° and the pen point of the device at isocentre pointing vertically downward. A piece of millimetre graph paper is taped to the table and the table is raised to contact the pen. The turntable can be rotated through its full range of motion, usually 180° or 360°, and the pen will again trace out an arc, the centre of which is the axis of rotation.

The technique of iteratively moving the pen to the centre of the arc will produce a minimum arc. The radius of this minimum arc is the 'zone of uncertainty' or the run-out on the bearing of the turntable. The run-out should be less than 1 mm. The axis of rotation of the turntable can be compared with the axis of rotation of the collimator by turning on the field light and observing the projection of the cross-hair. These two axes should agree to within 1 mm.

A check on the axis of rotation of the treatment table can be performed using a star shot. A ready-pack film should be taped to the table with the table at isocentre height. A pin prick should be made in the film pack at the position of the cross-hair projection. A long narrow field, for instance 0.2 × 20 cm^2, should be set on the collimators. With the collimator at 0°, an exposure to yield on optical density of approximately 0.3 should be made. The table should then be rotated through 40–50° and another exposure made without moving the film on the table top. Subsequent exposures should be made at angles in all quadrants. Angles in opposite quadrants should be carefully chosen so that they do not overlap.

A star pattern will be revealed on developing the film. The centre of this pattern is the axis of rotation of the table and should be within 1 mm of the pin prick denoting the axis of rotation of the collimator.

6.1.10 Motion of treatment table

The treatment table should move in a true vertical plane and laterally and longitudinally in true horizontal planes. The vertical motion can be verified by taping a piece of millimetre graph paper to the table top, raising the table to its highest position, and placing the gantry at 0°. The field light is turned on and the cross-hair projection is marked on the graph paper. The table is adjusted to its lowest position. The cross-hair projection should remain on the same point it was with the table in its highest position. Any deviation should be less than 2 mm.

To check the horizontal motion, the gantry is rotated to 90° and a plastic block with a piece of millimetre graph paper taped to it is placed on the table which is positioned at a height such that the cross-hair will project on the graph paper. With the table at one extreme of its lateral motion and with the turntable at 0°, the cross-hair projection is marked on the block. The table is then moved to the other extreme of its lateral motion. The cross-hair projection should remain at the same position on the graph paper and any deviation greater than 2 mm should not be accepted. The longitudinal motion of the couch can be checked with the gantry at 90° and the pedestal of the table at 90°. Again, a piece of graph paper is taped to a block on the table and the table height is positioned such that the cross-hair projects on the graph paper. The cross-hair projection is marked on the graph paper and the table is then moved through its full longitudinal range. The cross-hair should remain on the mark on the graph paper. Again, a deviation of greater than 2 mm is not acceptable.

6.1.11 Alignment of sidelights

All sidelights should be in true horizontal and vertical planes and should pass through the isocentre. The clear acrylic cube illustrated in Figure 2.13 can be used for this alignment. The cube is constructed of 30 × 30 cm^2 sheets of acrylic, 6 mm thick, with a cross-hair etched in the centre of each face. This block should be carefully constructed to ensure that it is square and that all the cross-hairs are centred.

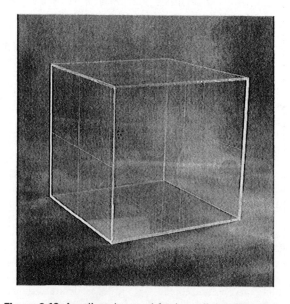

Figure 2.13 Acrylic cube used for laser light alignment.

The block is placed on the table and levelled. It is positioned by rotating the gantry to 0° and 270°, and iteratively shifting the block until the projection of the cross-hair from the accelerator aligns with the cross-hairs etched on the faces of the cube. The side lasers are then set up such that each laser is aligned with the cross-hair on the entrance and exit side of the cube. The sagittal laser can be aligned to pass through the cross-hairs etched in the top and bottom faces. The same alignment is performed for an overhead laser.

6.2 Radiation beam performance

6.2.1 Electron energy specification

Although we generally speak of the energy of an X-ray or electron beam, from a clinical standpoint, we are really interested in the depth dose characteristics. Measurement of the practical range is the most common technique of determining the energy of an electron beam in a clinical environment.

The practical range of an electron beam is usually measured in a water phantom using a thimble ion chamber. The surface of the water phantom is placed at the normal treatment distance and depth ionization measurements are made for a 15×15 cm^2 field size by moving the thimble ion chamber to subsequently greater depths while maintaining a constant SSD. When measuring electron depth ionization curves with an ion chamber smaller than the area of the beam, two corrections to the ionization readings are necessary. The first of these is the correction for the effective point of measurement. This correction is not significant for a parallel-plate chamber as the effective point of measurement is the inside surface of the entrance window. The correction for a cylindrical chamber is greater, with the effective point of measurement being shifted upstream from its axis. The amount of this shift has been debated to be from a half to three-quarters of the inner radius of the chamber, but the currently accepted best value is a half. For a 0.6 cm^3 Farmer-type chamber with an inner radius of a 3 mm, the effective point of measurement would be 1.5 mm upstream from its centre.

The second correction is required because ionization measurements at a constant SSD reflect not only the range of the electrons but also an inverse square effect. The inverse square law correction should be made from the effective point of measurement and is given by:

$$M_c = M \left(\frac{f_{vir} + d_{eff}}{f_{vir}} \right)^2 \qquad (4)$$

where M_c is the ionization measurement M after correction, f_{vir} is the SSD of the virtual source (see Chapter 4, Section 5.4) and d_{eff} is the effective depth of measurement.

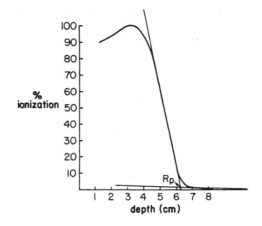

Figure 2.14 Definition of practical range for electrons.

The practical range, R_p, can then be found by plotting M_c on the y-axis versus depth on the x-axis, as shown in Figure 2.14. It is the depth where the linearly decreasing portion of the electron ionization curve intersects the ionization produced by the bremsstrahlung X-ray tail. The most probable energy at the surface of the phantom can be calculated as:

$$E_{p,0} = 0.0025R_p^2 + 1.98R_p + 0.22 \qquad (5)$$

where $E_{p,0}$ MeV is the most probable energy at the surface and R_p cm is the practical range. This energy is shown for a representative electron spectrum in Figure 2.15.

The most probable energy is one energy of clinical interest; another energy required by most dosimetry protocols is the average energy $\overline{E}_0$, which is also shown in Figure 2.15. It is discussed in detail in Chapter 3, Section 2.2.

The electron energy at the exit of the bending magnet system can be determined by adding the energy that the electrons lose in passing through all the components in the beam path between the exit window of the bending magnet and the phantom surface. These components include the scattering foils, monitor ion chamber, and air. The energy lost in each component equals the stopping power times the thickness of that component, and the total energy loss is given by:

$$\Delta E_T = \sum S_n T_n \qquad (6)$$

where S_n and T_n are the stopping power and thickness respectively of the nth component.

The most probable energy $E_{p,a}$ is shown in Figure 2.15. This energy, though not of immediate interest for treatment, is a useful analytical tool when correlated with the current through the bending magnet. Most accelerator manufacturers place a shunt resistor in parallel with the

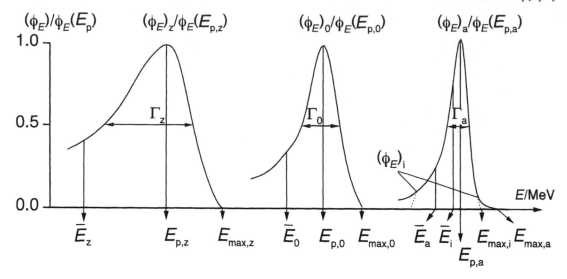

Figure 2.15 Representation of electron beam spectrum and energy definitions. The spectrum on the right represents the intrinsic accelerator beam (subscript a) and the initial electron beam (subscript i). Any difference is the result of energy-defining slits. The spectrum in the middle of the figure represents the electron beam at the surface of the phantom (subscript 0), while the left-hand-spectrum represents the spectrum at depth z (subscript z). The most probable energy in each case is indicated by E_p and the average energy by $\bar{E}$. (Redrawn from ICRU 1984.)

bending magnet. The current through this resistor can be plotted against $E_{p,a}$ to yield a calibration curve of the bending magnet. This curve serves as a quality assurance tool as it should remain constant. A change in the relationship between shunt current and energy may indicate problems in the bending magnet (e.g. a shorted coil).

6.2.2 Electron flatness and symmetry

Field flatness and symmetry are specified either over some region of specified beam profiles passing through the central axis at particular depths or in planes at stated reference depths (see Section 3.2).

If the specification is in terms of beam profiles, then these measurements should be made in a water phantom at the normal treatment SSD. The depth of measurement should be d_{max} or other relevant depth, such as the depth of the 90% dose (d_{90}), $[\frac{1}{2}]d_{80}$, etc., following the guidelines specified in the protocol being used. The profiles should be normalized to the central axis value at that depth.

Flatness and symmetry are specified over a central region that avoids the penumbra, which may be quoted as the central 80%, although this is actually over 50–60% of the area of the beam (see Section 3.2). One alternative method, which avoids the penumbra region, is to specify the flatness and symmetry inside the 50% dose values by some fixed distance, where, for example, 1.5 cm is a reasonable value. For a 10×10 cm^2 field this definition requires only the central 7 cm or 70% to meet the flatness

and symmetry specification; however, for a 30×30 cm^2 field this definition requires the central 27 cm or 90% to meet the flatness and symmetry specification. In addition to the two principal planes, the flatness and symmetry should also be specified along diagonals. In this case the distance from the 50% level should be increased, for example, to 2.5 cm because the penumbra regions join in the corner and allowance should be made for this. Alternatively, if following IEC guidelines (Section 3.2), part of the flatness criteria includes maximum distances between specified isodoses and the geometric field edge.

Within the central region, flatness should be specified to be within a certain percentage of the central axis value. Reasonable values would range from 3 to 4% less than the central axis value. Any flatness specification in terms of an average value in the central region, such as ±3% of the average value in the central region, should be avoided since the calibration is carried out on the central axis and not at some average value. If flatness is specified to an average value, then the dosimetry becomes ambiguous. The IEC recommendations define specific values relative to central axis values at stated depths (see Section 3.2).

The symmetry specifications should be that any two points equidistant from the central axis are within 2 to 3% of each other, depending on the recommendations being followed. Beam symmetry is verified by folding the plot of the beam profile about the centre of the beam. This is best accomplished by aligning the beam edges. The two halves can be compared with each other over the central region by viewing on a light box.

If the flatness is specified in terms of the uniformity index (Section 3.2), the data should be measured with a film exposed perpendicular to the central axis of the beam at the depth of the reference plane. The optical density can be converted to dose at that depth using a sensitometric curve determined at the reference depth. The position of the appropriate isodensity lines can then be determined with a densitometer. For example, if the sensitometric curve indicated that 45% density corresponded to 50% dose, and that 95% density represented 90% dose, the areas enclosed by the 95% and the 45% isodensity curves could be determined and their ratio would represent the uniformity index.

The IEC also recommend tests at various gantry and collimator angles, in addition to the standard settings.

6.2.3 Electron penumbra

The penumbra is variously defined as the distance between the 20 and 80% values or the 10 and 90% values of the beam profile, where 100% is the central axis value, or by distances between specified isodoses and the geometric field edge under stated conditions (IEC). The electron penumbra is generally specified at either d_{max} or half the therapeutic range. Generally, the distance between the 20 and 80% dose values is 10–12 mm for electrons below 10 MeV and 8–10 mm for electrons between 10 and 20 MeV, when the end of the collimation system is no more than 5 cm from the surface. If the final collimation is 10 cm or more from the surface, the distance between the 20 and 80% levels may exceed 15 mm.

The physicist should also note that the 90% dose contour becomes narrower at depth as illustrated by the dark area in Figure 2.16. This dark area is the margin between the 50 and 90% isodose values. The increase in penumbra width at depth with the concomitant narrowing of the 90% dose contour has significant treatment-planning implications (see Chapter 10).

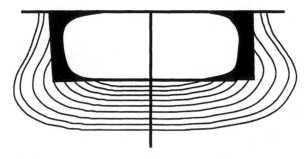

Figure 2.16 Constriction of the 90% contour for electron beams with depth.

6.2.4 Electron collimation

Whether cones or trimmers are used, electron collimation should be designed to reduce the dose outside the field to a clinically acceptable level. Some cones are designed to provide electron scatter to assist in flattening the field. These may be designed with thin walls to reduce the weight that the radiographers are required to lift. The cones produce an acceptable dose outside the field at the normal treatment distance; however, electrons may leak through the thin walls and produce significant dose levels on the cone surface. The collimator leakage on the cone surface should be specified to be less than 5% of the central axis dose at d_{max}. Measurements on the surface of the cone can be made using film.

6.2.5 X-ray energy specification

Energy specification for X-ray beams is not a straightforward matter. The depth–dose characteristics are not a function solely of maximum photon energy but also of target and flattening filter design. For instance, a 'thin' target design will produce an X-ray beam with a higher average energy and thus will be more penetrating than a 'thick' target design for the same maximum photon energy.

The thin target design consists of a thin layer of a material with a high atomic number Z, such as gold or tungsten, upstream followed by a low Z material such as carbon. The high-energy electrons encounter the high Z material first and produce bremsstrahlung X-rays as they slow down. After passing through the high Z material they are stopped by the low Z material. A thick target is composed of a high Z material only, with the electrons stopping in it. Since bremsstrahlung production increases with Z and with electron energy, fewer low-energy X-rays are produced in a thin target. The electrons, having lost some energy in the thin target, stop in a low Z material in which comparatively few low-energy X-rays are generated. Whereas with a thick target, the low energy electrons stop in the high Z material.

The design of the flattening filter can influence the depth–dose characteristics of a high energy beam because pair production increases with photon energy and with the atomic number of the material. Therefore a high Z filter may filter more high-energy X-rays than low-energy X-rays.

At one time, manufacturers specified their X-ray beams as the energy of the electrons on the target. Obvious deficiencies in this specification are that the depth–dose characteristics are not uniquely defined by this nomenclature, and that the electron energy could only be indirectly determined by the manufacturers from interpolation of various accelerator parameters.

A more direct means of determining the electron energy on target is to use the calibration curve of the bending magnet shunt current discussed in Section 6.2.1. The value of this current for the photon beam can be compared with the electron energy on target using this calibration curve.

In recent years, manufacturers have tended to quote photon energy as a 'nominal' value, but this specification is not always clear. Some manufacturers may quote a value based on a comparison with data in the British Journal of Radiology Supplement 25 (BIR 1996). They compare the central axis per cent depth dose at 10 cm depth of a 10 × 10 cm^2 field at 100 cm SSD. For example, this value is reported to be 83% for a 25 MV X-ray beam. In this case a manufacturer producing an accelerator with this depth dose might label the machine as a 25 MV machine. The scheme has some utility in that it addresses a clinically useful quantity, but the deficiency is that the match may only be at this one point and there may be significant differences between the machine in question and the data for other field sizes or depths.

The calibration protocols of the Nordic Association of Clinical Physics (NACP 1980) and the American Association of Physicists in Medicine (AAPM 1983) and others, offer other ways of defining photon energy that may be more appropriate (see Chapter 3, Section 2.1). To determine photon energy with the NACP protocol, the central axis percentage depth ionization for a 10 × 10 cm^2 field at 100 cm SSD is measured and the ratio of the ionization at 10 cm to the ionization at 20 cm is calculated. This ratio is then correlated with an 'acceleration potential' using a graph in the protocol. The AAPM adopted a similar approach, but in this case the measurements are made in a 10 × 10 cm^2 field at a constant source-chamber distance of 100 cm and the ratio of ionization at 20 cm depth to the ionization at 10 cm is calculated. This is a tissue–phantom ratio (TPR$_{10}^{20}$) and is often referred to as the Quality Index. The physicist can derive a 'nominal accelerating potential' from this ratio by using a graph in the protocol. The advantage of this scheme is that the energy depends on the beam penetration at more than one depth. The disadvantages are that the ratio of ionization is a very strong function of energy and the graphs have very steep gradients, which make it difficult to determine the energy accurately. For the purposes of these protocols this is not important because the stopping power ratios and mass energy absorption coefficients change very slowly with energy.

For acceptance testing, the energy of the beam should be determined by measuring the central axis percentage depth doses in accordance with the machine specification. A small volume ion chamber should be used in a water phantom for this measurement.

6.2.6 X-ray flatness and symmetry

The flatness and symmetry of photon beams are generally specified in similar ways as for electron beams,

except that for photons they are specified at a depth of 10 cm. Again, specific IEC recommendations are discussed in Section 3.2, being applicable to measurements at 90 cm SSD and 10 cm depth for a 100 cm isocentric unit. It is recommended that photon beams be specified at d_{max}, as well as at 10 cm. This specification prevents the off-axis peaking of the profiles from becoming too large at d_{max}. The off-axis peaking results from flattening filters being designed to produce a flat beam at 10 cm. The filter is cone shaped and centred on the central axis, and this produces differential hardening across the face of the beam with the centre of the beam having a higher average energy than the periphery and therefore the beam is more penetrating on the central axis. It follows that, if the beam is flat at 10 cm, then it must be peaked off-axis at depths shallower than 10 cm. The peaking of a 6 MV X-ray beam should be approximately 8% or less at d_{max} for a 40 × 40 cm^2 field at 100 cm SSD (see Section 3.2 for specific IEC recommendations). Higher energy beams should have less off-axis peaking. The IEC recommend tests at various gantry and collimator angles, in addition to the standard settings.

6.2.7 Photon penumbra

Most linear accelerator manufacturers specify the photon penumbra as the distance between the 20 and 80% points of a beam profile measured 10 cm deep in a water phantom. The penumbra is usually specified for a 10 × 10 cm^2 field with the surface of the phantom at 100 cm, resulting in a profile of 11 cm FWHM. The exact specification may vary somewhat from these conditions depending on the vendor, but in any event one can reasonably expect the penumbra to be 10 mm or less under these conditions. The IEC guidelines again recommend standard measurement conditions of 90 cm SSD and 10 cm depth and that penumbra be specified as the 20–80% distance. However, they do not provide tolerance values.

The penumbra for cobalt units is generally specified at depths of 7 or 10 cm for a 10 × 10 cm^2 field at 80 cm SSD. Because of the large source size and shorter SSD of cobalt units the penumbra will be larger than for linear accelerators. A typical penumbra for a cobalt unit is 15 mm.

6.3 General

6.3.1 Monitor linearity and end effect

The monitor ion chamber and associated electronics of a linear accelerator should provide a monitor unit setting linear with dose to better than 1%. This system should also have an end effect of less than 1 monitor unit (mu). Similarly, for cobalt units the timer should be accurate to better than 1% with an end-effect correction of less than 2 s.

The linearity and end effect can be determined by placing an ion chamber at a fixed depth in a water phantom and exposing it to different monitor unit settings over the range of the monitor system. The correlation coefficient of a linear regression analysis, where the ion chamber reading is the dependent variable and the number of monitor units is the independent variable, will demonstrate the linearity of the system. The value of this correlation coefficient should be at least 0.999. The intercept is a measure of the end effect with a zero intercept indicating that there is no monitor end effect. A positive intercept on the x-axis implies that less radiation was delivered than intended, while a negative x intercept implies that more radiation than intended was delivered. In each case the intercept should be less than 1 mu. In addition tests should be carried out on dose monitor reproducibility and stability with time and with gantry angle (IEC 1989a, 1989b; AAPM 1994a).

6.3.2 Wedges

Wedge angles and wedge factors should be compared with specification (see Chapter 4, Section 4 for methods). For dynamic wedges both the positional and dose performance should be tested by setting various irradiations and comparing actual positions and elapsed mu with the expected values.

6.3.3 Arc therapy

The demonstration of the arc therapy specification for either electrons or X-rays can be performed without an ion chamber or phantom in the beam. For this test a number of monitor units and a number of degrees for the arc are set and the radiation is initiated. Termination should be within both 1 mu and 3° of the set values. This test should be repeated over a number of arcs and monitor unit settings.

6.3.4 Other considerations

Computer control systems require their own specific acceptance testing (AAPM 1993). Other facilities, options and accessories, e.g. EPIDs, etc., may also require acceptance testing so that they meet their specification. The details of these tests are outside the scope of this chapter. However, a local test procedure should be drawn up to ensure that all relevant parameters are tested. In doing this, as in drawing up the acceptance test procedure (ATP) for standard parameters, it is useful to review relevant documents, e.g. manufacturer's own ATP, any relevant IEC guidelines (IEC 1989a, 1989b), model ATP, any relevant reports from professional groups (e.g. AAPM Task Groups 35, 40, 45: AAPM 1993, 1994a, 1994b; IPSM 1988; IPEM 1998, etc.). In addition, there is a growing body of publications which may not yet have been adopted in official guidance on the performance specification and acceptance of these newer technologies. Some guidelines have begun to incorporate some of this already (e.g. AAPM 1993), but the pace of technology development is faster than consensus guidelines can be developed.

6.4 Protection surveys

During installation it is important to conduct radiation measurements in the surrounding areas (adjoining rooms, corridor, control console, etc.), to make sure that the radiation levels are safe and meet all regulatory requirements.

As soon as the highest energy photon beam has been obtained and initially tuned with the flattening filter in place, a full protection survey of the building should be carried out. Such procedures are described in IPSM Report 54 (IPSM 1988). Barriers exposed to the direct radiation beam and to scattered and leakage radiation must be checked and the results compared with the values predicted by the calculations outlined in Section 5.3.

If it is found for a particular set of conditions that the radiation outside the room has not been reduced to a safe level then several procedures can be followed:

(1) add additional shielding to the barrier or fill voids if they exist;

(2) restrict access to the space where radiation levels are high;

(3) restrict the beam from operating under these conditions, which may mean not allowing the primary beam at a given energy to be directed against the barrier.

Options (2) and (3) should be avoided if at all possible since they limit the use of space and/or the equipment.

If the measurements are made for the highest photon beam energy available at the highest dose rate to be used clinically and the shielding is found to be adequate, then it can be assumed that the shielding is also adequate for all other photon energies and for all electron beams. However, it is prudent to test this assumption with spot checks.

In addition, for photon energies above 10 MV (generally 15 MV and above) a neutron survey must be performed. Outside the room a 'rem' survey meter may be used. Since neutrons are assumed to be produced isotropically, all barriers should be tested and, in particular, the entrance way must be measured. If the maze is not adequate, steps can be taken to reduce the neutron dose as described in NCRP Report 79 (NCRP 1984).

With the production of neutrons, induced radioactivity is possible either as a direct result of the (γ, n) reactions or by activation by the neutrons. This radioactivity is

Table 2.4 Average monthly total body and hand dose equivalents for radiation therapy techniques (adapted from Glasgow 1984)

Therapy unit	Average monthly dose equivalent (μSv)		Hand-body ratio	Probable source of hand exposure
	Total body	Hand		
Cobalt-60 (AECL)	200	300	3:2	Leakage radiation
4 MV linear accelerator (Varian CI–4)	150	300	2:1	^{234m}Pa in uranium collimators
25 MV linear accelerator (Varian CI-35)	150	450	3:1	(γ, n) in treatment aids

short-lived and the amount will depend upon the energy of the X-ray beam and the length of time that the beam has been on. There have been no reports indicating that this radioactivity is a hazard to the patients (although some will be produced in the patient) or to personnel who enter the room immediately after the treatment. Personnel monitors show some increase over those worn by people working on low-energy accelerators (Table 2.4). However, some care should be taken for long exposures such as those associated with whole-body irradiation for bone-marrow transplants, where it is sometimes found that enough radioactivity has been induced to trigger the radiation room monitor.

Leakage radiation from the treatment head with the primary beam blocked should generally be measured 1 m from the target and 1 m from the path of the electrons through the accelerator. Acceptable values are summarized in various publications (ICRP 1982; NRPB 1988). In some cases the leakage radiation in the plane of the patient at 1 m must also be measured (IEC 1981; CRCPD 1982). The measurement must be performed for both X-ray leakage and, if the photon energy is high enough, neutron leakage. Inside the treatment room it is not possible to use a 'rem' meter, and foil activation methods are used to measure the neutron dose. If there is excess leakage, inadequacies in the shielding can be found by wrapping X-ray films around the treatment head.

For cobalt treatment units leakage measurements must also be conducted with the source in the 'off' position. In this case a survey meter will be used to measure the radiation levels 1 m from the source in three orthogonal planes. The average of these readings should not exceed 20 μSv h^{-1} and the highest reading should not exceed 100 μSv h^{-1}.

6.5 Electrical and mechanical safety

The electrical and mechanical safety of the installation must also be considered. The Institute of Physical Sciences in Medicine (1988) has described these requirements in some detail. Three broad categories

under which the electrical and mechanical safety for linear accelerators should be considered were identified:

(1) pre-installation;

(2) installation;

(3) clinical use.

The electrical and mechanical specifications must meet all applicable regulations. In general, architectural engineers, building engineers, maintenance engineers, and physicists will work together with the manufacturers to make sure that the equipment is electrically and mechanically safe.

6.6 Warning lights, interlocks, and monitors

Each installation will have warning lights to indicate when the beam is on, interlocks on the entrance door and elsewhere to turn the beam off if the interlock is triggered, radiation room monitors to indicate the presence of radiation in the treatment room, and audio and video monitors to hear and see the patient under treatment. All these must be checked to verify that they are operating correctly as detailed in IPSM Report 54 (1988).

Computer record and verify systems, or computerized accelerator control systems generally, and how they should be tested have not been discussed. As these systems become more common these questions must be addressed, but at the present time there is no agreement on the procedures that should be adopted. The overall structure of the computer systems should be reviewed to ensure that the machine will not operate unless certain parameters are set, and to determine what the limits on these parameters are. It is relatively easy to determine for any given treatment that the information stored by the record and verify system is correct and, for a computer-assisted set-up, that the right parameters were set. However, it is not so easy to devise tests that will ensure that, for any computer-assisted set-up and treatment, the machine set the right parameters and recorded the right dose. Experience has shown that if the limits on the parameters are set too tightly, the computer will shut the machine down frequently; however, if the limits are set too wide then there will be uncertainty in the treatment. Record-and-verify systems are discussed in more detail in Chapter 11, Section 4.

7. Summary and conclusions

In this chapter some of the concerns associated with the planning and acceptance of megavoltage radiotherapy installations have been presented.

Although there are several types of megavoltage equipment, the majority of institutions will have linear accelerators producing X-rays and very often electrons as well. The majority of the information in this chapter deals with this situation, although all the information can apply to any type of megavoltage equipment.

In addition to guidelines and suggestions about equipment specification, criteria for selecting equipment, and treatment room design, detailed information is given on acceptance testing.

Although much of this information is quite detailed, it is expected that there will be variations in the approach based upon local conditions and individual preferences. However, the main features should always be covered. Great care should be taken in selecting, installing, and testing megavoltage equipment. The investment in time and money can be considerable, and errors and oversights can be costly and can produce extensive delays before patients can be treated. As a general rule, two years should be allowed from the time that the decision is made to proceed with the acquisition of a machine to the time that the first patient is treated.

There has been no discussion of the personnel requirements associated with the installation of this type of equipment, since this will vary greatly depending on how much of the work is contracted out, how much help the manufacturers give, how much input the architects require, etc. However, the medical physicist will help define the specifications for the purchase of the treatment units (as well as simulators and treatment planning systems), will be involved in the design of the facility, and will survey the environs after installation of the radiation treatment machines to ensure compliance with all applicable regulations. The medical physicist will also be responsible for acceptance testing, commissioning, calibration, and periodic quality assurance (QA) of the radiation equipment (AAPM 1994a, 1994b). Therefore, the overall supervision and monitoring of the acquisition and testing of megavoltage installations can best be done by an experienced medical physicist.

8. References

American Association of Physicists in Medicine (1983). A protocol for the determination of absorbed dose from high-energy photon and electron beams. Report of AAPM Radiation Therapy Committee Task Group 21. *Med. Phys.*, **10**, 741–77.

American Association of Physicists in Medicine (1993). Medical accelerator safety considerations. Report of AAPM Radiation Therapy Committee Task Group 35. *Med. Phys.*, **20**, 1261–75.

American Association of Physicists in Medicine (1994a). Comprehensive QA for radiation oncology. Report of AAPM Radiation Therapy Committee Task Group 40. *Med. Phys.*, **21**, 581–618.

American Association of Physicists in Medicine (1994b). AAPM code of practice for radiotherapy accelerators. Report of AAPM Radiation Therapy Task Group 45. *Med. Phys.*, **21**, 1093–121.

British Institute of Radiology (1996). Central axis depth dose data for use in radiotherapy. *Br. J. Radiol.*, Supplement 25.

Conference of Radiation Control Program Directors (1982). *Suggested state regulations control of radiation* (HHS Publ. FDA 83–8203). FDA, Rockville, MD.

Dudziak, D.J. (1969). Fast neutron biological dose attenuation by lead and polyethylene shields. *Nucl. Appl.*, **6**, 63.

Glasgow, G.P. (1984). Residual activity in radiation therapy treatment aids irradiated on medical linear accelerators. In *Radiotherapy Safety, American Association of Physicists in Medicine Symp. Proc. 4*. American Institute of Physics, New York, 54–63.

Institute of Physical Sciences in Medicine (1986). *Radiation protection in radiotherapy*. IPSM Report 46. IPSM, York.

Institute of Physical Sciences in Medicine (1988) *Commissioning and quality assurance of linear accelerators*. IPSM Report 54. IPSM, York.

Institute of Physics and Engineering in Medicine (1997). *The design of radiotherapy treatment room facilities*. IPEM Report 75. IPEM, York.

Institute of Physics and Engineering in Medicine (1998) *Physics aspects of quality control in radiotherapy*. IPEM Report 81. IPEM, York.

International Commission on Radiation Units and Measurements (1984) *Radiation dosimetry: electron beams with energies between 1 and 50 MeV*. ICRU Report 35. ICRU, Bethesda, MD.

International Commission on Radiological Protection (1982) Protection against ionizing radiation from external sources used in medicine. ICRP Report 33. *Ann. ICRP*, **9**, (1).

International Electrotechnical Commission (1981). *Safety of medical electrical equipment–part 2: Particular requirements for medical electron accelerators in the range of 1 MeV to 50 MeV* (IEC 601–2–1). IEC, Geneva.

International Electrotechnical Commission (1989a). *Medical electrical equipment – medical electron accelerators in the range 1 MeV to 50 MeV – functional performance characteristics*. IEC No 976. IEC, Geneva.

International Electrotechnical Commission (1989b). *Medical electrical equipment – medical electron accelerators – guidelines for functional performance characteristics*. IEC No 977. IEC, Geneva.

Kersey, R.W. (1979). Estimation of neutron and gamma radiation doses in the entrance mazes of SL75–20 linear accelerator treatment rooms. *Medicamundi*, **24**, 151–5.

National Council on Radiation Protection and Measurements (1976). *Structural shielding design and evaluation for medical use of X-rays and gamma rays of energies up to 10 MeV.* NCRP Report 49. NCRP, Bethesda, MD.

National Council on Radiation Protection and Measurements (1977). *Radiation protection design guidelines for 0.1 – 100 MeV particle accelerator facilities.* NCRP Report 51. NCRP, Bethesda, MD.

National Council on Radiation Protection and Measurements (1984). *Neutron contamination from medical accelerators.* NCRP Report 79. NCRP, Bethesda, MD.

National Radiological Protection Board (1988). *Guidance notes for the protection of persons against ionising radiations arising from medical and dental use.* HMSO, London.

Nordic Association of Clinical Physics (1980). Procedures in external radiation therapy dosimetry with electron and photon beams with maximum energies between 1 and 50 MeV. Recommendations of the NACP. *Acta Radiol. Oncol. Rad. Phys. Biol.,* **19**, 55–79.

Shure, K., O'Brien, J.A., and Rothberg, D.M. (1969). Neutron dose rate attenuation by iron and lead. *Nucl. Sci. Eng.,* **35**, 371.

Svensson, H. and Hettinger, G. (1971). Dosimetric measurements at the nordic medical accelerators. 1. Characteristics of the radiation beam. *Acta Radiol. Ther. Phys. Biol.,* **10**, 369–84.

9. Additional reading

In addition to the references the following further reading is recommended.

Green, D. (1986) *Linear accelerators for radiation therapy.* Adam Hilger, Bristol.

Horton, J.L. (1987) *Handbook of radiation therapy physics.* Prentice-Hall, Englewood Cliffs, NJ.

Hospital Physicists' Association (1970) *A suggested procedure for the mechanical alignment of tele-gamma and megavoltage X-ray beam units.* HPA Ser. 3. HPA, London.

National Council on Radiation Protection and Measurements (1989) *Medical X-ray, electron beam and gamma-ray protection for energies up to 50 MeV (equipment design, performance and use).* NCRP Report 102. NCRP, Bethesda, MD.

Starkschall, G. And Horton, J. (Eds) (1991). *Quality assurance in radiotherapy physics.* Medical Physics Publishing, Madison, WI.

Van Roosenbeek, E. (1984). Room design and radiation protection surveys for high energy medical electron accelerators. In *Handbook of medical physics,* Vol. 11. (ed. Waggener, R.G., Kereiakes, J.G., and Stalek, R.J.). CRC Press, Boca Raton, FL.

Chapter 3

Absolute dose determination for high-energy photon and electron beams

B.J. Mijnheer, D.I. Thwaites, and J.R. Williams

1. Introduction

The principal aim of absolute dose determination is to enable an ionization chamber to be used at a reference point in a phantom and, with the use of appropriate conversion and correction factors, to yield the absorbed dose to water at that point for the situation in which the chamber is replaced by water. Ideally chamber calibration factors need to be available for every radiation quality used in the radiotherapy centre. The objective is achieved through the use of an ionization chamber calibrated at an accredited standards laboratory and the application of an appropriate protocol. The following problems can be identified:

1. In general, standards laboratories do not have the same beam qualities as are used in radiotherapy centres. Therefore the calibration at one energy has to be transferred to other radiation qualities.

2. Although absorbed dose calibration standards based on calorimeters have more recently become available, most standards laboratories use primary standards that measure exposure and/or air kerma in free air. The conversion of this measurement to one of absorbed dose in a different medium to air is non-trivial.

3. When the ionization chamber is placed in the medium it alters the radiation field. Corrections have to be applied for this. These corrections differ for the beam in which the chamber was calibrated and the user's beam.

4. The reading of an ionization chamber is affected by ambient conditions and, therefore, measurement corrections have to be made for various influence quantities such as temperature, pressure, dose rate (or dose per pulse) and polarity.

5. The corrections and conversions implied in (1) to (4) depend on the chamber design and materials, on applied voltage and on beam type and energy.

6. Generally a radiotherapy centre will only have one dosimeter which will be sent for calibration at a standards laboratory for a stated range of radiation

qualities. This is usually referred to as a secondary standard or local reference instrument. The dosimeters used for routine measurements (field instruments) must be calibrated against the local reference for the particular range of radiation types and qualities available in the centre.

7. Systematic errors in dosimetry may be introduced due to differences in the primary standards in the different national standards laboratories. In addition there are a variety of national and international dosimetry protocols available, which may introduce further systematic differences.

The requirements for accuracy and precision in the dose delivered to a patient were considered in Chapter 1. This chapter is concerned with the measurement of absorbed dose at a reference point in a phantom. This measurement is limited in its accuracy by the uncertainties in measurement of the reference quantities at the standards laboratories and the transfer of calibration factors to the local instruments, in the uncertainties in the measurement in the user's beam, and in the uncertainties introduced in dosimetry protocols (and their application) used to convert the dosimeter reading to absorbed dose to a medium. The measurement of absorbed dose at the reference point is the first step in the clinical dosimetry chain and it is a measurement that affects the treatment of all patients. Great care should therefore be taken to ensure that no errors are introduced at this stage. This chapter discusses several different national and international dosimetry protocols for megavoltage photon beams and for electron beams. It should be emphasized that once a protocol has been chosen, it is important for the maintenance of consistency that it is followed in detail.

2. Specification of beam quality

The derivation of absorbed dose in the user's photon or electron beam, using a calibrated ionization chamber, requires the application of energy dependent factors, regardless of whether the calibration has been in terms of exposure, air kerma or directly in terms of absorbed dose. The first step in an absorbed dose determination is, therefore, to establish the energy distribution of the radiation beam, i.e. a specification of the beam quality. Other than the special case of a cobalt unit this is not a trivial exercise.

2.1 X-ray beams

X-rays are produced with a broad spectrum of energies, ranging up to the maximum energy of electrons that strike the target, with a peak at approximately half this maximum value. In principle, the full energy spectrum should be known in order to derive the energy-dependent factors necessary for the determination of absorbed dose. However, these factors, or ratios of factors, are slowly varying functions of energy, so that relatively large variations in spectrum have an insignificant effect on the final calculation. It is usually sufficient to use a single value parameter to describe the quality of the user's X-ray beam.

The parameter that is required to specify quality depends on the protocol to be used. Two parameters are described in this text but careful attention should be given to the protocol to ensure that the precise definition of the parameter is understood and is followed.

2.1.1 Nominal accelerating potential (MV)

The most important factor that influences the spectrum is the energy of the electrons striking the target. The traditional method of specifying quality is, therefore, to state the energy of the electron beam. The X-ray beam quality is given as a nominal accelerating potential expressed in the unit MV. This distinguishes it from the energy of the near mono-energetic beam of electrons that produced it, expressed in the unit MeV, although numerically they should be the same.

Manufacturers of treatment units generally state X-ray quality in terms of MV. However, for dosimetry purposes the user should establish this value independently. The energy of the electron beam is not easy to measure directly and MV is best derived by comparison with standard depth dose data. The *British Journal of Radiology* in its Supplement 25 (BIR 1996) has published depth–dose data for energies between 2 and 50 MV. In that publication, several methods for beam-quality specification are discussed. The method preferred is to apply the per cent dose at 10 cm deep (D_{10}) on the central axis of a 10×10 cm^2 field at 100 cm source-to-surface (skin) distance (SSD) as an index of beam quality. This method has not yet been generally adopted and as an additional index the depth of the 80% isodose (d_{80}) under the same conditions is also applied. BIR (1996) gives the relation between both these

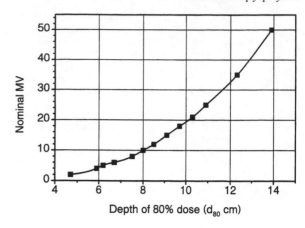

Figure 3.1 Variation of the depth of the 80% isodose along the beam axis (d_{80}) with nominal MV using data from BIR (1996).

quantities, as well as with other beam quality specifiers. Figure 3.1 shows the variation of d_{80} with nominal MV. At higher qualities, it varies more slowly with energy, which can lead to relatively large errors in the derivation of nominal MV. However, it will be seen in Section 3.1 that an error of 1 MV would lead to an error in dosimetry of 0.2% or less.

An example of the method for determining MV is:

1. Measure the central axis depth dose in water at 100 cm SSD and for a 10×10 cm^2 field. This should be done through the surface of the water phantom or through a thin window in the side of the water phantom.
2. Interpolate the depth of the 80% isodose from the data.
3. Use the data in Figure 3.1 to derive the value for the nominal MV.

It may be noted that in the specification of beam energy, manufacturers normally use this or an equivalent method to derive MV. This numerical value may differ quite significantly from the true accelerated electron energy, particularly at higher energies.

2.1.2 Quality index

The problem with the MV method is that the exact shape of the bremsstrahlung spectrum depends on a number of factors other than electron energy. This is the reason that the derivation of MV involves a rather circular route. Linear accelerators do not produce mono-energetic electron beams, so there is a further spread in the bremsstrahlung spectrum, which will depend on the design of the particular accelerating and beam-bending systems. Traditionally, thick tungsten targets have been used with linear accelerators. However, there have been investigations of thin targets, which produce more penetrating radiation, and of thick aluminium targets, which cause less self attenuation of the higher energy photons for accelerators operating at high energies (> 15 MeV). Beam quality is, therefore, dependent on target design. All accelerators have flattening filters, which have the secondary effect of altering the energy spectrum. The magnitude of this effect depends on the material used and its thickness. In addition to these factors affecting the primary spectrum, there are also factors that alter the spectrum and magnitude of secondary radiation in the treatment beam, such as the design of the collimation system.

For these reasons, most modern protocols have specified energy directly in terms of the attenuating properties of the beam. This eliminates the circularity involved in deriving MV by comparison with 'standard' sets of depth–dose data. One approach is to use d_{80} as the quality specifier directly rather than using it to derive the nominal MV (BIR 1996; IEC 1989). However, any such single parameter may be affected by high-energy recoil electrons reaching the surface, which could contribute to the dose at the depth of dose maximum and thus the value of d_{80}, etc. A recent suggestion (AAPM 1999) is to use the per cent depth-dose at 10 cm, but using a thin lead absorber in the beam to standardize and minimize the secondary electron effect on the value.

The parameter applied in most modern protocols, sometimes referred to as 'the quality index', is the ratio of the chamber reading at a depth of 20 cm in a water phantom, to the reading at a depth of 10 cm for the same fixed source to chamber distance (SCD) and for a field size of 10×10 cm^2 at the chamber. This is actually a tissue–phantom ratio (TPR$_{10}^{20}$). This quality index should be measured in a water phantom, which should extend at least 5 cm from the edges of the beam and by at least 5 cm beyond the chamber. In theory, the value of quality index is independent of SCD but in practice, it is generally measured at the position of the isocentre, that is at the source–axis distance (SAD).

An alternative quality index referred to in some older protocols is defined for a fixed source-to-surface (skin) distance (SSD = 100 cm), with the field size defined as 10×10 cm^2 at the surface. The quality index for this definition is, therefore, the ratio of the central axis depth doses at 20 cm and 10 cm (D_{20}/D_{10}). It may be noted that in some situations (NACP 1980) a beam specification parameter has been used which is the inverse of this ratio.

2.1.3 Comparison of specifications

Both quality index and nominal MV are derived from the attenuating properties of the beam. There is, therefore, a straightforward empirical relationship between the two. Table 3.1 compares nominal MV and quality index (TPR$_{10}^{20}$). In addition, other quality specifying parameters,

Table 3.1 A comparison of photon beam quality specification parameters. Data from BIR (1996)

MV (nominal)	TPR$_{10}^{20}$	d_{80} (cm)	%DD_{10}	%DD_{20}/%DD_{10}
4	0.626	5.9	63.0	0.541
5	0.646	6.2	65.0	0.557
6	0.677	6.7	67.5	0.582
8	0.713	7.5	71.0	0.611
10	0.731	8.0	73.0	0.625
12	0.748	8.5	75.0	0.639
15	0.763	9.1	77.0	0.649
18	0.775	9.7	79.0	0.658
21	0.789	10.3	81.0	0.669
25	0.798	10.9	83.0	0.676
(^{60}Co	0.57	5.1	58.7	0.50)

d_{80}, D_{10}, and D_{20}/D_{10}, are listed. These data have been interpolated from BIR 1996. The relative merits of different beam-quality specifiers are discussed in BIR (1996), ICRU (1999), and IAEA (2000).

2.2 Electron beams

As electrons are charged particles, the electron energy spectrum changes continuously as the beam passes through any material. The relatively narrow spectrum emerging from the accelerator is characterized by the most probable energy in front of the vacuum exit window, $E_{p,a}$. The spectrum is both decreased in energy and widened by passing through scattering foils, monitor chamber and air, along the path of the beam. At the phantom or patient surface, the spectrum is characterized by two parameters: the most probable energy at the surface, $E_{p,0}$; and the mean energy at the surface, $\overline{E}_0$. Because the electron energy loss interactions are such as to skew the spectrum towards lower energies, $\overline{E}_0$ is always less than $E_{p,0}$ and the difference increases with the energy spread of the spectrum. Thereafter, as the beam penetrates the phantom or patient, the energy continues to decrease and the mean energy $\overline{E}_z$ at depth z falls until the beam is completely stopped. Some of these energies are illustrated in Chapter 2, Figure 2.15.

Energy specification is obtained from empirical relationships between electron energy and the measured values of specific characteristics of the depth attenuation curves in water.

2.2.1 The mean energy at the surface, $\overline{E}_0$

The most significant energy parameter for dosimetry is $\overline{E}_0$, which is required in absorbed dose derivations to determine the appropriate correction/conversion factors required. It is obtained from the value of the 50% depth, R_{50}, taken from the measured curve of the attenuation characteristics of the beam in water. A number of slightly different approaches have been taken to this. The most commonly used relationship is:

$$\bar{E}_0 = 2.33 \times R_{50} \tag{1}$$

which is assumed to be valid for energies of around 5–35 MeV.

The factor 2.33 MeV/cm was originally obtained from Monte Carlo calculations of depth–dose curves and from measurements, essentially for mono-energetic broad parallel beams. Therefore, the relationship should strictly be:

$$\bar{E}_0 = 2.33 \times R_{50,d}^{\infty} \tag{2}$$

with the additional d indicating that the 50% depth is obtained from a depth–dose curve and the superscript implying that the curve is measured for a constant source-to-chamber distance (SCD). It is often more convenient to use measured values of R_{50} taken from depth–dose curves at a fixed SSD (f), usually 100 cm, to give $R_{50,d}^{f}$ or from depth ionization curves ($R_{50,i}^{f}$), also at fixed SSD.

There are differences between the R_{50} values obtained from these three approaches, which increase with energy, and strictly corrections should be made to equation (2) if either of the other two R_{50} values are used. Curves presented in the NACP protocol (NACP 1980) show the relationship between $\bar{E}_0$ and R_{50} obtained from depth–dose or depth–ionization curves at 100 cm SSD, illustrating the differences from equation (2). Table IV of the IAEA protocol (IAEA 1987) presents tabulated values of these data linking $\bar{E}_0$ to both $R_{50,d}^{f}$ and $R_{50,i}^{f}$. The IAEA parallel-plate chamber protocol (1997) and the IPEMB electron protocol (1996) provide fitted quadratic expressions to this data to link $\bar{E}_0$ to either the ionization or the dose R_{50} at fixed standard SSD.

The value 2.33 MeV/cm is an approximation of the available data for a derivation of $\bar{E}_0$ from depth–dose data. In general it underestimates $\bar{E}_0$. However, the use of this approach as the basis for the selection of stopping power ratios for beam calibration purposes produces values close to those obtained from accurate modelling of real clinical beam spectra (Andreo 1993; IPEMB 1996; IAEA 1997).

It may be noted that the corresponding representative constant linking $\bar{E}_0$ and $R_{50,i}^{\infty}$ is 2.38 MeV/cm. The older UK protocols (HPA 1985; IPSM 1990) use this value, rounding to 2.4, and recommending either measurements at fixed SCD, or appropriate corrections applied to fixed SSD measurements. It may be noted that the AAPM protocols (AAPM 1983, 1994) use equation (1) with the value 2.33 MeV/cm, but applied to $R_{50,i}^{f}$.

In recent recommendations for electron dosimetry (Burns *et al.* 1996; McEwan *et al.* 1998; AAPM 1999; IAEA 2000), the beam-quality specifier is simply taken

as the value of $R_{50,d}^{f}$ without a conversion to a nominal energy value.

For any of these approaches, the R_{50} determination, from depth–dose or depth–ionization curves, must be carried out in a sufficiently large field, such that the values are independent of field size. It should be stressed that $\bar{E}_0$ thus obtained must be applied to all field sizes with that beam, including smaller fields where the depth–dose curves are altered due to reduced scatter from the smaller irradiated area. Field sizes of at least about 12×12 cm^2 should be used for the determination of R_{50} for energies up to 15 MeV, and larger fields as appropriate at higher energies. All depths must be corrected to take account of the effective point of measurement of the chamber. Ideally, a suitable plane-parallel chamber should be used, to minimize positioning uncertainties and also typically minimizing the effects of recombination and polarity. In addition, the data should be converted to dose at each depth if depth–dose curves are required. If R_{50} is obtained in a material other than water, it must be scaled to water (see Section 5.4). Such a procedure increases the uncertainties and measurements in water are, therefore, recommended.

Although there are differences in the detail of method and application of these relationships in different dosimetry protocols, the net effect on absorbed dose determination is generally not large (typically within a few tenths of a per cent for beam energies up to about 20 MeV).

2.2.2 The most probable energy at the surface, $E_{p,0}$

$E_{p,0}$ is a useful parameter to characterize depth–dose distributions, as it is well related to the practical range, R_p. Practical range values can be determined from either depth–ionization or depth–dose curves at 100 cm SSD in water, also using sufficiently large fields and similar experimental conditions to those outlined above. It is defined as the depth of intersection of the tangent to the steepest part of the descending region of the curve with the extrapolation of the bremsstrahlung tail, (see Chapter 2, Figure 2.14). There are a number of empirical relationships in the literature linking $E_{p,0}$ and R_p. The most widely used expression is:

$$E_{p,0} = 0.22 + 1.98R_p + 0.0025(R_p)^2 \tag{3}$$

which is based on experimental measurements and Monte Carlo calculations. It is valid to within about 2% in the energy range 1 to 50 MeV.

2.2.3 The mean energy at depth z, $\bar{E}_z$

Although many of the factors required in absorbed dose determination are generally given as functions of $\bar{E}_0$ and z, some require an estimate of the mean energy at depth z. A widely used relationship, based on mono-energetic electron beams having a surface energy of $\overline{E}_0$, is:

$$\overline{E}_z = \overline{E}_0 \left(1 - \frac{z}{R_p}\right) \qquad (4)$$

where the depth of interest, z, and R_p are measured in the same material. This approximate relationship is close to the true values only for lower energy electron beams, or at depths close to the surface and close to R_p for higher energies. Monte Carlo calculations have been carried out on the realistic variation of $\overline{E}_z$ with depth. These data are summarized in table V of the IAEA protocol (1987) and are reproduced in IPEMB (1996) and IAEA (1997).

3. Calibration of ionization chambers

3.1 General

Every radiotherapy department should possess an ionization chamber with a calibration factor traceable to a primary or secondary standard dosimetry laboratory. Most standard laboratories provide an air kerma calibration factor N_k, (or an exposure calibration factor, N_x) at a single megavoltage quality, which is normally ^{60}Co gamma rays. At the standards laboratory, the chamber is calibrated in air with a build-up cap. The calibration factor gives the air kerma (or exposure) divided by the instrument reading corrected for the measurement conditions. It is determined at the position of the centre of the chamber in the absence of the chamber, i.e. it gives the exposure or air kerma for the situation in which the chamber is not present. The two calibration factors are related by:

$$N_K = N_X \frac{W}{e}(1 - g)^{-1}, \qquad (5)$$

where W is the average energy expended to produce an ion pair in dry air, e is the electronic charge and g is the fraction of energy of secondary electrons that is converted to bremsstrahlung in air. The currently accepted value of W/e is 33.97 J C^{-1} and for a ^{60}Co gamma-ray beam g is equal to 0.003.

In order to convert ionization chamber readings to absorbed dose values it is firstly necessary to apply a number of correction factors, k_i, to the calibration factor in air. These air calibration correction factors are needed because the presence of the chamber in the radiation field alters the field, i.e. the exposure or the air kerma at the position of the centre of the ionization chamber. The air calibration corrections are given by:

$$\Pi k_i = k_{\text{att}} \cdot k_{\text{m}} \cdot k_{\text{cel}} \cdot k_{\text{stem}} \qquad (6)$$

where k_{att} is a correction for absorption and scattering in the wall, build-up and central electrode of the ionization chamber; k_{m} is a correction for the difference in composition between the wall plus build-up cap and air and is given by:

$$k_{\text{m}} = [\alpha s_{\text{wall,air}}(\mu_{\text{en}}/\rho)_{\text{air,wall}} + (1 - \alpha)s_{\text{cap,air}}(\mu_{\text{en}}/\rho)_{\text{air,cap}}]^{-1} \qquad (7)$$

where α is the fraction of the ionization due to electrons set in motion in the chamber wall; $(\mu_{\text{en}}/\rho)_{\text{air,wall}}$ and $(\mu_{\text{en}}/\rho)_{\text{air,cap}}$ are the mass energy-absorption coefficient ratios air to wall and air to build-up cap, respectively; $s_{\text{wall,air}}$ and $s_{\text{cap,air}}$ are the mass stopping-power ratios wall to air and build-up cap to air, respectively; k_{cel} corrects for the difference in composition between the central electrode and air and k_{stem} corrects for the influence of the stem on the ionization.

It may be noted that in the IAEA protocol (1987), the definition of k_{m} differs in that the inverse ratios are used. However, the differences in the resultant values of this factor are small. Numerical values for $k_{\text{att}} \cdot k_{\text{m}}$ for various ionization chamber/build-up cap combinations can be found in dosimetry protocols and will be discussed in Section 5.2.

In a number of dosimetry protocols, the correction factors k_i are combined with exposure or air kerma calibration factors yielding the cavity-gas calibration factor N_{gas}, as defined in the American protocols (AAPM 1983, 1994) or absorbed dose to air chamber factor, N_D, (now generally written as $N_{D,\text{air}}$) as defined in the NACP (1980) and IAEA (1987) and related protocols:

$$N_{D,\text{air}} = N_K \cdot (1 - g) \cdot k_{\text{att}} \cdot k_{\text{m}}. \qquad (8)$$

It should be noted that, in these protocols, it is assumed that the value of k_{stem} is unity and that k_{cel} is combined with p_{cel} (see Section 4) into a global correction factor, which is taken into account during the measurements at the user's radiation quality. More recent protocols, following a similar formalism, such as the IPEMB electron protocol (1996) and the IAEA parallel-plate chamber protocol (1997), have used $N_{D,\text{air}}$ to designate this quantity to distinguish it from absorbed-dose-to-water calibration factors. In both the latter protocols, k_{cel} and p_{cel} are introduced separately, rather than as a global factor.

An increasing number of standards laboratories are now offering calibration services directly in terms of absorbed dose to water. Dosimetry based on absorbed dose standards has lower overall uncertainties than air-kerma based systems, is based on a more robust system of primary standards, and provides a simpler formalism. The National Physical Laboratory (NPL) in the UK provides absorbed dose to water calibration factors ($N_{D,\text{w}}$) directly for ^{60}Co gamma–ray beams and for 4–19 MV X-ray beams, with quality indices 0.57 to 0.79, based on a graphite calorimeter system (DuSautoy 1996). A UK protocol utilizing this service has been in clinical use since 1990 (IPSM 1990). Similarly, the Physikalisch Technische Bundesanstalt (PTB) in Germany has offered

$N_{D,w}$ values for a ^{60}Co gamma-ray beam for some time as the basis for dosimetry of a range of beam qualities (DIN 1997). A number of other protocols are under development to base dosimetry on absorbed dose standards, e.g. a new AAPM report (1999) intended to replace the existing North American air-kerma based protocols for high-energy photon and electron beams (AAPM 1994), a comprehensive new IAEA code of practice (2000) intended to cover all modalities, and a UK protocol (IPEM 2000) for electron dosimetry based on the recently developed NPL service for calorimetry-based direct electron absorbed dose standards (McEwan et al. 1998). It is expected that this approach will gradually become the norm over the next few years. It may be noted that where direct $N_{D,w}$ factors are available over an appropriately wide range of qualities, then the specific quality dependence of a particular chamber is directly obtained. When a single $N_{D,w}$ factor is available, generally for a ^{60}Co calibration beam, then either calculated or generic quality conversion or correction factors, k_Q, are required. Calculated k_Q are based on similar data, i.e. stopping power ratios and perturbation factors, as are used in current protocols, but used in the form of ratios between the user quality, Q, and the calibration quality, Q_0.

Using equations (12) and (13) in Section 4, it will be seen that the relation between $N_{D,air}$ and $N_{D,w}$ for the user beam quality, u, is given by:

$$N_{D,w} = N_{D,air} \cdot (s_{w,air})_u \cdot \left(\Pi p_i\right)_u \qquad (9)$$

with $s_{w,air}$ being the water to air mass stopping-power ratio and Πp_i the product of the correction factors to be applied to the measurements in the phantom.

It should be noted that N_K, $N_{D,air}$ and $N_{D,w}$ are all expressed in the same unit: Gy/scale division or Gy C^{-1}. It is, therefore, important that the various calibration factors, which may differ considerably in their absolute value, are not interchanged. In Section 5 numerical examples will be given to illustrate the conversion of one calibration factor into another and how to utilize in a hospital the various calibration factors for the determination of absorbed dose in radiation beams used for patient treatment.

It is recommended, even for small hospitals, that several ionization chambers should be available for absorbed dose determination. One of these chambers should have a calibration factor directly traceable to a standard dosimetry laboratory. This chamber, the secondary standard or local reference instrument, should only be used for special measurements, e.g. the calibration of field instruments that are used for the actual measurements in the beams of the treatment machines.

By comparing the readings of the local reference and the field instrument with their build-up caps in air in a

^{60}Co gamma-ray beam, the exposure or air kerma calibration factor of the field instrument can be determined directly. The $N_{D,air}$ calibration factor of the field instrument can then be obtained by applying the appropriate k_i values for that particular chamber.

If a ^{60}Co beam is not available, or if the calibration is directly in terms of absorbed dose to water, or if the dosimetry protocol specifies it, the comparison has to be carried out in a water or PMMA phantom irradiated by a photon or electron beam in the hospital. It is only in this way that $N_{D,w}$ for the field instrument can be obtained directly from known $N_{D,w}$ values for the local reference instrument. From equations (11) and (12) it will be seen that the assessment of N_K and $N_{D,air}$ calibration factors of the field instrument cannot be obtained simply from the ratio of the readings of both instruments in these circumstances. The determination of N_K and $N_{D,air}$ also requires the ratio of either the correction factors $(\Pi k_i)_u$ and $(\Pi p_i)_u$ or $(\Pi p_i)_u$ respectively, for both the local reference and field instrument. Therefore, it can be advantageous to use the same type of chamber as both reference chamber and as the field instrument, where possible, because the readings during these phantom measurements will then be directly proportional to the N_K, $N_{D,air}$ and $N_{D,w}$ calibration factors.

The number of chambers allowed as the local reference in a particular dosimetry protocol varies considerably (see Table 3.2). AIFB (Italy) applies only one, while AAPM (US), IAEA, etc., provide data for a large number of ionization chambers. Other protocols are based upon a limited number of commonly employed ionization chambers, e.g. IPSM/IPEMB (UK) and NCS (Holland, Belgium).

3.2   Parallel-plate ionization chambers

The use of parallel-plate ionization chambers is recommended in most dosimetry protocols for electron beams with mean energies below about 10 MeV. The calibration of these chambers in photon beams is not as simple as for cylindrical chambers because accurate theoretical values for $k_{att}.k_m$ or p_{wall} are not available. The Dutch code of practice (NCS 1989) applies measured $k_{att}.k_m$ data. Recent protocols for parallel-plate chamber use for electron beam dosimetry (AAPM 1994; IPEMB 1996; IAEA 1997) all recommend the preferred method of field instrument calibration to be by intercomparison with a suitably calibrated cylindrical chamber in a high-energy electron beam, although other methods are also discussed as less desirable alternatives.

IAEA (1997) deals specifically and comprehensively with the use of parallel-plate chambers and summarizes current knowledge on the various formalisms for their application in electron and photon beams. It presents details on design, construction, perturbation and other correction factors for available chambers, and provides

Table 3.2 Examples of local reference ionization chambers as recommended in various protocols[a]

Protocol	Photon beams	Electron beams[b]
AIFB (1988)	ENEA	ENEA (cyl)
DGMP (DIN 1997)	Six types of chamber	PTW 233641 (cyl)
		PTW 23343 (pp)
HPA (1983), IPSM (1990)	NE 2561	
HPA (1985)		NE 2571 (cyl)
		Vinten 631 (pp)
IPSM (1992)		NACP (pp)
		PTW 23343 (pp)
IPEMB (1996)		NE 2571 (cyl)
		NACP (pp)
		(Markus) PTW 23343 (pp)
		(Roos) PTW 34001 (pp)
NCS (1986, 1989)	NE 2505/3A	NE 2505/3A (cyl)
	NE 2561	NE 2571 (cyl)
	NE 2571	PTW 23343 (pp)
AAPM (1983, 1994)	Most commercially available	Most commercially available
IAEA (1987, 1997)	chamber types	chamber types

[a]NE, NE Technology; PTW, Physikalisch Technische Werkstätte.
[b]cyl, cylindrical chamber; pp, parallel-plate chamber.

practical recommendations and data as part of a code of practice and worked examples for their use. IPEMB (1996) provides some specific discussion of similar topics for the parallel-plate chambers and formalism adopted in that protocol for electron beam dosimetry. It may be noted that some of the numerical data given in IAEA (1997) are intended to replace the equivalent data in the earlier IAEA code of practice (1987), although it is stated that in no instance is the final dose determination significantly changed.

It should be stressed that parallel-plate chambers should generally not be used for absolute dose determinations in photon beams (where absolute is taken to mean the calibration of the dose per monitor unit or time) because of the relatively large uncertainties in some of the correction factors, such as p_{wall}.

4. Derivation of absorbed dose to water using calibrated ionization chambers

The formalism applied for dose determination in a high-energy photon or electron beam, using the ionization chamber method, is in principle the same in most dosimetry protocols. Firstly the field instrument is calibrated in terms of exposure, air kerma or absorbed dose to water, as discussed in the previous section. In some protocols, an intermediate step is then included in which an $N_{D,air}$ or N_{gas}, calibration factor is derived from

the exposure or air kerma calibration factor. The calibrated field instrument is then used to determine the absorbed dose to water, $D_{w,u}$, at a reference point in a phantom irradiated by the photon or electron beam.

Two basic assumptions underlie the formalism. Firstly it is assumed that W is constant for all photon and electron beam energies, i.e. the ratio between the reading M and the absorbed dose to the air inside the chamber is the same during the calibration and at the user's quality. The second assumption is that the Bragg–Gray equation can be used to derive the absorbed dose to water at the reference point from the absorbed dose to air inside the chamber volume.

The following equations are then valid:

$$D_{w,u} = M \cdot N_X \cdot (W/e) \cdot \Pi k_i \cdot (s_{w,air})_u \cdot (\Pi p_i)_u \quad (10)$$

$$D_{w,u} = M \cdot N_K \cdot (1-g) \cdot \Pi k_i \cdot (s_{w,air})_u \cdot (\Pi p_i)_u \quad (11)$$

$$D_{w,u} = M \cdot N_{D,air} \cdot (s_{w,air})_u \cdot (\Pi p_i)_u \quad (12)$$

$$D_{w,u} = M \cdot (N_{D,w})_u \quad (13)$$

where M is the corrected instrument reading, which is derived from the uncorrected instrument reading M_{uncorr} by applying a number of measurement corrections to take account of influence quantities:

$$M = M_{uncorr} \cdot p_t \cdot p_p \cdot p_{hum} \cdot p_{ion} \cdot p_{pol} \quad (14)$$

where p_t, p_p, p_{hum} are the air temperature, pressure and humidity correction factors, respectively; p_{ion} is the ion recombination factor and p_{pol}, is the correction factor for polarity effects in the user's beam. Application of these corrections will be discussed more fully in Section 5.1.

$(\Pi p_i)_u$ is the product of a number of phantom correction factors to be applied to the measurements in the phantom at the user's quality. The phantom corrections are given by:

$$\Pi p_i = p_{wall} \cdot p_d \cdot p_f \cdot p_{cel} \tag{15}$$

where p_{wall} corrects for the difference in composition between the ionization chamber wall and water; p_d corrects for the difference in ionization at the effective point of measurement and the depth at which the absorbed dose is stated; p_f corrects for the fluence perturbation due to the presence of the air cavity in the water phantom and p_{cel} corrects for the composition of the central electrode. Numerical values for these phantom correction factors will be given in Section 5.3.

Protocols have been developed and have evolved with time to indicate how equations (10)–(12) should be used, and in particular to provide values of the factors in these equations. The earliest protocols simplified equation (10) by combining all factors into a global correction factor, C_λ for photon beams and C_E for electron beams, which only depended on the energy of the user's beam:

$$D_{w,u} = M \cdot N_X \cdot C_\lambda \tag{16}$$

$$D_{w,u} = M \cdot N_X \cdot C_E. \tag{17}$$

These C_λ and C_E factors were intended to convert from exposure to absorbed dose calibration and had the unit, cGy R^{-1}. This method was introduced by the HPA in the UK and recommended by the ICRU (1964). One significant problem was that C_λ and C_E should depend on the size, shape and wall composition of the chamber, but only one set of values was supplied. At the time, various correction factors in equations (10)–(12) were either not fully understood or were ignored in the calculation of C_λ and C_E values. Therefore, the HPA introduced new values for C_λ in 1983 (HPA 1983), which were based on better data for the correction and conversion factors required in equation (11) and were specified only for one particular type of ionization chamber. For electrons, a somewhat modified approach was introduced in 1985 (HPA 1985) in which C_e was given for two designated chambers, supplemented in 1992 with additional recommendations (IPSM 1992). It should be noted that all these UK recommendations have now been superseded by newer protocols (IPSM 1990; IPEMB 1996). The NCS (1986, 1989) and others, simplified equation (11) into:

$$D_{w,u} = M \cdot N_K \cdot C \tag{18}$$

and provided C values for some types of commonly employed ionization chambers, which is similar to the procedure followed by HPA (1983, 1985).

The HPA, NCS and similar protocols all used an air kerma calibration factor in combination with a combined C factor for all conversion and correction factors for a limited number of ionization chambers. These protocols, which can be called N_K protocols, had the advantage of increasing the likelihood of dosimetric consistency between radiotherapy centres. They do not, however, permit a large choice of local reference chambers. It can also be argued that this approach does not encourage the hospital physicist to think about the steps that are being taken in the derivation of absorbed dose.

Other protocols (NACP 1980; AAPM 1983, 1994; IAEA 1987, 1997; AIFB 1988; IPEMB 1996) apply equation (12) and can therefore be called $N_{D,air}$ protocols. These protocols allow greater flexibility, in particular in the choice of the ionization chamber. In these protocols, no distinction is made between a local reference or field instrument – although exceptions include the Italian protocol (AIFB 1988), which is an $N_{D,air}$ protocol but allows only the use of one particular type of ionization chamber, and the UK electron protocol (IPEMB 1996), which allows only one transfer secondary standard instrument and then a limited number of designated field instruments. In this approach, all correction and conversion factors have to be calculated or looked up from tables, for each type of chamber and radiation quality, separately. For this purpose, worksheets can be filled in by the user. The advantage of this concept is that a large variety of ionization chambers can be used. Such a procedure requires, however, a thorough knowledge of the whole report, and is more time consuming and error prone than the use of an N_K protocol.

The current UK code of practice for high-energy photon dosimetry based on the NPL absorbed dose to water calibration service (IPSM 1990), uses equation (13). Its simplicity decreases the inherent uncertainties in photon dosimetry but a disadvantage is that a separate calibration factor for each ionization chamber at each photon radiation quality is required. The German practice of providing a ^{60}Co absorbed dose to water calibration (DIN 1997) requires a conversion of the ^{60}Co calibration factor to the user's quality, which can be derived from equation (9):

$$N_{D,w,u} = N_{D,w,Co} \frac{(s_{w,air})_u}{(s_{w,air})_{Co}} \cdot \frac{(\Pi p_i)_u}{(\Pi p_i)_{Co}} \tag{19}$$

where the ratio of factors converting from the calibration quality (^{60}Co) to the user's beam quality (u) is the k_Q factor mentioned in Section 3. This method improves the accuracy compared to starting with an exposure or air kerma calibration because only the ratios of conversion and correction factors are required and because any chamber-to-chamber variations in k_i and p_i are included in a direct $N_{D,w}$ calibration. In addition, where measured, k_Q over a suitable range of beam qualities (or individual $N_{D,w}$ factors, such as provided by the NPL calibration service) are available for a given instrument, the specific chamber's behaviour with beam quality is incorporated. All other approaches, including N_K, $N_{D,air}$ but also $N_{D,w}$ with calibration at a single quality require calculated or generic k_Q, which assumes all chambers of a given type behave in the same way and so cannot distinguish any chamber-to-chamber variations within a given chamber type. Whilst this gives rise to only small additional uncertainties for well-proven graphite-walled cylindrical chambers, such as the NE 2561 or 2571, it can give rise to much larger uncertainties for chambers using other materials (e.g. NE 2581) or for parallel-plate chambers. As noted above, it is expected that $N_{D,w}$ protocols, such as the current UK (IPSM 1990) and German (DIN 1997) examples, will gradually replace N_K and $N_{D,air}$ protocols, in response to developments in standards laboratories and the recent development of additional dosimetry protocols based on absorbed dose standards (AAPM 1999; IAEA 2000; IPEM 2000).

5. Practical application of protocols

The main factors influencing the selection of dosimetry equipment and dosimetry protocol are the type of calibration service provided by the national standard dosimetry laboratory and the availability of specific types of ionization chambers. Examples of the recommended local reference dosimeters for high-energy photon and electron beam dosimetry are given in Table 3.2. The reasons that those chambers were chosen are that they have a high stability of response and have well-known values of the correction factors k_i and p_i, although this is not necessarily so clear-cut for parallel-plate chambers. In addition, dose values determined with these chambers have generally been compared with data obtained with other independent methods of dosimetry (see Section 8).

A number of recommendations for ionization chamber design have been given in several dosimetry protocols (e.g. IAEA 1987, 1997; IPEMB 1996). Many commercially available ionization chambers fulfil these recommendations and the choice in buying a particular chamber is, therefore, mainly determined by other factors such as the availability in a particular country, applicability in both photon and electron beams as appropriate, and the price. In addition, the rigidity of the chamber wall might influence the decision. Graphite-walled chambers, such as the NE 2571, are much more fragile than chambers having a wall made from A-150 plastic, e.g. the NE 2581 chamber, or chambers made from PMMA having a thin layer of graphite as conductor, e.g. the PTW 23333 chamber. The latter two types of chamber have, however, rather large uncertainties in their k_i and p_i correction factors and are, therefore, not recommended as the local reference. They are, however, useful as field instruments, after suitable calibration,

although there would be increased uncertainties if they were used for electrons and, therefore, they are generally not recommended as first choice instruments in those beams.

Details of how to determine the absorbed dose at a reference point under reference conditions, i.e. the calibration of the dose monitor, will be discussed in Section 6. In this section the various correction factors will be discussed in more detail.

5.1 Measurement correction factors

The calibration factor for a chamber is the ratio of the true value of the best estimate of the stated dosimetric quantity being measured to the instrument reading under standard conditions. For measurements taken in non-standard conditions, various precautions and corrections may be necessary. Initial precautions include ensuring that the measurements are not significantly affected by: warm-up of the measuring system; thermal disequilibrium of the chamber and the phantom; drift; leakage currents with or without radiation present; stem effects; cable effects; etc.. Electrometer operating conditions should be checked. Initial irradiation may be advisable to provide charge equilibrium in the various chamber materials. Measurement correction factors, as introduced in equation (14), are then required:

(1) to correct for any difference between the ambient air conditions affecting the chamber reading at the time of measurement and the standard ambient air conditions for which the calibration applies (temperature, pressure, humidity); and

(2) to convert the measured charge to the induced charge, i.e. to correct for ion recombination and polarity effects in the user's beam.

When the ionization chamber is used at a temperature and pressure different from the calibration conditions its reading should be multiplied by:

$$\frac{P_0 \cdot (273.2 + T)}{P \cdot (273.2 + T_0)}$$

in which $T°C$ is the ambient temperature of the chamber taken as that of the phantom when in equilibrium, and P the pressure. P_0 is the reference pressure and its value is generally 101.33 kPa (1013.3 mbar). The reference temperature T_0 varies; some standard laboratories use 20°C, while others provide calibration factors at 22°C.

The effect of changes in air humidity on the response of an ionization chamber is small. If the chamber is calibrated for 50% relative humidity, then no correction is needed for measurements carried out in the range of relative humidities from 20 to 70%. It should be noted that some chamber wall materials (nylon, A-150 plastic) are hygroscopic. By water uptake the effective volume of these chambers will change, resulting in variations in calibration factor up to several per cent. These chambers should, therefore, be handled cautiously in high humidity conditions.

In dosimetry, the quantity of interest is the charge liberated in the chamber. The charge collection efficiency will, however, be less than unity if ion recombination occurs. The degree of ion recombination depends on the charge density (dose per unit time or dose per pulse) and the field strength. Ion recombination corrections vary, therefore, depending on whether the radiation is continuous, pulsed or pulsed-swept, and with the applied voltage between the electrodes. Correction factors can be determined by measurement or by calculation based on Boag's theories (reviewed and summarized in ICRU 1982). In general it is recommended that they be based on measurement to take account of variations between chambers. However, calculation can be used to check the magnitude of measured corrections and also to scale from the measurement conditions to other situations. Equations for calculating the ion recombination correction factor, p_{ion}, can be found in the various protocols (e.g. NCS 1989; DIN 1997; IPEMB 1996; IAEA 1997) and in ICRU (1982). An important parameter in these calculations is the field strength. The percentage loss of signal due to recombination is shown to be inversely proportional to the applied voltage, V, and proportional to the square of the (effective) electrode spacing, d. It is, therefore, necessary to check if this nominal spacing corresponds with the manufacturer's specification. This can be done by taking radiographs of the chamber. For cylindrical chambers, it is preferable to take two views at 90° to each other, to verify that the central electrode is completely parallel to the external wall. The other parameter required for these calculations for accelerator beams is the dose per pulse at the chamber, obtained from a knowledge of the dose rate at the chamber and the appropriate accelerator pulse repetition frequency (i.e. that describing the number of pulses per second of radiation produced, which is not always straightforward to obtain, depending on the operation of the accelerator).

The factor p_{ion} can be assessed experimentally by plotting the value of the inverse of the measured reading $(1/M)$ against $1/V$ over a range of voltage and extrapolating to infinite voltage, or by using the simpler two-voltage method, as described in most dosimetry protocols (e.g. AAPM 1983; IAEA 1987; NCS 1989; IPEMB 1996; IAEA 1997) and in ICRU (1982). It should be noted that some parallel-plate chambers exhibit behaviour indicating non-linear relationships between $1/M$ and $1/V$ at higher voltages, in which case lower voltages are preferred and special precautions may be required (IPEMB 1996; IAEA 1997). It should also be noted for these measurements (and for polarity measurements) that significant times (up to several minutes) may

be required before stabilization after voltage strength or polarity is changed.

For most ionization chambers, p_{ion} is close to unity for continuous radiation. For pulsed beams, the correction is generally less than 1% or so for X-ray beams and less than a few per cent for electron beams. These values are significant for dosimetry accuracy and should be checked, as above, for the particular beam, measurement conditions, chamber, and polarizing voltage. For pulsed-swept beams, the dose per pulse can be significantly higher, resulting in p_{ion} values up to 1.20. Ignoring ion recombination or its change when the pulse repetition frequency of these scanning beams is varied, can lead to large errors in output determinations and clinical doses. These errors have been observed during dosimetry intercomparisons between centres participating in clinical trials.

The polarity effect is the difference in readings obtained in the same irradiation conditions, but with the applied voltage polarity reversed and is due to directly deposited primary or secondary electrons in the chamber materials, essentially in the electrodes, adding or subtracting from the collected charge. It should be measured for each individual ionization chamber at the reference point by reversing the collection voltage. The magnitude of the polarity effect can be quite large for small ionization chambers at lower electron energies and it increases with field size. Stem and cable irradiation play an important role in the polarity effect, particularly for cylindrical chambers. If not taken into account, the polarity effect can lead to considerable errors in dose determination, although protocols often recommend not using chambers that are shown to have significant polarity effects (IPEMB 1996; IAEA 1987, 1997). However, the average of the absolute value of the two readings at each polarity is generally a good representation of the ionization in the air of the chamber cavity.

5.2 Air calibration correction factors

Values for the correction factors k_{att} and k_m are generally based on calculations. For a number of cylindrical chambers having different shape, size, and wall and build-up cap composition, calculated values for the product $k_{att}.k_m$ can be found in several protocols, e.g. IAEA 1987, 1997. The product varies between 0.95 and 0.997, e.g. for NE 2561 and 2571 chambers with graphite walls, aluminium central electrode and Delrin build-up cap the values are 0.979 and 0.985, respectively. Due to uncertainties in some of the calculated values, particularly of k_m, the NCS Codes of Practice (1986, 1989) applied average values of theoretical and experimental data.

In the first protocols to include k_{cel}, the value has been taken to be 1.008 for cylindrical ionization chambers with an aluminium electrode of 1-mm diameter and

1.006 for the NE 2561 chamber, which has a hollow aluminium central electrode. However, precise Monte Carlo calculations (Ma and Nahum 1993) have indicated that both have the same value, 1.006. These have been incorporated into more recent protocols (e.g. IPEMB 1996; IAEA 1997). It should be noted that for ionization chambers having an electrode made of a material identical to the wall of the chamber, k_{cel} will be unity.

Stem corrections are generally very small and k_{stem} is usually assumed to be equal to unity.

5.3 In-phantom correction factors

The influence of the wall material on the ionization in the air cavity, which arises if the walls have different composition than the medium, thereby changing the electron spectrum in the cavity, is taken into account by the factor p_{wall}. For electron beams it has been shown that the wall effect is usually less than 0.5% for common wall materials, at least for cylindrical chamber construction, and can therefore be ignored. For photon beams p_{wall} is given by:

$$p_{wall} = \alpha \cdot s_{wall,w} \cdot (\mu_{en}/\rho)_{w,wall} + (1 - \alpha) \quad (20)$$

with α having the same definition as in the air calibration correction factor k_m (equation 7); $s_{wall,w}$ is the wall to water mass stopping-power ratio; and $(\mu_{en}/\rho)_{w,wall}$ is the water to wall mass energy absorption coefficient ratio. For ^{60}Co gamma-ray beams p_{wall} values vary between about 0.985 and 1.01 for a number of commonly employed ionization chambers, being around 0.992 for a graphite wall of around 0.5 mm thick (IAEA 1987; NCS 1986). For high photon beam energies, p_{wall} values generally differ by less than 0.5% from unity because α becomes smaller.

For measurements in a water phantom, the chamber should be fitted with a thin waterproofing sheath, e.g. made of PMMA, preferably not thicker than 1 mm. If the PMMA holder is thicker, the formula for p_{wall} has to be extended to a three-component equation, yielding p_{wall} values that are up to 1.0% higher than values calculated using equation (20).

For plane-parallel chambers, p_{wall} values calculated using equation (20) will have large uncertainties because the influence of the side-wall on the total ionization and the contribution of the different wall materials are difficult to take into account. Experimental data or more sophisticated calculations of p_{wall} are required. At present, plane-parallel chambers are not recommended for the accurate determination of dose at the reference point in a phantom irradiated by a photon beam. For similar reasons the generally preferred method to transfer a calibration factor from an $N_{D,air}$ calibrated cylindrical chamber for use for electron dosimetry is to use a higher energy electron beam, rather than a photon beam.

The displacement correction, p_d, and the fluence correction, p_f, correct for the introduction of a cavity into the medium. One effect of a cylindrical cavity in a monodirectional beam is to move the point of measurement upstream from the geometric centre of the chamber. For ^{60}Co beams and electron beams the resulting effective point of measurement is about $0.5r$ upstream of the chamber centre and for high-energy photons it is about $0.75r$ upstream, where r is the cavity radius. These data result in p_d values varying between 0.985 and 0.990 for a number of ionization chambers for ^{60}Co beams. For higher photon energies, p_d is about 0.99 (NCS 1986). Another way of taking this displacement correction into account is by positioning the chamber with its effective point of measurement at the required depth and omitting p_d from equation (15). This is the procedure recommended in all dosimetry protocols for electron beams. A disadvantage of this procedure for photon beams is that positioning a chamber at a depth deviating from the reference values, i.e. at 5 or 10 cm, is more cumbersome and might lead to errors.

The factor p_f corrects for the change in the electron fluence due to the presence of the cavity in the medium. Fluence corrections are not required for photon dose determinations at the reference point because electron equilibrium exists. In electron beams there will be an imbalance between the number of electrons scattered from the adjacent phantom material into the air cavity and the number of electrons scattered out of the air cavity. Also, the overall track length of electrons in the air cavity volume will be different from the overall track length in a similar volume of phantom material. Because the inward scatter is dominant, p_f is less than one. For Farmer-type cylindrical chambers the correction varies between about 1% at 15 MeV to 4% at 4 MeV mean energy at depth (AAPM 1983; IAEA 1987, 1997; IPEMB 1996). For plane-parallel chambers with adequately designed guard rings, e.g. the NACP or the Roos chambers, p_f is unity. However, for other types of plane-parallel chambers, there may be a small but significant correction, e.g. it is about 2% at $E_z = 3$ MeV for the PTW/Markus chamber (NCS 1989; IPEMB 1996).

From theory and experiments it has generally been concluded that in electron beams there is little difference in response between chambers having graphite or aluminium central electrodes. Therefore, the value of p_{cel} for Farmer-type chambers has generally been taken to be unity in electron beams, although Monte Carlo calculations by Ma and Nahum (1993) have indicated a value of 1.002 in higher energy electron beams, with rather larger values at lower energies. The increase in response that can be observed in air if a graphite electrode is replaced by aluminium in a ^{60}Co gamma-ray beam will also occur in a phantom, i.e. p_{cel} has been taken to be 0.992 in line with k_{cel} being 1.008. Based on the same Monte Carlo calculations as previously mentioned, p_{cel} would become 0.994, in line with a k_{cel} value of 1.006 and there is evidence for slight variations in p_{cel} as photon beam quality varies. Most protocols that have included specific consideration of central electrode effects (AAPM 1983; IAEA 1987) have assumed that for these chambers the product of $k_{cel}.p_{cel}$ is unity for photon beams with maximum energy below 25 MeV. However, in electron beams this product has been taken to be 1.008 (IAEA 1987; NCS 1989) or less (IPEMB 1996; IAEA 1997) for a Farmer-type chamber having an aluminium electrode of 1 mm diameter, e.g. the NE 2571 chamber.

5.4 Non-water phantoms

All dosimetry protocols have the end result of calibrating a particular radiation beam in terms of absorbed dose to water, taking this as the reference material. Thus water is the phantom material primarily recommended for measurement. However, in some circumstances this can give rise to potential problems. Chambers require waterproofing sheaths, the water needs a container, and positioning uncertainties can be larger in areas of high dose gradient, particularly for lower energy electron beams and parallel-plate chamber use. In addition, solid phantoms can be quicker to set up for routine measurements. Therefore, a need arises for other phantoms to be recommended when these problems become significant.

For relative measurements, it is often convenient and it may be necessary, to use non-water phantoms, particularly solid plastics. ICRU (1989) reviews the data on some materials used. However, for absolute dose determination, which is the subject of this chapter, the use of non-water phantoms should be minimized, because additional correction factors need to be introduced and the uncertainties are, therefore, increased. As a general rule for beam calibration, it is strongly recommended that water phantoms should be used whenever possible.

For megavoltage photon beams, where protocols are based on the use of cylindrical chambers, no significant problems arise with water. The protocols all recommend water and discuss the waterproofing and positioning requirements to be followed. The AAPM protocol (1983) allows the use of polystyrene and acrylic plastics and discusses the necessary distance scaling factors, the transfer of dose from plastic to water, and the excess scatter corrections required. However, in view of the above recommendation, these are not discussed here. It may be noted that the various commercial water-substitute plastics are generally close to water in their performance in megavoltage photon beams (Tello *et al.* 1995; Allahverdi *et al.* 1999).

For medium and higher energy electron beams ($\overline{E}_0$ greater than around 10 MeV or $\overline{E}_z$ greater than around 5 MeV, depending on protocol), cylindrical chambers are primarily recommended for calibration and measurements. Therefore, water is a practical phantom material and its use is recommended even though some protocols allow the use of other materials.

For lower energy electron beams, however, different considerations can arise. Dose gradients are steeper and depth–dose distributions extend to smaller projected distances. Parallel-plate chambers are preferred in order to minimize the perturbation in the direction of the beam. For these chambers, positioning problems become more significant and some of them are more difficult to waterproof. Thus all protocols make some recommendations in recognition of the need for solid phantoms at these energies.

Certain standard industrial plastics have been used for this purpose, mainly PMMA (Perspex, Plexiglas, Lucite) and polystyrene. In older protocols, essentially pre-1981, no major differences were recognized between these and water, except for electron density differences. However, care must be exercised in their use. It is now accepted that four types of problem may arise:

1. Depths must be scaled to the equivalent depth in water. A number of approaches have been used including scaling by electron density, by stopping power or range, or by 50% depth. A discussion of some of these can be found in (AAPM 1991; IPEMB 1996).

2. Because of different scattering properties, electron fluence build-up changes with type of material. For polystyrene, this can result in measurement corrections of about 2.5 to 3% at an effective energy below about 3 MeV at the measurement point. This correction falls linearly with energy. PMMA has been considered in some protocols to exhibit negligible differences to water due to this effect. However, there is evidence to support corrections of up to about 1% at lower energies in some samples of Perspex.

3. For phantom materials that are insulators, 'charge storage' effects may occur that arise from the electrons stopped in the material. These are unable to disperse and the associated electric fields can modify the measured ionization at a cylindrical cavity during subsequent irradiation. These effects can be large, depending on the material, the accumulated dose, and the dose–time history of the phantom. Charge storage effects are minimized by using phantoms made of a number of sheets rather than being a solid block. Each sheet should be as thin as possible and no more than 2 cm. Charge storage effects do not appear to affect measurements made with plane-parallel chambers.

4. Sample variations can occur between different manufacturers, mixes or batches of the same nominal

plastic, due to differences in composition. For example, there are well-documented differences for electron beam measurements carried out in clear and white polystyrene, but other subtler batch differences can be present due to contaminants, density differences, etc.

Most modern electron dosimetry protocols take the first two of these effects into account, but use a variety of approaches and magnitudes of correction factors. Some protocols warn of the third and some of these give advice on how to minimize the effects. Some protocols point out the fourth problem and some recommend that the user check the density of the particular sample. It is clear that such differences between protocols increase inconsistency and uncertainties.

Alternatively, commercially available materials specifically formulated for dosimetric purposes are allowed in certain protocols. For example, A-150 plastic is included in IAEA (1987) and (1997). This material is electrically conducting, which eliminates charge storage problems. It is, on the other hand, hygroscopic and this may influence accurate dose determinations. Epoxy-based water-substitutes are included in AAPM (1991), IPEMB (1996), and IAEA (1997). They exhibit negligible charge storage effects and, depending on their formulation, may show only small effects of types (1) and (2) above. The variation in composition of these materials should be small, provided that quality control is applied at the manufacturing stage with dosimetry requirements in mind. However, there may be different formulations available under similar generic names. Thus the possibility of uncertainty in composition and, therefore, differences in factors (Tello *et al.* 1995; Nisbet and Thwaites 1998) should be considered. It may also be noted that these materials are significantly more expensive than the more standardly recommended plastics. The current UK electron dosimetry protocol (IPEMB 1996) contains a detailed discussion of the use of non-water phantom materials and provides scaling and fluence correction factors for a range of materials. IAEA (1997) has rather different scaling factors, but utilizes the fluence correction factors from IPEMB (1996).

Whatever non-water phantom is used when circumstances dictate that water is not appropriate, the choice and the method of use and the corrections to be applied must be within the framework of the selected dosimetry protocol. Again, this ensures consistency of the dose statement based on that particular protocol. It must be recognized that most investigations of the consistency between protocols have been carried out for graphite-walled chambers in a water phantom (see Section 8). Thus conclusions on the consistency of modern protocols (essentially within about 1%) apply to that situation. Using other chambers and other phantom materials can increase this difference significantly.

5.5 Worked examples

In this section, some examples will be given of how, in practice, the absorbed dose to water can be determined in a photon or electron beam by applying the equations given in Section 3 and 4. The numerical values for the conversion and correction factors applied in these worked examples are those recommended in a range of dosimetry protocols (NCS 1986, 1989; IAEA 1987) and belong to a consistent set that is also applied by the standards laboratories. A graphite-walled Farmer-type chamber, which is used in many hospitals for absolute dose determinations, is chosen in these examples. However, not all protocols give values for the physical quantities required for these calculations because they recommend other types of local reference chamber. Readers using other protocols are, therefore, referred to their specific codes of practice on how to calibrate and use their chambers, according to those recommendations. Due to the simplicity of the concept of N_K protocols, which specify only one or a few reference chambers and which provide combined factors for those chambers, no example of the use of these codes of practice are given. For similar reasons, no examples are given of the use of the UK $N_{D,w}$ approach (IPSM 1990). The $N_{D,air}$ protocols (AAPM 1983, 1994; IAEA 1987, 1997; IPEMB 1996) on the other hand can be quite complex to apply. A number of physical quantities have either to be calculated or looked up in tables or figures. For that reason the AAPM (1983), IAEA (1987, 1997) and related protocols have included worksheets with examples of how they should be applied. IPEMB (1996) follows a similar approach, but limits the number of chambers allowed, so is not as complex.

Example 1

A Farmer-type ionization chamber has an exposure calibration factor, N_x, of 1.300 R/scale division for $P_0 = 101.3$ kPa and $T = 20°C$. What are the values for the air kerma calibration factor, N_K, the absorbed dose to air chamber factor, $N_{D,air}$, and the absorbed dose to water calibration factor, $N_{D,w}$? The chamber has a graphite wall of 0.065 g.cm^{-2} thickness, an aluminium central electrode with diameter equal to 1.0 mm, and a PMMA build-up cap of 0.558 g.cm^{-2} thickness.

(a) Equation (5): $N_K = N_x.W/e.(1-g)^{-1}$.
Substitution of $N_x = 1.300$ R/scale division, 1R = 2.58×10^{-4} C.kg^{-1}, $W/e = 33.97$ J.C^{-1} and $g = 0.003$, yields $N_K = 1.143$ cGy/scale division.

(b) Equation (8): $N_{D,air} = N_K.(1 - g).k_{att}.k_m$.
Substitution of $k_{att}.k_m = 0.981$ yields $N_D = 1.118$ cGy/scale division.

(c) Equation (9): $N_{D,w} = N_{D,air}.(s_{w,air})_{Co}.(p_{wall})_{Co}.(p_d)_{Co}$.
Subsitution of $(s_{w,air})_{Co} = 1.133$, $(p_{wall})_{Co} = 0.993$,

and $(p_d)_{Co} = 0.987$, yields $N_{D,w} = 1.241$ cGy/scale division.

The data used in this example are taken from the IAEA protocol (1987) and NCS Code of Practice (1986). Other protocols may give rather different factors and final dose.

Example 2

The same chamber as in Example 1 has been used for the determination of the absorbed dose to water at 5 cm depth in a water phantom when irradiated with a 6 MV X-ray beam (quality index 0.68). The average reading for 100 monitor units, corrected for leakage and polarity, is 73.41 scale divisions at $P = 101.1$ kPa, $T = 23.5°C$ and 50% relative humidity. The ion recombination correction factor, p_{ion}, amounts to 1.005. The corrected reading is:

$$73.41 \cdot \frac{101.3}{101.1} \cdot \frac{273.3 + 23.5}{273.2 + 20.0} \cdot 1.005$$

$$= 74.80 \text{ scale divisions.}$$

The absorbed dose can now be calculated using the different calibration factors.

(a) Equation (10): $D_{w,u} = M.N_X.W/e. \, \Pi k_i.(s_{w,air})_u.(\Pi p_i)_u$.
Substitution of $N_X = 1.300$ R/scale division; 1 R $= 2.58 \times 10^{-4}$ C kg^{-1}; $W/e = 33.97$ J C^{-1}; $k_{att}.k_m = 0.981$; $k_{cel} = 1.008$; $(s_{w,air}) = 1.119$; $p_{wall} = 0.995$; $p_d = 0.988$; and $p_{cel} = 0.992$, yields $D_{w,u} = 92.0$ cGy.

(b) Equation (11): $D_{w,u} = M.N_K.(1 - g).\Pi k_i.(s_{w,air})_u.(\Pi p_i)_u$.
Substitution of $N_K = 1.143$ cGy/scale division; $(1 - g) = 0.997$ and the other values as given above, yields $D_{w,u} = 92.0$ cGy.

(c) Equation (12): $D_{w,u} = M.N_{D,air}.(s_{w,air})_u.(\Pi p_i)_u$.
Subtitution of $N_{D,air} = 1.118$ cGy/scale division and the other values as given above, yields $D_{w,u} = 92.0$ cGy.

Remember that k_{cel} is not included in $N_{D,air}$ and that the product $k_{cel}.p_{cel}$, which is 1.000 for this chamber, is applied in equation (9) in the IAEA protocol (1987) approach being followed in this example. If k_{cel} and p_{cel} are included explicitly, or if the newer values of these quantities are used, they would still cancel each other in the final calculation, so the dose obtained would be unchanged.

In some protocols (NACP 1980; IAEA 1987), p_{wall} is given the symbol p_u. Applying equation (12) and the recommended value of $p_u = 0.995$, would yield $D_{w,u} = 93.1$ cGy. In these protocols the dose is, however, calculated at the effective point of measurement i.e. at $0.75r = 2.4$ mm in front of the geometrical centre for this chamber. The dose at 5.0 cm depth in the phantom will

then be: $D_{w,u}$ (5.0 cm) $= D_{w,u}$ (4.76 cm). $p_d = 93.1 \times 0.988 = 92.0$ cGy.

(d) Equation (18): $D_{w,u} = M.N_K.C$.
Substitution of $N_K = 1.143$ cGy/scale division, and $C = 1.077$ as can be derived, for example, from NCS (1986), yields $D_{w,u} = 92.1$ cGy.

Example 3

The same chamber as in Examples 1 and 2 is used for the determination of absorbed dose to water in a water phantom irradiated with an electron beam with a mean energy at the surface, $\bar{E}_0$ of 12 MeV. The chamber is positioned with its effective point of measurement, which is located at half the chamber radius (1.6 mm) in front of the geometrical centre, at the depth of dose maximum, which is 2.0 cm. The mean energy at the depth of dose maximum is 8.0 MeV. The reading corrected for leakage, polarity, ion recombination, temperature and pressure is 89.6 scale divisions for 100 monitor units. The absorbed dose can now be calculated using the different calibration methods.

(a) Equation (10):
$D_{w,u} = M.N_X.W/e.\Pi k_i.(s_{w,air})_u \, .(\Pi p_i)_u$.
Substitution of $N_X = 1.300$ R/scale division; 1 R $= 2.58 \times 10^{-4}$ C.kg^{-1}; $W/e = 33.97$ J.C^{-1}, $k_{att}.k_m = 0.981$; $k_{cel} = 1.008$; $(s_{w,air})_u = 1.008$; $p_f = 0.973$; and $p_{cel} = 1.000$, yields $D_{w,u} = 100.0$ cGy (again taking values from the NCS (1986, 1989) or the IAEA (1987) Codes of Practice, other protocols may give somewhat different values).

(b) Equation (11): $D_{w,u} = M.N_K.(1 - g).\Pi k_i.(s_{w,air})_u.(\Pi p_i)_u$.
Substitution of $N_K = 1.143$ cGy/scale division; $(1 - g) = 0.997$ and the other values as given above yields $D_{w,u} = 100.0$ cGy.

(c) Equation (12): $D_{w,u} = M.N_{D,air}.(s_{w,air})_u.(\Pi p_i)_u$.
Substitution of $N_D = 1.118$ cGy/scale division; $(s_{w,air})_u = 1.018$; $p_u(= p_f) = 0.973$ and $p_{gbl,cel}(= k_{cel}) = 1.008$, yields $D_{w,u} = 100.0$ cGy.

Note, here the example follows IAEA (1987) in applying a global $p_{gbl,cel}$, i.e. the combination of k_{cel} and p_{cel}, where for electron beams, p_{cel} is taken as unity. This is used with an $N_{D,air}$, which has no k_{cel} included. If later protocols are used (IPEMB 1996; IAEA 1997), which include k_{cel} in $N_{D,air}$, then this would look rather different, but the outcome would be the same except for the slightly different recommended values. This illustrates the importance of becoming familiar with the detailed terminology and content of the particular protocol being used and of then applying it carefully.

(d) Equation (18): $D_{w,u} = M.N_K.C$.
Substitution of $N_K = 1.143$ cGy/scale division and $C = 0.977$, yields $D_{w,u} = 100.1$ cGy.

As another example of the dangers of mixing codes unthinkingly, equation (18) cannot be applied in combination with the C_e values provided in the older UK Code of Practice (HPA 1985; IPSM 1992), as the calibration route and the calibration quantity for electron field instruments is different in the two approaches. In any event, those older protocols have been superseded by the current UK electron dosimetry protocol (IPEMB 1996), based on an $N_{D,air}$ approach.

6. Calibration of the dose monitor

The most critical dose measurement for external beam therapy is that which is generally referred to as the calibration of the dose monitor, i.e. the measurement of the absorbed dose under reference conditions per monitor unit of an accelerator, or the measurement of the absorbed dose rate for a cobalt unit. Great care is required to ensure that the calibration is carried out correctly. The basic dosimetric calibration of the treatment unit should be repeated at least once and should also be verified by a second physicist independently of the first. This should involve a completely new set-up of all equipment, preferably with a second calibrated ionization chamber. If that is not possible, there should be an independent check of the calibration factor of the chamber in the user's beam. Patient treatment should not be started until these independent checks have been satisfactorily completed.

The dose monitor is generally calibrated in terms of the ratio of monitor units to the absorbed dose on the central axis at the depth of dose maximum, d_{max}, for a $10 \times 10 \ cm^2$ field and for the standard SSD, generally 100 cm. It is common practice to adjust the calibration of the monitor so that this ratio is equal to 100, i.e. one monitor unit (mu) is equivalent to an absorbed dose of 1 cGy at this position in these conditions. This position is chosen because it is the point to which the dose data for fixed SSD treatments are generally normalized. This calibration is performed at an SSD equal to the source-to-axis distance (SAD), usually 100 cm, but with the chamber not necessarily at the position of d_{max}, but at a stated reference depth. Alternatively, the chamber can be placed at the reference depth, but with the source-to-chamber distance equal to the SAD. When an SSD set-up is used, the reference field size is defined at the surface of the phantom, but for an SAD set-up it is defined at the measurement position.

For photon beams, the calibration must be performed through a measurement at the reference depth, defined in the dosimetry protocol. The dose at d_{max} may then be calculated by dividing the dose at the reference depth by the per cent depth dose at that depth using the depth–dose data or the tissue-phantom ratios (or specifically

TMR) that are to be used for clinical dosimetry. The reason that dose is calibrated at a reference depth is that the dose at d_{max} may be influenced by electrons originating outside the phantom. The dose may, therefore, be affected by the presence of accessories or other materials in the beam in a way that is not reflected in a change in dose at greater depths. In addition, the depth of the dose maximum varies with field size at high energies. It is, therefore, more reliable to use a greater depth for the reference calibration. In the past, various reference depths have been used in the different protocols. In ESTRO recommendations for monitor unit calculations (ESTRO 1997) the use of a single reference depth (10 cm) was recommended for all high-energy photon beam qualities, for calibration as well as for the determination of other beam parameters, to ensure that the measurement point is beyond the range of the most energetic secondary electrons originating outside the phantom for the usual range of beam qualities encountered. Chamber calibration factors for these beams are generally assumed to be independent of depth, at least over the variation of depths normally of concern.

This fundamental calibration of the dose monitor should be referenced to the weekly/daily calibration consistency measurements. For photons, these latter measurements may be made either in air with the chamber held in a rigid jig which is attached to the face of the accelerator, and using a build-up cap, or in a solid phantom (see Chapter 5, Section 9). For electrons, measurements in a solid phantom are recommended for consistency checks, with attention paid to possible phantom problems (see Section 5.4). The chamber used for the weekly/daily calibration is normally different from the one used for the reference point measurement. It does not necessarily need to be calibrated in terms of absorbed dose. The chamber used for the reference point measurement can be the chamber which was calibrated at a standards laboratory or preferably a field instrument calibrated against this local reference chamber.

6.1 Photon beams

The following procedure should be adopted for the calibration of the dose monitor for X-rays:

1. Select the reference depth in accordance with the protocol in use. This will depend on the quality index of the beam. Alternatively a value of 10 cm may be used, if following the recommendations of ESTRO (1997) in conjunction with a national or international protocol.

2. Place the chamber in its waterproof sheath at the reference depth in the water phantom. The protocol recommendations should be followed carefully to ensure that an appropriate sheath is used. The majority of protocols recommend a thin protective

cap. Adjust the phantom height to 100 cm SSD, if using an SSD set-up, and the field size to 10×10 cm^2. (Alternatively, an SAD setup may be used.) It should be noted that the IAEA and related protocols specify that the centre of the chamber is displaced from the position of measurement. If these protocols are followed, the chamber centre should be positioned at a depth equal to the reference depth plus the displacement distance (see Section 5.3 and Section 5.5, Example 2).

3. Record the reference chamber reading for a known monitor unit setting. Apply correction factors to the reading for temperature, pressure and other appropriate influence quantities and convert to absorbed dose at the reference depth, D_r, following the detailed recommendations of the protocol being used:

$$D_r = M \cdot N \cdot \Pi c_i$$

where M is the corrected reference chamber reading, N is the appropriate chamber calibration factor and Πc_i is the product of correction/conversion factors required, which depend on the details of the protocol and the particular chamber calibration method.

4. Correct to absorbed dose at d_{max}, D_d:

$$D_d = D_r \cdot (100/\%DD_r)$$

where $\%DD_r$ is the per cent depth dose at the reference depth. Thereby establish the link between monitor units (mu) and absorbed dose at the normalization point, i.e. d_{max}. Alternatively TPR (or TMR) data may be applied to convert from the reference depth to the normalization point, depending on local practice.

5. If necessary adjust the monitor calibration factor to 100 mu Gy^{-1} and repeat the measurement.

6. Remove the water phantom and position the chamber used for weekly/daily checks in its normal position and follow the normal weekly/daily consistency check procedure. Measure the ratio of monitor units to the corrected chamber reading, M_D. The daily consistency factor (DCF) is given by:

$$DCF = mu / M_D$$

For the daily monitor checks, this factor multiplied by the corrected reference chamber reading per monitor unit should be equal to unity, within the tolerance set locally. Alternatively M_D represents the reference daily chamber reading (after correction) for a specified number of monitor units.

7. This set of measurements should be independently checked and any discrepancies greater than the experimental errors (approximately 0.3%) should be reconciled.

Similar measurements should be made for a cobalt unit, except that the output of the unit should be measured in terms of absorbed dose per unit time. This measurement should also be repeated independently by a second physicist. At the same time the normal quality control test of the timer should be made to ensure its correct adjustment. The output measurement should be compared with the calibration certificate issued by the supplier of the source. After correction for decay, differences in excess of 5% should be investigated and if possible reconciled.

6.2 Electron beams

For calibration of the dose monitor for electron beams, the exact details of recommended procedures will vary with the dosimetry protocol or code of practice selected. In some protocols, the sequence of some steps is changed. It is important that there is strict adherence to the protocol and that recommendations from different sources are not mixed together. A general scheme emphasizing the main points is given below.

1. Determine $\overline{E}_0$ from depth–dose or depth–ionization curves as required (see Section 2.2).

2. Select the reference depth in accordance with the protocol. This will generally be the depth of dose maximum (d_{max}) for the beam and field size to be used. In some circumstances it may be a fixed depth, or a depth related to R_{50}, e.g. $0.5.R_{50}$, chosen to be close to d_{max} and increasing with $\overline{E}_0$.

3. Position the effective point of measurement of the chamber at the reference depth in the phantom. Adjust the phantom height to be the normal treatment distance, normally 100 cm SSD, and select a field size of 10×10 cm^2. The protocol recommendations on phantom and sheath materials and sizes should be followed carefully.

4. Take repeated chamber readings for known monitor unit settings, correcting for pressure, temperature, recombination, and polarity. Using information on $\overline{E}_0$, depth of measurement and chamber used, select the appropriate calibration, correction and conversion factors for the measurement situation and the protocol followed. Convert the measurement to absorbed dose. Include any phantom correction factors necessary if phantom materials different to water have been used (see Section 5.4).

5. If measurements have not been carried out at d_{max}, for reasons complying with protocol recommendations, corrections may be required to convert to d_{max} from the measurement position, based on measured depth dose information.

6. Express the results in the form required by local planning procedures, generally the ratio of mu to

dose at d_{max}. If necessary, adjust the ratio to 100 mu/Gy and repeat the measurements.

7. Remove the phantom and position the chamber and phantom to be used for weekly/daily output consistency checks in their normal positions and follow the normal weekly/daily measurement procedure. Establish the link between absolute absorbed dose calibration and weekly/daily consistency check measurements.

8. The whole set of measurements should be repeated and independently checked by a second physicist. Any discrepancies greater than the experimental errors (approximately 0.5%) should be reconciled.

7. Quality control of calibration

The main steps leading up to the dose monitor calibration are the calibration of a local standard dosimeter either at a national standards laboratory or at a secondary standards laboratory, the calibration of field instruments against the local standard and the calibration of the beam under reference conditions using recommended procedures.

This calibration chain ensures traceability of dosimetry to primary standards in each centre. At each stage, careful application of recommended procedures and data from protocols and codes of practice ensures accurate and consistent dosimetry in the transfer from the standards (primary or secondary) to the absorbed dose calibration of each beam in the radiotherapy centre. In order to ensure continuing quality of dosimetry, a suitable quality control programme must be established, encompassing each part of this chain. It should, therefore, include consideration of both the output calibration of the treatment unit and the dosimetric equipment used in that calibration.

7.1 Calibration of instruments

The calibration of local standards has been discussed in Section 3. It must be repeated at regular intervals. Calibration of field instruments against local standards must similarly be repeated at frequent intervals. Any national or protocol recommendations should be observed. For example in the UK the 'secondary standard' system must be calibrated every 3 years at the NPL and field instruments should be calibrated at least annually against this local standard system. For field instrument calibrations, any national or other appropriate guidelines must be carefully followed, particularly if linked to the dosimetry protocols used. In addition to regular chamber calibrations, further calibrations must be carried out following significant repair, or if there is any suspicion that the response of the system may have changed.

Typical variations from one calibration to the next should always be within 1% and, generally, within a few tenths of a per cent, provided that there has been no major repair or change to the system.

Calibrations should include checks on the linearity of response, scale factors and leakage where appropriate. Other tests on the systems should also be carried out, as recommended by the manufacturers. All dosimeter checks and tests and calibration measurements must be recorded in a designated logbook.

7.2 Check-source measurements

Between chamber calibrations, a regular pattern of check-source measurements should be carried out to ensure constancy of response of the system. For example, for local standards that are to be used infrequently, checks should be done at least once every 3 months and also before and after any major use of the equipment for beam or chamber calibration. Similar check-source measurements should be carried out at more frequent (e.g. monthly) intervals on field instruments, which have more frequent routine use. Checks should also be done on the local standard before and after it is sent for calibration to a primary or secondary standards laboratory, to ensure its response is unchanged as a result of transport.

The usual check-source is a ^{90}Sr source, contained in a housing that ensures that the chamber and source are positioned in a fixed geometry relative to each other. Frequently for cylindrical chambers these are in a relatively massive shielding container and care must be taken to ensure that temperature equilibrium has been reached and that the temperature at the chamber position is correctly measured. For parallel-plate chambers, small planar ^{90}Sr sources can be used placed in a plastic housing constructed to reproducibly and closely site the source and the chamber together. These present a more significant radiation protection problem in use than the contained sources. An alternative method for institutions having a cobalt unit is to position the chamber in a rigid jig, which can be attached, in a simple and reproducible way, to the face of the cobalt unit. For both methods, chamber readings should be obtained for a number of irradiation times and, after correction for temperature and pressure, can be converted to the time to give a certain reading. Correcting this for source decay to some chosen reference time allows a standard measurement to be compared to previous values. If no damage or modifications have occurred in the system, then typical variations should always be within 1% and generally within a few tenths of a per cent. If significant variations are seen, then further investigations are required and ultimately a full recalibration of the system may be needed. It should be noted that a specific change in check-source reading should never be used to change the calibration factors by a similar amount; the chamber will generally respond differently to the beta radiation from the check-source compared to the photons of the calibration beam. Again all measurements must be recorded in a suitable log-book. If a cobalt unit has been used and significant changes measured, the possibility of a fault which could have altered the output should be investigated. An example of such a fault is a change in the shutter opening speed. This can be checked with a second dosimetry system.

7.3   Reference-point checks

As part of the quality assurance of the absolute absorbed dose calibration, all measurements, correction and conversion factors must be recorded. All distances, field sizes and depths should be checked and double-checked. Independent verification of the calibration should be carried out (Section 6). Immediately after the absolute calibration, a set of simpler and easily reproducible quality control measurements should be made, so that they can be referenced to the calibration.

These quality control measurements on the absorbed dose calibration must then be carried out at regular and frequent intervals throughout the lifetime of the machine, to ensure consistency in output of the treatment unit in terms of dose per unit time or monitor setting. These may be at two levels:

(1) a weekly check on the calibration consistency, using a field class ionization chamber; and

(2) a daily consistency check relative to that, using another chamber or a diode.

These measurements are discussed in Chapter 5, with suitable tolerance and action levels. Any variations outside these levels must be investigated and rectified. All regular calibration consistency checks must be recorded in a suitable log-book.

Finally, it is recommended that a repeat of the absolute absorbed dose calibrations be carried out at least once a year, following the full procedures outlined in Section 6.

7.4   Accessory equipment

Besides the dosimeter systems used in monitor calibration, other equipment is necessary and must be included in the quality control programme. In particular, pressure and temperature measuring devices must be checked at yearly intervals and more frequently for electronic devices. For thermometers, it is sufficient to compare the response of a number of instruments, in order to ensure no single instrument is out of line. For barometers, a check against locally available pressure standards is required. If this is from a local airport or weather station, for example, it is important to ascertain whether the quoted pressure is the local pressure or has

been corrected to sea level, and appropriate corrections may then be made. Any such equipment must have any checks and tests carried out that are recommended by their manufacturers. Phantoms, build-up caps and sheaths must be regularly inspected for damage that could distort the depths or the dosimeter responses.

7.5   Dosimetry intercomparison or audit

One final step in a quality assurance programme concerned with beam calibration is to participate in dosimetry intercomparisons, where available, where dose measurements are compared between different centres or to an assessment by a separate institution. Where these are carried out by independent personnel, who are not responsible for – or involved in – the local procedures, they may be regarded as a form of quality audit of these aspects of dosimetry.

8.   Accuracy of the absolute dose determination

The accuracy in the absolute dose determination using an ionization chamber is determined by many factors. Firstly, the chamber and its electrometer, including the cables and connectors, should be well designed and behave according to their specifications. Guidance is given in IEC (1997). Important characteristics are a small polarity effect, low ion recombination, and a low leakage. In order to determine these effects, it is necessary to have a variable high-voltage supply with two polarities. The electrometer reading should have enough digits to reduce its rounding error, while the long-term stability should be good. It is essential that the materials and dimensions of the wall, central electrode, and build-up cap are known in order to determine the conversion and correction factors required for the absorbed dose calculation from its reading. The uncertainty in the calibration factor obtained from, or traceable to, the standard dosimetry laboratory is the second important contribution to the overall accuracy. Finally, the correction and conversion factors required in the computation of the absorbed dose from the ionization chamber reading introduce additional uncertainties.

An important question is, what differences in dose values can be observed if different dosimetry protocols are used? For photon beam measurements with an NE 2561 chamber, the different recommendations can be compared, as data for this chamber is included in most protocols. Some small adaptations of particular protocols are necessary to perform this intercomparison, e.g. for the movement of the effective point of measurement to the reference point, the conversion between different beam quality specifiers, or the extraction of effective k_Q

Table 3.3 Uncertainties in absolute dose determination using an ionization chamber at the reference point in a phantom irradiated at the user's quality by applying equation (11); the values correspond to one standard deviation (taken from Brahme *et al.* 1988)

Physical quantity	Uncertainty		
	^{60}Co	Photon beams	Electron beams
M (corrected reading)	0.5	1.0	1.0
M (long-term stability of timer or monitor)	0.5	1.5	1.5
N_K	1.0	1.0	1.0
$k_m.k_{att}$	1.6	1.6	1.6
$s_{w,air}$ (theoretical values)	1.5	1.5	1.5
$s_{w,air}$ (quality specification)	–	1.0	1.5
p_{wall}	0.5	–	–
$p_{wall}.p_d.p_{cel}.k_{cel}$	–	1.0	–
$p_f.p_{cel}.k_{cel}$	–	–	1.5
Overall uncertainty	2.3	3.1	3.6

from $N_{D,w}$ calibrations. Older protocols, such as AAPM (1983) and HPA (1983) gave rather higher estimates of dose, generally by about 1%, compared with more recent N_k or $N_{D,air}$ protocols, such as NCS (1986) and IAEA (1987). Differences of the same order of magnitude can be observed for other chambers, where comparisons can be made, such as the NE 2505/3A, NE 2571 and PTW 23332 chambers. It should be noted here that the older N_K based UK protocol (HPA 1983) was superseded in 1990 by an $N_{D,w}$ based protocol (IPSM 1990) and that this approach is increasingly being adopted internationally. The IPSM (1990) protocol gives estimates of dose that are rather higher than the $N_{D,air}$ protocols. Considering all these comparisons, it can be generally stated that the agreement of all modern high-energy photon protocols, for graphite-walled chambers in water phantoms is within around 1%.

The results of similar comparisons (Thwaites 1994a) for electron dosimetry for an NE 2571 chamber using pre-1993 protocols, and (Nisbet *et al.* 1998) for a NE 2571 chamber, and also for Markus and NACP parallel-plate chambers using more recent electron dosimetry protocols (AAPM 1994; IPEMB 1996; IAEA 1997), show that differences are also generally within around 1% between recent electron protocols.

It can, therefore, be concluded that the consistency between recent protocols, and even between recent and older protocols, is good for graphite-walled chambers in a water phantom. This good agreement does not imply, however, that the absolute accuracy is also satisfactory because all protocols, other than the direct $N_{D,w}$ protocol (IPSM 1990), use basically the same approach, although somewhat different values for the physical quantities. It is important, therefore, also to estimate the overall uncertainty in the absolute dose determination.

The various factors contributing to the overall uncertainty in the absolute dose determination at the reference point in a phantom irradiated by a megavoltage photon or electron beam are presented in Table 3.3, with data taken from Brahme *et al.* (1988) and quoted as one standard deviation (1 SD). More recent analyses have reduced these overall uncertainties a little (Andreo 1990; Thwaites; 1994b). It is assumed here that the ionization chamber has an air kerma calibration factor traceable to a standard dosimetry laboratory. The uncertainty in the ionization chamber reading is determined by the uncertainty in the various reading correction factors (equation 14) but, in addition, by the long-term stability of the timer or monitor. The uncertainty in the stopping-power ratio $s_{w,air}$ also has two components: the uncertainty in the theoretical values; and the uncertainty in the input values, i.e. the beam quality specification. The uncertainty in the in-air correction factor k_{cel} is correlated to that in p_{cel}, to be applied during the measurements in the phantom, and are therefore given as a combined uncertainty in the table.

It can be seen that the stopping-power ratio and, to a lesser degree, the air and phantom correction factors, make the largest contributions to the overall uncertainty in absolute dosimetry. Reducing these uncertainties requires major efforts, both theoretical and experimental, and is the limiting factor on the overall uncertainty. An alternative way to reduce uncertainties is to base dosimetry on an absorbed dose-to-water calibration, particularly if it provides directly measured calibration factors for the user's chamber over an appropriate range of qualities. As discussed above, such an approach has been in use for some time in the UK (IPSM 1990) and in a rather more limited way in Germany (DIN 1997), and there are other developments internationally in standards laboratories and protocols indicating that this will be the general basis for dosimetry within a short time (AAPM 1999; IAEA 2000; IPEM 2000). The UK standards laboratory quote an uncertainty of 0.7% (1 SD) on the photon $N_{D,w}$ factors and a recent analysis of the uncertainties up to clinical beam calibration indicates an overall uncertainty of 1.3% (1 SD) (Allahverdi and Thwaites 1999) for photon beams. Similar uncertainties are expected for electron beam dosimetry based on directly measured $N_{D,w}$ factors (McEwan *et al.* 1998). Other $N_{D,w}$ approaches, using a one-point ^{60}Co calibration and calculated k_Q will have rather greater uncertainties, but less than the N_K based approaches. As these newer protocols are introduced, careful comparisons are required between such a measurement procedure and those currently recommended in dosimetry protocols before hospitals change their procedures.

In order to judge the value of the overall uncertainty in absorbed dose determinations using an ionization chamber, this method can be compared with other methods of absolute dose determination. Figure 3.2 shows the result of an intercomparison of absorbed dose to water determinations in photon beams using an NE 2561 ionization chamber and a graphite calorimeter (Aalbers *et al.* 1988). As can be seen from this figure, the differences are rather small, 1.0% at maximum. Similar differences have been observed in comparisons during the clinical introduction of the graphite-calorimeter based $N_{D,w}$ protocol in UK hospitals and between the varying approaches to absorbed dose standards taken by different standards laboratories, including ionization methods, albeit that this last is only for ^{60}Co (Boutillon *et al.* 1994).

A second independent method of absolute dosimetry is the use of a ferrous sulphate dosimeter (Fricke dosimetry). A comparison of absorbed dose determinations using ionization chamber and Fricke dosimetry is given in Figure 3.3. Again, maximum differences of about 1% can be observed (Wittkämper *et al.* 1991).

Another facet of the overall uncertainty in absorbed dose determinations is the precision achieved in clinical practice. From a number of recent dosimetry intercomparisons performed in radiotherapy centres in various countries, a standard deviation of about 1–1.5% was observed in the frequency distribution describing the difference between the measured and stated dose values under reference conditions for megavoltage photon beams and electron beams as discussed, for instance, in (Thwaites *et al.* 1992; Nisbet and Thwaites 1997).

These findings provide evidence that consistent results can be achieved by applying ionization chambers in combination with recent dosimetry protocols.

9. Summary and conclusions

In this chapter, some of the practical and theoretical aspects related to absolute dose determination have been discussed. Although ionization chamber theory has been well developed over a number of decades, it is only more recently that accurate and consistent values for the various conversion and correction values for individual types of ionization chamber became available.

The most important conclusion of the comparison of the various dosimetry protocols is that, despite the many differences between these protocols or codes of practice, the final result is closely similar. Obviously the differences in data for the various conversion and correction factors compensate each other, or have only

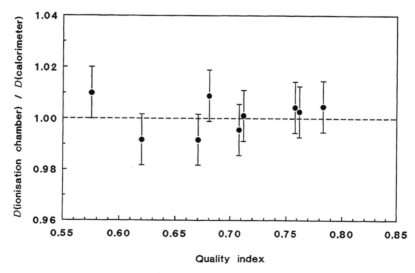

Figure 3.2 Ratio of absorbed dose (*D*) to water determined with an NE 2561 ionization chamber and with a graphite calorimeter, as a function of the quality index of photon beams using data from Aalbers *et al.* (1988).

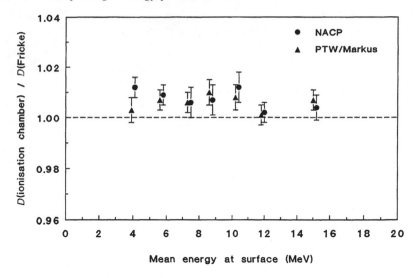

Figure 3.3 Ratio of absorbed dose (*D*) to water determined with the NACP and Markus plane-parallel chambers and with Fricke dosimetry, as a function of the mean electron energy at the surface of the phantom using data from Wittkämper *et al.* 1991.

a minor influence on the final dose calculation, at least for a graphite-walled ionization chamber in a water phantom. It can also be concluded that the care with which measurements are performed and the proper application of a protocol are as important as the choice of a particular protocol. The correct understanding of a complex protocol, or the use of a simple code of practice, are prerequisites for the avoidance of errors in the dose calculation from ionization chamber readings. The use of a particular protocol, or code of practice, will largely depend on local factors, such as the calibration service provided by the national standard dosimetry laboratory, the availability of particular types of ionization chambers and recommendations given by national organizations of medical physicists. It is expected that the gradual dissemination and adoption of $N_{D,w}$ protocols will further improve the accuracy and consistency of radiotherapy dosimetry.

10. References

Aalbers, A.H.L., Van Dijk, E., Wittkämper, F.W., and Mijnheer, B.J. (1988). Determination of absorbed dose to water in clinical photon beams using a graphite calorimeter and a graphite-walled ionization chamber. In *Dosimetry in radiotherapy, Volume 1*, pp. 37–48. IAEA, Vienna.

Allahverdi, M. and Thwaites, D.I. (1999). An experimental assessment of achievable accuracy in the basic radiotherapy dosimetry chain for megavoltage photon beams. *Phys. Med Biol.* (In press.)

Allahverdi, M., Nisbet, A., and Thwaites, D.I. (1999). An evaluation of epoxyresin phantom materials for megavoltage photon dosimetry. *Phys. Med. Biol.*, **44**, 1125–32.

American Association of Physicists in Medicine (1983). A protocol for the determination of absorbed dose from high-energy photon and electron beams. Report of AAPM Radiation Therapy Task Group 21. *Med. Phys.*, **10**, 741–77.

American Association of Physicists in Medicine (1991). Clinical electron beam dosimetry. Report of AAPM Radiation Therapy Task Group 25. *Med. Phys.*, **18**, 73–109.

American Association of Physicists in Medicine (1994). The calibration and use of parallel plate ionization chambers for dosimetry of electron beams: an extension of the 1983 AAPM protocol. Report of AAPM Task Group 39. *Med. Phys.*, **21**, 1251–60.

American Association of Physicists in Medicine (1999). Protocol for clinical reference dosimetry of high-energy photon and electron beams. Report of Task Group 51. *Med. Phys.*, 26, 1847–70.

Andreo, P. (1990). Uncertainties in dosimetric data and beam calibration. *Int. J. Radiat. Oncol.*, **19**, 1233–47.

Andreo, P. (1993). The status of high-energy photon and electron beam dosimetry five years after the publication of the IAEA code of practice. *Acta Oncol.*, **32**, 483–500.

Associazione Italiana di Fisica Biomedica (1988). Protocollo per la dosimetria di base nella radioterapia con fasci di fotoni ed elettroni con E_{max} fra 1 e 40 MeV. *Fisica Biomedica*, **6**(2), 1–40.

Boutillon, M., Coursey, B.M., Hohlfeld, Owen, B. and Rogers, D.W.O. (1994). Comparison of primary water absorbed dose standards. In *Measurement assurance in dosimetry*, pp. 95–111. IAEA, Vienna. See also, Allisy-Roberts, P. *Comparisons and calibrations at the BIPM*. Report CCEMRI(I)/99-1. BIPM, Sèvres.

Brahme, A., Chavaudra, J., Landberg, T., McCullough, E.C., Nüsslin, F., Rawlinson, J.A. et al (1988). Accuracy requirements and quality assurance of external beam therapy with photons and electrons. *Acta Oncol.* 27 Suppl. 1, 1–76

British Institute of Radiology (1996). Central axis depth dose data for use in radiotherapy. *Br. J. Radiol.*, Supplement 25. BIR, London.

Burns, D., Ding, G., and Rogers, D. (1996). R_{50} as a beam quality specifier for selecting stopping power ratios and reference depths for electron dosimetry. *Med. Phys.*, **23**, 383–8.

Deutsches Institut für Normung (1997). *Dosismessverfahren nach der Sondenmethode für Photonen- und Elektronenstrahlung; Teil 2 Ionisationsdosimetrie. DIN-6800-2.* DIN, Berlin

DuSautoy, A.R. (1996). The UK primary standard calorimeter for photon-beam absorbed dose measurement. *Phys. Med. Biol.*, **41**, 137–51.

European Society for Therapeutic Radiology and Oncology (1997). *Monitor unit calculation for high-energy photon beams.* Booklet 3 (Dutreix, A. Bjärngard, B.E., Bridier, A., Mijnheer, B.J., Shaw, J.E. and Svensson, H.). Garant, Leuven.

Hospital Physicists' Association (1983). Revised code of practice for the dosimetry of 2 to 35 MV X-rays and of caesium-137 and cobalt-60 gamma-ray beams. *Phys. Med. Biol.*, **28**, 1097–104.

Hospital Physicists' Association (1985). Code of practice for electron beam dosimetry in radiotherapy. *Phys. Med. Biol.*, **30**, 1169–94.

Institute of Physics and Engineering in Medicine (2000). Code of practice for electron beam dosimetry based on absorbed-dose-to-water standards. (In preparation.)

Institute of Physics and Engineering in Medicine and Biology (1996). The IPEMB code of practice for electron dosimetry for radiotherapy beams of initial energy from 2 to 50 MeV. *Phys. Med. Biol.*, **41**, 2557–603.

Institute of Physical Sciences in Medicine (1990). Code of practice for high-energy photon therapy dosimetry based on the NPL absorbed dose calibration service. *Phys. Med. Biol.*, **35**, 1355–60.

Institute of Physical Sciences in Medicine (1992). Addendum to the code of practice for electron beam dosimetry for radiotherapy (1985): interim additional recommendations. *Phys. Med. Biol.*, **37**, 1477–83.

International Atomic Energy Agency (1987). *Absorbed dose determination in photon and electron beams.* Technical Report Series no. 277. IAEA, Vienna.

International Atomic Energy Agency (1997). *The use of plane parallel ionization chambers in high-energy electron and photon beams: an international code of practice* . Technical Report Series no. 381. IAEA, Vienna.

International Atomic Energy Agency (2000). *Absorbed dose determination in external beam radiotherapy based on absorbed-dose-to-water standards: an international code of practice for dosimetry.* IAEA, Vienna. (In press.)

International Commission on Radiation Units and Measurements (1964). *Radiation dosimetry: X-rays and gamma-rays with maximum photon energies between 0.6 and 50 MeV.* ICRU Report 14. ICRU, Bethesda.

International Commission on Radiation Units and Measurements (1982). *The dosimetry of pulsed radiation.* ICRU Report 34. ICRU, Bethesda.

International Commission on Radiation Units and Measurements (1989). *Tissue substitutes in radiation dosimetry and measurement.* ICRU Report 44. ICRU, Bethesda.

International Commission on Radiation Units and Measurements (1999). *Dosimetry of high-energy photon beams based on standards of absorbed dose to water.* ICRU, Bethesda. (In press.)

International Electrotechnical Commission (1989). *Medical electrical equipment: medical electron accelerators; functional performance characteristics.* IEC no 976. IEC, Geneva.

International Electrotechnical Commission (1997). *Medical electrical equipment: dosimeters with ionization chambers as used in radiotherapy* IEC no 60731. IEC, Geneva.

Ma, C.M. and Nahum, A.E. (1993). Effect of the size and composition of the central electrode on the response of cylindrical ionization chambers in high-energy photon and electron beams. *Phys. Med. Biol.*, **38**, 267–90.

McEwan, M., DuSautoy, A., and Williams, A. (1998). The calibration of therapy level electron beam ionization chambers in terms of absorbed dose to water. *Phys. Med. Biol.*, **43**, 2503–19.

Nederlandse Commissie voor Stralingsdosimetrie (1986). Consistency and simplicity in the determination of absorbed dose to water in high-energy photon beams: a new code of practice. *Radiother. Oncol.*, **7**, 371–84.

Nederlandse Commissie voor Stralingsdosimetrie (1989). *Code of practice for the dosimetry of high-energy electron beams.* NCS Report 5. NCS, Bilthoven.

Nisbet, A. and Thwaites, D.I. (1997). A dosimetric intercomparison of electron beams in UK radiotherapy centres. *Phys. Med. Biol.*, **42**, 2393–409.

Nisbet, A. and Thwaites, D.I. (1998). An evaluation of epoxy resin phantom materials for electron dosimetry. *Phys. Med. Biol.*, **43**, 1523–28.

Nisbet, A., Thwaites, D.I., Nahum, A.E., and Pitchford, W.G. (1998). An experimental evaluation of recent electron dosimetry codes of practice. *Phys. Med. Biol.*, **43**, 1999–2014.

Nordic Association of Clinical Physics (1980). Procedures in external beam radiation therapy dosimetry with electron and photon beams with maximum energies between 1 and 50 MeV. Recommendations of the NACP. *Acta Radiol. Oncol.*, **19**, 55–79.

Tello, V.M., Tailor C., and Hanson, W.F. (1995). How water equivalent are water equivalent solid materials for output calibration of photon and electron beams? *Med. Phys.*, **22**, 1177–89.

Thwaites, D.I. (1994a). Current status of dosimetry protocols for megavoltage electron beams. In *Measurement assurance in dosimetry*, pp. 395–409. IAEA, Vienna.

Thwaites, D.I. (1994b). Uncertainties at the end point of the basic dosimetry chain *Measurement assurance in dosimetry*, pp. 239–55. IAEA, Vienna.

Thwaites, D.I., Williams, J.R., Aird, E.G., Klevenhagen, S.C., and Williams, P.C. (1992). A dosimetric intercomparison of megavoltage photon beams in UK radiotherapy centres. *Phys. Med. Biol.*, **37**, 445–61.

Wittkämper, F.W., Thierens, H., Van der Plaetsen, A., de Wagter, C., and Mijnheer, B.J. (1991). Perturbation correction factors for some ionization chambers commonly applied in electron beams. *Phys. Med. Biol.*, **36**, 1639–52.

Appendix I.

Abbreviations of national and international organizations involved in the development of dosimetry protocols

AAPM	American Association of Physicists in Medicine (US)
AIFB	Associazione Italiana di Fisica Biomedica (Italy)
CCEMRI	Comité Consultatif pour les Etalons de Mesure des Rayonnements Ionisants
CFMRI	Comité Français 'Mesure des Rayonnements Ionisants'
DGMP	Deutsche Gesellschaft für Medizinische Physik (Germany)
HPA	Hospital Physicists' Association (UK)
IAEA	International Atomic Energy Agency
ICRU	International Commission on Radiation Units and Measurements
IPSM	Institute of Physical Sciences in Medicine (UK)
IPEM(B)	Institute of Physics and Engineering in Medicine (and Biology) (UK)
NACP	Nordic Association of Clinical Physics (Nordic countries)
NCS	Nederlandse Commissie voor Stralingsdosimetrie (the Netherlands)
SEFM	Sociedad Española de Fisica Medica (Spain)
SSRBRP	Swiss Society of Radiation Biology and Radiation Physics (Switzerland)

Chapter 4
Relative dosimetry

J.L. Horton

1. Introduction

After a therapy machine is accepted and before it can be placed in clinical service the physicist must acquire an extensive set of radiation measurements that characterize its performance. All measurements discussed in this chapter will be relative to the calibrated output that is described in Chapter 3. This chapter will discuss relative measurements that are required before a high-energy linear accelerator with photons and electrons can be placed in clinical service. A high-energy linac has been chosen because it demands the most measurements, but this schema can easily be modified for low-energy photons-only linacs or cobalt units.

2. Dosimetry equipment

The purchase of a high-energy linear accelerator is not undertaken lightly. The hospital administration knows it is an expensive piece of equipment that is required for the optimal therapy of many cancer patients. The physicist must convince the administration that the timely commissioning of the unit, as well as continuing physics quality assurance and possible recommissioning measurements, demand a large armamentarium of dosimetry equipment. Although the cost of the dosimetry equipment may be large in absolute terms, it is a small fraction of the linac cost, usually 5–10%, about the same as a 1-year service contract for a high-energy machine. It is a cost-effective investment because proper dosimetry equipment not only shortens the time required to commission the machine and place it in clinical service but it also speeds the process of returning the linac to clinical service following a major repair such as waveguide or bending magnet replacement.

2.1 Ionometric dosimetry

The most expensive piece of dosimetry equipment will be a water phantom that permits ion chambers to be scanned through the radiation distribution. Although a two-dimensional scanner will suffice, a three-dimensional scanner is very helpful because one can scan both in-plane (that plane defined as passing through the gun and between the pole face of the bending magnet) and cross-plane (the horizontal plane orthogonal to the in-plane) and change depths without changing the set-up. In addition to a scanning water phantom, a scanning densitometer is needed to read films. Many manufacturers use the carriage of the scanning water phantom to move the densitometer. This permits the acquisition of a scanning densitometer for a small increment in cost. Regardless of the arrangement, both the scanning water phantom and densitometer should have an accuracy of movement of 1 mm and a precision of 0.5 mm. The water phantom should be able to scan 50 cm in both horizontal dimensions and 40 cm in the vertical dimension. The water tank should be at least 10 cm greater in each dimension than the scan. A window in the vertical direction in one side of the phantom and in the horizontal direction in another side will permit scanning in-plane and cross-plane when the gantry is at 90° or 270°. This window can be milled in the side of the tank and closed by Mylar. It should be just large enough to permit ion chamber access, otherwise it will flex under hydrostatic pressure.

A polystyrene or water-equivalent plastic phantom should be obtained for ionometric dosimetry. This phantom should consist of 10 blocks of dimensions $25 \times 25 \times 5$ cm^3. One block should be drilled to accommodate a Farmer or Farmer-type ion chamber with the centre of the hole 1 cm from one surface. A second block should be machined for a parallel plate chamber with the entrance window at the level of one surface of the block. This block permits measurements with the parallel plate chamber with no material between the window and the radiation beam. Sheets of build-up material should be 25×25 cm^2 with thicknesses of 0.5, 1, 2, 4, 8, 16 and 32 mm. These build-up sheets, combined with the 5-cm thick blocks, permit measurement of depth ionisation in 0.5 mm increments to any

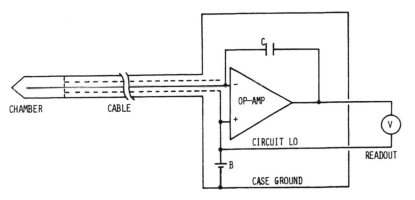

Figure 4.1 Schematic diagram of ion chamber connected to an electrometer with total capacitive feedback (from Humphries and Slowey 1987).

depth from the surface to 40 cm with the parallel-plate chamber, and from 1 cm to 40 cm with the Farmer chamber. The depth of 40 cm is the limit because 10 cm of backscatter should be maintained downstream from the measurement point.

The ion chamber inventory should consist of at least one chamber–electrometer system for calibration, two small volume thimble chambers for relative measurements, and a parallel-plate chamber for transition zone dosimetry. A Farmer or Farmer-type chamber is recommended for calibration, a thimble chamber with an inner diameter of 5 mm or less and a length of not exceeding 15 mm is recommended for relative measurements, and a parallel-plate chamber with a thin window and a plate separation of no more than 2 mm, and preferably no more than 1 mm, is recommended for transition zone dosimetry.

The thimble chambers to be used for relative measurements should be easily waterproofed. However, care must be taken with chambers that are permanently encapsulated in waterproof rubber tubing. Some of these chambers are not vented to air. These chambers should never be used for calibration as the pressure is indeterminate. They are neither sealed nor vented and behave as though they have a slow leak.

This inventory should be considered an absolute minimum. One should have at least one additional ion chamber–electrometer system for calibration. This system serves as back-up. With two calibrated systems a physicist can have one system calibrated in even-numbered years and one in odd-numbered years. If one system fails, then the other system is available with a calibration factor less than 2 years old. Additional electrometers, small thimble chambers for relative measurements, and one additional parallel-plate chamber are strongly recommended.

The most common electrometer currently used for dosimetry purposes is the negative feedback operational amplifier (op-amp) type shown schematically in Figure 4.1. The op-amp, represented by the triangle in the figure, has a high open-loop gain and high input impedance that permit it to maintain a potential in the 20–100 mV range between its positive and negative input. The positive input is referred to as the non-inverting input and the negative input is the inverting input. Negative feedback indicates some of the output of the amplifier is fed back to its negative input.

Figure 4.1 represents a total capacitive feedback circuit. All of the output is fed back through the capacitor C to the op-amp's input. Total feedback results in unity gain, so the charge Q on the capacitor C is the total charge collected by the ion chamber. If the capacitance of the capacitor is known to be C and if the voltage across the capacitor is measured to be V, then the charge Q is equal to CV. This is the charge collected for radiation exposure X.

If the capacitor were replaced by a resistor with a known resistance R, the voltage V across the resistor could be measured and the current I could be determined from $I = V/R$. This current could be related to the dose rate. This circuit is called total resistive feedback.

If a fraction of the op-amp's output is fed back to its negative input, the op-amp will produce a gain. This gain is approximately the reciprocal of the fraction of the signal fed back. By choosing the proper gain, some manufacturers produce a direct-reading electrometer for a given chamber.

It should be noted in Figure 4.1 that three leads go to the electrometer. The outer braid connects the thimble to case ground, which is connected to one side of the bias battery. The innermost cable, called the collector, connects to the negative input of the op-amp and the conductor between the outer braid and inner cable is connected to the positive input of the op-amp. Since the positive and negative inputs of the op-amp are at the same potential, within 100 mV, the inner cable and the conductor connected to the positive input are at essentially the same potential. The conductor connected to the positive input of the op-amp is the 'guard'. The volume enclosed by the thimble is the active volume and ionization created in this volume is collected between the thimble and the collector. Ionization created in the cable is collected between the outer braid and the guard because these two conductors have the same potential difference as the outer braid and collector. No current is collected between the guard and collector because they are at the same potential. The charge collected between the guard and the outer braid does not flow to the measurement capacitor C, so this signal is not measured. In this way the guard shields the collector from ionisation created in the cable.

An electrometer should have the following properties:

(1) a fast warm-up time (5–10 min);

(2) small pre- and post-irradiation background current (zero drift of op-amp less than 10^{-13} A);

(3) linear scales;

(4) consistency between scales;

(5) negligible leakage across the feedback capacitor (reading changes less than 0.05% min^{-1} after radiation is terminated);

(6) insensitivity to ambient conditions (zero drift less than 150 μV°C^{-1});

(7) an ability to accommodate changes in bias voltage in polarity and magnitude.

The voltage across the feedback element should be read out with a $4\frac{1}{2}$ digit voltmeter. The triaxial cable should be pliable, have a low radiation-induced signal, low microphonic noise, low leakage, low capacitance and come to rapid equilibration following any voltage change.

Further details of ionometric dosimetry equipment may be found in articles by Spokas and Meeker (1980), Humphries and Slowey (1987), and Humphries (1991).

2.2 *Diode dosimetry*

Over the last two decades, physicists have attempted to use silicon diodes for relative dosimetry measurements with varying degrees of success. Diodes promise several advantages. Because their sensitivity is approximately 18 000 times as great as an ion chamber of equal volume, very small volume diodes (typically 2.5 × 2.5 × 0.4 mm^3) may be used. The small volumes yield high spatial resolution. Other advantages include a signal independent of barometric pressure changes, negligible recombination effects, and a rapid rise time of the signal leading to short measuring times. In spite of these advantages early investigators found problems with the energy dependence of diodes in photon beams and the

sensitivity of the diode changing as a result of radiation damage.

More recently, Rikner (1983) has shown that p-type diodes are less sensitive to radiation damage than the n-type diodes that had been used previously for dosimetry. He also found that, with properly designed shielding, p-type diodes may be energy compensated to reduce greatly their photon energy dependence.

Several firms now offer diodes and diode readers for relative dosimetry. When purchasing these devices, p-type diodes should be specified. The manufacturer should also supply the energy and angular dependence characteristics of the diodes for evaluation before purchase.

Diode readers are basically electrometers with low dynamic impedance for pulses as short as a microsecond and a low input offset voltage that is stable with time and temperature. These electrometers are usually operated in the short circuit mode with zero external voltage across the diode.

Before using diodes clinically one should compare photon central axis per cent depth doses measured with the diodes to those measured with an ionization chamber. These measurements should be performed over the range of field sizes and energies for which the diode will be used. The absolute sensitivity of the diode should also be determined in a cobalt teletherapy beam or in a linear accelerator beam by comparison with an ion chamber measurement. This sensitivity should be checked periodically to assess whether radiation damage is adversely affecting the diode. Prior to clinical use, it is also important to check that the diodes have no dose rate dependence. This is important for linear accelerator beams that have high dose pulses of short duration, especially swept electron beams.

Because the ratio of the stopping power of silicon to water is essentially constant over the electron energy range of 5–25 MeV, several investigators have found good agreement between diodes and corrected ion chamber measurements of electron central axis depth doses particularly at depths greater than the maximum dose. For depths shallower than d_{max} diodes typically underestimate the dose compared to ion chamber measurements. Of course, each diode should be compared to corrected ion chamber measurements of electron central axis depth dose over the range of energies in one's clinic prior to clinical use.

Diode detector arrays are commercially available. These arrays feature several diodes positioned in a plastic or epoxy mount with each separated from its nearest neighbour by a fixed distance. This array allows simultaneous accumulation of data at several points in the beam. The resolution of the device may be increased by performing another exposure after repositioning the array by some fraction of the distance between diodes.

For example, if the diode spacing were 2 cm, a 5-mm resolution can be achieved by performing a minimum of three irradiations with the array moved 5 mm between each irradiation.

The use of these arrays can greatly reduce the time necessary to acquire beam data. This situation is particularly true for irradiation techniques involving dynamic fluence modulation, such as dynamic wedges (see Section 4.11.2). When using these devices, the sensitivity of each detector must be established. These sensitivities are expected to change with time as the detectors suffer radiation damage. The change in sensitivity may differ from diode to diode as the total dose to individual diodes may vary. A good quality assurance check during data collection is to compare the sensitivity of each diode to its nearest neighbour. Using the example in the previous paragraph of a diode detector array with 2 cm spacing, if a fourth irradiation were performed with the array shifted another 5 mm each diode would be in the same position as its nearest neighbour during the first irradiation. The sensitivities of the two diodes could then be compared.

2.3 Film dosimetry

X-ray film can be a useful tool, particularly for electron measurements and for quality assurance tests. The dose can be related to the darkening of the film, which is referred to as optical density. Optical density (OD) is defined as

$$OD = \log_{10}(I_o/I_t) \tag{1}$$

where I_o is the intensity of light incident on a region of film and I_t is the intensity of light transmitted through that region.

The optical density is measured with a densitometer, which consists of a light source on one side of the film and a receptor on the other side of the film to measure the light transmitted. After processing, even unirradiated film will attenuate some incident light due to the base. This attenuation of the incident light is referred to as fog. It should be subtracted from the OD in the irradiated areas to yield the net OD. The fog can be determined from unirradiated areas of a film or preferably from an unirradiated film from the same box processed at the same time.

The quantity of radiation required to produce an optical density of 1 depends on the film emulsion. Some emulsions are fast; these require a small amount of radiation to darken the film. Other emulsions are slow requiring high doses. The emulsion chosen depends on the application. A slow film using longer exposures allows better stability of the radiation beam.

Ideally the relationship between dose and optical density would be linear, but unfortunately this is not

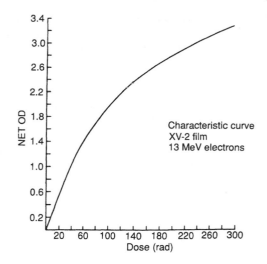

Figure 4.2 Characteristic curve for Kodak X-Omat V film plotting OD against dose in cGy(rad). (Reproduced with permission from Horton, J.L. (1987) *Handbook of radiation therapy physics*. Prentice–Hall, Englewood Cliffs, NJ).

always the case. Some emulsions are linear, some relatively linear over a limited range, others non-linear.

To use film for dosimetry, it is necessary to know the relationship between dose and OD. This can be determined by exposing several films of the type being used to known graded doses of radiation. These films can be processed at the same time as the experimental films. The net OD can then be plotted against dose as shown in Figure 4.2 to yield a characteristic curve. Chemistry changes during processing have a significant effect on the characteristic curve therefore, for accurate dosimetry, it is good practice to measure it each time film is used.

The uniformity of the emulsion varies slightly across the film and accounts for about a 2% difference in optical density on a given film. Dutriex and Dutriex (1969) concluded that a variation of 3% may be expected on films of the same batch processed simultaneously, and a variation of 5% on films of the same batch processed at different times.

Because the statistical fluctuations in the number of grains developed in 1 mm^2 of film for OD of 1 is much less than the variation in the uniformity of the emulsion, one should choose a densitometer with a 1 mm^2 aperture for high spatial resolution. If a higher spatial resolution is needed, then a rectangular aperture (0.1×10 mm) can be used to improve resolution along its short axis. The densitometer should read OD in the range 0–4, although films should not be used above 2.5 without determining the amount of radiation required to saturate the film, as some will saturate at approximately 3. The precision of the densitometer should be 0.01 OD units.

A plastic phantom for film dosimetry is needed. A convenient phantom can be designed with one section

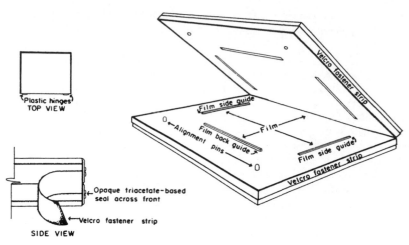

Figure 4.3 Water equivalent plastic phantom for film dosimetry in a plane parallel to the central axis of the radiation beam (from Bova (1990)).

serving as a film cassette holder. One design of cassette holder section (Bova 1990) is illustrated in Figure 4.3. This design is convenient for irradiating films parallel to the central axis of the beam. It consists of two sections of water equivalent plastic hinged on one side and with that side permanently covered with black photographic tape. Black Velcro is placed on the other three sides to permit opening and closing the cassette with a light tight seal. On the inside surface of one piece are plastic guides that position a bare 25×30 cm^2 film, such that the upper edge of the film is at the top surface of the cassette (the hinged side). The inside surface of the other piece of plastic has recesses to accept the plastic guides when the cassette is closed. Alignment pins on one side of the cassette mate with holes in the other side. After the film is sealed in the cassette, additional water-equivalent-plastic sheets can be placed on both sides of the cassette to provide full scattering.

If ready-pack film is used, a number of precautions are required if it is planned to irradiate the film parallel to the central axis of the beam. The edge of the film should be identified by carefully feeling through the paper, then the excess paper is folded down such that the edge of the film can be placed at the edge of the phantom. Holes should be placed in a corner of the downstream edge of the paper package, so that air can be squeezed out before placing the ready pack in the phantom; otherwise, air bubbles will be trapped between the film and the paper. These air bubbles transmit the radiation unattenuated, resulting in hot spots.

In recent years, radiochromic film has been used for a variety of dosimetric measurements (McLaughlin *et al.* 1996; Reinstein and Gluckman 1999). The film consists of monomer crystals in a gel bound to a Mylar (polyethylene terephthalate) substrate. The crystals are

partially polymerized by irradiation and change colour from light to a darker blue, the optical density increasing approximately linearly with dose. Like radiographic film, radiochromic film provides a two-dimensional dose distribution with high spatial resolution. It has been used for measurements around brachytherapy sources, for interface dosimetry, and for small field dosimetry.

There are differences in the handling and analysis of the two type of film.

1. Radiochromic film is much more tissue equivalent than silver halide radiographic film.

2. Radiochromic film may be handled in visible light, although it exhibits some sensitivity to ultraviolet light. Some users have covered the room lights with UV filters to minimize this effect.

3. Radiochromic film requires no post irradiation processing.

4. The absorption spectrum of the film exhibits two peaks, a smaller one at about 618 nm and a large one at 676 nm. The wavelength of the peaks shift slightly with irradiation. Thus, unlike radiographic films that have a neutral density response, the response of radiochromic film is a function of dose and of the wavelength of the transmitted light. This feature requires different readout devices than the standard film densitometer.

5. Radiochromic film requires a higher dose than radiographic film. Generally measurements are made in the range 10–2500 Gy depending on the type of film and the wavelength of the readout device.

6. The optical density of the film increases post-irradiation with the rate of change being dependent on storage temperature. Since the greatest post-

irradiation changes occur in the first day, it is generally recommended that the film is not read until 24 hours post-irradiation.

7. The response of the film may vary by up to 15% depending on the position on the film due to non-uniformity in the emulsion.

2.4 Quality control

To generate meaningful data, dosimetry equipment must be subjected to stringent acceptance tests and periodic quality control checks. The acceptance tests should be designed to verify that new equipment conforms to the purchase specifications. The quality control checks verify that the equipment continues to meet these specifications with use and to elucidate any problems that may occur. The quality control tests should be designed so that they can be performed in a relatively short time.

The quality control tests required depend on the particular piece of dosimetry equipment and its intended application. For instance, an ionometric dosimetry system used for calibration should be checked monthly in a radioisotope source to verify the constancy of its calibration factor. If the radiotherapy centre has a cobalt unit, then its monthly calibration check can serve as a verification of the dosimetry system. If the output of the cobalt unit varies from the expected value by more than 1% further investigation is required to determine the source of this variation. The first check should be a measurement of the output with a second calibrated dosimetry system. If this system indicates a variation from the expected value, then the problem is probably with the cobalt unit. However, if measurement with the second dosimetry system indicates agreement with the expected output, a problem with the first dosimetry system is indicated. If the centre does not have a cobalt unit, then a ^{90}Sr check-source should be used.

Thimble ion chambers should also be checked for mechanical integrity by lightly pulling axially on the thimble. Movement of the thimble may indicate it is broken and additional checks are required. Visual inspection of the window of parallel-plate chambers can reveal wrinkling that can change chamber sensitivity. The mechanical soundness of cable connectors should be inspected. These connectors should neither rotate about the cable nor exhibit any motion in the longitudinal direction relative to the cable.

Problems with microphonics can be revealed by slapping the side of the electrometer and moving the cable. If an integrated reading changes after either of these tests, a problem is indicated. Leakage can also be checked by observing the rate of change of an integrated signal. System leakage should not exceed the range of 5×10^{-13}–10×10^{-13} A. The source of any leakage may be found by checking each component. The electrometer is checked by acquiring a reading then disconnecting the cable. The rate of change of the electrometer reading should correspond to a leakage of between 10^{-13} and 10^{-14} A on any scale checked. If the electrometer is not leaking, the cable is checked by acquiring an integrated reading and then disconnecting the chamber. The leakage of the electrometer and cable should be in the range of 5×10^{-13}–5×10^{-14} A. Finally, if the cable and electrometer do not exhibit leakage problems but the system does, then the source of the problem is the ion chamber.

The mechanical accuracy and precision of a scanning water phantom must be verified before initial use and on a periodic basis. The vertical movement can be tested by attaching millimetre ruled graph paper to one side of the tank with the rulings parallel to the orthogonal sides. A pointer can be fixed to the ion chamber carriage. The carriage can be moved a given distance with the controls of the water phantom. The accuracy of this movement can be determined by noting the distance the pointer travelled along the graph paper. The precision can be checked by repeating this test numerous times. Accuracy of movement in the horizontal planes can be similarly checked by taping graph paper to the bottom of the tank with rulings parallel to the sides of the tank.

For the initial commissioning of a scanning water phantom, one should compare representative depth doses and beam profiles determined with the new phantom to data measured with another phantom. The comparison data should be performed as soon as possible before or after the scanning phantom measurements to assure there have been no changes in the radiation beam. Also, the comparison data should be taken for a large number of monitor units at each point to verify that the scanning speed of the water phantom is not introducing errors. Obviously the ionometric dosimetry of the scanning water phantom system should be subjected to the same tests as outlined above. Any data processing and data analysis routines supplied with the water phantom should be verified against other data before initial clinical use.

Scanning film densitometers should be subjected to the same type of mechanical tests as a scanning water phantom, although the exact details depend on the design of the densitometer. One method of verifying the accuracy of movement is to transfer the rulings of millimetre graph paper to a clear sheet of plastic and to scan this in the densitometer.

The densitometer linearity can be checked with a calibrated film strip containing a series of steps of known OD. As an alternative to the calibrated film strip, a series of films can be exposed to different doses and their ODs can be measured with a laboratory grade densitometer that is known to be accurate. These measurements can be compared with the results from the scanning densitometer. The accuracy of the densitometer's ability to subtract the OD resulting from the film base plus fog should also be checked. This is done with an unirradiated film developed at the same time as the irradiated films. This film can be used to set the scanning densitometer to read zero at this OD. The net OD of other films determined with the scanning densitometer can be compared to measurements with the laboratory grade densitometer. As with a scanning water phantom, a check of any data processing and data analysis routines for the scanning densitometer should be made before placing them in clinical service.

Further details of specification and quality control of dosimetry equipment can be found in Holmes and McCullough (1983), Mellenberg *et al.* (1990), and Humphries (1991).

3. Dosimetry notebook

Upon completion of the commissioning measurements, the data will be prepared for entry into a treatment-planning computer and collation into a dosimetry notebook. The format of the data for the treatment-planning computer depends on the computer software (see Chapter 8, Section 5.2). The style of the dosimetry notebook depends on the individual preparing it, but a few general comments can be made. A loose-leaf notebook is useful, so that the notebook can be updated as the data changes with machine modifications or added to as data required for new procedures is measured. The notebook should contain a section on photon dosimetry, organized by energy, including central axis per cent depth doses and tissue–maximum ratios as a function of depth and field size over the range of interest, surface doses with and without the blocking tray, output factors, wedge transmission factors as a function of field size if necessary, blocking tray transmission factors, and half-value layers for lead and other materials used for blocking and construction of compensators. A separate section for electrons should include central axis per cent depth doses for all energies as a function of field size over the range of interest, surface doses as a function of energy, cone ratios as a function of energy for open cones, as well as, for cones with secondary blocking, thickness of lead for constructing lead masks as a function of electron energy, and air gap factors. These data can be arranged as either tables or graphs or both, depending on the user's choice.

Other useful tables to include would contain the machines capabilities, such as range of field sizes and electron cones, range of field sizes that wedges cover, treatment table capabilities, such as size of opening in table, weight limits, and height limits above and below isocentre. An abbreviated table of electron beam characteristics is convenient for treatment planning

purposes. In this table one may include the depth of d_{max}, depth of proximal and distal 90% values, and depth of 80–10% central axis per cent doses in 10% increments. The photon section should include surface dose, depth of 50% dose and per cent depth dose for a 10×10 cm^2 field at 100 cm FSD.

The data placed in the dosimetry notebook should be strictly controlled to prevent the inclusion of incorrect information. Each page should be initialled and dated by the individual who prepared the information and verified its accuracy. It is also helpful if code numbers relating the data to the log-book or computer files containing the original data are included at an appropriate place on the page. In a large department it is important that all copies of the data book are the same. This uniformity may be accomplished by assigning the task of issuing new dosimetry notebooks and updates to one individual. The appropriate individual for this responsibility would be the department head or chief medical physicist.

4. Photon measurements

4.1 Central axis per cent depth dose

The first group of measurements should be the central axis per cent depth dose values. The terminology 'central axis' will be used in this chapter to designate the axis of rotation of the collimator, whereas 'central ray' will be used to indicate the centre of an X-ray field formed with asymmetric collimators. The surface of the water phantom should be placed at the normal SSD or at the isocentre. In measuring the vertical depth of an ion chamber in a water phantom, one should measure from the bottom of the meniscus of the water. This is best performed by holding a ruler vertical with the end of the ruler at the centre of the chamber and sighting along the bottom surface of the meniscus to read the ruler. An alternative method is to place the centre of the ion chamber at the surface of the water. When properly positioned at the surface, the chamber, viewed end-on from beneath the water, will appear to be a complete circle because of internal reflection in the water.

The central axis per cent depth dose values should be measured over the range of field sizes from 4×4 cm^2 to 40×40 cm^2 in increments no greater than 5 cm. Measurements should be made to 35 or 40 cm in depth. Field sizes smaller than 4×4 cm^2 require special attention. Although 0.1 cm^3 chambers typically have diameters of 3–4 mm, the length is of the order of 1.5 cm. Because of lack of lateral electron equilibrium and penumbral effects for field sizes smaller than 4×4 cm^2, the dose can vary significantly across the length of the chamber. This situation requires detectors of small dimensions. When it is necessary to measure small field sizes three possible solutions are available. A 0.1 cm^3 chamber, positioned so that the central axis of the beam is parallel to the central electrode of the chamber, or a diode may be used in a water phantom. Alternatively, it is possible to use a parallel-plate chamber that has a small collecting electrode. Any of these techniques should be validated by measuring a central axis depth dose for a 10×10 cm^2 field first and comparing the results to those determined with conventional measurements. In addition, this comparison provides an estimate of the effective point of measurement of the diode or of the chamber irradiated parallel to its long axis.

When measuring central axis per cent depth dose, the physicist should be aware that the depth of maximum dose will shift toward the surface as the field size increases. This effect results from an increasing number of secondary electrons in the beam generated from the increasing surface area of the collimators viewed by the detector.

4.2 Output factors

A linear accelerator is typically calibrated by measuring the ionization per monitor unit at the reference depth specified by the appropriate calibration protocol (see Chapter 3). This measured ionization is converted to dose and is then divided by the appropriate central axis per cent depth dose to determine dose at d_{max} for a standard field size and standard SSD. The monitor calibration is adjusted to yield 1 cGy per monitor unit for these reference conditions. The standard SSD is normally 100 cm and the standard field size is usually 10×10 cm^2. As the field size changes the radiation output changes. This change is quantified by measuring the output at d_{max} on the central axis for each field size and dividing that output by the output at d_{max} on the central axis for the 10×10 cm^2 field. These ratios are referred to as output factors. It is important to remember, as pointed out in Section 4.1 on central axis per cent depth dose, that d_{max} changes with field size. Therefore, the output for each field at its particular d_{max} should be measured at the standard SSD. An alternative method is to measure ionization at a constant reference depth (e.g. 5 cm) for all field sizes and divide by the central axis per cent depth dose of the given field size to relate the measured ionization back to d_{max}. The ratios of the calculated ionization at d_{max} for the given field to the calculated d_{max} ionization for a 10×10 cm^2 field will also yield output factors.

Output factors are usually given as a function of equivalent square field as shown in Figure 4.4. This approach is valid if the output for rectangular fields is equal to the output of its equivalent square field. However, it should never be assumed this is true and it should always be verified by measuring the output for a number of rectangular fields at the d_{max} for each of these

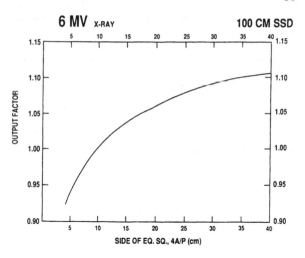

Figure 4.4 X-ray output of a linear accelerator as a function of the equivalent square field size. The data are normalized to a 10×10 cm^2 field.

fields. Outputs for rectangular fields with high- and low-aspect ratios should be measured. If the output of the rectangular field varies from the output of its equivalent square field by more than 2% it may be necessary to have a table of output factors for each rectangular field. This matter can be further complicated because some accelerators exhibit a dependence on jaw orientation. For example, the output of a rectangular field may depend on whether the upper or lower jaw forms the long side of the field. This machine characteristic should be investigated. If this is the case a family of output curves may be required similar to that shown in Figure 4.5 (Coffey *et al.* 1980). If the machine does display this dependence, a protocol on designation of the jaw settings for patient treatments should be developed to assure the correct output factor is used for patient dosimetry.

If the linear accelerator has asymmetric jaws, it will be necessary to determine the output factors for fields formed by these jaws. These output factors should be stated at d_{max} on the central ray of the asymmetric field. The output factors for asymmetric fields can usually be approximated by:

$$[OF(r)]_{a,y} = [OF(r)]_s OAR(d_{max}, y) \qquad (2)$$

where $[OF(r)]_{a,y}$ is the output factor for an $r \times r$ field formed with asymmetric jaws. The central ray of this field is y cm from the central axis of the beam at d_{max}; $[OF(r)]_s$ is the output factor for an $r \times r$ field formed with symmetric jaws; $OAR(d_{max},y)$ is the off-axis ratio measured at d_{max} and y cm from the central axis of the beam.

This model should be verified by spot-check measurements of the output factors for several asymmetric fields.

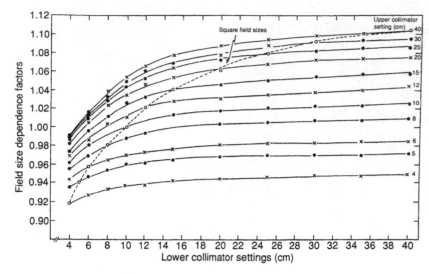

Figure 4.5 Variation in output factors as a function of upper and lower jaws settings (from Coffey *et al.* 1980).

Generally the change in output with change in field size can be modelled as arising from photon scatter from the collimators plus photon scatter in the phantom. The output increases with field size because as the collimators are opened they present more surface area to the beam with concomitantly more radiation being scattered from these surfaces. Likewise, as more phantom volume is irradiated, more scatter occurs in the phantom. Scatter from other head components and scatter back into the monitor chamber also contribute to the measured changes for accelerators.

This construct is analogous to dividing the output of a cobalt unit into the peak scatter factor and the field-size dependence of the output measured 'in-air' with a build-up cap. The idea of the 'in-air' measurement is to measure only the 'primary' radiation. In this sense, primary radiation means radiation not scattered by the phantom; however, it will contain photons scattered by the collimators and air.

As with ^{60}Co, the collimator scatter and the phantom scatter may be measured separately in higher energy beams. Analogously, the collimator scatter correction factor is determined by measuring the change in output versus field size 'in-air' with a build-up cap large enough to provide electronic equilibrium. These values are normalized to a 10×10 cm^2 field. However, a problem arises with high-energy beams and small fields. From an operational standpoint the field must be larger than the build-up cap. If a standard plastic build-up cap is used, it may be 6 cm or more in diameter for high-energy beams. This precludes measurement of the collimator scatter correction factor for fields below 7 or 8 cm.

The large build-up cap also prevents a measurement of the 'primary' dose because of scatter occurring in the build-up cap. This scatter has been estimated to be in the range of 1–10% for X-ray energies between 2 and 30 MV.

Two solutions to the problem are possible. The collimator scatter correction factor can be measured by using a build-up cap constructed of higher density material such as aluminum or copper. This will reduce the size of the cap permitting measurement of fields down to 4 cm. The other approach is to measure the collimator scatter correction factor by placing the ion chamber at an extended SSD but with the field defined at the normal SSD. For instance with the chamber at 200 cm one can measure the collimator scatter correction factor down to fields with dimensions of 4 cm at 100 cm. Since these are relative measurements, they should all be made under the same conditions. In other words, if a high density build-up cap is used, measurements for all field sizes should be made with the same cap.

The phantom scatter correction factor can be determined from measurements of collimator scatter correction factor and output factors. The phantom scatter correction factor is equal to the ratio of the output factor to the collimator scatter correction factor:

$$S_{p}(r) = \frac{OF(r)}{S_{c}(r)} \qquad (3)$$

where $OF(r)$ is the output factor measured at d_{max} in-phantom for field size $r \times r$; $S_{c}(r)$ is the collimator scatter correction factor measured 'in air' for field size $r \times r$; $S_{p}(r)$ is the phantom scatter correction factor for field size $r \times r$.

It should be noted that the phantom scatter correction factor is the same quantity as the normalized peak scatter factor defined in BIR (1996).

Alternatively, the phantom scatter correction factor may be measured. In this case the output at d_{max} in phantom is measured for a given field size. The field is then blocked to the reference field size, usually 10×10 cm^2, without changing the collimator opening. For fields smaller than the reference field size, the geometry is reversed. The collimator is set for the reference field and measurements are made for the smaller field defined by blocks. In these geometries the collimator scatter remains the same for both measurements but the phantom scatter changes. The ratio of the output at d_{max} for the field of interest to the output at d_{max} of the reference field size is the phantom scatter correction factor.

It may be noted that because of secondary electron effects, some recent guidelines have opted for normalization at 10 cm depth rather than at d_{max}, with 'mini-phantom' measurements rather than the build-up cap for the collimator scatter determination (Dutreix *et al.* 1997). The approach to the separation of the head and phantom scatter is the same. Output factors and other parameters are then referenced to the selected normalization depth (e.g. 10 cm). These measurements link to TPR approaches (see next section).

4.3 Tissue–maximum ratios

Tissue–maximum ratios (TMRs) are an extension of the tissue–air ratio concept. A tissue–air ratio (TAR) is the ratio of dose at some depth in phantom to the dose in air. The measurements are made at that same point in space for the same field size defined at the point of measurement. A TMR is the ratio of dose at some depth in phantom to the dose at d_{max} in phantom. These measurements are also at the same point in space for the same field size defined at the point of measurement. The TMR is a special case of the tissue–phantom ratio (TPR), which is the ratio of dose at some depth in phantom to the dose at a reference depth in phantom. The measurements are made at the same point in space with the same field size defined at that point. In the case of TMRs, the reference depth is d_{max}. Since the depth of d_{max} is dependent on field size for high energy X-ray beams, the deepest d_{max} should be chosen. In general this will be for the smallest field size. Although TARs, TMRs, and TPRs were originally conceived for calculating dose at the isocentre for rotational therapy, they are now used for static isocentric treatments and treatments at extended SSD. In the latter case they are useful because, to the first order, they are independent of SSD.

TMRs can be calculated from per cent depth doses and phantom scatter correction factors:

$$\text{TMR}(d, r_d) = \left(\frac{\%\text{DD}(d, r, f)}{100}\right)\left(\frac{f + d}{f + d_{max}}\right)^2\left(\frac{S_p(r_{d_{max}})}{S_p(r_d)}\right) \quad (4)$$

where r is the field size defined at the surface; $r_d = r(f + d)/f$ is the field size at depth d and at SSD f; $r_{d_{max}} = r(f + d_{max})/f$ is the field size defined at depth d_{max} and SSD f, $\%\text{DD}(d, r, f)$ is the central axis percentage depth dose for $r \times r$ field at depth of d and SSD f; and $S_p(r_{d_{max}})$ and $S_p(r_d)$ are the phantom scatter correction factors for field sizes $r_{d_{max}} \times r_{d_{max}}$ and $r_d \times r_d$, respectively.

The calculated values of TMRs should be verified with measurements at several depths and several field sizes over the entire range of both these parameters. These measurements are time consuming because the ion chamber remains at the isocentre and the depth of the water above the ion chamber is changed. One possible solution to automating these measurements has been suggested by Reinstein and McShan (1982). They designed a system with the ion chamber at the isocentre fixed with a rigid rod to the collimator face plate. The treatment table supports a large water phantom and the depth of the ion chamber in the water phantom is changed by changing the height of the table under computer control.

A concise summary of the formulae linking TMR and %DD to each other and to the other parameters can be found in Appendix B of BIR (1996).

4.4 Scatter–maximum ratios

Analogous to the extension of the TAR concept to TMRs, the scatter–air ratio (SAR) concept was extended to scatter–maximum ratios (SMR) to calculate scatter dose. SMRs are useful for calculations that require the radiation field to be divided into a primary and a scatter component. The two most widely encountered examples are highly irregular fields and tangential fields that extend beyond the patient resulting in a lack of scatter. The definition of SMR can be written mathematically as:

$$\text{SMR}(d, r_d) = \text{TMR}(d, r_d)\left[\frac{S_p(r_d)}{S_p(0)}\right] - TMR(d, 0) \quad (5)$$

where $S_p(0)$ is the phantom scatter correction factor for zero field size determined by extrapolating $S_p(r_d)$ and TMR$(d,0)$ is the tissue–maximum ratio at depth d for the primary beam. The TMR for the primary beam at depth d may be found by extrapolating measured TMR versus field size data for depth d to zero area field size.

An alternative method of finding the TMR of the primary beam is to determine an effective linear attenuation coefficient for each field size. Best results are obtained by fitting an exponential attenuation curve to TMR data beyond a depth of 10 cm. The effective linear attenuation coefficients for each measured field size can then be extrapolated to yield an attenuation coefficient for zero field size. The primary TMR beyond d_{max} is then given by:

$$\text{TMR}(d, 0) = \exp[-\mu(d - d_{max})] \quad (6)$$

where μ is the effective linear attenuation for zero field size found by extrapolation.

The effective attenuation coefficient in narrow-beam geometry can be measured by placing the ion chamber with an appropriate build-up cap 200 cm from the source on the central axis and opening the collimators wide enough to cover the build-up cap. A narrow column of water is placed on the central axis at 100 cm. By varying the depth of water between the source and the ion chamber the attenuation coefficient for the primary beam can be determined.

These three techniques should yield similar values for the TMR of the primary beam. The SMRs are easily calculated with equation (5) once TMR(d,0) is known.

4.5 Block and blocking tray transmission ratios

Most linacs have collimators that form rectangular fields. Because treatment volumes are rarely rectangular, the radiation oncologist frequently requires blocks to shield critical structures within the irradiated area. The blocks are either individually designed and fabricated locally of a low melting-point alloy, such as Lipowitz's alloy, or standard 'library' blocks may be purchased from the vendor of the treatment machine. In most instances these blocks are five half-value layers thick along the direction of the beam and it is frequently assumed that they reduce the dose in the shielded area to 3% of the unshielded dose. This assumption is incorrect. The five half-value

layers may reduce the primary beam to 3% of its unattenuated value but because of scatter in the patient, the dose in the shielded area depends on the size of the field, the depth of interest, the size of the block, and its position in the field. A very small block surrounded by a very large radiation field may only reduce the radiation to 20–30% of the unshielded dose on the central axis at d_{max}. A large block at the edge of a small field may reduce the dose to 5% of the d_{max} dose.

As a general rule, five half-valve layer blocks will reduce the dose to 10–15% of the dose at d_{max} in the unshielded field. This reduction is relatively constant with depth. At shallow depths, where scatter is minimal, the dose will be approximately 10%; however, as the depth increases the primary is attenuated in the patient but the scatter builds up yielding a dose in the shielded region of approximately 15% of the d_{max} dose. At greater depths the further attenuation of the primary will reduce the dose in the blocked area back to approximately 10% of the d_{max} dose in the unshielded beam. Figure 4.6 displays beam profiles normalized to the central axis d_{max}, measured at several depths in a 25 × 25 cm^2 field under two 'library' blocks in a 6 MV X-ray beam. One of these blocks is somewhat larger than the other. Under the larger block, the dose is reduced more than under the smaller block, and for both blocks the dose is reduced more at d_{max} than the intermediate depths, which show the highest doses. As the depth increases the doses decrease from their values at intermediate depths.

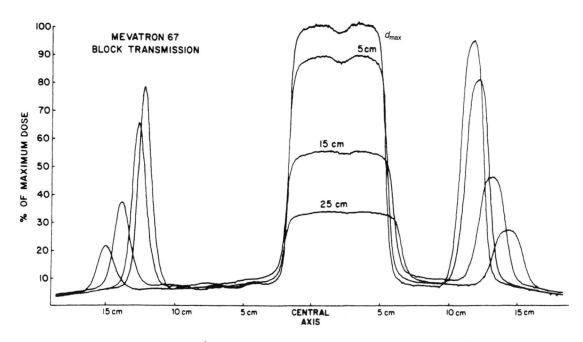

Figure 4.6 Beam profiles for a 25 × 25 cm^2, 6 MV X-ray beam at four depths in a water phantom with shielding blocks either side of the central axis. (Reproduced with permission from Horton, J.L. (1983) *Int. J. Radiat. Oncol. Biol. Phys.*, **9**, 1217).

The dip in the beam profiles near the central axis results from the tray on which the blocks are resting. This tray consists of a plastic plate containing several large holes that permit the block to be attached to the tray. The tray decreases the transmitted beam, resulting in the dip relative to the direct beam passing through the holes in the tray. The amount of beam attenuation provided by the tray must be known, so the number of monitor units can be increased to given the correct dose. For solid trays, this attenuation is easily measured by placing an ion chamber on the central axis of the beam at 5 cm depth in phantom in a 10×10 cm^2 field. The ratio of the ion chamber signal with the tray in the beam to the signal without the tray is the blocking tray transmission factor. For trays with holes, the measurement should be made under the solid part which will yield the tray transmission factor under the solid region of the tray. The area of the holes and the area of the solid part can be used to get a weighted average of the tray transmission factor:

$$T_T = \frac{A_H}{A_T} + \frac{A_s}{A_T} T_s \qquad (7)$$

where T_T is the tray transmission factor, T_S is the transmission factor under the solid part of the tray, A_H is the area of the tray occupied by holes, A_S is the area of the solid tray, and A_T is the total area of the tray.

Although the tray transmission factor should be measured for several depths and field sizes, it usually has only a weak dependence on these variables and a single value can generally be used for all depths and field sizes.

4.6 Central axis wedge transmission ratios

The central axis wedge transmission ratio is the ratio of the dose at a specified depth on the central axis of a specified field size with the wedge in the beam to the dose for the same conditions without the wedge in the beam. Central axis wedge transmission ratios are usually called 'wedge factors'. Frequently, wedge factors determined for one field size at one depth are used to calculate beam-on time or monitor unit settings for all wedged fields and depths. This practice is not recommended because the wedge factor is generally a function of both depth and field size.

The field size variation may depend not only on the width of the field along the gradient of the wedge but also on its length. In other words, the central axis wedge transmission factor for a given wedge for a 10×10 cm^2 field may differ from a 10×20 cm^2 field even when the 10 cm is along the wedge gradient in both cases. These dependencies mean that central axis per cent depth doses must be measured with the wedge in the beam for the range of field sizes. The dose with the wedge in the beam can then be related to the calibrated dose rate by measuring the wedge transmission ratio at one depth for each field size.

To measure the central axis wedge transmission ratio for a given field size at one depth, the ion chamber should be placed on the central axis of the beam with its axis parallel to a constant thickness of the wedge. Two sets of measurements should be performed with the wedge position rotated 180° between them to verify that the position of the wedge and ion chamber is correct. The wedge is turned by rotating the collimator or by rotating the wedge itself. Rotation of the wedge itself will indicate whether the side rails are symmetrically positioned about the collimator axis of rotation. Rotation of the collimator verifies that the ion chamber is positioned on the collimator axis of rotation. The measured values should be the same for the two wedge orientations. If they vary by more than 5% for a 60° wedge or 2% for a 30° wedge, then either the chamber or the wedge is not positioned correctly and the situation should be corrected. Otherwise it is usually adequate to take the average value of the two wedge orientations as the correct value.

4.7 Beam profiles

Treatment planning in two or three dimensions requires a knowledge of the dose off-axis, as well as on the central axis. This information is usually obtained by measuring radiation profiles transverse to the central axis at several depths in a water phantom. These beam profiles can be combined with the central axis per cent depth dose values to generate isodose curves.

The number of profiles and the depths at which they are measured will depend on the requirements of the treatment-planning system. Some require profiles at a few equally spaced depths, others require several profiles at specified depths, and some require only one off-axis profile for the largest field size measured 'in-air' with a build-up cap. Regardless of the requirements of the planning system, data should be measured in addition to that required as computer input. This allows checks of the calculation algorithm for fields intermediate to those measured. In particular, full isodose curves should be acquired and retained as reference data.

Of course, profiles should be measured for both open and wedged fields. The profiles of the wedged field can then be combined with the central axis per cent depth dose values for wedged fields to generate wedged isodose curves. Any change in wedge factor with depth is then included in the isodose curves.

Another problem that was not adequately addressed by some commercial treatment-planning systems is asymmetric collimators. This was an example of linear accelerator development outpacing the development of treatment-planning algorithms. Several techniques have been proposed. One approach proposed by Khan *et al.* (1986) to the calculation of dose at depth *d* in the field $r \times r$ at a point *x* cm off axis is:

$$D(d,x,r) \approx D(d_{\max},r)\text{mu}[S_c(r)]_s[S_p(r)]_s$$
$$\times \frac{[\%\text{DD}(d,r,f)]_s}{100}\text{OAR}(d,x) \qquad (8)$$

where $D(d_{\max},r)$ is the dose per monitor unit, mu is the number of monitor units, $[S_c(r)]_s$ and $[S_p(r)]_s$ are the collimator and phantom scatter correction factors on the central axis of a symmetric field of size $r \times r$, $[\%\text{DD}(d,r,f)]_s$ is the central axis per cent depth dose at depth *d* for the symmetric field at SSD *f*, and OAR(*d,x*) is the off-axis ratio at distance *x* from the central axis of the symmetric field at depth *d*.

This does not take into account the change of collimator scatter for the position of the asymmetric jaws.

For isocentric treatment equation (8) becomes:

$$D(d, x, r) \approx D(d_{\max},r)\text{mu}[S_c(r)]_s[S_p(r)]_s$$
$$\times [\text{TMR}(d, r)]_s \text{OAR}(d, x)\left(\frac{\text{SCD}}{\text{SAD}}\right)^2 \qquad (9)$$

where $[\text{TMR}(d,r)]_s$ is the tissue–maximum ratio on the central axis at depth *d* for the symmetric field $r \times r$, and SCD and SAD are the source–calibration point and source–axis distances, respectively.

OAR(*d,x*) is well approximated by the off-axis ratio at depth *d* and off-axis distance *x* for the largest symmetric field size available for points well removed from the penumbra. This model is but one of several suggested for dealing with asymmetric jaws. An evaluation of the approach that best fits the local requirements should be made to define the necessary measurements.

A final caveat must be given for measurement of the penumbra region. The changing dose gradients in this region require a small-volume detector. Some situations may even demand corrections to measurements with a small detector. For fields less than 3 cm along the measurement axis, the penumbra region becomes a significant fraction of the total profile measured. In this case a correction may be warranted.

Dawson *et al.* (1986) employed a system of ion chambers with different internal diameters and extrapolated their results to a zero-volume detector. Their results indicated that neither beam energy nor depth significantly changed the dependence of the 20–80% or 10–90% penumbral width on the internal diameter of the chamber. On the basis of their data, they recommended a procedure for correcting the penumbra. To employ this correction, the distances of the 90% and 80% levels from the central axis are increased by half the internal radius of the ion chamber, and the distance of the 20% and 10% levels from the central axis are decreased by the same distance.

Sibata *et al.* (1991) have modelled the measured spatial dose distribution as a convolution of the true spatial dose distribution and the detector response function. This approach is reasonable, but a response function has to be assumed as it is not known.

It should be noted that careful consideration should be given to the length of the detector as well as the width for very small field sizes.

4.8 Transition zone dosimetry

Knowledge of the dose at the interface of two media is important in a variety of clinical situations. The most common of these is the entrance dose region between the patient surface and $d_{\max}$. Other areas that have been studied are interfaces at small air cavities, such as nasopharynx, at the exit surface of the patient, at bone–tissue interfaces, and between a metallic prosthesis and tissue.

These measurements are usually time consuming because they are not easily automated with a water phantom and scanner. The rapidly changing dose gradient demands measuring with a thin-window parallel plate chamber. The requirement for a thin window makes water phantom measurements difficult because of the need to waterproof the chamber and to avoid deformation of the window by hydrostatic pressure.

Measurements are typically performed in a polystyrene phantom or water-substitute phantom. In a constant SSD geometry, measurements should begin with the block containing the chamber upstream, backed by two 5-cm blocks of backscattering material. The build-up sheets can be placed downstream from these blocks for this initial set-up. The first measurement is made with no build-up material upstream from the chamber. The next depth is measured by moving the appropriate sheet of build-up material from the bottom to the top of the phantom. This scheme maintains a constant SSD as build-up material is added.

For every experiment in any transition zone, the initial measurements should always be repeated at the same depths but with the opposite polarity on the entrance window. Large differences in the signal at the interface may be observed when the polarity is reversed. Measurements made further from the interface exhibit smaller differences than those nearer the interface. For depths beyond the transition zone, readings with either polarity should be the same. The true value is frequently said to be the average of the signals of the two polarities. This statement is almost correct, although in fact the true value is:

$$Q_T = \frac{Q_+ - Q_-}{2} \qquad (10)$$

where the positive and negative signs refer to the polarity of the signal and the sign of each signal is maintained in this calculation.

The value computed with this operation is the same as the average of the absolute magnitudes unless $Q+$ and Q_- have the same sign. This occurs in low signal-to-noise situations, where the cable or stem contribute a significant spurious current that does not change sign with a change in polarity, while the true signal from the sensitive volume of the chamber does change sign with change in polarity.

Another correction to be made accounts for the spacing of the two electrodes in a parallel-plate chamber. Of course, an extrapolation chamber could be used to make a series of measurements at each depth with different plate separations. Then the readings could be extrapolated to zero volume, but this is a time-consuming process. Gerbi and Khan (1990) have developed a technique that corrects fixed separation parallel-plate chamber data to extrapolation chamber values. They demonstrated that this correction is a function of beam energy, depth, plate separation, and guard ring width. The relationship of the corrected value to uncorrected value is:

$$\%DD(d, E) = [\%DD(d, E)]_1 - \xi(0, E)L \exp[-\alpha(d/d_{max})] \quad (11)$$

where $\%DD(d,E)$ is the corrected per cent depth dose at depth d in the build-up region for a beam of energy E, $[\%DD(d,E)]_1$ is the uncorrected per cent depth dose for the same conditions, L is the plate separation in mm, α is a constant equal to 5.5, and $\xi(0,E)$ is a variable equal to $a(E) + b(E)C$, in which $a(E)$ equals $27.19 - 32.59IR$, $b(E)$ equals $-1.666 + 1.982 \, IR$, C is the collector edge to sidewall distance in mm, and IR is the ionization ratio, i.e. ionization at 20 cm depth in water to 10 cm depth in water with both measurements made at the SAD of the machine (this is equivalent to the quality index, TPR_{10}^{20}).

4.9 Beam quality and field flatness

The energy of the X-ray beam decreases as the distance off-axis increases. This energy decrease is the product of two physical processes. For thin, high, Z targets bremsstrahlung energy increases with increasing angle, but for thick, high, Z targets bremsstrahlung energy decreases with increasing angle. Most accelerator manufacturers employ a thick-target design but some use a thin, high, Z target followed by a low-Z electron stopper to increase the average photon energy. The second process that contributes to the off-axis energy change is the differential hardening of the beam by the conically shaped flattening filter. This second process is more important as all present accelerators demonstrate a decrease in photon energy with increasing distance off-axis. Accelerator manufacturers are giving more attention to this problem by designing composite filters that demonstrate less change in energy with distance off-axis.

The 'horns', or off-axis peaking, in transverse profiles at shallow depths are a result of this change in energy with off-axis distance. Manufacturers typically design flattening filters to yield a flat profile at 10 cm depth. Because the energy in the periphery of the beam is less than the energy on the central axis, the penetration in the periphery is less. Therefore, the profile must be peaked off-axis at d_{max} to yield a flat profile at 10 cm depth.

This problem becomes important for irregular field calculations at off-axis points where the primary is multiplied by an off-axis factor before being added to the scatter. Many irregular field algorithms require the off-axis profile at d_{max} and then make corrections to this profile at other depths. It is incumbent upon the physicist to understand this algorithm for the computer that is used. Some computers use an empirically determined correction factor.

Other computers use a physical model, such as proposed by Hanson *et al.* (1980), in which the primary TMR is not only a function of depth but also of off-axis distance. They described a technique for measuring the half-value layer (HVL) in a narrow-beam geometry for several points off-axis. However, Kepka *et al.* (1985) give a method to extract the HVL in water from the large field beam profiles at several depths, so that additional HVL measurements are not required.

The reader must determine what algorithm is used in his/her treatment-planning computer to determine what data are necessary.

4.10 Distance correction

Certain treatments require larger field sizes than the maximum field of 40×40 cm^2 at 100 cm found on most linear accelerators. This situation requires that patients are treated at extended distances. For these cases, the applicability of the inverse square law (ISL) dependence of output should be verified.

The standard technique is to make 'in-air' ion chamber measurements over a range of field sizes and distances. For each field size, the data for the range of distances can be plotted as the reciprocal of the square root of the reading on the y-axis versus the distance on the x-axis. If these data form a straight line, ISL is applicable, and if the straight line passes through zero, the virtual source is at the same position as the target. If the straight line has a positive x-intercept the virtual source is downstream of the target, while a negative x-intercept implies that the virtual source is upstream of the target. For instance, if on a 100 cm machine the x-intercept were $+1$ cm, then the virtual source would be 99 cm from isocentre. In this case, the ISL applies but the calculation should be from 99 cm rather than 100 cm. As mentioned, this analysis should be performed for the range of field sizes as collimator scatter may change the virtual source position. Of course, if the data do not follow a straight line the ISL is not applicable and special calibrations will be required at each point.

A second less commonly used technique to verify ISL is to examine the beam divergence. For a given field size, films can be exposed perpendicular to the central axis at d_{max} at several distances from the source. The distance between the 50% density values, or full-width at half-maximum (FWHM), is then determined at each distance. These values can be plotted on the y-axis against distance on the x-axis. If ISL is valid, these data should yield a straight line and the x-intercept will again represent the position of the virtual source. All the films should be irradiated to yield approximately the same OD on the central axis. This can be done by assuming a priori that the ISL applies. One problem with this technique is that the range of field sizes and distances where it may be used is limited by the size of the film.

4.11 Asymmetric collimators, dynamic wedges, and multi-leaf collimators

Many new accelerators are equipped with either asymmetric collimator jaws or multi-leaf collimators (MCL) or both. Accelerators equipped with asymmetric collimators may also have a dynamic wedge option. These options require additional time to commission the machine for clinical practice. Typical accelerator designs allow for the upper set of collimator jaws to travel past the collimator axis of rotation by at least 10 cm and the lower set to travel past the same axis by 2 cm, both distances projected to isocentre. A dynamic wedge option usually allows for at least 15, 30, 45 and 60° wedge fields up to 20 cm in the wedge direction and 40 cm in the unwedged dimension. It is theoretically possible to form wedge fields for any arbitrary wedge angle with appropriate software. An MLC permits the formation of irregularly shaped fields, usually up to 40 cm in length with a 1 cm resolution at the isocentre.

4.11.1 Asymmetric collimator

One of the benefits of asymmetric collimators is the possibility of abutting adjacent fields with identical field divergence. Uniform dose at the field abutment demands highly accurate and precise placement of the collimator jaws. The dose gradient of the 50% decrement line is typically 15–20% per mm. As the readout resolution of collimator position is 1 mm, the abutment of two fields could theoretically produce a 30–40% over or under dose at the abutment. In practice, the non-uniformity of dose is less than this value and will vary on a daily basis due to the lack of precision in the set-up of both the jaws and the patient. However, it is highly recommended that the characteristics of each machine be tested for different jaw abutments on multiple days. One technique is to place a film oriented perpendicularly to the collimator axis of rotation. A double exposure is made by irradiating with two abutting fields. Typically the processed film demonstrates either a lighter or darker line along the abutment edge. This procedure should be performed for different field sizes with the abutment region at varying distances from the collimator axis of rotation to determine this effect. Also, this procedure should be repeated a few times to determine if the pattern of over or under dose is consistent. Another test is to rotate the gantry between irradiations to determine the effect of gantry flexing. An example of similar tests may be found in Zacarias *et al.* (1993) and in Chapter 5, Section 11.1.4.

Output factors for asymmetric fields were discussed in Section 4.2 above.

4.11.2 Dynamic wedges

Independent collimator jaws may be used to create wedged-shaped isodose distributions by moving one of the independent collimator jaws, while the other remains stationary during irradiation. This technique is referred to as a dynamic wedge. Clinical implementation of dynamic wedges requires measurement of central axis per cent depth doses, central axis wedge transmission factors, and transverse beam profiles of the dynamic wedges. These measurements are more complicated than profile measurements for standard physical wedges because of the dynamic modulation of the photon fluence during the delivery of the radiation field. The central axis per cent depth dose may be measured by integrating the dose at each point over the entire irradiation of each dynamic wedge field measured. The central axis wedge transmission ratios can be determined from the central axis per cent depth dose measurements. In this instance the ratio of the collected ionization at a specified depth for the dynamic wedge field is compared to the collected ionization at the same specified depth for the open field with the same collimator settings. The field size dependence of the central axis wedge transmission ratio for physical wedges was discussed in Section 4.6. It is important to note that the central axis wedge transmission ratios for dynamic wedges typically have a much large field size dependence than physical wedges. Also, it is important to note that this field size dependence may not be smooth. Some implementations of the dynamic wedge technique show a significant change in the trend of the central axis wedge transmission factor as the field width changes between 9.5 and 10 cm. This change has been demonstrated to approach 20% (Klein *et al.* 1995a). This characteristic should be carefully investigated on each machine. Transverse beam profiles are measured with an array of detectors, an integrating dosimeter such as X-ray or radiochromic film, or a commercial beam imaging system. When a detector array is used the sensitivity of each detector must be determined. Both ion chamber and diode detector arrays are commercially available. When using film, its energy dependence as a function of position in the beam is required.

4.11.3 Multi-leaf collimators

Multi-leaf collimators (MLC) are finding widespread application for conventional field shaping as a replacement for shaped blocks constructed of low melting-point alloy. The advantages of an MLC include a reduction in the amount of storage space in the treatment room, elimination of the need for the treatment technologists to lift heavy blocks, and the ability to treat multiple fields without re-entering the treatment room. Disadvantages include the discrete step size of the leaves and additional quality assurance requirements. Additional data is also required to characterize the output factors, central axis per cent depth doses, and penumbra of the MLC fields and the leakage through and between the leaves.

Typically, the central axis per cent depth dose of MLC defined fields is not significantly different from fields defined with the collimator jaws. The penumbra of MLC defined fields should be measured for both the leaf ends and the leaf edge considering also the effective penumbra for field edges formed by a series of MLC leaves at an angle and changes at various distances from the central axis. The penumbra will depend on the leaf design and whether the leaves are singly or doubly focused, but generally the MLC penumbra is within 2 mm of the penumbra of fields defined with the collimator jaws with the greatest difference being for singly focused MLC fields not centered on the collimator axis of rotation. It has been reported (Boyer *et al.* 1992) that for MLC systems added downstream from a conventional four-jaw collimator system, the output factors for MLC shaped fields are closely approximated by the product of the collimator scatter correction factor for the collimator setting and the phantom scatter correction factor for the irradiated area. This relation is the same as for fields formed with conventional lead or low melting-point alloy blocks. However, for MLC systems that replace at least one set of conventional jaws, Palta *et al.* (1996) report that the output factor is approximated by the product of the collimator scatter correction factor and phantom scatter correction factor, where both are for the irradiated area. Of course, the physicist should verify these relationships for central axis per cent depth dose, isodose shape, and position, penumbra and output factors on each machine during commissioning (Klein *et al.* 1995b).

Leakage through the MLC consists of transmission through the leaves and leakage between the leaves. Leakage between the leaves is easily demonstrated by exposing a film perpendicularly to the collimator axis of rotation with the leaves fully closed. Leakage through the leaves can be determined by comparing transverse beam profiles measured for fields collimated with the MLC to fields collimated with the collimator jaws. Typical values of MLC leakage are in the range of 3–5% of the isocentre dose, but with significantly higher values where the two rounded ends of opposite leaves meet.

5. Electron measurements

5.1 Central axis per cent depth dose

Electron central axis per cent depth dose values have been measured with both cylindrical and parallel-plate ion chambers. The effective point of measurement for parallel-plate chambers is usually taken to be the inside surface of the entrance window. For cylindrical chambers, the effective point of measurement is shifted forward of the centre of chamber. The amount of this displacement has been a subject of much discussion, but most medical-physics organizations are converging to a value equal to half the inside radius of the chamber toward the source. Cylindrical chambers also perturb the electron fluence more than parallel-plate chambers. To correct for this perturbation, one must apply a replacement, or perturbation, correction factor. This factor is less than unity for cylindrical chambers, and it decreases (i.e. diverges further from unity) as the energy of the electron beam decreases and the depth in phantom increases. Further details are given in Chapter 3, Sections 4 and 5.

Thin-window parallel-plate chambers with a plate separation of 2 mm or less are generally accepted to have a replacement correction of unity. However, the replacement factor is dependent on guard-ring design, as well as plate separation distance. Chambers with narrow guard rings tend to have replacement factors further removed from unity than those with wider guard rings. Some parallel-plate chambers can also be difficult to waterproof if used in a water phantom, and hydrostatic pressure can deform the thin entrance window if a thin waterproof sheath is used. This deformation changes the chamber's sensitivity. Use of a parallel-plate chamber in phantom can lead to a dosimetric mismatch if the phantom material differs from the material of the chamber. This mismatch can result in either an increase or decrease in the number of backscattered electrons with the chamber in place than would occur in a homogeneous phantom, depending on the materials involved.

With these caveats, most medical-physics societies recommend calibration of low-energy electrons with specially designed parallel-plate chambers because the replacement correction factor deviates significantly from unity for cylindrical chambers in these cases. Higher energy electrons, with a mean surface energy above 10 MeV, can be measured with cylindrical chambers.

Allied with the choice of ion chambers is the choice of phantom material. Water is generally recommended for high-energy electrons because it is nearly tissue equivalent and is readily available in high purity. Plastic phantoms are recommended for low-energy electron measurements with a thin-window parallel-plate chamber that cannot be readily waterproofed to prevent hydrostatic deformation of the window. Plastic phantoms are also useful for film dosimetry.

Several plastic materials are acceptable for phantoms. However, these plastics are not exactly water equivalent, i.e. they do not have the same linear collisional and radiative stopping powers and the same linear angular scattering power as water. This lack of exact water equivalence requires that depths of measurements made in plastic phantoms be corrected to water equivalent depths by scaling. The American Association of Physicists in Medicine (AAPM 1991) recommends a scaling factor based on the ratios of the depth of the 50% ionization measured in the two materials, i.e.:

$$d_{\text{water}} = d_{\text{med}}\left(\frac{R_{50}^{\text{water}}}{R_{50}^{\text{med}}}\right) \qquad (12)$$

where d_{water} is the depth in water equivalent to the actual depth d_{med} in phantom material, and R_{50}^{water} and R_{50}^{med} are the depths of the 50% ionization in water and phantom medium, respectively.

The ICRU (1984) makes similar recommendations but based on a ratio of continuous slowing down approximation (CSDA) ranges. In their notation this is:

$$\frac{d_{\text{P}}(m)}{d_{\text{P}}(w)} = \frac{(r_o/\rho)_{\text{m}}}{(r_0/\rho)_{\text{w}}} \qquad (13)$$

where $d_{\text{P}}(m)$ and $d_{\text{P}}(w)$ are the depths of per cent dose P in the phantom medium and water, respectively, and $(r_o)_{\text{m}}$ and $(r_o)_{\text{w}}$ are the CSDA ranges in phantom material and water, respectively. The CSDA ranges are expressed in units of mass per area and so must be divided by the densities ρ of the respective media for use in the scaling equation. More detail can be found in the appropriate protocols and in Chapter 3.

Two cautions are necessary. The first is that polystyrene is an ambiguous term. Some medical physicists refer to clear polystyrene as polystyrene, and to white polystyrene, which has a 3% loading of TiO_2, as 'high-impact' polystyrene. Others refer to the white polystyrene as polystyrene and the clear version as 'clear' polystyrene. When using tables for depth-scaling factors, it should be ascertained which polystyrene is listed. The second caution is that the density of a given plastic may vary with batch and manufacturer. It should be verified that the plastic used has the same density as the plastic referred to in the dosimetry protocols.

Although the phantom and ion chamber are set up in the same way for measuring electron central axis per cent depth dose as for photons, it must be remembered that unlike photons, electron per cent depth ionization curves are not equivalent to per cent depth dose curves. It should be recalled from Chapter 3 that ionization measurements must be multiplied by two factors, the restricted stopping power ratio and the replacement factor to convert to dose. These factors are energy dependent and thus depth dependent because the electron beam loses energy as it penetrates the phantom.

The method to convert depth ionization measured in water to electron per cent depth dose may be summarized as follows:

1. Shift the effective point of measurement at each depth, as detailed in Chapter 3, Section 5.3. If a parallel-plate chamber is used, the effective point of measurement is the inside surface of the front window.

2. Determine the range from depth–ionization measurements for a sufficiently large field, as detailed in Chapter 2, Section 6.2.1.

3. Find the average energy at the surface based on half-value depth (Chapter 3, Section 2.2.1) again using a sufficiently large field.

4. Find the average energy at each depth z from:

$$\overline{E}_z = \overline{E}_0(1 - z/R_{\text{P}})$$

where R_{P} is the practical range. This may preferably be done using Monte Carlo tabulated values of $\overline{E}_z/\overline{E}_0$ given in some protocols (see Chapter 3).

5. Obtain the appropriate factors to convert from ionization to dose at each depth based on the protocol chosen.

6. Normalize these values to the maximum value and multiply by 100 to find per cent depth dose.

The 90% dose is usually taken to be the therapeutic dose. For fields with dimensions similar to or smaller than the range of the electrons, loss of side scatter equilibrium will result in a decrease in the depth of the therapeutic dose, although the range will remain approximately the same as for larger fields. For field sizes larger than the range the depth of the therapeutic dose remains constant. This field size dependence is illustrated in Figure 4.7. Electron per cent depth dose should be measured in field size increments small enough to permit accurate interpolation of other field sizes. Surface dose is a significant factor in many electron treatments and is best measured with a thin-window parallel-plate ion chamber. Depth dose should be measured to depths great enough to determine the X-ray contamination in the beam.

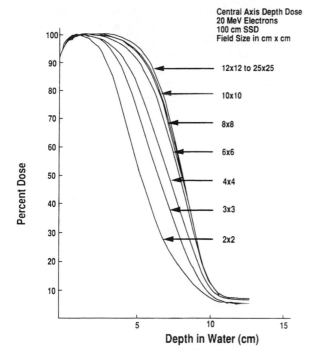

Central Axis Depth Dose
20 MeV Electrons
100 cm SSD
Field Size in cm x cm

12x12 to 25x25

10x10

8x8

6x6

4x4

3x3

2x2

Figure 4.7 Depth–dose curves for 20 MeV electrons showing the lack of variation for field sizes greater than the practical range (approximately 10 cm).

5.2 Output factors

5.2.1 Secondary collimators

Like photons, the output (in cGy per mu) is a function of field size and should be determined at d_{max} at the standard SSD. The output should be measured with a small volume ion chamber at d_{max} for each field size as discussed in the output factor section for photons. The output depends on the method used to define the field. Four types of collimation are used to define an electron field. These are:

(1) X-ray jaws;

(2) secondary collimators (cone or trimmers);

(3) irregularly shaped lead or low melting-point alloy metal cutouts placed in the secondary collimators;

(4) collimation, usually lead, placed directly on the patient's skin.

Trimmers, which are continuously variable collimators, are attached to the X-ray jaws and the two move as a unit. The position of the trimmer projected to the isocentre usually 'trims' 5 cm per side from the X-ray field. The trimmer serves to reduce the penumbra that would otherwise be very broad from the electrons scattering in air through distance from the X-ray jaw. As a result, the output factor for rectangular fields is

dependent on which set of X-ray jaws forms the width and which forms the length.

Mills *et al.* (1985) have shown that rectangular field output factors for Therac 20 trimmer-defined electron fields can be calculated within 1.5% using the expression:

$$OF(x, y) = [OF(x, 10)\ OF(10, y)] + CF(x,y) \quad (14)$$

where $OF(x,y)$ is the output factor for field $x \times y$ cm and $CF(x,y)$ equals 0 for D less than or equal to zero, and equals C for D greater than zero with D given by:

$$D = \frac{(x - 10)(y - 10)}{|(x - 10)(y - 10)|^{1/2}}$$

where x and y are the X-ray jaw settings of the machine and C is a constant of proportionality that must be determined for each energy on each machine.

Mills *et al.* (1985) state that this behavior of the output factor for rectangular fields is due to the X-ray jaws because the x and y jaws are at different distances from the patient. They give the square root method as an alternative technique:

$$OF (x, y) = [OF(x, x)\ OF(y, y)]^{1/2} \quad (15)$$

where $OF(x,x)$ and $OF(y,y)$ are the output factors for the square fields with sides of x and y, respectively. For their machine, this formula predicts the output factors to within 3%. These models must be verified by the physicist for each accelerator before it is used clinically.

Cones are usually available in a limited number of square fields typically 5×5 cm² to 25×25 cm² in 5-cm increments. Circular and rectangular cones are available but are not as common as the square cones.

The purpose of the cone depends on the manufacturer. Some use cones only to reduce the penumbra as trimmers do, while in other cases cones are used to scatter electrons off their sides to improve field flatness and symmetry. If cones are used, the output for each cone relative to the output at d_{max} for the 10×10 cm² cone must be determined at each energy. Frequently the values are referred to as cone ratios rather than output factors.

5.2.2 Metal cut-outs

Metal cut-outs of lead or low melting-point alloy can be placed in the end of the cone nearest the patient to define irregular fields. These cut-outs yield essentially the same penumbra as the cones themselves. A thickness of 12 mm of the low melting-point alloy Lipowitz's metal is adequate for electrons up to 20 MeV. The output factor for fields defined with these cut-outs depends on the electron energy, the cone, and the area of the cut-out. The dependence of output should be determined for square field inserts down to 4×4 cm² for each energy and each

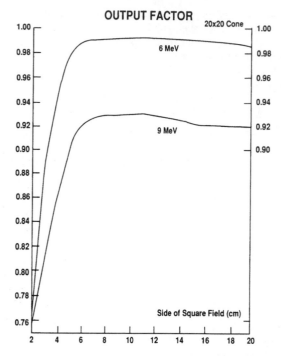

Figure 4.8 Electron output factors for a 20×20 cm^2 cone with square field inserts of different sizes.

cone during commissioning and plotted as a graph as shown in Figure 4.8.

Fields smaller than 4×4 cm^2 require special precautions because the size of the ion chamber may begin to approach the size of the field. Lack of lateral electron equilibrium and penumbral effects may result in a large variation in dose across the length of a 0.1 cm^3 thimble chamber, which may be 1.5 cm and, depending on the situation, smaller detectors may be required. A parallel-plate chamber with a small collecting electrode may be used in a polystyrene phantom or a diode can be used in a water phantom. In either case, the small field and the 10×10 cm^2 field should be measured with the same set-up. The shift toward the surface of d_{max} for small electron fields necessitates searching out d_{max} for the small field. The output factor should be the ratio of dose at d_{max} for the small field to dose at d_{max} for the 10×10 cm^2 field. For an ion chamber, this means the ionization must be converted to dose at the appropriate d_{max} before determining the output factor. If central axis per cent depth dose data measured with diodes have been shown to agree with similar data measured with corrected readings from an ion chamber, then the diode data can be used directly.

Film may be an alternative solution. Film could be exposed in a polystyrene or water-equivalent-plastic phantom, such as described in Section 2.3, with the film parallel to the central axis of the beam. One film should

be exposed to a 10×10 cm^2 field; the other film, to the smaller field. The films should be scanned to find the central axis d_{max} for each field. The ratio of the dose at d_{max} of the small field to the dose at d_{max} of the large field is the output factor. In this discussion it is assumed that the dose has been correctly determined from the net optical density with a characteristic curve and that good agreement has been demonstrated between per cent depth dose measured with film to that determined from corrected ion chamber data for a 15×15 cm^2 field. Even then these measurements require great care and it is advisable to use other methods for additional comparisons.

The output factor or cone ratio is a function of energy, cone size, and insert size. An open 10×10 cm^2 cone should still be used as the calibration field and all other values can be stated relative to this calibration field. For rectangular fields formed by placing inserts in cones the equivalent square field concept is usually valid. The equivalent square can be approximated with the equivalent square tables of BIR (1996) or as four times the area divided by the perimeter. However, the validity of this should be checked on each machine.

5.2.3 Skin collimation

Skin collimation is used to minimize penumbra for very small electron fields, to protect critical structures near the treatment area, and to restore the penumbra if treatment at extended distance is required (see Section 5.4). When designing skin collimation, the cone chosen should be larger than the area to be treated. The skin collimation then collimates this larger field to the treatment area and provides protection from scatter by extending a distance outside the treatment area. The thickness required for any electron shielding can be estimated by:

$$t_{Pb} \text{ (mm)} = 0.5 \, E_{p,0} \text{ (MeV)} + 1 \text{ for lead}$$

and

$$t_{LM} \text{ (mm)} = 1.2 \, t_{Pb} \text{ (mm) for Lipowitz's metal}$$

where $E_{p,0}$ (MeV) is the most probable electron energy at the surface of the patient and t_{Pb} and t_{LM} are thicknesses of lead and Lipowitz's metal.

For some clinical situations it may be necessary to minimize the weight of the skin collimation on the patient and somewhat thinner masks may be considered. In these situations it is recommended that the degree of shielding provided be assessed. This can be accomplished with a thin-window parallel-plate chamber in a polystyrene phantom at a depth of 1 mm.

Skin collimation effects the per cent depth dose as well as the penumbra. The field size dependence of the per cent depth dose is principally a result of scattering in the patient. The per cent depth dose for a field defined by skin collimation can be approximated as the per cent depth dose of the same size field determined by secondary collimation, such as a cone. The field size dependence of the output results from air scattering and the X-ray jaws. In most cases, for cones that are 5 cm or more from the skin, the output for a field defined with skin collimation is the same as the output defined by the secondary collimator for that treatment. For example, a 15×15 cm^2 cone that contains a 12×12 cm^2 Lipowitz's metal cut-out is used to treat a patient with 6 MeV electrons and an 8×9 cm^2 field defined by skin collimation. The output can usually be approximated as the output of a 6 MeV electron beam for the 15×15 cm^2 cone with a 12×12 cm^2 cut-out. However, for cones that contact the skin the output may be closer to the cone ratio of the 8×9 cm^2 field defined by skin collimation.

If the skin collimation defines a field so small that the per cent depth dose changes, then the output will be affected and another approach is required. In this case output can be estimated from the size of the secondary blocking (trimmers, cones, cut-outs placed in cones) and the per cent depth dose of the area defined by the skin collimation. The output with extensive collimation can be approximated as:

$$D(E, C_s, A_B) = D(E, C_s, A_o) \% DD(E, C_s, d_{max}, A_B) \quad (16)$$

where $D(E,C_s,A_B)$ is the dose for energy E, cone C_s, and blocked area A_B, $D(E,C_s,A_o)$ is the dose for energy E, cone C_s, and open area A_o, and $\% DD(E,C_s,d_{max},A_B)$ is the per cent depth dose for energy E, cone C_s, at d_{max} for the blocked field.

This formula can be clarified with the following example. A 6×6 cm^2 field of 13 MeV electrons is defined by a cone without a cut-out. The patient is treated with a 3×3 cm^2 field size defined by skin collimation. The per cent depth dose is that of the 3×3 cm^2 field. The output is the product of the output for the 6×6 cm^2 cone times the per cent depth dose of a 6×6 cm^2 field at the depth of d_{max} for the 3×3 cm^2 field. The depth of d_{max} for the 3×3 cm^2 field is 1.3 cm. At 1.3 cm the 6×6 cm^2 per cent depth dose is the proximal 94%. The output for this example is 94% of the output for the 6×6 cm^2 cone.

The models presented in this section for estimating output are dependent on machine and applicator design as well as air gap between the patient and the cone. Sufficient measurements must be performed to validate whatever model is used for a particular machine.

5.3 Beam profiles

Information about the off-axis dose distribution is required for treatment planning. These data are usually measured as transverse beam profiles for input to a computerized treatment-planning system. The profiles are combined with central axis per cent depth dose to yield the isodose curves. This information is generally used for treatment planning in the format of isodose curves. The number of transverse profiles and depths at which they must be measured depends on the treatment-planning system.

The profiles are measured in a water phantom with a small volume ion chamber. The surface of the phantom is placed at 100 cm or the normal SSD and the ion chamber is scanned perpendicularly to the central axis.

Electron transverse profiles can also be measured with film dosimetry techniques. Shiu *et al.* (1989) recommend combining profile information determined with film with central axis per cent depth doses measured ionometrically. In this case, the film is placed perpendicular to the central axis of the beam at the depth of interest. Conversion of optical density to dose is required as described in Section 2.3.

An alternative film dosimetry technique is to measure isodose curves rather than beam profiles. The film is exposed parallel to the central axis of the beam. Optical isodensity is converted to isodose. Shiu *et al.* (1989) discourage this technique because the per cent depth dose determined with film is typically 1 mm shallower than ionometric determination for depths greater than 10 mm. For depths shallower than 10 mm, the differences observed were as great as 5 mm. A better alternative for isodose measurements is to use small volume ion chambers or diodes.

5.4 Air gaps

It is frequently necessary to treat electron fields at an extended SSD because the surface shape prevents close positioning of the electron cone. The extended distance affects the electron dose distribution because of the additional scattering in the longer air path. The most obvious difference is decreased output. Another change is increase in the penumbral width. This, of course, may be important for abutting fields. The position of a virtual point electron source is a key piece of information needed to predict the changes in the electron dose distribution caused by extended treatment distances. The virtual source position is the point which is closest to intersecting the back projections of the mean directions of motions of electrons passing through a plane perpendicular to the central axis at the isocentre.

The methods of determining the position of the virtual source are similar to those discussed for verifying inverse square law for photons (Section 4.1). A field of 20×20 cm^2 or greater should be used to minimize the effect of collimator scatter for either technique used. The virtual source position is useful in treatment planning to predict the beam divergence at extended SSDs. However, to correct the output at an extended SSD, the inverse square dependence must also be modified because of collimator and air scatter. The correction factor for output at an

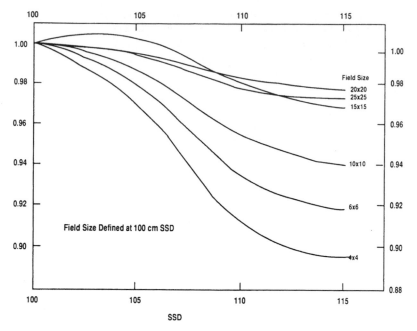

Figure 4.9 The air-gap correction factors for 20 MeV electrons measured for a range of field sizes and air gaps up to 15 cm.

extended SSD is a product of the inverse square factor and an air-gap factor. The air-gap factor corrects for deviations of output from inverse square law. The air gap factor may be either greater or less than unity as the output may either increase or decrease at extended distances depending on collimator design, electron energy, field size and air gap. The equation to calculate output at extended SSD is:

$$D(E, C_s, f) = D(E, C_s, f_0)\left(\frac{f_{vir} + d_{max}}{f_{vir} + d_{max} + h}\right)^2 \phi_h \quad (17)$$

where $D(E, C_s, f)$ is the dose for energy, E and cone, C_s; at extended SSD f, $D(E, C_s, f_0)$ is the dose for energy, E and cone, C_s; at calibration SSD f_0, f_{vir} is the virtual SSD, h is the air gap, and ϕ_h is the air-gap correction factor.

This air-gap correction factor should be measured in phantom at d_{max} using all the cones and energies available over a range of extended SSDs. The data can be plotted as the family of curves shown in Figure 4.9. Air-gap factors for rectangular fields can be approximated by the square root formula previously discussed for output of rectangular fields. In this instance the formula is:

$$\phi_h(E, x, y, h) = [\phi_h(E, x, x, h)\phi_h(E, y, y, h)]^{1/2} \quad (18)$$

where $\phi_h(E, x, y, h)$ is the air-gap correction factor for energy E, rectangular field with sides x and y cm, and air

gap h, and $\phi_h(E, x, x, h)$ and $\phi_h(E, y, y, h)$ are the air-gap correction factors for energy E for square fields with sides x and y, respectively, with air gap h.

Khan *et al.* (1978) have suggested an alternative approach to the virtual source position – the effective point source position. This technique simulates the clinical situation with measurements at d_{max} in phantom, as a function of air-gap between the end of the cone and phantom surface. Khan *et al.* (1978) recommend making these measurements every few centimetres, out to 10–15 cm from the cone. If inverse square law is assumed:

$$\frac{Q_0}{Q_h} = \left(\frac{f_{eff} + d_{max} + h}{f_{eff} + d_{max}}\right)^2 \quad (19)$$

or

$$\left(\frac{Q_0}{Q_h}\right)^{1/2} = \frac{h}{f_{eff} + d_{max}} + 1 \quad (20)$$

where Q_0 is the collected ionization with no air gap, Q_h is the collected ionization with air gap h, and f_{eff} is the effective SSD. If $(Q_0/Q_h)^{1/2}$ is plotted on the y-axis versus air gap h on the x-axis, m, the slope of the resulting line, is the reciprocal of $f_{eff} + d_{max}$ or:

$$f_{eff} = \frac{1}{m} - d_{max}. \quad (21)$$

The output at extended SSD may be calculated with the effective SSD formalism without an air-gap correction. In this case the formula is:

$$D(E, C_s, f) = D(E, C_s, f_0) \left(\frac{f_{eff} + d_{max}}{f_{eff} + d_{max} + h} \right)^2. \quad (22)$$

Depending on energy, field size, and collimation, $(Q_0/Q_h)^{1/2}$ may vary from a straight line if the air gap becomes too large. A special calibration will be required if this deviation from the inverse square law becomes too great. Also the effective SSD may change with field size for a given energy. In this case a table of effective SSDs as a function of field size and energy will be required.

Because of the limited penetration of electron beams with energy less than 25 MeV, the change in per cent depth dose with change in SSD is not significant for most situations. Some authors recommend the use of the Mayneord F-factor (simple ISL) to correct per cent depth dose for extended SSD. However, for SSDs up to 110 cm and energies up to 25 McV this correction is less than 2%.

There can be significant changes in the per cent depth dose at extended SSD if the electron beam is flattened with collimator scatter as is the case for some accelerator models. The per cent depth dose of a 6×6 cm^2, 20 MeV beam at 100 and 110 cm SSD is shown in Figure 4.10. The decrease in scattered electrons at 110 cm decreases the surface dose and increases the depth of the 95% dose. For these machines it may be necessary to measure isodoses over a range of SSDs.

Treatment at an extended SSD will also increase the penumbra width. At lower energies, the width of the penumbra (80–20%) increases approximately propor-tionally with the air gap. As energy increases, this increase in the penumbra is less dramatic at depth than for lower energies, but at the surface the increase in penumbra remains approximately proportional to the air gap. Because a large number of clinical situations demand treatment at an extended SSD, it is recommended that a sample of isodose curves at an extended SSD is measured to evaluate the algorithms in the treatment-planning system. The penumbra can be restored when treating at extended distances by use of skin collimation (see Section 5.2.3).

6. Summary

This chapter has provided an introduction to the relative dosimetry measurements required to place a high energy linear accelerator in clinical operation. The dosimetry equipment and its quality assurance have been reviewed, as well as the electron and photon measurements needed for standard treatments. Techniques and methodologies required for specialized treatments, such as stereotactic radiosurgery and intra-operative radiotherapy, have not been presented.

7. References

American Association of Physicists in Medicine (1991). Clinical electron-beam dosimetry. Report of AAPM Radiation Therapy Committee Task Group No. 25. *Med. Phys.*, **18**, 73–109.

Bova, F.J. (1990). A film phantom for routine film dosimetry in the clinical environment. *Med. Dosim.*, **15**, 83–5.

Boyer, A.L., Ochran, T.G., Nyerick, C.E., Waldron, T.J., and Huntzinger, C.J. (1992). Clinical dosimetry for implementation of a multileaf collimator. *Med. Phys.*, **19**, 1255–61.

British Institute of Radiology (1996). *Central axis depth dose data for use in radiotherapy*. Br. J. Radiol., Supplement 25. BIR, London.

Coffey, C.W., Beach, J.L., Thompson, D.J., and Mendiondo, M. (1980). X-ray beam characteristics of the Varian Clinac 6-100 linear accelerator. *Med. Phys.*, **7**, 716–22.

Dawson, D.J., Schroeder, N.J., and Hoya, J.D. (1986). Penumbral measurements in water for high-energy X-rays. *Med. Phys.*, **13**, 101–4.

Dutreix, J. and Dutreix, A. (1969). Film dosimetry of high-energy electrons. *Ann. N.Y. Acad. Sci.*, **161**, 33–43.

Dutreix, A., Bjärngard, B., Bridier, A., Mijnheer, B., Shaw, J., and Svensson, H. (1997). *Monitor unit calibration for high energy photon beams*. Physics for Clinical Radiotherapy, Booklet No. 3. ESTRO/Garant, Leuven.

Gerbi, B.J. and Khan, F.M. (1990). Measurement of dose in the buildup region using fixed-separation plane-parallel ionization chambers. *Med. Phys.*, **17**, 17–26.

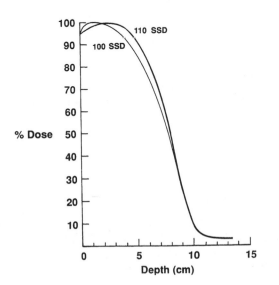

Figure 4.10 The effect of extended SSD on the per cent depth doses for a 6×6 cm, 20 MeV electron beam.

Hanson, W.F., Berkley, L.W., and Peterson, M. (1980). Off-axis beam quality change in linear accelerator X-ray beams. *Med. Phys.*, **7**, 145–6.

Holmes, T.W. and McCullough, E.C. (1983). Acceptance testing and quality assurance of automated scanning film densitometers used in the dosimetry of electron and photon therapy beams. *Med. Phys.*, **10**, 698–700.

Humphries, L.J. (1991). Quality assurance of dosimetry equipment. In *Quality assurance in radiotherapy physics* (ed. G. Starkschall and J. Horton), pp. 197–205. Medical Physics Publishing, Madison, Wisconsin.

Humphries, L.J. and Slowey, T.W. (1987). Dosimetry instrumentation. In *Radiation oncology physics* (ed. J.G. Kereiakes, H.R. Elson, and C.G. Born), pp. 110–38. American Institute of Physics, New York.

International Commission on Radiation Units and Measurements (1984). *Radiation dosimetry: electron beams with energies between 1 and 50 MeV.* ICRU Report 35. ICRU, Bethesda, MD.

Kepka, A.G., Johnson, P.M., and David, J. (1985). The effect of off-axis quality changes on zero area TAR for megavoltage beams. *Phys. Med. Biol.*, **30**, 589–95.

Khan, F.M., Sewchand, W., and Levitt, S.H. (1978) Effect of air space on depth dose in electron beam therapy. *Radiology*, **126**, 249–53.

Khan, F.M., Gerbi, B.J., and Deibel, F.C. (1986). Dosimetry of asymmetric X-ray collimators. *Med. Phys.*, **13**, 936–41.

Klein, E.E., Low, D.A., Meigooni, A.S., and Purdy, J.A. (1995a). Dosimetry and clinical implementation of dynamic wedge. *Int. J. Rad. Onc. Biol. Phys.*, **31**, 583–92.

Klein, E.E., Harms, W.B., Low, D.A., Willcut, V., and Purdy, J.A. (1995b). Clinical implementation of a commercial multi-leaf collimator, dosimetry, networking, simulation, and quality assurance. *Int. J. Rad. Onc. Biol. Phys.*, **33**, 1195–208.

McLaughlin, W.L., Puhl, J.M., Al-Sheikhly, M., Christou, C.A., Miller, A., Kovacs, A. *et al.* Novel radiochromic films for clinical dosimetry. *Rad. Prot. Dosim.*, **66**, 263–8.

Mellenberg, D.E., Dahl, R.A., and Blackwell, C.R. (1990). Acceptance testing of an automated scanning water phantom. *Med. Phys.*, **17**, 311–4.

Mills, M.D., Hogstrom, K.R., and Fields, R.S. (1985). Determination of electron beam output factors for a 20-MeV linear accelerator. *Med. Phys.*, **12**, 473–6.

Palta, J.R., Yeung, D.K., and Frouhar, V. (1996). Dosimetric considerations for a multi-leaf collimator system. *Med. Phys.*, **23**, 1219–24.

Reinstein, L.E. and McShan, D.L. (1982). Computer-controlled direct TMR measurement. *Med. Phys.*, **9**, 917–9.

Reinstein, L.E. and Gluckman, G.R. (1999). Optical density dependence on post-irradiation temperature and time for MD-55-2 type radiochromic film. *Med. Phys.*, **26**, 478–84.

Rikner, G. (1983). Silicon diodes as detectors in relative dosimetry of photon, electron, and proton radiation fields. Doctoral thesis. Uppsala University.

Shiu, A.S., Otte, V.A., and Hogstrom, K.R. (1989). Measurement of dose distributions using film in therapeutic electron beams. *Med. Phys.*, **16**, 911–5.

Sibata, C.H., Mota, H.C., Beddar, A.S., Higgins P.D., and Shin, K.H. (1991). Influence of detector size in photon beam profile measurements. *Phys. Med. Biol.* **36**, 621–631.

Spokas, J.J. and Meeker, R.D. (1980). Investigation of cables for ionization chambers. *Med. Phys.*, **7**, 135–40.

Zacarias, A.S., Lane, R.G., and Rosen, I.I. (1993). Assessment of a linear accelerator for segmented conformal radiation therapy. *Med. Phys.*, **20**, 193–8.

8. Additional reading

American Association of Physicists in Medicine (1998). Radiochromic film dosimetry: recommendations of AAPM Radiation Therapy Committee Task Group 55. *Med Phys* 25, 2093–2115.

Hogstrom, K.R. (1991). Treatment planning in electron beam therapy. *The role of high energy electrons in the treatment of cancer: Frontiers of radiation therapy and oncology*, Vol. 25. (ed. J.M. Vaeth and J.L. Meyer), p. 30. Karger, New York.

Horton, J.L. (1987). *Handbook of radiation therapy physics.* Prentice–Hall, Englewood Cliffs, NJ.

McKerracher, C., and Thwaites, D.I. (1999). Assessment of new small-field detectors, against standard–field detectors for pratical stereotactic beam data acquisition, *Phys. Med. Biol.*, 44, 2143–2160.

Thwaites, D.I., Burns, D.T., Klevenhagen, S.C., Nahum, A.E., and Pitchford, W.G. (1996). The IPEMB code of practice for electron dosimetry for radiotherapy beams of initial energy from 2 to 50 MeV based on an air kerma calibration. *Phys. Med. Biol.*, 41, 2557–603.

Chapter 5

Quality control of megavoltage therapy units

K.-A. Johansson, G. Sernbo, and J. Van Dam

1. Introduction

Every radiotherapy department must have a quality assurance (QA) programme, including all the different steps in the radiotherapy process, in order to ensure safety and quality of treatments. One of the elements of such a general programme is devoted to the equipment used for radiotherapy. Components in a QA programme for therapy equipment include planning for installation, acceptance tests, commissioning, training, quality control (QC), and preventative maintenance. This chapter deals with a QC protocol for megavoltage equipment (i.e. electron accelerators and cobalt units).

The term 'quality control', is defined as a regulatory process through which the actual performance is measured, compared with existing standards, reference values, etc., and the actions necessary to keep or regain conformity with these standards (IOS 1977). A quality control protocol is a series of planned activities.

The question of what constitutes acceptable quality of a certain treatment unit must be left to the professional judgement of the senior staff concerned. The requirements will usually depend upon the particular use of the equipment, taking into account the local conditions and methods, and the knowledge of what is technically achievable. Nevertheless, certain basic requirements for therapy units have been identified which guarantee an acceptable level of quality and safety in the routine use of the unit.

Modern megavoltage units (machine and accessories) are complex and require that due attention is paid to performance throughout their lifetime, in particular to ensure that the commissioning performance is maintained. The superior performance of the units cannot be fully exploited unless a high degree of quality and consistency is reached, and this is possible only through quality control. The quality of the treatment of a patient can be compromised or completely lost by gross equipment failure, as well as by the undetected deviation

of a single parameter. Every parameter affecting patients and staff has to be included in the QC protocol. Some of these have to be measured daily, others weekly, monthly or yearly. QC activity should ensure that the therapy unit performs according to specifications, and that the unit is safe to use for both patients and staff. Moreover it should guarantee the accuracy of the dose delivered, prevent major errors, minimize treatment machine downtime, and promote preventative maintenance procedures.

In shaping this chapter, we were guided in part by national and international recommendations (Brahme 1988; IPSM 1988; WHO 1988; IEC 1989a, 1989b; SFPH 1989; AAPM 1994a, 1994b; IPEM 1999), by recently published QC procedures for new technology, such as multi-leaf collimators, dynamic wedges, and electronic portal imaging devices (Thompson *et al.* 1995; Klein *et al.* 1995, 1996; Chui *et al.* 1996; Rajapakshe *et al.* 1996; Hounsell and Jordan 1997; Ma *et al.* 1997), but mainly by our own experience. Currently there are no national or international QC recommendation for these new modalities in radiotherapy. This chapter is concerned with QC protocols for the main types of megavoltage therapy units. These may not be satisfactory for all types of machines and will, to some extent, depend on the type of unit, intended clinical use, treatment technique, and the resources (such as personnel, test equipment, etc.) available in a given department. No single QC protocol is suitable for all radiotherapy departments world-wide. While the practice of weekly checks only on the dose output is no longer accepted as adequate QC, checks that are too extensive and time consuming may represent a costly effort with limited benefit to the patient.

An important aspect of a QA programme for high-technology devices is continuous training of the operators. By giving only an initial training at the beginning of the clinical use of the unit, incorrect use is likely to develop over its lifetime. Feedback from operators is essential in evaluating the need for changes

Table 5.1 Criteria for the different tests

	Daily	Basic	Extended
Number of parameters	Few	Some	All
One check including several parameters	Some	Few	None
Mainly observation (O) or quantification (Q)	O	O/Q	Q
Comparison (C) or independent (I) test	C	I	I
Results in arbitrary (A) or SI-units (S)	A	A	S
Duration of test	Short	Limited	Long

in written procedures, designing QC, and handling other problems. All operators must fully understand the modes of operation and the procedures used in patient treatment. Performance information collected and documented by operators is vital for the QA of dynamic mode treatments.

A specific QC protocol should be written for each treatment unit and should specify:

(1) test method;

(2) test equipment;

(3) parameters to test;

(4) frequency of measurement;

(5) responsibilities for different groups of staff;

(6) reference values;

(7) tolerances;

(8) actions to be taken;

(9) rules for documentation.

Each of these will be considered in the following sections. QC tests must be designed to be simple and quick to implement if they are to be accepted and properly performed.

In this chapter, an appropriate and practical QC protocol for typical megavoltage units is presented. It is hoped that it will prove useful in modifying or establishing a suitable quality control protocol for any radiotherapy centre.

Special treatment techniques carried out on a particular unit require specific, locally designed QC procedures of their dosimetry. Examples of such techniques are total body irradiation, stereotactic brain therapy, intraoperative treatment These are not dealt with here. However, QC of intensity modulated radiotherapy is included due to the expected potential and future common use.

2. General methods and test materials

Adequate and efficient methodology is a prerequisite for successful quality control. This section is intended to provide guidelines for the general methods and test equipment to be used for the different checks. Detailed methods are presented in Section 9–12.

This QC protocol has been designed for four categories of tests:

(1) patient-specific;

(2) daily;

(3) basic, with weekly to monthly frequency;

(4) extended, with a time interval of 6 months to 2 years.

Checks of certain parameters of particular interest may be included in more than one of the different categories. Some of the requirements for these tests are shown in Table 5.1.

Patient-specific tests are discussed in Section 9. They do not replace the other tests, but they are a sensitive tool to identify machine malfunctions and may be used to determine a suitable frequency for the other tests.

2.1 Methods

The many different types of therapy units available make it difficult to design a set of tests applicable to all units. The methods vary in sophistication, depending on the purpose of the measurements, and the time and resources available. All checks and measurements must be made when the treatment unit is used in the same way as for patient treatment. Although some parameters are adjusted in maintenance mode (e.g. flatness) they *must* be checked in therapy mode. If the therapy unit is computer controlled, then the patient treatment mode should be used for all routine dosimetry checks. The tests are designed for isocentric units and may need modification for other units.

Patient-specific tests may involve *in vivo* dosimetry, visual checks of field shape, use of electronic portal imaging devices (EPID), etc..

The daily-test method is mainly a series of comparisons between two or more parameters or subsystems forming part of the therapy unit. When a deviation is observed it is not easy to identify which individual parameter is in error, it can only be concluded that the system is not working properly. An independent test method must then be used to identify the error. A computer self-test should be run every morning before the other daily checks.

For the basic tests, absolute test methods are proposed but in some cases several parameters are included in the same test set-up. This method is time saving, but the interpretation of the result can be somewhat difficult when one or more parameters deviate. The basic test is mainly an accurate constancy check capable of detecting significant deviations from the expected performance. It is not a 'calibration'.

The extended tests should include most parameters, be accurate, and should measure each parameter independently, but they are more limited than the commissioning measurements. The methods and test equipment used for the acceptance and commissioning procedures are often suitable for the extended tests. The results of the tests should usually be given in absolute terms.

The results obtained from the daily and basic tests may be stored on computer. In particular, when using computer-controlled equipment for static and dynamic treatments, the number of tests, and consequently of results, increases greatly. The benefits of a well-structured data base for the storage of results becomes substantial. Short-, medium- and long-term variations of the parameters are then easily analysed and presented.

2.2 Test instrumentation

It is important that every department has an adequate set of test equipment, some of which should, if possible, be dedicated to QC. To ensure quality it is important to carry out constancy checks and calibration of the dosimetry test equipment. These topics are covered in Chapter 3.

There are now a number of systems commercially available that are specially designed for multiple checks. Five detectors within the field give information about dose and beam symmetry, another four detectors at the edges of the beam assess field size accuracy, and one detector under some special build-up material gives information about energy. Such a system can be used for different beam energies just by adding build-up material. This device may easily be adopted for daily and basic

tests. Electronic portal imaging devices (EPIDs) have the potential to be used for flatness and symmetry checks.

2.2.1 Instrumentation for patient-specific test

An *in vivo* dosimetry system is necessary for these tests, at least one diode for each photon beam quality and one for electron beams (see Chapter 11, Section 2.3).

2.2.2 Instrumentation for daily test

Equipment should be dedicated to this test and, for convenience, should be left in the treatment area.

Daily-test dosimeter

This should be a semiconductor detector (*in vivo* dosimetry system) or a field class ionization chamber with a suitable electrometer. A diode is much more robust than an ionization chamber.

Daily-test phantom

A solid plastic phantom about $200 \times 200 \times 50$ mm^3 with a 100×100 mm^2 field and a central cross marked on the surface. If an ionization chamber is used then a suitable hole should be made to accommodate it.

Fixation for phantoms

It should be possible to attach the daily-test phantom (and the basic-test phantoms, and preferably also the film phantom) to the radiation head by means of a quick release mechanism to allow positioning on the accessory mount. This reduces set-up time and can be used at any gantry angle.

2.2.3 Instrumentation for basic test

The equipment should be dedicated to this type of test and should preferably be kept on a trolley. This enables easy transportation to the different units, and ensures that all test equipment and documentation are kept together.

Ionization chamber

This should be a cylindrical field class instrument with an electrometer. For checks of low-energy electron beams it is desirable to have a plane-parallel ionization chamber. Different chambers must be used for daily and basic tests to allow independent measurements.

Basic-test phantom

This should be a simple block of plastic, $200 \times 200 \times 70$ mm^3 with a hole 50 mm and 20 mm from the two surfaces that can accommodate an ionization chamber. In addition, separate solid plastic ($200 \times 200 \times 5$–50 mm^3) sheets are required for measurements of beam quality in electron and photon beams.

Beam-alignment test frame

This consists of a sheet of semi-transparent paper marked with a centre cross and a 200×200 mm^2 square mounted

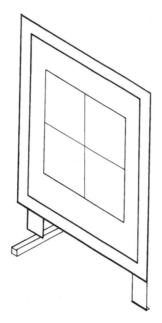

Figure 5.1 Test frame for beam alignment, a semi-transparent screen on an aluminium frame.

on an aluminium frame. To keep the frame in a vertical position it can be mounted on a stand, or simply supported by lead blocks. A typical frame is shown in Figure 5.1.

Film phantom

This is a sheet of 5 mm polystyrene (white), about 250×370 mm^2 (depending on film size) with a centre cross and a square 200×200 mm^2 engraved on the top side. The corners of the 200-mm square and a coaxial 190-mm square are fitted with 1-mm diameter $\times$ 5 mm lead markers in drilled holes. A ninth marker, 20 mm in from one corner, is used for orientation, (see Figure 5.2).

Film envelope

A number of double black plastic envelopes of the actual film size to be used for exposing photographic film should be available.

Film type

Film should be selected that has a low background optical density and a linear dose–density curve over a reasonable dose interval. Certain types of graphic film (e.g. Agfa Gevaert RA711p) are used in many institutions; the linearity in the dose range 0.3–1.5 Gy is good and the background density is low when developed in a standard X-ray film processor. (In some processors, the thin graphic film sheet must be attached to a piece of X-ray film, otherwise it may get lost.) Alternatively, treatment verification film (e.g. Kodak X-Omat V) can be used, but it has a small linear range and a high

background density. The film should be placed in the phantom in the double envelopes and compressed to avoid air cavities, which would affect the amount of scattering. For these measurements, the film is used perpendicular to the beam axis. It should be noted that the sensitivity of film varies non-linearly with energy. Because of this, and the limitations in linearity of response, the density profile is not exactly equal to the dose profile and the dose–density relation should be checked regularly. To do this an envelope-wrapped film can be irradiated with small field sizes of increasing dose distributed over the film area.

2.2.4 Other dosimetric instrumentation

For QC activities and other dosimetry purposes it is necessary to have additional equipment including:

(1) film dosimetry system (processor and scanning densitometer);

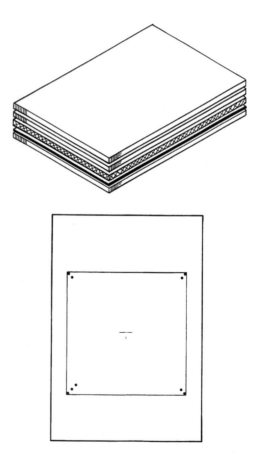

Figure 5.2 Film phantom. The small dots are lead markers corresponding to square 200×200 mm^2 and 190×190 mm^2, one lead marker is for orientation. Above is shown a typical set-up with backscattering and build-up material surrounding the film and the film phantom sheet.

(2) radiation field scanning system;

(3) other equipment to include: thermometer, barometer, stop-watch, rulers, sliding callipers, spirit level (sensitivity better than 0.3 mm/m) for horizontal and vertical use, a small plumb line with a conical tip and a straight, conically tipped rod with a diameter of 6–10 mm.

3. What should be tested

The performance of all parameters that are important to quality and safety must be checked regularly, although not necessarily with the same frequency. The selection of parameters to be monitored is mainly based on experience with different types of accelerator and should reflect the treatment techniques used routinely. Some examples of what to consider when designing a QC protocol are presented below.

Additional items will need consideration for those units that carry out certain specialized treatments, such as stereotactic brain therapy, total body irradiation, or intraoperative radiotherapy.

3.1 Optical and mechanical systems

Even quite new units may have some optical and mechanical defects that will, over a period of time, result in the accuracy of the beam-directional system or in the patient set-up system falling below an acceptable level. A quick basic beam-alignment check should detect problems, such as instabilities in lamp filaments, lamp holders, lasers and laser fixtures. Minor collision damage and wear in the collimating system will cause fewer problems if they are detected early, preferably at the basic test. Isocentric treatments need a well-adjusted and stable laser system, while multi-field SSD techniques use extensive couch movements. An extended beam-alignment check should detect most errors.

Asymmetric fields have a number of uses including the provision of non-divergent field edges and the reduction in interleaf leakage for multi-leaf collimators (MLC). Asymmetric collimators are also commonly used for segmented radiotherapy. The alignment of the collimator jaws must be accurate, particularly for matching non-divergent fields with a common isocentre. Details of the QC programme for asymmetric jaws depend on clinical use.

3.2 Dose monitor

Modern accelerators have dual dose-monitoring systems, but the two monitors are not completely independent of each other. They are usually located close to each other in the accelerator head and integrate over a similar area of the fluence. A mechanical change in the position of the scattering foil or of the flattening filter may, in the worst case, result in a small change in the signal from the monitor chamber causing only small changes in the dose to the patient at the centre of the field. However, there may be a significant change in the dose uniformity.

3.3 Beam symmetry

Beam asymmetry sometimes occurs between two halves of the field due to imperfections and instabilities of the beam symmetry servo system. This asymmetry is common in some types of accelerators and varies with time, beam energy, gantry orientation, etc. For other accelerators the symmetry is stable and seldom needs adjustment.

3.4 Multi-leaf collimator (MLC)

Commercial MLCs are reliable, well-engineered devices that allow simple blocking, conformal therapy or ultimately intensity modulated radiotherapy (IMRT) to be carried out. For some accelerators the MLC replaces one pair of the collimator jaws. For others the MLC is a device attached to the accelerator head, with the two pairs of collimator jaws being retained. Currently, the main role of the MLC is to replace beam-shaping blocks, but its great potential lies in dynamic use for creating IMRT. A computer is used for the control of the leaves for static, as well as for dynamic, treatments. MLCs are relatively new in routine use and hence the QC procedure is either not covered or is only briefly mentioned in the literature. QC should mainly be concerned with positional accuracy, leaf motion integrity, leaf leakage, interlocks, networking, and data transfer. The dynamic use of MLC is discussed in Section 3.5.4.

3.5 Computer-controlled systems

Hardware and software problems and human errors in the use of computers may potentially result in large errors in modern radiotherapy units. Computer-controlled therapy units can have very elaborate software packages, capable of controlling many parameters that are difficult for the user to test extensively. One way of doing this is to run a set of well-known reference 'test cases' of varying complexity. Unfortunately, independent test methods are not yet well developed, and more effort is required in this area.

Conventional QC programmes are inadequate for this new computer-controlled technology. New QC procedures are, therefore, needed. Some major areas of computer controlled radiotherapy can be identified as follows.

3.5.1 Console computer and software

For modern accelerators some of the modalities are under computer control. The console computer and the computers dedicated to different services must be part of a QC programme. Inherent computer self-tests are effective for regular checks. They must, however, be invoked manually and must be complemented by inspection of check sums and the print out of data and calibration files. When new computer software is installed, it is mandatory to perform at least a basic QC programme. The physicist responsible should gain knowledge of the software package and its influence on the accelerator performance.

3.5.2 Computer-controlled wedged field

Computer-controlled jaw movement during irradiation is possible with some linear accelerators. In this way, angled isodoses that mimic wedged fields can be produced. For example, Varian described this as a dynamic wedge (DW) or enhanced dynamic wedge (EDW); Siemens use the term 'virtual wedge' (VW). Stored computer files and computed data are used to control the movable jaw position in relation to the portion of treatment delivered. Due to the criticality of the dynamic jaw movement, it is important to check periodically both 'wedge' factors and isodose angles. Errors in the calibration of the collimator jaw movements or in the computer files, which control the movements, will have a great effect on the delivered dose for computer controlled wedged fields.

3.5.3 Auto set-up

Modern computer-controlled radiotherapy equipment offers the possibility of delivering complex, multiple-field treatments with minimal operator intervention. Parameters such as gantry angles, collimator angles, field sizes, MLC, and couch positions can be set-up, delivered, and monitored by the computer-controlled system. The parameters are transferred from either a simulator and/or from a treatment-planning system and are then stored in the auto set-up computer. The auto set-up system has often replaced the so-called check and confirm (record and verify) system. This means that the human operator has to perform the check and verification of the set-up. This change in check and verification from manual set-up and computer verification to the reverse situation requires detailed training of the accelerator operators. To achieve good quality, the security of file transfer and file storage, as well as the movement calibration of computer-controlled parameters, have to be checked on a regular basis.

More complex non-coplanar field arrangements composed of multiple segments may be automatically set-up and treated without interruption. Each segment may have a different beam mode and energy, gantry and collimator angle, couch orientation, and MLC shape. This is one step towards IMRT.

3.5.4 Intensity modulated radiotherapy

IMRT to generate optimized dose distributions can be created by using a scanning beam, a dynamic MLC, a field composed of multiple segments or by using irregularly shaped 3D compensators. The main method considered in this chapter will be IMRT created by dynamic MLC. IMRT using dynamic MLC movements is being developed and has been clinically tested in a few institution around the world. A common approach is to use a number of static field positions, with dynamic MLC motion on each field to create the required intensity modulation.

Human limitations in detecting malfunctions in complex arrangements requires stringent QC procedures, to ensure the safe delivery of the intended intensity modulated dose distribution to the patient. QC is necessary throughout the whole treatment. Semi- or fully-automated mechanical, as well as dosimetric, tests have to be performed. In this test, the total performance of the accelerator and its accessories involved in the IMRT has to be checked. A separate test computer, independent from the control computer that governs the delivery of the treatment, may be a suitable method. Co-operation with the manufacturer in order to design a suitable QC procedure is advisable for IMRT. This type of test can never replace a QC programme that includes a conventional test of each subsystem of the accelerator in a static situation.

3.6 Accessories

Accessories such as mechanical wedge filters, shadow trays, lead blocks, and similar devices are attached to the unit. These devices must be positioned and safely locked in the correct position in order not to injure staff or patients. Particular attention must be paid to units with external wedge filters, such as most cobalt units, where damage is more likely. Small positional errors will significantly change the dose to the patient.

3.7 Interlocks

The only way to check an interlock is to interrupt or disturb the normal conditions that it is monitoring. Some interlocks, like entrance-door switches and collision-protection devices on the treatment head and collimators, are obvious candidates for checking. However, care must be taken not to overlook less obvious ones such as the symmetry/flatness detector and the excess dose-rate detector. Some of the interlocks are checked by the console computer software before the beam is switched on. Co-operation with the manufacturer regarding these checks and necessary information are essential for the design of the QC procedure.

3.8 *Electronic portal imaging device (EPID)*

An on-line EPID is a test instrument that plays an important role in improving radiotherapy. However, as these systems become part of regular clinical practice, it becomes necessary to ensure their correct and reliable operation. Therefore, EPID is included in this chapter. Specifying QC of EPID is not an easy task, due to the limited routine clinical experience. The test must be an objective, quantitative, reproducible and simple measurement of the image quality, as well as of the geometrical accuracy. A test object that only provides a subjective impression of the quality of the image is not acceptable as a sufficient QC procedure.

4. Test frequencies

The QC programme for each treatment unit should be initiated at the time of installation and continue throughout the working life of the equipment. The frequency of the tests of a particular unit should be based on the following:

(1) the severity (grade) of risk for patient and staff in case of malfunction;

(2) the probability of an error that will affect the performance;

(3) the probability of an error that will affect the safety of the patient or staff;

(4) the expected life of the unit, including different subsystems;

(5) the expected long-term stability of the unit;

(6) the age of the unit;

(7) the complexity of the unit;

(8) the experience gained from using this unit;

(9) experience gained by other users.

Taking these criteria into account, suitable frequencies and intervals for planned checks are:

(1) daily checks;

(2) weekly to monthly (here called basic) check;

(3) extended checks, with an interval between 6 months to 2 years.

It should be pointed out that some flexibility should be applied to this classification. Special attention should be given to parameters that have shown large deviation from the expected value during the previous checks. The frequency of checks on those parameters could be increased. On the other hand, if previous measurements have indicated few and slow changes, some decrease in the frequency may be satisfactory. Critical parameters should have a fixed frequency, since the risk for patient and staff is large.

For safety checks, the intervals recommended by the manufacturer of the unit should be followed closely and can be linked to a planned preventative-maintenance programme. In addition, checks of all related parameters must be performed whenever an adjustment, alteration or repair of the machine is made (e.g. new field light bulb, new magnetron) as sometimes a repair that seemingly should not affect the characteristics of the unit could well do so. Upgrades or new releases of software packages are also a reason to perform a QC procedure of related parameters. Assistance by electronics and mechanical specialists is essential for a successful QC programme.

5. Responsibilities

Quality control involves a co-operation between several staff groups including physicists, radiation oncologists, radiographers (radiotherapy technologists), dosimetrists (physics technicians), and engineers, but a physicist must have the ultimate responsibility and co-ordinate the work of the different groups who may perform different activities. The physicist responsible delegates certain responsibilities to other individuals in the department who have appropriate professional skills and knowledge of the specific unit. The exact distribution of the tasks is not critical, but it is essential that each individual performs and records the results of the tests on a regular basis. When deviations larger than the tolerance level appear, action must be undertaken after agreement with the physicist responsible.

The physicist responsible must be personally convinced that the test is conducted to a standard that is acceptable at the local, national or international level, and ascertain whether, and when, a certain task has been performed. It is also incumbent on the physicist responsible for QC to inform the radiation oncologist regularly about the QC results, and to report immediately when any major deviations are detected (e.g. dose error or more than 10%, beam alignment error of more than 5 mm, as agreed locally and defined in the local protocol; see Section 7), and to decide whether the machine should be taken out of use. The judgement regarding the clinical relevance of a malfunction is usually the decision and responsibility of the radiation oncologist with the support of the physicist.

6. Reference data set and standard values

Measurements made during commissioning and after acceptance of the equipment and other similar measurements, like extended checks, made subsequently, serve as the basis for a reference data set. QC activities are intended to ensure that the performance of the unit always complies with the reference data set. If any deviation is detected, then action must be taken to ensure that the performance is restored to comply with the reference data set. If this is not possible, then the data set must be updated, both for reference purposes and for treatment planning and delivery, if appropriate. A degradation in the performance of certain parameters of a treatment unit is unavoidable, and from time to time the reference data set must be changed. The data used for treatment of patients is directly derived from the reference data set and if the reference data set is changed, then the data used at the treatment unit and for planning must also be changed. The unit should still comply with the relevant standards and fulfil clinical requirements.

The most frequent checks (daily and basic) of a therapy unit are made with a designated set of test equipment. The monitor calibration should be checked every week with the same ionization chamber and electrometer. To save time, and to reduce the risk of erroneous calculation, the expected values for the daily tests should be corrected readings in arbitrary units and not the calculated dose values. These expected values must be determined for the actual instrumentation designated for the QC checks, at the same time as the absolute measurements, under reference conditions (i.e. calibration), are carried out. This ensures direct linkage between the expected values and the reference data.

Measurements of symmetry and flatness are often made with photographic film or with a scanning device used in air. The profiles obtained in these measurements are, however, not identical to the profiles put into the treatment-planning system (TPS), but are merely a constancy check of related parameters. Using these simplified methods will thus require a set of reference data that relate to the particular measurement rather than any treatment parameter. This data set must be obtained at the same time as the data for the TPS and both must be updated whenever the standard reference data set is updated. The tolerances for such simplified measurements are often the same as for the standard data set, but every physicist using a simplified method must review the method and then set the appropriate tolerance.

The expected values for the daily test are regularly verified by the basic test procedure. In a similar way the basic test values are verified by the extended test procedure.

Intercomparison between institutions, quality audit, or similar comparative measurements, are a useful way of detecting systematic errors in the reference data sets (Chapter 14, Section 7).

7. Tolerance, action, and incident levels

Most of the parameters vary to a certain extent due to electrical and mechanical instabilities, but the average value should be close to the expected value or standard. Brahme (1988) defined two different performance descriptors:

(1) tolerance level (TL): when a parameter is in the range below the TL, the equipment is suitable for high-quality radiation therapy;

(2) action level (AL): when the action level is reached for any parameter, it is essential that appropriate corrective action is taken. The value of the AL is generally about double that of the TL.

It is also stated in Brahme (1988) that the action levels might be regarded as a more relevant level for use in the QC protocol during the serviceable life of the equipment. The values quoted are often defined as one standard deviation, and somewhat larger values may, therefore, be observed occasionally and be considered to be acceptable.

For larger deviations, it may be appropriate to define an incident (or reporting) level, IL. The clinical impact of a malfunction should be the basis for the selection of the IL. ILs should be agreed locally at every institution by the responsible staff. Generally, the IL is about 2–3 times the action level. An IL report should be prepared and presented to the staff responsible immediately after the malfunction is detected. The report should be stored and all IL reports over a limited time should be evaluated and suitable actions should be taken.

When QC programmes are drawn up these considerations must be incorporated in the QC protocol. It is recognized that inaccuracies and variations in the test method must be allowed for when assessing the tolerances. This is considered when the TL and AL values are established. An isolated deviation, somewhat larger than TL, is accepted without any action. However, if a series of measured values, over a limited time, stays close to one tolerance level, the parameter should be adjusted. A test yielding a value between TL and AL should be repeated within a shorter time interval than required in the QC protocol and it is essential to keep this particular parameter under continued observation. If the value remains between these levels a corrective adjustment should be made. Any value greater than the AL demands immediate corrective action. Some parameters are not easily and quickly corrected or repaired, some may be almost impossible or very expensive to restore. In such cases the responsible physicist should inform the radiation oncologist and they should decide on suitable action together. The action could be replacement or increase in the TL and AL. This can affect treatments and clinical decisions, e.g. if it is a geometric factor, the margin in the periphery of the clinical target volume may have to be increased.

8. Instructions and documentation

A description of the methods for each test must be written in a clear, concise, and easy to use form. All checks performed frequently (daily or basic checks) should have detailed written instructions. These written instructions will ensure consistency in the way in which checks are performed. The instructions should include expected values with tolerances, and specify what action should be taken at different deviations from the expected value. The instructions should stipulate the way in which malfunctions are to be reported.

The results of every daily check must be recorded together with the daily technical maintenance in a designated book, which should be kept in the control room of the unit. The radiographers should write down in this report book all problems encountered and questions about the machine. Thus it will serve as an important communication link between the operators of the therapy unit and the engineers and physicists.

All other checks and actions, as well as all acute and preventive maintenance, should be recorded in a separate log-book. Although separate data sheets are very convenient when making checks, they are not always sufficient for legal purposes. A dated report in a register is a well-defined link in the time chain of the QC actions of the department, but such a log-book will be difficult to use. The best policy is to use separate preprinted data sheets for writing down the results of the measurements, but to write and date the final conclusions of the checks and actions undertaken in the log-book. The results of the measurements, and of course the log-book, must be kept for an appropriate length of time (for follow-up and to avoid possible litigation).

Instructions and records of tests should be preferably be combined on the same page. Recording the results in chronological order on one page allows the detection of trends over time, as well as variation of the parameters. All actions taken should also be carefully noted. Storing the results in a computer makes it easier to detect even small potential problems. Our experience clearly shows the importance of proper recording and organization of test data. Information from different tests must be put together to create a true picture of machine performance. it must, however, be stressed that not all checks can be separated from each other because they may be interdependent.

9. Patient-specific test

Treatment verification and *in vivo* dosimetry are described in Chapter 11. Some of the tests routinely performed to verify patient treatments can also serve as checks on certain accelerator parameters and accessories. When a new accelerator, new accessory, or other new technology is commissioned and taken into routine clinical service, it is advisable to perform patient-specific tests prior to the first treatment and during the treatment sessions. With the clinical use of sophisticated techniques, such as IMRT, the patient-specific tests should be mandatory at least at the first fraction. The frequency of these tests may change depending on the accumulating experience of the equipment and treatment technique. The patient-specific tests are mainly intended to detect gross deviations in accelerator performance, in computer control, and in computation errors without delay. If patient-specific tests are performed, malfunctions are unlikely to persist for more than a short part of the day.

In vivo dosimetry with entrance measurements with one diode on the central axis or a few diodes inside the field are an effective way to check the delivered dose to the patient for different field sizes, wedges, etc.. The signal from the diode is, however, dependent on field size, obliquity, wedge, SSD, etc. If the diode is calibrated for only one field size and no corrections are applied, it can be recommended that a variation of $\pm 5\%$ from the expected value is accepted.

For computer-controlled wedged fields it is advisable to confirm the movements by checking the end position of the movable collimator after the treatment.

Illumination of the irregular-shaped field onto the original simulator film, beams-eye view (BEV), or digital reconstructed radiographs (DRR) at the therapy unit is a test of the set-up of the MLC and block and blocking tray, etc. This method allows a visual check of each field shape on the machine prior to the first treatment. Matching of the light field and the intended shaped field must be maintained to within 2 mm for all boundaries at the level of the isocentre.

With the introduction of a new modality, especially with dynamic radiotherapy, it is advisable to perform patient-specific tests. Prior to the first treatment, the operator should step through the computer-controlled set-up of each segment. Once this is accomplished, an irradiation is performed, in which the machine components are moved through all segments of the actual treatment. Films are irradiated separately for each field at the reference depth in a solid homogeneous phantom. The dose distributions are evaluated from the films and compared with the dose distributions for the actual patient field arrangement, but with computed dose distribution separately for each field in a similar homogeneous phantom at reference depth. Entrance *in vivo* dosimetry should be used at the first treatment.

10. Daily test

The aim of a daily test is to discover, without delay, deviations of parameters that would constitute a hazard to the patient or to the staff, or would lead to suboptimal treatments. Therefore, it should be performed before the first patient is treated each morning. The daily test must be straightforward, with detailed instructions both for the test method and for any consequent actions, and it must be easy to record. No matter how well a machine appears to perform, the frequency of this test should never be less than once a day.

The daily test is more an observation of the constancy than a quantification of the parameters. One effective and easy way to observe changes in any parameter is to compare complementary devices, such as the dose-monitor system with a diode or a separate ionization chamber, or the optical-distance indicator with the laser-alignment system. It is assumed that at least one of them is working properly, and all will be checked independently in the basic test. While small deviations of parameters close to the tolerance level will probably not be discovered by this type of measurement, it does form a basic overall performance check, even if only on a limited number of preselected parameters.

The test described here is designed for linear accelerators. For cobalt units a simple timer check and relevant parts of the gross beam alignment check is recommended. Table 5.2 gives a typical daily QC protocol with suggested action levels. if there is any deviation greater than the action level, the unit should not be used for treatment, and a basic check procedure should be done.

The daily protocol consists of three main tests:

(1) dose-monitor check;

(2) gross beam-alignment checks;

(3) for computer-controlled equipment (e.g. MLC), the 'daily check' self-checking/calibration procedure recommended by the manufacturer.

Table 5.2 A typical QC protocol for the daily test of an accelerator

Check	Action level
Dose monitor relative to the test-dose meter	±5%
Optical-distance indicator relative to the laser beams at isocentre	±3 mm
Cross-hair position relative to laser beams at isocentre	±3 mm
Field-size indicator relative to light field-size at isocentre for 10 × 10 cm^2	±3 mm
Symmetry of the light beam relative to the cross-hair position at isocentre	±3 mm
Collision protection devices	Functional test
Signals/lamps	Functional test
Entrance door interlock (optional)	Functional test
Console computer	Self-test
MLC unit	Self-test and calibration

A detailed procedure for the test is presented below. With this daily-test protocol it is expected that any gross malfunction of the unit, which could cause the patient injury, cannot continue for more than one full day, even in the worst situation.

In some centres, depending upon local practices, the technical knowledge of the radiographers, and the workload of the physicists, these daily checks may be performed by the radiographers who usually run the unit. This QC will be recognized as beneficial for the patient and easy to integrate into the daily routines. Experience indicates that the radiographers' interest in the general quality of the unit will increase when they participate directly in the QC work.

10.1 Dose-monitor check

This check is mandatory. Either a method with the daily-test phantom at the normal treatment distance on the couch or with it attached to the collimator by a fixation device may be applied. The gantry angle is usually 0° (easiest and quickest set up) but with the block fixed to the collimator alternative angles can be used. For accelerators with dual (or more) photon beam energies, the monitor should be checked every day for each energy. When electrons are available, select at least one energy per day by permutation, check every energy at least twice a week. If the unit is equipped with an *in vivo* dosimetry system with diodes or a similar device, this system may be used for the dose monitor check. Perform output measurements for a limited number of combinations of field size and wedge angle.

For units that use computer-controlled wedged fields, a few combinations of field size and wedge angle should be included every day. Both the dose-monitor check and the final position of the jaws must be correct.

10.2 'Gross' beam-alignment check

This test is recommended. With the daily-check phantom still at SSD, a number of 'gross' alignment checks may be performed simultaneously. The major advantage of this method is that it enables the check to be made without requiring a change in set-up.

10.3 Computer self-test

For computer-controlled units, a console computer self-test should be carried out at start-up or before the daily test. Also, for other equipment, such as the MLC unit, self-test and standard automatic-calibration procedures should be performed prior to the daily test. If available, review the print out of the computer-controlled wedged field from the morning run (see Section 10.1).

10.4 Daily-test procedure

A typical procedure for the daily test is shown below. Start with a computer self-test.

1. Adjust the gantry and collimator angles to zero degrees. Position the daily-check phantom at the normal SSD using the distance indicator.

2. Set a 10×10 cm^2 field size using the normal field size indicator.

3. Adjust the phantom, so that the cross-hair coincides with the central cross on the phantom.

4. The edge of the light field should agree with the marked 10×10 cm^2 field within ± 3 mm.

5. The lateral laser beams should touch the surface of the phantom within ± 3 mm, the vertical laser line should be within ± 3 mm of the central cross, and the sagittal laser should coincide with the central cross also within ± 3 mm.

6. Position the photon beam *in vivo* detector on the surface of the phantom in the centre of the beam, or the ionization chamber in the phantom.

7. Start the irradiation with a preselected number of monitor units, e.g. 100, using the lowest photon beam energy and repeat the procedure once. For a multi-photon beam energy unit, repeat the irradiation once for the other photon beam energies. Include also, if available, a few fields with the computer controlled wedge.

8. Change to the electron beam *in vivo* detector, or use a suitable depth for the ionization chamber and measure again.

9. Record the reading of the *in vivo* device in the report book. It should be within 5% of the expected reference value. For an unsealed air ionization chamber, the reading has to be corrected for temperature and pressure. For the daily test a look-up table for the correction factors is sufficient.

10. Check the instruments and the lamps on the control panel before and during the irradiation. The indication of these has to work properly.

In addition to the daily QC checks, it is advisable to perform a few preventive-maintenance checks on the unit. The engineer should visit the unit each day to check technical parameters, such as condition and frequency of the microwave system, vacuum, power supply, bending currents, etc. This visit should not take more than 10 minutes and should be recorded in the report book.

For some types of linear accelerators, the symmetry of the beam is not very stable. A quick check on this has now become more practical thanks to the availability of commercial systems with off-axis detectors. However, it

will prolong the time needed, and has therefore been left to the basic test protocol.

The energy of the beam and the depth–dose characteristics are usually stable and close to the preselected value. A change of the energy is also unlikely to occur without being discovered, since an energy change will usually result in a change of dose monitor factor. For some types of accelerators, the beam deflection current is very critically related to energy, which allows a check of energy constancy through the check on this current. A separate depth–dose check has, therefore, a low priority for the daily-test protocol.

11. Basic test

The basic tests should be performed with high-precision dosimetry equipment, which has not been set aside for the specific therapy unit. This test is a constancy check without any calibration of the unit, and is mainly a quantification of the status of the different parameters (see Table 5.1). Field-class instrumentation should be used. The QC tests must be performed with good precision and accuracy so that small deviations may be readily detected.

A preselected number of parameters should be tested. This test can be performed by either a physicist, a dosimeterist or an engineer, but it is important that the person is fully trained in the relevant methods, is well aware of all the characteristics of the unit involved, and knows about the methods for set-up and irradiation of patients. A permutation of individuals performing the check may be advisable. Fresh approaches may discover new problems and question possibly entrenched assumptions or misunderstandings. The test can be performed at any time of the day, but preferably with some permutation from week to week, since some of the parameters could vary during the day. This test requires only a limited amount of time: weekly test, 1–2 hours, and monthly tests, 2–3 hours.

The basic test is divided into three main parts:

(1) beam alignment;

(2) dosimetry;

(3) safety.

It is advisable to start with the beam-alignment check, since deviations discovered can influence the dosimetry. Table 5.3 shows a typical basic-test protocol.

The basic frequency of these checks for all parameters is weekly. However, with experience gained of the stability of the unit, some of the parameter checks may have a lower frequency. The absolute minimum frequency is monthly, but some of the parameters should be checked once a week independently of the results. Such parameters are: dose-monitor constancy, distance

Table 5.3 Typical QC protocol for basic tests of an accelerator

Check	Interval	Tolerance level	Action level
Optical distance indicator			
at isocentre	w	±2 mm	±3 mm
at 200 mm shorter and longer	m	±3 mm	±4 mm
Laser beams relative to isocentre	w	±2 mm	±3 mm
Field size indication relative to light field size, 20 × 20 cm² at isocentre	w or m	±2 mm	±3 mm
Coincidence radiation-light beam 20 × 20 cm² at isocentre	w or m	±2 mm	±3 mm
Congruence of opposed horizontal light beam	m	±3 mm	±4 mm
Dose monitor	w	±2%	±3%
Depth dose			
5/15 cm (photons)	m	±1.5%	±2%
$d_{max}/\sim$50% (electrons)	m	±6%	±8%
Beam profile symmetry 20 × 20 cm² at 7 cm off-axis	w or m	±2%	±3%
Daily dosimetry test system	w	±2%	±3%

NB: To achieve the full potential from the new modalities available on modern machines e.g. asymmetric jaws, MLC, etc., the mechanical positional accuracy should be better than 2–3 mm generally used in current practice. The tolerances specified here are those general values. However, for such facilities, the intended clinical use and the specification from the manufacturers may lead to a QC programme with tighter tolerances.

indicator, and safety aspects. It is proposed that a number of parameters are checked once every week, with some additional parameters each month.

The basic-test procedure should be instituted at the time of the acceptance tests, continued during the commissioning period and go on for the remaining lifetime of the unit. During the initial period it is preferable for the checks to be performed even two or three times a week in order to investigate the stability and any weak points of the unit as soon as possible prior to clinical use. During part of this period, the expected test values cannot be defined, the results should be recorded and evaluated later.

The basic test is also the proper moment to follow up the results of the daily tests for the previous week. It is important that the person performing the basic test inspects the report book for the daily test before carrying out the basic test.

There have been reports of instances in which the monitor response and beam symmetry vary with gantry angle. The test should therefore be performed with the gantry and collimator angles permutated weekly in steps of 90°.

11.1 Beam-alignment test (optics and mechanics)

The beam-alignment test should be performed for both accelerators and cobalt units.

For all measurements of field size and light field, the cross-wire centre is assumed to be at the rotation centre of the X-ray head, as described in Sections 11.1.1 and 12.1.2.

11.1.1 Cross-hair, lamp, field size indicator, sagittal laser

Set the gantry to the vertical position and the field size to 20 × 20 cm². Put the semi-transparent screen described in Section 2.2.2 horizontally on the couch and adjust the surface approximately to the source–axis distance (SAD). Position the screen centre cross on the light field cross-hair. The sagittal laser should now hit the screen centre cross. Rotate the collimator 180°, the cross should then remain inside a 2-mm diameter circle, and the light field borders coincide with the screen markings within 3 mm at each 90° orientation. This is a test of the lamp position and of the associated optics. If asymmetric fields are used clinically, with one of the jaws crossing the collimator axis, it is recommended that the light field and field-size indicator for sizes up to maximum asymmetry are checked (also see Section 11.1.4).

11.1.2 Distance indicator, collimator angle, opposed beams

Set the collimator to the selected angle, which should be incremented by 90° each week. Set a field size of 20 × 20 cm. Put the semi-transparent screen vertically and longitudinally on the couch. Adjust the couch until the screen centre cross coincides with the left and right lasers when the cross-hair from above hits the screen edge. The screen centre should now be close to the isocentre. Rotate the gantry to a horizontal position. If the lasers are well adjusted, the light field cross-hair should hit the screen centre. The light field edges should coincide with the 20 × 20 cm² drawing on the screen.

Note the optical distance meter reading and the positions of the field edges. Rotate the gantry 180° and again note the distance meter reading and the position of the cross-hair and edges of the light field.

This test gives a lot of information in a single set-up. Some common results are:

(1) different readings of the optical distance meter for the opposed gantry positions – adjust the screen position and try again;

(2) equal readings, but different from the expected reading – adjust the optical distance meter if the difference is greater than 2 mm;

(3) the field light edges should be parallel to the screen markings at both gantry angles. If not, tilt the screen to halve the discrepancy, adjust the collimator angle and rotate the gantry again – check the collimator angle. The error should be less than 0.5°.

If the result is difficult to interpret then a full mechanical alignment test should be performed.

If sag in the collimator blocks is suspected, then rotate the collimator to 90° and 180°. Any shortening of the edges probably indicates a lamp position problem or that there is sag in the collimator or radiation head.

Return the gantry to 0°. With a piece of paper close to the screen at the height of the central cross, try to read the distance indicator. This should be equal to SAD. It may be noted that sometimes a unit has both mechanical and electronic scales. One scale, usually the mechanical, has to be regarded as the main scale and the others as slave scales. All tolerances, etc., are set according to the main scale and the slave scales are then adjusted for best fit. This difference between master scales and slave scales must be known by everyone using the unit.

11.1.3 Coincidence between radiation field and light field

1. Set the field size to 20×20 cm^2 on the indicators.

2. Put a film on some backscattering plastic material on the couch. Locate the film phantom (Section 2.2.2) on top and fix them together.

3. Adjust to the normal SSD at the phantom surface, orientate the phantom so that the light field cross-hair coincides with the phantom centre cross.

4. Note any difference between the light field edges and the square engraving.

5. Put on more plastic material up to the depth of dose maximum for electrons and to 50 mm for photon beams.

6. Make an exposure.

The film is positioned at a distance of SSD plus the thickness of the film phantom (5 mm), and the size of the beam in the film plane must be corrected for divergence. The film can be judged by eye for the relationship between the radiation field and the light field shown by the small dots from the lead markers in the phantom. Compare the image with the measurement already noted of the light field position and the calculated field size. The misalignment should be less than 3 mm at each edge and the field centre should be no more than 2 mm from the light field centre. If any asymmetry or misalignment is detected and then adjusted, remember to go back in the test scheme to an appropriate level. If the film is of a satisfactory quality and a suitable depth has been used, it can be used for the beam-symmetry check (Section 11.2.2).

11.1.4 Asymmetric jaws

Each independent jaw should be checked by comparing jaw setting versus the 50% radiation edge and field light for four fields designed as quadrant (two non-divergent edges). Jaw positions are set, and the light field illuminated onto graph paper. A superimposed film is exposed four times with the four quadrant fields. Ideally the composite film should exhibit no distinct regions of overlap or gap. A film with the four quadrants exposed separately is shown in Figure 5.3. In order to demonstrate the resolution of the technique, two of the fields have been modified. One of the fields has been set too large by 2 mm to give an overlap. A second field has been set too small by 2 mm to give a gap. These two regions compared to the perfect matched non-divergent

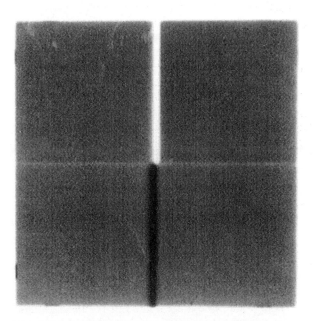

Figure 5.3 Exposed film, four asymmetric non-divergent fields superimposed. Two of the fields intentionally exposed with 2-mm gap and 2-mm overlap, respectively.

regions demonstrate that a mismatch of 0.5–1 mm will easily be seen on the film. This film has been exposed with the same collimator angle for all fields. If it is a common technique to match fields with different collimator angles, this test has to be repeated with different collimator angles for the four fields. Furthermore, a similar four-field test is advisable if adjacent non-divergent fields are created with a combination of one pair of asymmetric jaws and asymmetric MLC. For clinical use of adjacent non-divergent fields, the mismatch of fields at isocentre level should be less than 1 mm. It should be noted that the accuracy of movement of the asymmetric jaws will also affect the performance of computer-controlled wedged fields. A QC procedure for asymmetric jaws has been proposed by Klein *et al.* (1996).

11.1.5 Multi-leaf collimator

The QC procedure must be designed somewhat differently for the different types and commercial versions of MLC. The test presented here is common for all types. The range of clinical use may determine the frequency and scope of tests. Most MLC systems have a self-test and calibration-set procedure contained within the MLC unit, which is often performed automatically. The self-test is often both optical and electrical, and enables an individual leaf reproducibility of less than 0.5 mm at the isocentre. If possible, visually inspect the leaf edges when they are fully retracted. All edges must be in line.

Design three different MLC patterns. All pairs of leaves should have a gap of 5 mm, but use a different location of the gaps for the three patterns. Pattern 1 should have a small gap off-set by 10 cm in one direction. Pattern 2 has a gap off-set 10 cm in the other direction, and in the last pattern the gap is in the centre of the field. Expose one film at the depth of dose maximum with the three fields superimposed without moving the phantom. The SSD is unimportant, but the whole length of the gap must be inside the film. The collimator jaw perpendicular to the leaf motion must be fully opened. If there is another collimator jaw (for external MLC) it should be opened as much as possible. It is important to expose the film in the same order as the patterns were defined. These exposures are a test of leaf calibration in different locations, hysteresis effects, and inter-leaf leakage. Figure 5.4 shows a film exposed with these three patterns. This test should be performed at various gantry and collimator angles. QC procedures for different types of MLC have been proposed by Hounsell and Jordan (1995) and Klein *et al.* (1997).

Many steps are involved in the shaping process (TPS, digitizer, network, controller, etc.) to set the leaf pattern. A check of the pattern at the end of this chain must also be integrated into the QC process. If MLC files are transferred from one MLC machine to another this should be checked on a monthly basis.

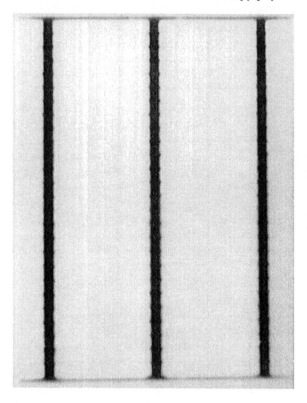

Figure 5.4 Exposed film, three fields superimposed different location of MLC gap.

11.2 Dosimetry test

11.2.1 Cobalt unit

For cobalt units the basic-monitor test consists of a check of the timer with an independent stop-watch and a check of the *in vivo* dosimetry system. In addition, it is advisable to check the output monthly with ionization chamber measurements.

11.2.2 Accelerator

Dose-monitor calibration check

All modern accelerators have dual dosimetry systems, however, they are not completely independent of each other and do not really measure the dose at the position of the patient. Use the basic-test phantom and a field-class ionization chamber and electrometer. A suitable measurement depth for all photon beam energies is 50 mm, and 10–30 mm for electron beams, close to the depth of dose maximum. The irradiation should be performed twice with a fixed dose monitor value. The reading should be corrected for the temperature in the phantom and for air pressure and should then be within 2% (TL) and 3% (AL) of the expected value. Fixation of the phantom to the treatment head (Section 2.2.2) will reduce the set-up time, particularly for gantry angles other than zero. This device is necessary for checking moving-beam mode when this technique is used clinically. Check that the second dose-monitor system is working properly.

At the same time as the basic test, the daily dose-monitor check should be performed in order to verify the agreement of the two methods. Position the daily-test instrumentation in the beam and irradiate according to the instructions. Take into account the deviation obtained in the dose-monitor check, note the daily-instrument reading and, if necessary, adjust the expected value of the daily check to give agreement.

Beam-quality check

A change of the beam quality, caused by malfunction or instabilities in the accelerator, will have effects on the dose distribution, particularly the dose along the beam axis. The usual way to estimate the beam quality and to take account of changes is to perform measurements at two different depths. Sequential measurements for the dose-monitor and beam-quality tests are recommended. The check on beam quality is performed by ionization chamber measurements at one other depth, which for photon beams could be 150 mm for a 10×10 cm field size. The second depth for electron beams should be at about the 50% dose level.

Beam-symmetry check

Beam symmetry may be checked relatively easily by densitometric evaluation of the film used for the congruence of light and radiation field (Section 11.1). Densitometric measurements along the major axes of the film are needed for the determination of field symmetry. Any difference in the symmetry of the beam profile should not exceed 2% (Table 5.3). Film measurements are not accurate enough for evaluation of the beam flatness. Measurements made with a scanner along two axes of the radiation beam can be used for both symmetry and flatness evaluation.

11.3 Safety checks

Open the door to the treatment room during irradiation, and check that the radiation is switched off. The function of any radiation warning system should also be checked.

Try all movements, look and listen for any problems. Gently rock the couch top and the collimator to detect play and loose brakes. Inspect the shadow tray holder, the lead-block holders, the wedges and wedge holder for wear and damage. If time is available, press one of the main emergency switches.

11.4 Computer-controlled systems

Restart all computers and observe them perform their built-in self-test and communication tests. To perform this test completely, the accelerator may have to be shut down and restarted. This procedure is also part of the morning check and takes some time. If it is routinely performed and properly recorded every morning, then the frequency could be monthly. In this case, the physicist or engineer should occasionally attend the morning run-up and observe the self-test and calibration run.

11.4.1 Computer-controlled wedged field

Once a month check the files and programs used for controlling the jaw movements, make checksums and compare to reference data. Permutation of the check file set is advisable. Check that all files are write protected. These procedures must be carried out in a controlled manner and set up and supervised by a person familiar with the software structure and the potential consequences of modification in this structure.

A check of the collimator jaw positioning servo, movement servo, and the dose-rate servo, as well as the computer file, are performed by output measurements. Place an ionization chamber on the collimator axis at the reference depth in a phantom. Measure weekly the wedge factor for 10×10 cm^2 and 20×20 cm^2 field sizes, minimum to maximum wedges angles, and all wedge directions. Select an appropriate frequency for these combinations, so that these fields are checked once a month. The wedge factor should deviate less than 2% from the expected value. A QC procedure for computer-controlled wedged fields has been proposed by Klein *et al.* (1996).

11.4.2 Auto set-up

If an auto set-up procedure is used clinically, the parameters in each part of the basic check should be automatically set-up. Check that the parameters are within the tolerance level. If the set-up is not performed correctly, make the necessary adjustments of the parameters and continue. Use auto set-up for the next check and so on. The basic check can be performed in a way that allows verification of scales, indicators, etc., as it proceeds. Nevertheless, for some units with auto set-up, the basic maintenance must contain parts of the scale/position test. For auto set-up all scale calibration is important. Auto set-up check of complex segmented treatment is checked as IMRT.

Security of file transfer and file storage must be checked. Once every month an active patient record should be printed and compared to the input data.

11.4.3 Intensity modulated radiotherapy (IMRT)

Thompson *et al.* (1995) proposed that the QC programme be divided into two parts. The test of the movements, scales, and alignment of a combination of the dynamic movements of the MLC, gantry, collimator, table, and collimator jaws can be performed using a film in a phantom in a fixed position on the treatment couch. The combination of the fields is delivered by the accelerator and controlled by the computer without intervention of the operator. To check the dosimetric accuracy and reproducibility, output and beam performance with changing gantry angle, collimator angle, etc., to stimulate a multiple-segment treatment, the multiple irradiation is then carried out with an integrating detector, (e.g. film, detector array, portal imaging device), attached to the head.

An alternative method is that the test phantom may consist of the standard-film phantom or the ionization-chamber phantom, supplemented with sheets or blocks of plastic. The results must be compared to calculated values and data from calculations on the TPS. Dose measurements in a 3-D water phantom are an excellent but time-consuming method. However, this may be used when establishing references for some IMRT cases for the solid phantom. If IMRT is performed with dynamic leaf motion, the QC must also confirm parameters such as leaf speed. QC procedures for IMRT are also presented by Chui *et al.* (1996) and Ma *et al.* (1997).

11.5   Electronic portal imaging device (EPID)

A QC phantom, for quantitative measurements of image quality, has been proposed by Rajapakshe *et al.* (1996), which uses high contrast bars with a spatial frequency of 0.1–0.7 lp/mm. The phantom is about 15 mm thick. The phantom has to be supplied with geometrical well markers in order to check the geometry. During the test, the phantom should be placed on the top of the detector in order to acquire test images. Placing the phantom at the isocentre will give more blurring of the image due to the scattered radiation and the effect of the linac source size. The test is intended to monitor the performance of the EPID rather than that of the accelerator. Some EPIDs have a gantry angle dependence; therefore the test with the phantom has to be performed at different gantry angles.

The most common use of EPID is to compare the verification image with a reference image from either the simulator or a digitally reconstructed radiograph. The software often has tools for measurements of displacement between these images. These tools have also to be checked regularly. In addition, EPID can be used for exit dosimetry. A specific QC programme has to be designed for such measurements. Rajapakshe *et al.* (1996) and Klein *et al.* (1996) have proposed QC procedures for EPIDs.

12.   Extended tests

The extended tests are fairly comprehensive and time consuming and include most parameters. The extended-test set is a selection of checks from the original

acceptance test, the commissioning phase, and the calibration procedure. The methods used for extended tests are similar to, or may be the same as, those used at the initial stage (see Chapter 2). Therefore, only limited information is given in this chapter about the methods and test instrumentation, with the exception of beam alignment.

The extended test presented is divided into three parts:

(1) beam-alignment test;

(2) dosimetry test;

(3) safety test.

The intervals between extended tests may be quite long, about 6 months to 2 years, but every part of the complete extended test programme must be carried out at least once biannually. The intervals for the different parts are usually not fixed, because the timing of the test may be affected by other factors, such as extra tests following repairs, deviations discovered in other tests, and any relevant local circumstances. Shorter intervals may also be used if the basic tests indicate any problems.

It is essential to compare the results of these tests with the set of reference data used in routine clinical practice (tables, graphs, computer data sets, etc.), as well as standards. When significant deviations between these are discovered, action should be taken. The first action is to restore the unit. If this is not possible the second step is to introduce new reference data for subsequent clinical use. The monitor calibration factor and beam symmetry are usually easy to restore, but this is not normally possible for changes in the field-size dependence of the monitor calibration and, therefore, new data should be introduced for clinical use in such cases. Whenever significant deviations are discovered in these tests, a second person should verify the deviation, preferably with independent test equipment. Errors in test equipment and human mistakes should not be discounted.

The test should not be performed in a continuous test period, since it will be very time consuming and actions that interrupt the test procedures often have to be taken. Probably the most convenient time for these tests is just after the extensive preventive technical maintenance of the unit.

12.1   Beam alignment

The complete test on beam alignment is usually performed prior to the extended dosimetry checks. Interactions between various parts of the unit makes it advisable to perform the tests and, if necessary, to make adjustments in the order set out below.

12.1.   Mechanical pointer

To visualize the axis of rotation of the collimator system, a mechanical front pointer on the collimator rotational axis should be used. The pointer holder must allow the pointer rod some axial movement. Marks on the rod indicate the position of the conical tip at the source–axis distance (SAD) and SSD (SSD in this case means the normal fixed treatment distance). Two rods may be needed if the axial movement is limited and in this beam-alignment protocol it is assumed that two rods are used. Mark the position of the holder on the head and always attach it in that position. The pointer rod must be straight. Check it by rotating in its holder.

If no pointer is available, the cross-hair on the light field centre may be used as a substitute (with a modified procedure), only if the field lamp rotates with the collimator. Optical distance indicators mounted at an angle to the beam direction cannot be used.

12.1.2 Axis of rotation of collimator system

1. Set the gantry to the vertical position and check this with the spirit level.

2. Attach the mechanical pointer to the head.

3. Fix a sheet of graph paper on the couch.

4. Adjust the height for the longer mechanical pointer, rotate the collimator and mark the position of the pointer tip on the paper for different collimator angles.

5. If the collimator has a locking device, mark when the lock is engaged. Any defects in the collimator bearings may show up as jumps in the marked position.

6. Adjust the pointer holder so that the tip, when rotating with the collimator, describes a circle with a diameter less than 2 mm.

7. Put the shorter pointer into the holder, adjust the couch height and rotate the collimator. The tip should again give a circle with a diameter of less than 2 mm. If not, the upper position of the rod is not on the axis. The holder must be adjusted and the action repeated, starting with the long rod. When both rods give a circle of less than 2 mm, the pointer rod defines the rotational centre of the collimator.

12.1.3 Distance indicator

All distance indicators should be checked.

1. Place the semi-transparent screen (Section 2.2.2) vertically on the couch, so that it can be viewed from both sides.

2. Move the gantry to 90° and attach the front pointer with the SAD rod to the head.

3. Adjust the couch until the pointer just touches the screen.

4. Read the pointer setting, rotate the gantry 180°, and check the pointer reading.

5. Adjust the screen position and repeat the test until both readings are equal, then read and adjust both the optical distance indicator and, if necessary, the mechanical pointer to show the correct distance, i.e. SAD.

6. If the normal fixed-treatment distance (SSD) differs from the SAD, put the SSD rod in the holder. Set the screen to the tip and read the optical-distance meter. If the measured value differs from the expected value by more than 2 mm, the reasons for this must be carefully considered and reconciled.

7. Check the linearity of the optical-distance meter by comparing measurements from the optical indicator and the mechanical pointer rods. The optical-distance indicator should be correct within 2 mm over the range SSD+100/–200 mm.

12.1.4 Head pitch and roll angle

Head pitch and roll movements are usually available only on cobalt units.

1. Put in the SAD rod and set the couch to 10 mm below the isocentre.

2. Turn the gantry to 90° and draw a line on a sheet of paper on the couch using the pointer rod as a ruler.

3. Turn the gantry to 270° and draw another line. These lines should form one straight line.

4. On a cobalt unit, adjust the head pitch and repeat the action until the lines coincide. Read the head pitch scale, if possible adjust to 0°.

5. On an accelerator, estimate the maximum distance between the pointer tip and the correct point at the isocentre. It should be less than 2 mm.

6. Set the gantry to give a vertical beam, and attach the SAD rod.

7. By eye, position the second front pointer rod on the couch in a horizontal position on the rotational axis of the gantry. The marker tip should point to the tip of the SAD pointer at a distance of a few mm.

8. Rotate the gantry ± 180° without moving the marker and check for any difference in the relative position between the two tips in the rotational plane.

9. If any difference is observed, adjust the marker rod and, on a cobalt unit, the head roll angle. Repeat until the difference is minimized.

12.1.5 Mechanical isocentre

The sphere that surrounds all possible positions of the tip of the SAD pointer rod, when rotating the gantry and the collimator through 360° (if possible), describes the 'mechanical isocentre' of the unit. The diameter of this sphere should be less than 2 mm. Note that to meet this tolerance level means that it is not possible to allow the maximum deviation of every one of the parameters that influence the isocentre position.

12.1.6 Symmetry of collimator jaws

Accelerators usually have a focusing-type collimator. To check the mechanical symmetry, access must be gained to the collimator jaws. If the collimators have light-field trimmers, mark their positions and remove them. Carefully observe the two collimator pairs while changing the field-size settings. The movements must be smooth and without jumps.

Fasten a sheet of paper on the couch. Set a square field size of about 25×25 cm^2, rotate the gantry through $90°$, and attach the pointer. Set a straight ruler to the inner surface of the collimator, in contact with the collimator surface, and draw a line representing the continuation of the collimator inner surface on the paper (see Figure 5.5). Repeat for the opposite collimator jaw. Finally draw lines along the mechanical pointer. Rotate the collimator $180°$ and repeat the procedure. The lines should be symmetrical with respect to the pointer lines, and these should coincide. Any deviation greater than 1 mm requires adjustment.

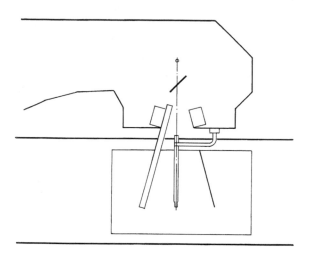

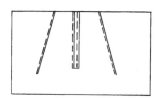

Figure 5.5 Set-up for test of collimator jaw symmetry. Gantry angle $90°$. Full lines for collimator angle $0°$, dotted lines for collimator angle $180°$.

Rotate the collimator through $90°$ and repeat the check for the second collimator pair. Repeat the check for a 10×10 cm^2 field size, in order to verify the linearity of the collimator movements.

12.1.7 Position of field-defining lamp

With the gantry at $0°$, adjust the field lamp until the light field at normal SSD is symmetrical, with respect to the centre of the field (defined by the pointer tip) at all collimator angles. X-ray trimmers must not interfere with the light beam. If the lamp rotates with the collimator, fix an object in space close to the head. The shadow of the object should not move when the collimator rotates. Adjust the cross-hair to the centre of the light field.

Repeat the test 250 mm above and 500 mm below the normal SSD. The virtual positions of the cross-hair and the lamp are now centred on the rotational axis of the collimator.

This alignment is essential for accuracy in the set-up of the patient and deviations from this test should be less than 2 mm in diameter.

12.1.8 Radiation field and light-fields symmetry

The radiation beam is assumed to be reasonably flat. Set the field size to 20×20 cm^2 on the field-size indicator. Orientate the film phantom (Section 2.2.2) at normal SSD, and set the light field symmetrically to the markings on the phantom. The cross-hair should then coincide with the centre cross. Add some build-up, expose the film, turn the collimator $90°$, and expose another film. The developed films can be judged by eye for symmetry of the radiation-field versus the indicator-spot positions. If any asymmetry in the spot positions is observed, and the asymmetry remains in the same direction on both films, it is due to the radiation source not being on the rotational axis of the collimator. If the asymmetry is rotated by $90°$, it is due to asymmetry in the collimator jaws. Compare the results with the results of the mechanical symmetry check of the collimators.

These checks may be made with a detector scanned along the major axes of the irradiation beam. The measurements are evaluated in a similar manner.

If any asymmetry is detected, make the necessary adjustments and go back in the test scheme to an appropriate level. The remaining asymmetry should be less than 2 mm at the isocentre.

12.1.9 Light-field size and radiation-field size

Set the gantry to the vertical position. Fix a sheet of paper on the couch, set it to the normal fixed-treatment distance with the mechanical pointer and check the optical indicator. Mark the cross-hair and the light-field edges. Measure with a ruler the field sizes for several field settings, from the minimum to maximum size (NB Before using graph paper, first check its accuracy against a ruler.)

Use a dose-plotting device with the detector at the normal fixed-treatment distance (SSD) and then add water to a depth corresponding to maximum build-up. Measure dose profiles for the same settings as above. The field sizes correspond to the 50% level of the profiles. Compare the set of measurements of the radiation-field sizes with the set of light-field sizes. For an accelerator with dual photon beam energies, this method for field-size determination will sometimes make it difficult to adjust the indicators to fit the field sizes for both energies. The exact method depends on the field-size definition adopted in the centre. In particular, it will be different if the IEC definition is used that specifies field size at a depth of 10 cm.

If a scanner is not available, then film can be used. However, in the penumbra region the 50% dose level does not exactly coincide with the 50% optical density level, as the energy in the beam penumbra differs from that in the beam centre and the film sensitivity varies with energy. The expected deviation in a field-size measurement using a graphic film can be about 1 mm, but this should be checked for the actual film used.

If the radiation and light beams do not match, one or more of three remedies should be considered:

(1) adjust the lamp along 'the beam axis';
(2) attach low-density light-field trimmers to the collimators;
(3) adjust the field-size indicator.

Whatever action has been taken, go back in the test scheme and restart at an appropriate level. The light field and the radiation field should correspond within 2 mm.

In the case of a unit equipped with asymmetric jaws and/or MLC, similar measurements have to be performed using these modalities. For asymmetric fields, the non-divergent jaw position is important, but the linearity over the range of movements from maximum to minimum has also to be checked. These tests must be customized to any specific collimator design. After calibration and checking of field-limiting devices, actual field shapes and sizes must be compared to shapes and sizes of fields presented from the treatment-planning system for the actual unit. The test must be performed at the four major gantry angles.

Expose a film to check the interleaf leakage and closed-position leaf transmission. The closed-leaf separation should be small at isocentre level. The gap between opposing leaves is to avoid mechanical collision.

12.1.10 Penumbra trimmer

If the collimators are equipped with penumbra trimmers, determine the penumbra from the above measurements and compare to previous records. To reduce the penumbra, try very small adjustments of the trimmers, remeasure and fix the trimmers in the optimum position. Adjustment of the trimmers should not change the field size, but it is advisable to check two field sizes.

12.1.11 Couch

All tests on the treatment couch should be performed with a load of 75 kg distributed evenly along its length. Adjust the gantry to $0°$ and the couch height to the normal SSD. Put a sheet of paper on the couch and mark the position of the cross-hair or the tip of the pointer, while rotating the turntable isocentrically. The 'completed' circle should have a diameter of less than 3 mm.

To test the vertical movement of the couch, attach a V-shaped steel wire (bent paper clip) to the radiation head. Move the couch to its highest position and run a plumb line through the V. Set the tip of the plumb bob just above the couch surface, and mark its position when the couch is moved down to its lowest position and back up again. Any fault in the vertical movement of the couch can easily be detected.

At table heights of 200 and 400 mm below the isocentre, use the spirit-level to check the slope of the couch for different lateral and longitudinal positions. For a fixed SSD technique, the lateral and vertical movements are particularly important. For an SAD technique, the isocentric movements are important.

12.1.12 Indicators

With the help of the spirit-level and the rulers, test all indicators not previously checked (gantry, treatment couch, floor rotation, etc.).

12.2 Extended dosimetry test

For all of the extended dosimetry checks a water phantom should be used together with a calibrated reference ionization chamber and electrometer. A suitable dosimetry protocol should be followed, see Chapters 3 and 4. Evaluate the records of the results obtained from the basic tests prior to this test.

12.2.1 Dose-monitor calibration

It is necessary to calibrate the dose monitor under reference conditions every year for all beam qualities used routinely. If any change is noted in the calibration factor of the dose monitor, it should be restored to the reference value. Changes to the dose-monitor calibration may have occurred because the basic tests are performed under non-reference conditions and the change to the reference calibration may be due to problems with the basic test methods, e.g. the influence of the accumulated electrical charge ('charge storage' effect) in the basic phantom   (see Chapter 3, Section 5.4). If such changes are noted, new reference values for the basic tests should be determined and it may be necessary to revise the basic calibration method.

1. Check the calibration at the reference depth for a field size of 10×10 cm^2. A repeat of this measurement, including set-up, is recommended. This is the normalization value for the output factors, etc.

2. Test different monitor settings (corresponding to about 0.2–6 Gy) for linearity and for shutter end time of the cobalt unit.

3. Test the dose-rate dependence of the dose monitor.

4. Test gantry-angle dependence for comparison with results from the basic checks.

12.2.2   Relative dose-monitor factors

A selected number of combinations of beam sizes, accessories, beam qualities, etc., should be measured at the reference depth in water. Preferably use blocks and irregular shaped devices for a specific patient in order to verify the field size corrections routinely used in clinical practice.

1. Check field-size dependence for square fields (6×6 cm^2, 10×10 cm^2, 20×20 cm^2, and maximum), rectangular fields (6×30 cm^2, 30×6 cm^2) and a few typical irregularly shaped fields.

2. Check the wedge filter and other filter factors. Use field sizes 6×6 cm^2, 10×10 cm^2, and 20×20 cm^2 for all filters. Measure the wedge-filter factor with the wedge in two orientations 180° apart (see Chapter 4, Section 4.6).

3. Check the shadow tray factor and other plates used routinely for a field size of 10×10 cm^2.

In addition, the output 15 cm off-axis at the reference depth with the upper jaws positioned at −10 cm (i.e. 10 cm over centre) and at 20 cm should be checked to ensure that the head scatter component is constant.

12.2.3   Depth dose

Measure the depth–dose distribution on the beam axis for all beam qualities and with a combination of field sizes and accessories.

Use different field sizes, 6×6 cm^2, 10×10 cm^2, and 20×20 cm^2, without a wedge filter and with a 45–60° wedge.

12.2.4   Dose profiles

The symmetry, flatness, and penumbra should be determined for all beam qualities at a few field sizes (at least maximum and 10×10 cm^2) and at more than one gantry angle. Restore any symmetry of the beam, and evaluate the flatness, symmetry, and penumbra. Simultaneously check the expected values of the basic-symmetry check.

Spot-checks of profiles in phantom and comparison with computer-calculated profiles should also be performed. This check should include all wedges.

12.2.5   Isodose distribution

The isodose distribution can only be tested satisfactorily if an automatic isodose plotter is available. Select a combination of a few field sizes and wedges filters and compare the measured isodose distribution with that computed by the treatment-planning system.

12.3   Extended safety test

An extended safety test is difficult to specify in detail as it must incorporate safety controls required by the manufacturer of the treatment machine and special checks to meet national regulations. Thus the QC protocol presented below should be modified to include any other test required by national regulations.

An extended safety check must not only test the function of individual systems, but also the second level of a double-security system. Failing components of the safety system should be detected during maintenance and not in the safety test. The extended safety check should be performed after corrective maintenance and after the safety check specified by the manufacturer.

12.3.1   Safety interlocks

The following items should be checked:

(1) door switches in the treatment room and the equipment room;

(2) emergency switches in the treatment room and control room;

(3) anti-collision devices;

(4) limit switches for moving parts, including back up systems;

(5) dosimetry systems, including back up systems;

(6) computer-controlled interlocks in maintenance mode and in treatment mode;

(7) excess dose-rate detector;

(8) flatness-fault detector;

(9) wedge identification and position;

(10) wedge field-size interlock;

(11) emergency-shutter system for cobalt units;

(12) MLC malfunction interlock.

An excess dose-rate interlock should halt the accelerator if treatment is started in photon mode without the target and flattening filter in position. Such a combination can cause an extremely high dose rate and can almost instantly injure the patient severely. Testing the excess dose-rate interlock is difficult, as some dismantling is normally necessary. Details of the test procedure must come from the accelerator manufacturer or from the service engineer.

The emergency-shutter system for cobalt units must be checked. When the emergency-shutter system is activated and the shutter is closed, it should not be possible to open the shutter again without a reset operation. This reset operation should prohibit regular use of the emergency switch as the standard shutter-closing device.

Certain treatment units may have safety interlocks not on this list. Several of the interlocks are probably already in the safety check specified by the manufacturer or otherwise described in the service manual for the unit. If not, the user must call upon the manufacturer to provide information about test methods for these interlocks.

12.3.2 Electrical safety

The following items should be checked for electrical safety:

(1) treatment unit;

(2) light installation;

(3) *in vivo* dosimetry system;

(4) emergency light;

(5) auxiliary equipment.

It is important to check that the protective earth is connected to all equipment not marked as doubly insulated. All equipment in the treatment room and the control room should be connected to one common three-phase distribution panel with a common protective earth rail. The *in vivo* dosimetry system must be checked in both these aspects. The instrument is located in the control room and the detector is in direct contact with the patient in the treatment room. Pay special attention to new wiring and new equipment.

12.3.3 Safety of auxiliary devices

The following items should be checked:

(1) lead-block holders;

(2) block-transporting devices;

(3) patient-lifting devices;

(4) patient-supporting devices;

(5) heavy doors, motorized doors;

(6) radiation monitors for cobalt units.

Check the maximum permissible load on the treatment head and the lead-block holders against the heaviest lead blocks used. A change in treatment technique can radically change the weight of the lead blocks used. Any change in the manufacturing process for individual lead blocks calls for a control, not only of mechanical strength in fixation, but also of accuracy in positioning. In the case of a motorized door, check all safety functions, all limit switches, and the emergency-opening system.

Use a small field size and direct the beam away from the detector when checking the function and the sensitivity of radiation monitors for a cobalt unit.

12.3.4 Radiation protection

The following items should be checked:

(1) any changes in the building affecting the treatment room;

(2) treatment unit (patient protection);

(3) cobalt units (patient and staff protection);

(4) lasers (patient and staff protection).

A survey must be carried out following any changes to the treatment room to ensure that the radiation protection barrier is intact and sufficient in all possible conditions of machine usage.

A check of the leakage radiation from the treatment head should detect any lead shielding missing or damaged after maintenance. Use film in envelopes to completely cover the treatment head, having marked their position. Close the collimator and run the unit. Specialized large-volume chambers are needed to quantify leakage radiation. Ionization chambers for radiation therapy measurements are too insensitive for this purpose.

All lasers should have appropriate warning labels and care should be taken not to look directly into the laser beam.

13. References

American Association of Physicists in Medicine (1994a). Comprehensive QA for radiation oncology. Report of AAPM Radiation Therapy Task Group 40. *Med. Phys.*, **21**, 581–618.

American Association of Physicists in Medicine (1994b). AAPM code of practice for radiotherapy accelerators. Report of AAPM Radiation Therapy Task Group 45. *Med. Phys.*, **21**, 1093–121.

Brahme A. (ed.) (1988). Accuracy requirements and quality assurance of external beam therapy with photons and electrons. *Acta Oncol.*, 27 Suppl. 1. 1–76

Chui C.-S., Spirou S., and LoSasso T. (1996). Testing of dynamic multileaf collimation. *Med. Phys.*, **23**, 635–41.

Hounsell A.R. and Jordan T.J. (1997). Quality control of the Philips multileaf collimator. *Radioth. Oncol.*, **45**, 225–33.

Institute of Physical Sciences in Medicine (1988). *Commissioning and quality assurance of linear accelerators.* IPSM Report 54. IPSM, York.

Institute of Physics and Engineering in Medicine (1999). *Physical aspects of quality control in radiotherapy*. IPEM Report 81. IPEM, York.

International Electrotechnical Commission (1989a). *Medical electrical equipment – medical electron accelerators in the range 1 MeV to 50 MeV – guidelines for functional performance characteristics*. IEC No 977. IEC, Geneva.

International Electrotechnical Commission (1989b). *Medical electrical equipment – medical electron accelerators – functional performance characteristics*. IEC No 976. IEC, Geneva.

International Organization for Standardization (1977). *Statistics, vocabulary and symbols*. ISO No 3534. ISO, Geneva.

Klein E., Harms W., Low D., Willcut V., and Purdy J. (1995). Clinical implementation of a commercial multileaf collimator, dosimetry, networking, simulation, and quality assurance. *Int. J. Radiat. Oncol. Biol. Phys.*, **33**, 1195–208.

Klein E.E., Low D.A., Maag D., and Purdy J.A. (1996). A quality assurance programme for ancillary high technology devices on a dual energy accelerator. *Radioth. Oncol.*, **38**, 51–60.

Ma L., Geis P.B., and Boyer A.L. (1997). Quality assurance for dynamic multileaf collimator modulated fields using a fast beam imaging system. *Med. Phys.*, **24**, 1213–20.

Rajapakshe R., Luchka K., and Shalev S. (1996). A quality control test for electronic portal imaging devices. *Med. Phys.*, **23**, 1237–44.

Société Francaise Des Physiciens d'Hopital (1989). *Quality control of electron accelerators for medical use*. SFPH, Paris.

Thompson A.V., Lam K.L., Balter J.M., McShan D.L., Martel M.K., Weaver T.A. *et al.* (1995). Mechanical and dosimetric quality control for computer controlled radiotherapy treatment equipment. *Med. Phys.*, **22**, 563–6.

World Health Organization (1988). *Quality assurance in radiotherapy*. WHO, Geneva.

14. Further reading

American Association of Physicists in Medicine (1982). *Proceedings of symposium on quality assurance of radiotherapy equipment*. Symposium proceedings No 3. AAPM, New York.

American College of Medical Physics (1991). *Quality assurance in radiotherapy physics* (ed. G. Starkschall and J. Horton). Medical Physics Publishing, Madison.

DIN-Standard 6847, part 5 (draft) (1986). *Medizinische elektronen-beschleuniger-anlagen; konstanzprüfungen apparativer qualitätsmerkmale*. Beuth–Verlag, Berlin.

First International Symposium on Quality Assurance in Radiation Therapy (1984). *Int. J. Radiat. Oncol. Biol. Phys.*, **10**, Suppl. 1.

Horton J.L. (1987). *Handbook of radiation therapy physics*. Prentice–Hall Inc., New Jersey.

Johansson, K-A., Horiot, J.C., Van Dam, J., Lepinoy, D., Sentenac, I., and Sernbo, G. (1986). Quality assurance control in the EORTC co-operative group of radiotherapy. 2. Dosimetric intercomparison. *Radioth. Oncol.*, **7**, 269–79.

Rassow J. (1988). Quality control of radiation therapy equipment. *Radioth. Oncol.*, **12**, 45–55.

Chapter 6
Kilovoltage X-rays

S.C. Klevenhagen, D.I. Thwaites, and R.J. Aukett

1. Introduction

Kilovoltage X-ray equipment has been widely used, and many older texts discuss equipment and techniques extensively. In recent years its use has diminished as megavoltage X-rays and, more recently, electrons have replaced it for most clinical applications. However, kilovoltage X-rays still have a role to play in the range of modalities available in radiotherapy. Their advantages are generally those of low cost compared with megavoltage units, because of the relative simplicity of design and operation, and the use of simple collimation and field shaping.

X-ray therapy in the kilovoltage range is conventionally divided into a number of areas depending on the accelerating potentials and other general characteristics of the treatment beams. They are summarized below.

1. Grenz rays, of around 10–20 kV. These are now infrequently used.

2. Contact therapy using potentials of around 40 or 50 kV and very short source–surface distance (SSD) of a few centimetres or less. These provide a very rapidly falling depth–dose and are useful for treatment depths of only 1–2 mm.

3. Superficial therapy, using potentials of around 50–150 kV. With typical filtration, these provide beams with half-value layers (HVL) in the range of 1–8 mm Al. The SSD is normally in the range 10–30 cm. Typical beam characteristics are suitable for treatment of lesions up to about 5 mm deep, in terms of delivery of 90% of the incident (surface) dose.

4. Orthovoltage therapy ('deep' therapy) with X-ray beams generated between 150 and 500 kV. The majority of current clinical sets are operated at 200–300 kV. With typical filtration, these provide beams of 1–4 mm Cu HVL. The treatment distance is usually about 50 cm SSD with the 90% dose within about 2 cm of the surface.

Planning and acceptance testing of therapy installations, absolute dose calibration, relative dosimetry, and quality control of treatment equipment have been dealt with in previous chapters. These have concentrated on megavoltage applications, since this accounts for the vast majority of treatments. Much of this can be applied with suitable modification to the kilovoltage range. However, there are a number of significant differences between the two areas. These include the equipment, beam-quality specification, beam characteristics, use of filtration, scatter effects, and practical approaches to acceptance, dosimetry, and quality control. Most kilovoltage beam treatments are applicator defined and use a single field. Treatment planning is, therefore, relatively straightforward, but it is important to remember the differences due to scatter and to relative bone absorption.

Partly for the reasons outlined, and partly due to local preference, clinical practice can vary considerably between one country and another, or one centre and another. In some cases, tumours at intermediate depths, such as spinal metastases and sarcomas, are commonly treated with orthovoltage. In others, megavoltage photons or electrons are always used. The choice of qualities for superfical therapy also varies widely, as does the use of contact therapy. The way in which measurements are carried out should reflect local clinical practice. Where compromise is unavoidable, those components that directly affect treatment delivery will require the greatest accuracy. Where data is not clinically relevent, less accuracy may be acceptable.

This chapter is intended to summarize some of the specific characteristics and problems associated with kilovoltage X-ray beam use, stressing differences from megavoltage therapy, and drawing attention to some recent work on kilovoltage X-rays which is relevant to practical procedures.

2. kV X-ray equipment

Design criteria and operation of conventional kilovoltage therapy X-ray sets, which are based on standard stationary anode therapy tubes and the associated circuitry, are covered in detail in many texts and will not be repeated here. The weakest link in these systems has generally been the glass envelope-design tube. A more recent development has been the metal-ceramic tube, resulting in a compact, constructionally simplified lightweight X-ray source.

An example of a practical version of the metal-ceramic tube (Philips) is shown in Figure 6.1. The anode, kept at earth potential, is directly welded onto the external metal envelope of the tube, facilitating simple water cooling arrangements. The accelerating voltage, or high tension (HT) is provided to the cathode by means of a cable, which fits into a metal-ceramic connector. This design prevents discharges ('flash-over') via the insulator surfaces. Only a single HT cable is required and this, together with relatively small diameters of about 10 cm, makes the tube very easy to manipulate. The focus-to-window distance is short, enabling relatively long applicators to be used, which is a convenient feature in setting up patients.

Metal-ceramic X-ray sources are provided with a beryllium window, which is integrally welded to the steel tube giving an inherent filtration of 2.2 mm Be (maximum). The emission characteristics are, therefore, very different to those from the glass tube. Because of the high radiation output, they can be operated at 50% of the conventional tube current and down to 20% of the rated HT value, without adversely affecting the beam quality.

In summary, the metal-ceramic tube has the following general advantages compared with glass envelope tubes:

(1) reduced weight of about 25–35% of that of a conventional tube for the same kilovoltage range;

(2) reduced physical dimensions;

(3) increased reliability of operation;

(4) lack of electrical discharges;

(5) insensitivity to mechanical shock.

3. Specification of beam quality

3.1 Quality parameters

As with megavoltage X-ray beams, a practical method of specifying beam quality is required to predict the penetrative characteristics of the beam and to select appropriate factors for dosimetry, etc. Radiation quality cannot be described simply by a statement of accelerating potential (kV). The more rapidly the penetration of the beam varies with energy, the more detailed the knowledge of radiation quality is required. Ideally, a complete knowledge of the spectral distribution of the beam would provide all the information required, but such distributions are not easy to measure and anyway have more physical than clinical significance. For kilovoltage beams, it has generally been the accepted practice to express quality in terms of half-value layer (HVL), i.e. the thickness of a specified absorber that reduces the beam intensity to half its original value. Because this parameter describes the ability of a beam to penetrate material, it is directly linked to the characteristic of most clinical significance. For most clinical purposes, a statement of at least kV and HVL is recommended as a quality specifier. Beams of the same HVL can be produced from different combinations of kV and filtration. Generally ionization chamber calibration factors for these beams would be similar (Section 5), but the beams could exhibit differences in some

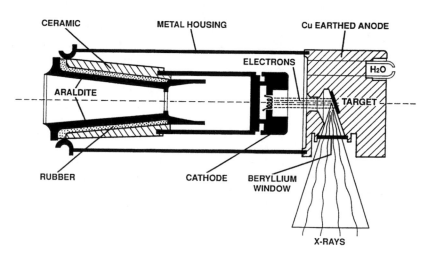

Figure 6.1 Schematic cross-section of a metal-ceramic tube.

parameters, such as backscatter factor and depth dose (Section 4).

The HVL is obtained by measuring an absorption curve of the radiation in the specified material and interpolating the thickness corresponding to 50% absorption (Section 3.2). Where appropriate, the second HVL may also be quoted. This is the additional layer required to reduce the intensity from 50 to 25% of the initial value. Although radiations of different spectral distributions can have the same first HVL, their second HVLs will not be the same. The ratio of first to second HVL is termed the homogeneity coefficient and is unity for monoenergetic photon beams and less than one for heterogeneous beams.

The usual materials for specifying HVL are aluminium for superficial X-ray beams and copper for orthovoltage. It may be noted that in some situations for low-voltage X-ray treatments, the concept of half-value depth in millimeters of tissue has been used as a quality specifier because it has a direct meaning to the clinician. However, this is only valid for a given field area and SSD and does not have an unambiguous physical meaning.

One concept that has been used for some descriptive purposes is the equivalent (or effective) energy, the single photon energy having the same attenuation properties as the heterogeneous beam of interest. From HVL measurements, the effective linear attenuation coefficient can be found, $\mu = 0.693/\text{HVL}$, and the equivalent energy can be found from tables of μ or μ/ρ, the mass attenuation coefficient, against energy, such as in Hubbell (1982) or ICRU (1992). The equivalent energies for therapy beams are typically 30–50% of the maximum energy in the spectrum, where the latter corresponds to the peak kilovoltage applied to the tube.

For megavoltage beams, the Quality Index now generally used to specify beam quality is TPR_{10}^{20}, the ratio of the TPRs at 20 and 10 cm depth (see Chapter 3). A similar index for kilovoltage X-rays, the ratio between the TPRs at 5 and 2 cm depth, has recently been suggested by Rosser (1998). However, it is too early to evaluate the practical usefulness of this quantity compared with HVL.

3.2 Half-value layer measurement (HVL)

Determination of HVL involves the repeated measurement of exposure at a selected point in a beam, for increasing thicknesses of the appropriate attenuating material placed between the source and the detector. A monitoring chamber may be useful to permit correction for variations in exposure rate, provided that it is placed so that its readings are independent of the amount of absorbing material placed in the beam and its presence does not affect the measurements. The chamber used for the attenuation measurements should be selected to have a minimum quality dependence over the range concerned. For lower energies, for which aluminium is generally used, particular attention should be given to the purity of the material. Standard grades of aluminium contain a significant proportion of copper, as well as other higher atomic number materials. These can significantly affect the results at lower energy, so that high purity material (>99.5% and, ideally, >99.9%) is recommended below about 100 kV.

Excessive scatter will result in an overestimate of HVL, therefore, so-called 'good geometry', i.e. narrow-beam and scatter-free conditions, must be employed (Figure 6.2). Limiting the field size as much as possible reduces the amount of scattered radiation reaching the detector, but the field must be large enough to encompass the whole of the sensitive volume of the chamber. Care must be taken with the alignment of the tube, the beam diaphragm (which must be sufficient thickness to absorb the primary beam), and the ion chamber; it is best to use a radiographic method to ensure alignment. It is also necessary to minimize scatter from room walls, etc. This is achieved by positioning the chamber at least 40 cm away from any potential scattering material. As a general rule, the attenuating material can be placed close to the beam diaphragm and approximately midway between the source and the chamber, provided reasonably long distances are being used. A source–chamber distance of about 100 cm is preferable. This ensures the chamber is at least 50 cm or so from the metal sheets and so avoids any significant scatter contribution from the attenuator or the diaphragm. It also positions the attenuators at a reasonable distance from any monitor chamber. For very

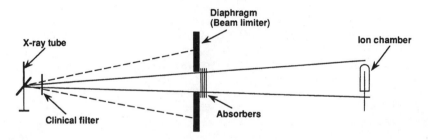

Figure 6.2 Experimental arrangement for HVL measurement.

low energy beams, distances should be kept as short as practicable, as air attenuation can affect results in these cases (ICRU 1970), requiring correction if significant. For shorter distances, keeping the attenuators as close to the source as possible will minimize the scatter contribution to the detector, however, scatter effects on the monitor chamber, if present, must then be carefully assessed (Carlsson 1993). Plotting transmission against absorber thickness on either semi-logarithmic or linear graph paper, enables the HVL and second HVL to be obtained.

For clinical purposes, HVL derived in this way will generally be of sufficient accuracy because the per cent depth–dose data are not critically dependant on HVL. However, if greater precision in the specification is required, the zero field size HVL can be obtained by extrapolation (Trout *et al.* 1960).

When measurements are performed at energies below 100 kV, particular attention should be given to the energy dependence of the chamber. Significant corrections to the measured HVL may be required in the 0.5–2 mm Al HVL range for certain chambers, particularly for lightly filtered beams.

3.3 Filtration

Radiotherapy tubes are normally operated with external metal filters positioned in the beam in order to modify the radiation quality. They preferentially remove the softer photon components, which would simply irradiate the most superficial layers and produce an undesirably rapid attenuation through those layers. An example of the effect of filtration on the spectral distribution of a 220 kV X-ray beam is illustrated in Figure 6.3, whilst Figure 6.4 shows an example of the relation between HVL and increasing filtration.

The choice of filter material is a compromise between a number of requirements:

(1) the filter thickness should be neither too thin for mechanical stability nor too thick for convenience;

(2) the hardening of the beam should be appreciable without an unacceptable reduction in intensity;

(3) the atomic number of the filter should be such that no absorption edge occurs within the useful spectral range of the beam.

Requirement (2) depends on the atomic number (Z) of the filter. In general, the higher the atomic number, the more efficient is the filter in hardening with minimum loss of intensity. However, the other requirements imply the use of filters of lower atomic number at lower energies. At superficial energies, aluminium filters are almost invariably chosen, typically having a thickness within the range 0.5–3 mm. For orthovoltage beams, composite filters are necessary to remove the character-

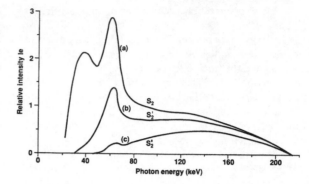

Figure 6.3 The effect of filtration on a 220 kV X-ray beam: (a) no filtration; (b) 1 mm Cu; (c) 2 mm Cu filtration.

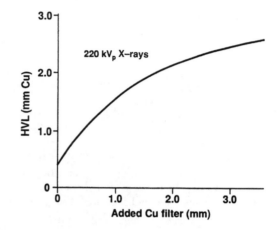

Figure 6.4 Relationship between HVL and filtration for a 220 kV beam: initial filtration 1 mm Al only.

istic X-rays of a higher Z filter by a subsequent layer of lower Z material. Typical filters are of copper 0.5–2 mm thickness, followed by 1 mm of aluminium. Alternatively, a Thoraeus filter of typically 1 mm tin, 0.25–0.75 mm copper and 1 mm aluminium may be used.

In practice, sets often have a number of filters for different kilovoltage settings. Care must be taken to ensure correct combinations are used in order to prevent errors in incident dose rate and penetration. This is generally achieved by interlocks, but their operation must be regularly checked. It is important that all staff are aware of the necessity of checking the selection of the correct filter–kV combination, particularly after changes in operating conditions, such as modality changes or non-standard use.

It must only be possible to insert composite filters in the correct orientation, with the highest Z component towards the X-ray source. As filters are designed to alter the beam quality, any quality specification measurements and dosimetry for clinical use must only be carried out with the appropriate filter in place. Clinical filters are added close to the exit window of the tube. When specifying filtration, a clear distinction should be made between inherent filtration and added filtration.

3.4 Spectral distribution in a phantom

As a beam penetrates the phantom or patient its spectral distribution is altered by scattering and absorption. In the kilovoltage range the response of dosemeters can have a significant energy dependency, so that these changes may need to be considered. For example, Greening and Wilson (1951) reported measurements in a 250 kV beam, with an equivalent primary energy of 97 keV, carried out using a method based on double ionization chambers of different energy responses. At the surface of the phantom, softer scattered radiation reduced the equivalent energy to about 84 keV. This progressively decreased with depth in the phantom to 68 keV at 15 cm, because of the increasing scatter component. However, for superficial X-rays, differences in quality with depth are small due to the relatively small difference in the energy of the scattered radiation. In addition to these changes there are differences in quality across the beam because of differential filtration, particularly along the anode–cathode axis.

4. Beam characteristics

4.1 Radiation distribution in air

The distribution of radiation intensity from a reflection target, such as that in an X-ray tube, is neither symmetrical nor uniform and cannot be easily corrected with a flattening filter because of the limited radiation output available. The largest changes in the beam

intensity are observed in the distribution along a line parallel to the tube axis (Figure 6.5). The exposure rate does not usually decrease symmetrically on either side, but falls off more rapidly in either the cathode or the anode direction, depending on the target angle of the tube and hence on the balance between the 'heel effect' and the initial spatial distribution of the X-rays. The target angle is defined as the angle between the direction of the electrons emitted from the cathode and the normal-to-the-target surface. It is chosen roughly to balance the two effects, but since other considerations need to be taken into account, some asymmetry is always present. Typical target angles are 30° for orthovoltage energies and 45° for superficial. If a single X-ray tube is used over a wide range of voltages, e.g. 100–300 kV, the tube should have a target angle appropriate to the lower voltage, i.e. about 45°.

The exposure distribution along a line perpendicular to the tube axis is more favourable. It usually decreases symmetrically on either side of the central ray due to several effects, including inverse square law (ISL), obliquity of filtration, and the design of the tube and the windows of the tube and housing. Tubes of different makes may vary in this respect, so appropriate data must be obtained for the particular set.

4.2 Radiation distribution in phantom

The requirement for data on radiation distributions, particularly depth doses, is different for kilovoltage than for megavoltage therapy. Moreover, the requirements may vary depending on the beam quality to be employed. At low beam qualities up to about 150 kV, the clinical interest is in treating superficial layers of tissue, hence the information on dose distributions at greater depth is less important, unless there is a need to avoid the irradiation of the underlying tissues or organs. However, the beam

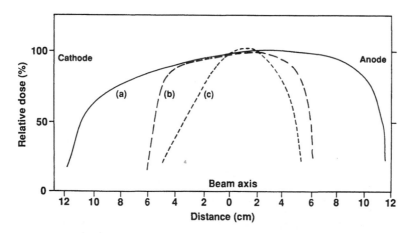

Figure 6.5 Radiation distributions across an X-ray beam in the direction of the tube axis at a depth of 2 cm, with no equalizing filter present, for field sizes of: (a) 20 cm; (b) 10 cm; and (c) 6 cm.

flatness is of interest if a uniform dose is to be delivered, as is the information on the distribution at the beam edges if protection of sensitive organs, such as the eyes, is required.

When the clinical intention is to treat deeper tissues using higher energies, it may be necessary to have more detailed information on the particular depth–dose distribution and isodose curves, as well as the cross-beam uniformity and the penumbra width for each beam and treatment condition used.

The specific requirements on the range of measurements to be taken, the exact data required for treatment planning, and the accuracy acceptable for each set of parameters will depend on local clinical practice and treatment planning approaches.

4.3 Backscattered radiation

4.3.1 The backscatter factor

Scatter effects are very significant for kilovoltage beams. One particularly important parameter to describe these effects is the backscatter factor (BSF), which quantifies the increase in radiation dose at the surface due to the radiation scattered from the phantom or patient.

BSF is defined as the ratio of an appropriate quantity of radiation at the reference point, i.e. on the surface of the patient or phantom and on the central axis of the beam, to the equivalent quantity at the same position in the absence of the phantom, i.e. in the primary incident beam. The radiation quantity used in this definition has varied over the years. Older definitions have used the ratio of exposure (ICRU 1973) or the ratio of absorbed dose (BIR 1983), with and without the phantom present. A more recent definition by the IPSM (1991) adopted the ratio, B_w, of water collision kerma on the surface of a large water phantom to the same quantity in the absence of the phantom. The IAEA dosimetry code of practice (IAEA 1987) specifies a ratio of air kerma.

For the X-ray energies considered here, the quantities water kerma, collision water kerma, and absorbed dose to water, all have effectively the same values and will result in the same values of backscatter factor whichever quantity is specified.

In the experimental determination of B_w, it is convenient to use ionization chambers. If these are air-equivalent, the result is a ratio of exposures (or air kerma). Using the relationship between exposure and water kerma (or absorbed dose to water), B_w can be written as:

$$B_w = \frac{[X \cdot (\mu_{en}/\rho)_{w,air}]_{z=0}}{[X \cdot (\mu_{en}/\rho)_{w,air}]_{air}} \qquad (1)$$

in which X is the exposure, and $(\mu_{en}/\rho)_{w,air}$ is the average ratio of the mass energy absorption coefficients for water and air. The subscripts 'z = 0' and 'air' indicate that the

measurements are at the surface of the phantom and at the same point free-in-air, respectively. The average energy per ion pair (W/e), which usually appears in the conversion from exposure into kerma, has cancelled and the small differences between the chamber wall and water have been disregarded. Usually the ionization chamber will not be exactly air-equivalent. Therefore, in converting each measurement to exposure, different chamber calibration factors should strictly be used, as the X-ray spectrum is different in the two situations. It is also necessary to apply a perturbation correction to allow for the effects of the displacement of the phantom by the chamber and its stem. In addition, the ratio of mass energy absorption coefficients will be different in numerator and denominator, one being averaged over the spectral energy fluence distribution applicable to the beam at the phantom surface and the other over that applicable to the primary photons in the absence of the phantom.

Thus, B_w determined from the ratio of exposure measurements will have a number of systematic errors, which are difficult to quantify. However, the theoretical data show overall variation of the coefficient ratio of only 10% for photon energies from 10 keV to 10 MeV. The discussion in Section 3.4 indicates only small differences in beam quality on going from free-in-air to surface irradiation. In the absence of more precise data, it is normally assumed that $(\mu_{en}/\rho)_{w,air}$ and the various other terms cancel. Thus, within these experimental uncertainties, B_w is simply taken as the ratio of the chamber readings after correction for any temperature difference between the in-air and the phantom surface measurements.

For many years, Supplement 17 of the *British Journal of Radiology* (BIR 1983) and its forerunners have been the main source of backscatter data for low- and medium-energy X-rays. In 1984, Grosswendt (1984) used Monte Carlo methods to calculate backscatter factors for X-rays generated at voltages between 10 and 100 kV, which were subsequently used in the IAEA code of practice (IAEA 1987). These new values differed considerably from those in BIR (1983), particularly in the range 0.1–1.0 mm Al HVL. Later, Grosswendt (1990) repeated the calculations, extending the X-ray energy range upwards to 280 kV and including a range of SSDs from 10 to 100 cm and also short SSDs from 1.5 to 10 cm, and field sizes from 1 to 20 cm diameter. Similar calculations were also made by Knight and subsequently appeared in 1992. These newer theoretical data have been experimentally verified (Klevenhagen 1989; Harrison *et al.* 1990) and on this basis a new set of BSFs was recommended for routine use in radiotherapy (IPSM 1991), in place of the older data in BIR (1983). Some selected values are shown in Figure 6.6. These are valid for thick, full size phantoms, i.e. under full scattering conditions, and are presented to illustrate the variation of BSF with beam quality and field size.

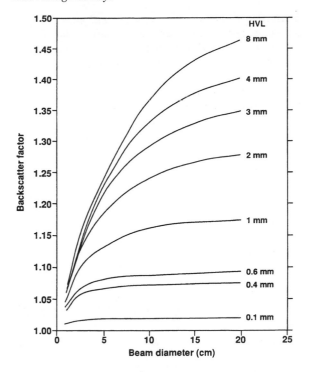

Figure 6.6 BSFs for 0.1–8 mm Al HVL X-ray beams and field diameters of 1–25 cm, using the recommended data from IPSM (1991).

The newer values of BSF have been incorporated into the more recent series of tabulations in BIR (1996), which superseded BIR (1983). Both IPSM (1991) and BIR (1996) provide discussion of, and data on, the variation of BSF with beam quality, field size and, where appropriate SSD. In addition, BIR (1996) provides discussion of, and references for, the small changes in BSF that can occur for different kV values for the same HVL and for different designs of beam collimation, e.g. for diaphragm-limited or closed-applicator units.

The experimental determination of B_w is not a trivial exercise (Klevenhagen 1989; Harrison *et al.* 1990) and it is easy to introduce systematic errors. For example, the use of a parallel-plate ionization chamber, rather than a thimble chamber, may reduce the effect of the displacement of the phantom by the chamber and its stem at low energies. However, for many commercially available parallel-plate chambers there is a significant difference between the calibration factors in phantom and in air. Because of such practical difficulties, and in order to promote consistency in dosimetry at these qualities, it is recommended that tabulated values are used in clinical practice rather than those measured locally.

4.3.2 Backscatter build-up with phantom thickness

One other less appreciated parameter that can influence backscatter significantly is the thickness of underlying tissue. The dependence of BSF on this and on surface beam area is shown in Figure 6.7 for a 2 mm and an 8 mm Al HVL beam taken from Klevenhagen (1982). The relative amount of backscatter, expressed as a fraction of the full backscatter, increases with the thickness of underlying material. Thin layers give rise to a reduced BSF and this should be considered when calculating dosage in radiotherapy, e.g. in areas such as the nose or the ear.

The build-up to full backscatter depends on beam area and quality. It is most rapid for small field sizes (see Figure 6.7) with a decreased dependence on field size above about 50 cm². It is also more rapid for lower energy beams. The curves may be described by the following relationship:

$$FFBS = 1 - \exp(-t/k) \qquad (2)$$

where FFBS is the fraction of the full backscatter, t cm is the thickness of the underlying material, and k is a constant, which describes the slope of the scatter build-up curves; k depends on beam quality and the surface

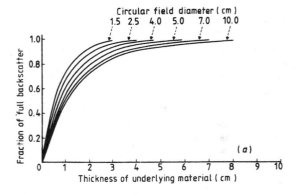

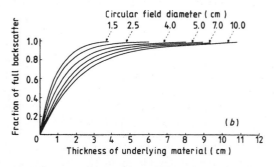

Figure 6.7 Dependence of backscatter build-up on the thickness of underlying material and surface beam area for: (a) a 2-mm Al HVL; and (b) an 8-mm Al HVL beam.

area of the beam. Information on constants for a range of radiation qualities can be found in Klevenhagen (1982).

4.4 Surface dose

The dose at the skin surface is arguably the most significant quantity in kilovoltage therapy and yet it is rather ill-defined, both as to where it should be measured and how this should best be done. Although the term 'surface dose' implies a quantity determined precisely at the skin surface, this is a somewhat misleading term since such a determination is virtually impossible to make and, even if made, would need to be interpreted with caution from the clinical point of view.

In terms of the radiation effect, the dose measured at the true surface has little meaning because of the insensitivity of the superficial skin layers. Therefore, the specification of the entrance dose needs to be related to the depth at which the radiation-sensitive layer begins. This is below the epidermis at a depth of about 0.1–0.15 mm. Thus the term 'skin dose' is best taken as meaning the dose to the dermis and, in order to estimate the skin dose, a layer of absorber equivalent in thickness to the epidermal thickness is required for incorporation in the entrance window of the dosemeter, which should be a plane parallel chamber.

In considering this thickness, a minimum figure of 7 mg cm^{-2} has often been assumed, based on earlier estimates of the range of epidermal thicknesses. However, more recent work has shown that the thickness varies significantly with body site, being approximately 5 mg cm^{-2}, 7 mg cm^{-2}, and 40 mg cm^{-2} on the body trunk, the arms and legs, and the fingertips, respectively, with no dependence on sex or on age between 15 and 89 years. The relevance of this in dosimetry is that the ionization chamber window thickness becomes an important issue when measuring surface dose on the grounds of radiobiology as well as physics. Lack of appreciation of this problem may lead to serious dosimetric errors (Klevenhagen *et al.* 1991). To standardize dosimetric procedures in these situations, IPSM (1991) suggested that a depth of 8.5 mg cm^{-2} is taken as the reference depth in kilovoltage X-ray dosimetry, whilst some other suggestions have been to take a depth equivalent to 100 μm of tissue, i.e. 10 mg cm^{-2}. Thus the chamber front window should be at least equal to the lower of these thicknesses. This is sufficient to provide electronic equilibrium for superficial qualities even at 150 kV. To achieve this depth some parallel-plate ionization chambers may require the use of additional material on top of the front wall

For orthovoltage therapy, a greater thickness is required to achieve electronic equilibrium. Since thimble ionization chambers are normally used, this is provided inherently by the chamber wall, which is typically 40–65 mg cm^{-2} thick. The additional attenuation provided by this thickness is small and can generally be ignored, even at the lower end of the superficial range (50 kV), which can be demonstrated by examining the variation in calibration factor with HVL for any typical chamber.

4.5 Central axis depth doses

Depth doses vary with beam quality, beam area, SSD, and field shape.

4.5.1 Beam quality

Figure 6.8 shows typical curves for 50 kV, 100 kV, and heavily filtered 300 kV beams under the conditions specified. For these qualities the dose maximum lies on, or close to, the surface. The 300 kV curve, with an effective energy of 164 keV, displays a slight build-up effect, with a region of almost constant dose for the first 2 or 3 mm from the surface. In this case, the scattered radiation building up over the first few mm compensates for the attenuation of the primary photons. Where the build-up of scattered radiation is greater than the primary radiation attenuation, an initial rise in per cent depth dose will be produced. In general, for this reason at qualities greater than around 150 kV, 0.7 mm Cu HVL, the dose maximum does not lie exactly on the surface. This scatter build-up effect is greatest at about 200 kV, HVL around 1–2 mm cu. Build-up then decreases as energy increases, until above about 500 kV it begins to increase again due to the increased path lengths of secondary electrons (i.e. above these energies, it begins to exhibit 'megavoltage-type' electron transport build-up).

As scatter is field-size dependent, scatter build-up is most marked for larger field sizes. In addition, it may be noted that these scatter build-up effects will be more

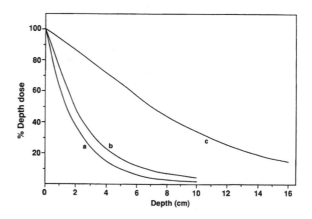

Figure 6.8 Depth–dose curves for three kilovoltage therapy X-ray beams: (a) 50 kV, 1 mm Al HVL, 6 cm diameter field, 10 cm SSD: (b) 100 kV, 2 mm Al HVL, 6 cm diameter field, 10 cm SSD; (c) 300 kV, 3 mm Cu HVL, 10 × 10 cm^2 field, 50 cm SSD. (Data from BIR (1996)).

marked in diaphragm-limited beams than for closed-end applicators, because in the latter a significant amount of the build-up takes place in the plastic of the applicator end, and therefore, the starting point of the depth–dose curve in tissue or phantom is much closer to the peak value of the curve.

This same effect can also result in higher per cent depth dose values being observed over the first few cm at lower beam qualities than at higher beam qualities, e.g. 2 mm Cu HVL rather than 3 mm Cu HVL, particularly at larger field sizes and more significantly for diaphragm-limited beams. Therefore, per cent depth dose does not increase continuously over the whole quality range, other parameters being equal. The detail of the variations with quality depend on scatter and therefore on field size and depth, as well as collimation design.

BIR (1996) provides discussion and extensive tables of depth doses for a wide range of beam qualities (specified by HVL), field sizes and, for superficial quality beams, SSDs. This illustrate the points discussed above. In addition, it provides discussion of, and references for, the variations in depth doses than can occur:

(1) for different beams of the same HVL, but produced from different kV and filtration combinations;

(2) for different designs of beams collimation, e.g. for diaphragm-limited or closed-applicator units;

(3) and for different designs of applicator.

For example, the tabulations of orthovoltage per cent depth doses indicate that the values of diaphragm-limited beams are typically a few per cent greater in equivalent conditions of beam quality, field size, and depth (or the equivalent per cent depth dose is typically at a greater depth) than for closed-end applicators.

For lower energy beams, it is easy to introduce systematic errors into depth–dose measurements unless very careful attention is given to selection of equipment and to technique (see Section 6). This is due to the steep dose gradients involved, the often significant energy dependence of the dosimeters available, and the difficulties of assessing the surface dose. Accurate measurements depend on the availability of appropriate equipment and expertise. Therefore, it is often preferable to use published tabulations of depth-dose data for beams of the same HVL and similar accelerating potential and filtration as the user's beam. Suitable tabulations can be found in BIR (1996).

4.5.2 Beam area

Variations with beam area are significant at kilovoltage energies due to the significant scatter contribution, the degree of change depending also upon the quality. Figure 6.9 shows typical variations at a number of depths for a radiation beam of HVL = 2 mm Cu. It can be seen

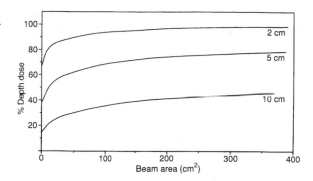

Figure 6.9 Dependence of depth dose on area for a diaphragm-limited beam of 2 mm Cu HVL at 50 cm SSD and depths 2, 5, and 10 cm. (Data from BIR (1996)).

that the per cent depth dose increases with the area as the scatter contribution increases. The change is more marked at small field sizes. The depth–dose values at a given depth change less rapidly with increasing area for the large field sizes, because the scatter contribution to the central axis approaches saturation.

4.5.3 Source–surface distance

Per cent depth doses at a given depth increase with SSD because of the effect of beam divergence with distance from the source, which is governed by inverse square law (ISL). At increased SSD, the distance from the phantom or patient surface to the point of interest is a smaller proportion of the total distance from the source and, therefore, the relative attenuation from the surface to that depth is reduced. Thus, although the absolute intensity at the surface falls as SSD increases, the per cent of the surface dose that is transmitted to a given depth is increased. The significance of this effect diminishes with increasing SSD and is, therefore, more marked for superficial sets, which typically have SSDs in the range of 10–20 cm, than for orthovoltage sets with SSDs between 30 and 50 cm.

Taking the ISL effect alone, a rough estimate of the change in depth dose can be obtained from the simple formula:

$$\frac{D_{d,f_2}}{D_{d,f_1}} = \frac{(f_1 + d)^2}{(f_1)^2} \cdot \frac{(f_2)^2}{(f_2 + d)^2} \tag{3}$$

which can be written as F^2, where $F = \left[\frac{(f_1 + d)}{f_1}\right] \cdot \left[\frac{f_2}{f_2 + d}\right]$.

Here $D_{d,f}$ is the per cent depth dose at depth d and at SSD f. Subscript 1 refers to the SSD for which the data were measured or specified, and subscript 2 is for the SSD of interest.

This expression should be used with caution since it is only valid for the primary beam. Generally, when SSD is increased the improvement in the depth dose is less than F^2 due to the effects of scatter, which produces discrepancies between the real situation and the predictions from equation (3). The degree to which scatter has an influence depends on the field size and the radiation quality. The simple expression above is strictly only useful for small changes in SSD from the standard values.

For a more accurate prediction, Burns has given a comprehensive general set of expressions to convert between various dosimetric quantities and to convert depth doses between different SSD. These are concisely summarized in Appendix B of BIR (1996). For kilovoltage beams the maximum dose is on, or close to, the surface. Therefore, the general expression for depth dose conversion simplifies to:

$$D_{d,f_2,S} = D_{d,f_1,S/F} \cdot \frac{\text{BSF}(S/F)}{\text{BSF}(S)} \cdot F^2 \qquad (4)$$

in which $D_{d,f,S}$ is the per cent depth dose at depth d, SSD f, and for a field size $S \times S$, which for kilovoltage beams is defined at the surface. The other parameters are defined above.

Most kilovoltage sets have applicators providing two or more SSDs and also treatments may often be carried out at non-standard SSD. In many situations, such changes in SSD can have a more significant effect on the depth dose than changes in the quality of radiation and the changes must be taken into account for accurate dosimetry. BIR (1996) provides tabulations of per cent depth doses for superficial beams for a range of SSD from 10 to 30 cm.

4.5.4   Field shape

Depth–dose tables are generally presented for square or circular fields and for specific beam areas. Intermediate depth–dose values can be obtained by linear interpolation. Values for rectangular fields are not usually listed. They give smaller depth doses than square or circular fields of the same area, because the scatter from the more distant parts of the rectangular field is attenuated relatively more as it travels towards the central axis. Generally, therefore, a conversion must be made by finding an equivalent square or circle for each size and shape of a rectangle which has the same depth–dose values. Tables of equivalent squares and equivalent diameters of rectangular fields are presented in BIR (1996), with a good review of the different approaches to obtaining equivalence. A reasonable approximation for an estimate of the length of the side of the equivalent square (L) for a rectangular field of moderate elongation, is:

$$L = \frac{2ab}{(a+b)} \qquad (5)$$

where a and b are the lengths of the sides of the rectangular field. An approximate relationship for quick estimations of equivalence between square and circular fields is:

$$\frac{L}{D} = 0.9 \qquad (6)$$

where L is the equivalent square field side and D is the equivalent circular field diameter.

Although there are more exact relationships on which the tabulations to be found in BIR (1996) are based, the above expressions will often be sufficiently accurate.

4.6   Isodose curves

In clinical treatments performed with X-rays in the orthovoltage range, it may be necessary to consider the doses to many other points within the treated volume. This information is facilitated by isodose charts.

A typical isodose distribution for a 200 kV X-ray beam is given in Figure 6.10. The beam distribution for this radiation quality differs considerably from a distribution for megavoltage radiation (see Chapter 8, Section 2.1.1). For example, the penetration with depth is poorer; there is little absorbed dose build-up, resulting in the maximum dose appearing at, or close to, the surface; and there is a relatively wide penumbra with a sharp discontinuity at the geometric edge of the beam. Both the build-up effects and the distinctive wide penumbra are due to scattered radiation. Isodose lines are noticeably rounded, reflecting the radiation distribution across the beam as discussed in Section 4.1.

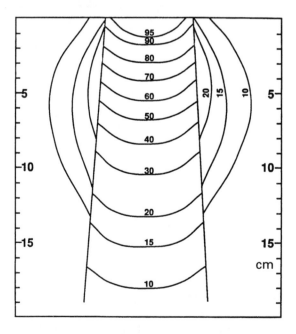

Figure 6.10 Isodose distribution across the short axis of a $15 \times 6 \text{ cm}^2$ field for a 200 kV (1.4 mm Cu HVL) beam at 50 cm SSD.

When using superficial beams for treatment there is seldom a need for isodose curves, since only the superficial tissue layers are to be treated. This may also be the case for higher energy beams, depending on clinical requirements and local practice.

4.7 Absorption in other materials

Photoelectric effect interactions make a significant contribution to the absorption from kilovoltage X-ray beams, increasingly so for lower energies such that they are the dominant interaction for beams of approximately 100 kV and below in water or soft tissue. Therefore, the same X-ray beam incident on tissues of different effective atomic number will give significantly different absorbed doses. These differences can be estimated compared to the absorbed dose to water by considering the ratio of mass energy absorption coefficients between the specific tissue and water. This approach assumes that the photon fluence in the tissue is the same as in water and, therefore, ignores any differences in scatter and absorption up to the point of interest in the two materials. The simplest approach would be to compare the coefficient ratios for the tissue of interest and for water, using tabulated values selected for the single equivalent energy, representative of the spectrum. More complete approaches include integration of the coefficients over the photon spectrum and Monte Carlo simulation of the spectra at different depths, if required (Ma and Seuntjens 1999). For muscle tissue, the differences are small (typically about $\pm 1\%$ in the orthovoltage range and $+2/-3.5\%$ in the superficial range), since the effective atomic numbers are similar. However, for bone there is a marked increase in absorbed dose as energy decreases, reflecting the increased absorption in the higher atomic number material. For example, below approximately 100 kV (3 mm Al HVL) the energy absorption in bone is as much as 4.5 times higher than in muscle. Even at orthovoltage energies around 200–250 kV (2–2.5 mm Cu HVL), the difference is still significant, at approximately 1.5 times higher, falling to a few per cent for harder beams, e.g. 1.05 at about 300 kV (4–5 mm Cu HVL). Smaller differences will be present for other body tissues such as cartilage.

5. Absorbed dose determination

5.1 Background

Beam calibration requires a precise determination of the quantity of radiation in terms of absorbed dose at a reference point in the beam under standard conditions. Since direct measurement of absorbed dose is seldom possible, indirect methods are usually employed. In the case of low- and medium-energy X-rays, the determination of absorbed dose is based on the use of air-filled cavity ionization chambers. At present a number of approaches are recommended for dose determination at these radiation qualities. They differ in several ways.

1. They may be based on a calibration in terms of either air kerma or exposure.

2. Each component of the conversion to dose may be expressed separately or they may be combined in a single factor.

3. Measurement may be made in air or at depth in a phantom.

4. The kilovoltage qualities may be broken up into a number of smaller ranges. These may differ from one code to another and may overlap.

In addition, the intercomparison between the field instrument and the local reference instrument may take place either in the user's beam or at a standards laboratory. This varies from one country to another, according to local circumstances, and is reflected in some of the different codes of practice.

Exposure and absorbed dose are related by the following general expression:

$$D_{\mathrm{w}} = X(W/e)_{\mathrm{air}}(\mu_{\mathrm{en}}/\rho)_{\mathrm{w,air}} \qquad (7)$$

in which D_{w} is the absorbed dose to water, X is the exposure, $(W/e)_{\mathrm{air}}$ is the quotient of the average energy expended to produce an ion pair in dry air by the electronic charge and $(\mu_{\mathrm{en}}/\rho)_{\mathrm{w,air}}$ is the ratio of the mass energy absorption coefficients of water to air averaged over the photon spectrum at the point of measurement.

If an air kerma calibration is used then:

$$D_{\mathrm{w}} = K(1 - g)(\mu_{\mathrm{en}}/\rho)_{\mathrm{w,air}} \qquad (8)$$

in which K is the air kerma and g is the correction due to bremsstrahlung. For kilovoltage beams, g can be considered to be zero and, therefore, this factor can be ignored.

The two measurement techniques, with the chamber in phantom or in air, deal with the scatter contribution to the point of measurement in a different way. When the measurement is made at a depth in a phantom, the scatter component is automatically included in the measurement and the derived output is valid for the beam quality and field size used at the time. The output for any other field size must be derived by a separate measurement.

When the measurement is made in air, the backscatter component must be separately included, by multiplying the in-air output by BSF. Therefore, it is useful to have information on the relative variation of BSF with field size at given beam qualities. In-air outputs also vary due to collimator or applicator scatter and these field size settings or applicator factors should be determined at installation and periodically checked thereafter.

All protocols are based on the use of ionization chambers calibrated against national standards. Since the aim is to measure exposure or air kerma at a point, the ionization chamber must be small, particularly for short SSD measurements where there may be very high dose gradients. The chamber should have an energy response as independent as possible of radiation energy, not varying by more than 5% within the 100–300 kV radiation range. It must have air equivalent walls of sufficient thickness to ensure that secondary electrons produced in interactions in materials outside and surrounding the chamber cannot enter the collecting volume. This requirement is dependent on radiation energy. For X-rays generated at 300 kV, a wall thickness of about 0.5 mm of unit density material (50 mg cm^{-2}) is sufficient. There are several commercial chambers available, such as the Farmer-type chamber, which meet these requirements.

Currently, the main accessible kilovoltage beam dosimetry protocols are IPEMB (1996) and IAEA (1987). There are other relatively recent codes, such as the Dutch protocol (NCS 1997), which has elements common to both the above. Older protocols, such as ICRU (1973), are still in use in many centres. A new AAPM code is also in preparation. The various methods will be outlined below, retaining the symbols of the original publications.

5.2   ICRU method

Two approaches are recommended in ICRU (1973). These depend on beam quality.

5.2.1   150–400 kV

For these qualities, absorbed dose to water is derived from a measurement of exposure with the ionization chamber placed on the beam axis at a depth of 5 cm in a water phantom irradiated with a 10×10 cm^2 field. Absorbed dose to water is given by:

$$D = Rk_1k_2NF \qquad (9)$$

in which D cGy (rad in the original) is absorbed dose to water at the position of the centre of the chamber when the chamber is replaced by water, R is the instrument reading, and N is the exposure calibration factor, determined by the standardizing laboratory at stated radiation qualities and under specified ambient conditions; k_1 is the factor to correct for differences in temperature and pressure from those specified (see Chapter 3, Section 5.1); k_2 is a factor to correct for differences such as in beam quality of the radiation field used for calibration and that of the hospital treatment machine; F cGy R^{-1} is a composite factor to convert from exposure (in Roentgens) to absorbed dose to water, which is listed in the report against beam quality specified by HVL.

Following the measurement at 5 cm, as specified in the recommendations, the dose is converted to a surface dose using the appropriate depth–dose data.

5.2.2   Below 150 kV

For these qualities, measurements should be made with a chamber positioned free-in-air on the central axis of the beam. The absorbed dose, D, at the phantom surface is then related to the ionization chamber reading, R, by the same formula and multiplying by the backscatter factor:

$$D = Rk_1k_2NF\frac{(f + x)^2}{f^2}\text{BSF} \qquad (10)$$

in which D, N, k_1, k_2, F, and BSF have the same meaning as above; f is the SSD; and x is the distance between the end of the applicator or treatment cone and the chamber centre. It may also be necessary to involve a correction for the deviation from the ISL due to possible scatter production from the applicator walls or other effects (see Sections 6.3 and 6.4). Values of BSF were discussed in Section 4.3.1 and the data from IPSM (1991) shown in Figure 6.6 may be used.

5.3   IAEA method

The code of practice of the International Atomic Energy Agency for the determination of absorbed dose to water in electron and photon beams (IAEA 1987) also divides kilovoltage dosimetry into two ranges depending on beam quality.

5.3.1   100–280 kV

Between these generating potentials (0.17–3.37 mm Cu HVL) a similar experimental procedure as that in ICRU (1973) should be used but employing a chamber calibrated in terms of air kerma. The absorbed dose to water, D_w, Gy, at the position of the centre of the chamber when it is replaced by water is given by:

$$D_w = M_uN_Kk_u(\mu_{en}/\rho)_{w,air}p_u \qquad (11)$$

in which M_u is the instrument reading in the user's beam corrected to the same ambient conditions as the calibration factor, N_K is the air kerma calibration factor of the chamber for the radiation quality of the incident beam in air, k_u is a correction factor taking into account the change in response of the ionization chamber due to the change in the spectral distributions between the in-air calibration and the measurement at the reference depth in water, and p_u is the perturbation correction factor for the replacement of water by the ionization chamber; $(\mu_{en}/\rho)_{w,air}$ has been defined previously. The values of these quantities are all tabulated in the code, against HVL alone or against HVL and kV. However, amended values of p_u have since been issued (IAEA 1993) and these should be used in place of the original ones.

5.3.2 Below 100 kV

In this range, the IAEA recommends that absorbed dose to water should be calculated from a measurement with the chamber in air, together with the application of a backscatter factor. The perturbation correction p_u is not required. The surface absorbed dose in a phantom is then related to the ionization chamber reading M_u by:

$$D_w = M_u N_K k_u (\mu_{en}/\rho)_{w,air} BSF \qquad (12)$$

in which BSF is the backscatter factor and other parameters have the same meaning as in the previous equation.

D_w in equations (11) and (12) represents the same quantity, absorbed dose to water, as in the ICRU equations 9 and 10, and the corrected reading, M_u, is the same as the product of the reading R and the correction factor, k_1. It may be noted that recombination corrections (see Chapter 3, Section 5.1) are generally not required for measurements in kilovoltage beams, using typical chambers at typical polarising voltages and for typical dose rates. However, they should be considered if dose rates are very high, for example in lightly-filtered low-energy beams and/or for very short SSD.

5.4 IPEMB method

In the 1996 UK code of practice (IPEMB 1996), the determination of absorbed dose is based on the air-kerma method. The use of composite conversion factors is abandoned and each component of the conversion to dose is expressed separately. Three separate energy ranges are defined, with specific procedures for each range: medium energy (0.5–4 mm Cu HVL), low energy (1.0–8 mm Al HVL), and very low energy (0.035–1.0 mm Al HVL).

The very low energy range extends the previous codes downwards. It is introduced as a separate range because of the need to use a parallel-plate chamber.

In addition to presenting the formalism, the code recommends the types of ionization chambers to be used. It also recommends in detail the techniques for intercomparing the field instrument with the local reference (secondary standard) chamber. This ensures that dose determined in the user's beam with the field instrument is traceable to a national standard. The intercomparison is carried out using the same X-ray facilities and radiation qualities that will subsequently be measured by the field instrument.

5.4.1 Medium energy

This covers half-value layers in the range 0.5–4 mm Cu (approximately 160–300 kV). Measurement is made with a thimble ionization chamber in a full-scatter water phantom at a depth of 2 cm. The chamber is placed on the central axis of the beam using a field size of approximately 10×10 cm and the standard SSD. The equation for calculating absorbed dose at the reference depth is:

$$D_{w,z=2} = M N_K k_{ch} \left[(\overline{\mu}_{en}/\rho)_{w,air} \right]_{z=2,\phi} \qquad (13)$$

where $D_{w,z=2}$ is the dose to water at the position of the chamber centre at a depth $z = 2$ cm, when the chamber is replaced by water; M is the ionization chamber reading corrected to standard pressure and temperature; and N_K is the chamber calibration factor to convert the instrument reading at the HVL concerned to air kerma free in air at the reference point of the chamber with the chamber assembly replaced by air; $[(\overline{\mu}_{en}/\rho)_{w,air}]_{z=2,\phi}$ is the mass energy absorption coefficient ratio, water to air, averaged over the photon spectrum at 2 cm depth of water and field diameter ϕ is tabulated in the code against HVL and field size; k_{ch} is the factor that accounts for the change in the response of the ionization chamber between calibration in air and measurement in a phantom.

k_{ch} corrects for the combined effect of the change in quality between the in-air and in-phantom measurements, for displacement due to the wall and air cavity and for the chamber stem. For the NE2561 and NE2571 ionization chambers used as local reference chambers, its value (tabulated in the code) varies between 1.023 at 0.5 mm Cu HVL, and 1.018 at 4.0 mm Cu, k_{ch} for the field instrument does not need to be known.

5.4.2 Low energy

This covers half-value layers in the range 1.0–8 mm Al (approximately 50–160 kV). Measurement is made with a thimble chamber free in air. The chamber is placed on the central axis of the beam close to the standard SSD and using a field size of approximately 7 cm diameter. The equation for the calculation of absorbed dose at the phantom surface is:

$$D_{w,z=0} = M_{air} N_K B_w \left[(\overline{\mu}_{en}/\rho)_{w,air} \right]_{air} \qquad (14)$$

where $D_{w,z=0}$ is the absorbed dose to water at the surface of a water phantom, when the surface of the phantom material is positioned at the same level as the chamber centre; $[(\overline{\mu}_{en}/\rho)_{w,air}]_{air}$ is the mass energy absorption coefficient ratio, water to air, averaged over the photon spectrum in air; B_w is the back scatter factor, defined as the ratio of the water collision kerma at a point on the beam axis at the surface of a full scatter water phantom, to the water collision kerma at the same point in the primary beam with no phantom, for the field size and SSD concerned. These are both tabulated in the code against HVL and the values of the mass energy absorption coefficient ratio are shown in Figure 6.11.

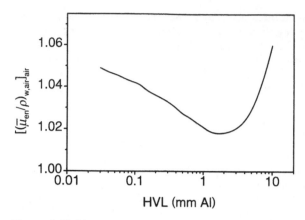

Figure 6.11 Mass energy absorption coefficient ratios, water to air, averaged over the photon spectrum in air, as a function of HVL. The data is taken from IPEMB (1996).

5.4.3 Very low energy

This covers half-value layers in the range 0.035–1.0 mm Al (approximately 8–50 kV). Measurement is made with a designated parallel-plate ionization chamber with the front face of the chamber at the surface of a full-scatter phantom. The chamber is placed on the central axis of the beam using the standard SSD and a field size sufficient to allow a 2 cm margin around the chamber. The equation for calculating absorbed dose at the reference depth is:

$$D_{w,z=0} = M_{air} N_K k_{ch} \big[(\overline{\mu}_{en}/\rho)_{w,air} \big]_{z=0,\phi} \qquad (15)$$

where $D_{w,z=0}$ is the absorbed dose to water at the phantom surface at the position of the front face of the chamber when the chamber is replaced by phantom material; $[(\overline{\mu}_{en}/\rho)_{w,air}]_{z=0,\phi}$ is the ratio of mass energy absorption coefficients between water and air, averaged over the photon spectrum at the surface of the water phantom, for a field diameter ϕ and is tabulated against HVL in the code; k_{ch} is the factor that accounts for the change in response of the ionization chamber between the calibration in air and measurement at the surface of a full-scatter, water-equivalent phantom.

There was little information available on the values of k_{ch} for parallel-plate ionization chambers at the time the code was published. Historically it has implicitly been assumed to be equal to unity. The code therefore recommends that this practice should continue until more information is available.

5.5 Comparison of methods

In all dosimetry methods, the calibration factor of the instrument must be applicable for the radiation quality of the beam concerned, and is obtained by intercomparison with exposure (or air kerma) standards during free-in-air calibrations at a standardizing laboratory. The primary

standards for medium-energy X-ray dosimetry are free air ionization chambers, designed to measure exposure. Air kerma is derived indirectly by multiplying the exposure (in C kg^{-1}) by $(W/e)_{air}$. At the time of the publication of the ICRU report, a value of 33.7 J C^{-1} was recommended for dry air. The currently recommended value is 33.97 J C^{-1}. This change results in an increase of 0.8% in the calculation of absorbed dose to water using the newer (e.g. IAEA and IPEMB) codes, as compared to the ICRU procedure.

The codes construct the formalism for deriving the final value of the absorbed dose in two different ways. The ICRU use the F conversion factor from exposure to dose and the IAEA and IPEMB use the explicit ratio of mass energy absorption coefficients of water to air averaged over the photon fluence spectrum at the point of measurement. This ratio is a component of the F-factor.

If the ratio of the mass energy absorption coefficients is derived from the F-factor by assuming that the replacement correction is unity and $(W/e)_{air}$ is 33.7 J C^{-1}, as used in ICRU (1973), it is found that there are differences from the values given in the later codes. These differences are as great as 2.5% at 0.17 mm Cu HVL. The mass energy absorption coefficient ratios given in both the IAEA and the IPEMB codes have been calculated using recent Monte Carlo techniques (Seuntjens *et al.* 1988; Knight and Nahum 1994; Ma and Seuntjens 1999) and the two sets of values agree within 0.4%. Therefore, one can expect to obtain somewhat different absorbed dose values during a therapy machine calibration depending on whether the protocol followed is an older one or one of the more recent ones.

The factors used for the derivation of dose at a depth for either the exposure or the kerma calibration methods are dependent on the specified depth and field size. The values given in ICRU (1973), IPEMB (1996), and IAEA (1987) are to be applied to measurements in a water phantom at a single depth (5 cm or 2 cm) and to a single field size (10 × 10 cm^2). The IAEA report also provides values of $(\mu_{en}/\rho)_{w,air}$ at the phantom surface and at depths of 0, 2, and 5 cm in water for an 11.3-cm diameter circular field and for X-ray generating potentials between 50 and 280 kV. The variation over this depth range for any given beam quality is not greater than 0.7%. The IPEMB protocol provides values at 2 cm depth for 1 and 40 cm square fields, as well as for the standard 10 × 10 cm^2 fields, for beam qualities of 0.5–4 mm Cu. The maximum variation over this field size range for any given beam quality is +1.1/–0.9%, compared to the 10 × 10 cm^2 field.

The Dutch code of practice for kilovoltage beam dosimetry (NCS 1997) is similar in approach to the IPEMB code, using a 2-cm reference depth for medium energy X-rays, which are defined by the NCS as 100–300 kV. It utilizes similar input data to the IPEMB and IAEA codes. It provides mass energy absorption coefficient ratios at 2-cm depth and for a 10×10 cm field, but also for a number of different generating potentials for each value of HVL (Seuntjens *et al.* 1988). The largest spread reported is at 0.4 mm Cu HVL (7.8 mm Al), where the values differ by around 1% when the beam is generated by potentials varying from 100 to 150 kV.

One further source of difference is that the IAEA equation incorporates a perturbation correction factor, p_u, ranging from 1.01 to 1.10 for cylindrical chambers of similar design to the Farmer chamber, and for HVLs between 3.37 and 0.17 mm Cu, respectively. It may be noted that these relatively large corrections, as given in the original IAEA code (1987), have since been revised (IAEA 1993) to lie in the range 1.01–1.03. The values of the factor k_{ch} given in the IPEMB (1996) protocol for the NE 2561 chamber (and taken to be the same for the NE 2571 Farmer chamber) range from 1.018 to 1.023 for HVLs between 4.0 and 0.5 mm Cu, respectively. In contrast, a corresponding correction (designated as a displacement correction, r) in ICRU (1973) is of insignificant magnitude, being less than 1%. Thus, again, the newer protocols (IPEMB and corrected-IAEA) are in close agreement with each other, but somewhat different to the older ICRU (1973). The Dutch protocol (NCS 1997) provides k_{ch} factors for the NE 2571 for some different generating potentials for the same HVL, showing only small differences, less than 0.5% for any given HVL.

The NCS protocol also provides correction factors to account for the presence of a water-proofing PMMA sheath of various thicknesses at qualities ranging from 0.1 mm Cu HVL (2.8 mm Al) to 5 mm Cu. The PMMA sheath increases the instrument reading. Corrections are within 0.3% of unity for a 1-mm sheath and within 1% for a 3-mm sheath. The IPEMB code recommends a PMMA sheath of less than 1.5-mm thickness for the medium-energy range (down to 0.5 mm Cu HVL), implying a sheath correction of no more than 0.25%. It may be noted that the use of rubber sheaths, which are frequently coated with fine talcum powder, is to be discouraged for chambers that may be used in kilovoltage beams, as contamination by the powder can lead to significant response changes.

Considering all these factors, it can be predicted that doses determined using the IPEMB, NCS or the (corrected) IAEA codes would agree to within ±1% for a wide range of commonly used beam qualities (medium energy and low energy in the IPEMB or NCS terminology). Comparing the older ICRU approach to the IPEMB code would indicate larger discrepancies, of up to around –4% for medium-energy (orthovoltage) beams, i.e. with the newer code producing larger dose values. For low-energy beams, considering only the basic

data involved in the in-air dose determination, differences could be up to +2% and –5%. Differences would then be modified if different sets of BSF were being used to convert from the in-air dose to a surface dose. A preliminary experimental comparison of orthovoltage protocols (Nisbet *et al.* 1999), taking account of the whole of the various recommendations, including the differences in calibration depths, has supported these figures.

All the three codes considered in detail here (ICRU 1973; IAEA 1987 and IPEMB 1996) use a calibration at depth in phantom in the orthovoltage range, either at 5 or 2 cm. There are other protocols that follow a similar approach, e.g. NCS. However many centres are still using older protocols, based on calibration in air, at these energies. It is expected that the forthcoming AAPM code is also likely to continue to accept calibration in air. However, the major source of uncertainty in treatment delivery is in the values of the depth doses. The difficulties in obtaining accurate measurements of these, particularly between 2 cm and the surface, has already been discussed. Therefore, there are advantages in using a protocol in which the dose is determined as close as possible to the depth of clinical interest. Where this point is at the surface, the corresponding dose determination would be in air, with the use of BSF to then convert to the dose on the surface.

Finally, it may be noted that, as for megavoltage photon and electron beams (see Chapter 3), there are developments in progress that will eventually lead to recommendations based on direct absorbed dose-to-water standards and calibrations, and these concepts are already being included in developing protocols (IAEA 2000).

6. Measurement of radiation distributions

6.1 Depth dose

Measurement of kilovoltage depth–dose distribution is not easy and requires a careful choice of equipment. The difficulties are due to the relatively steep gradient of the depth doses and the fact that the maximum dose for most energies is at, or close to, the surface of the phantom.

Ionization chambers are the most suitable devices for these measurements at kilovoltage energies. They can be obtained with a flat energy response and they have excellent precision and instantaneous read-out. Film dosimetry, although potentially offering excellent resolution, cannot be used with X-rays of this quality because of the strong dependence of film response on radiation energy. Diodes are generally not recommended for kilovoltage beams for similar reasons. Experimental assessment (Li *et al.* 1997; Ma *et al.* 1999) for medium-energy (orthovoltage) X-rays supports this. However, the same work has shown that reasonably accurate results are obtained using commercial p-type diodes, rear-shielded with a tungsten/epoxy mixture, for beams of 100 kV (2.4 mm Al HVL) and below, down to 50 kV (0.3 mm Al HVL). Li *et al.* (1997) and Ma *et al.* (1999) have shown that, by applying small (less than 2%) Monte Carlo calculated depth-dependent corrections to the results obtained with these diodes, accurate depth doses may be obtained. Diamond detectors may be suitable for measurements in medium-energy X-ray beams, with similar testing before use to verify their applicability. However, they may be less suitable for lower energy beams (NCS 1997).

TLD could be considered because it offers good resolution. An appropriate choice of TLD material has to be made, such that the energy dependence and the measurement precision is acceptable. However, TLD imposes a limitation on phantom type since the dosemeters cannot be used in water. In addition, the uncertainties are significant even in the best circumstances and the method is time consuming if many points are required.

When measuring the depth–dose distribution, the main problem is to determine the value at the dose maximum. For orthovoltage qualities, a thimble chamber is suitable. For superficial and softer qualities, the best method is to use a parallel-plate chamber with a thin sensitive volume of no more than 2 mm in depth, in order to provide good measurement resolution. A thin entrance window facilities measurement at the phantom surface. To avoid distortion of measurement by photoelectrons generated in the X-ray tube collimating system (Klevenhagen *et al.* 1991) sufficient build-up should be provided to bring the wall thickness to 8.5–10 mg cm^{-2}. The IAEA code of practice (IAEA 1987) lists the required characteristics for chambers to be used in softer X-ray beams, whilst IPEMB (1996) designates certain specific chambers and discusses their characteristics. These requirements are equally applicable to depth–dose measurements as to absorbed dose calibration of these beams. Some commercial parallel-plate chambers are available, which have been specifically designed for lower quality kilovoltage X-rays and have quite flat energy responses down to low energies. Others, particularly those which have been specifically designed for electrons, may have energy responses that are far from flat. The ideal ionization chamber for depth–dose measurements should be water equivalent. However, measurements with chambers that are air equivalent will be within about 3% of the true local value. Those chambers that deviate from water equivalence by more than this, in either direction, should be treated with caution.

The choice of phantom material must also be carefully considered. Water is preferred but it presents difficulties for measurements close to the surface and there may be problems associated with the water tightness of ionization chambers. A phantom made of a solid water equivalent material can be very convenient, particularly with a flat chamber that can be precisely positioned at any required depth using sheets of the phantom material. In selecting a water substitute material for a phantom, consideration should be given to the absorbing and scattering properties which ought to be similar to those of water for the X-ray spectrum of interest. If this is not the case, then corrections will be required to the measured depth doses. Information on the interaction properties of some materials can be obtained from ICRU (1989). Epoxy based water-substitutes are generally suitable. In every case the properties of the particular material should be checked by measurement, comparing it with water at convenient selected points.

6.2 Isodoses

If isodoses are to be measured, the considerations are similar to those for megavoltage beams, as discussed in Chapter 4. Measurements must be made in a water phantom, through the open surface, with careful alignment on setting up. The detector requirements for the depth direction have already been discussed. Ionization chambers may be used in both directions, but must be of small volume to give acceptable spatial resolution laterally as well as with depth. Diodes have generally not been recommended at these qualities. However, there are some reports (Li *et al.* 1997), using p-type, rear-shielded diodes that indicate that they may be used with caution for profile measurement, provided that they have first been checked by comparison with ionization chambers, to ensure that they are not significantly affected by the variation of quality across the beam. Their advantage in profile measurement is their good spatial resolution. However, they do not generally produce accurate profile tails due a significant part of the radiation being large angle scatter and the significant variations in angular response.

6.3 Determination of SSD

It is necessary to know the SSD exactly, particularly in superficial or contact therapy where short, or very short, SSDs are used and small changes can alter doses very significantly. The information provided by the manufacturer should always be verified, as the SSD can differ from the nominal SSD and can vary from applicator to applicator, subject to length tolerances. In addition, whenever a tube is changed the SSD should be remeasured. A convenient method of SSD determination is by means of a double pinhole camera in which the distance of the pinholes from the focus can be calculated from the separation of the two images of the focal spot and the physical distance between the holes. Alternatively, ISL extrapolation can be made from measurements at a number of different distances from the applicator end. However, ISL can be subject to uncertainty, particularly at low energies, and such measurements must be interpreted with care, as discussed in the following section.

6.4 Stand-off correction/ISL applicability

Under certain conditions, treatments need to be performed at non-standard SSD, i.e. with the tube applicator (cone) being at some stand-off distance from the patient surface. In addition, measurements often need to be carried out with the chamber's point of measurement not exactly at the applicator base. In these situations, corrections to output or to measurement are required and the obvious approach is to employ an inverse square correction.

However, there may be deviations from the ISL for a number of reasons. These include:

(1) a very short SSD combined with a finite source size;

(2) the applicator may produce scatter causing deviations close to its end, which would normally be in contact with the skin surface under standard conditions;

(3) the effective SSD may differ from the physical SSD;

(4) air attenuation may be significant at low energies, particularly if larger changes in SSD are involved.

One method of assessing these effects is to make measurements at a number of distances between the applicator end and the effective point of measurement. Plotting $(1/\text{reading})^{\frac{1}{2}}$ against these distances gives the required information. A linear regression analysis of the data indicates whether ISL is applicable or alternatively whether further investigation is required. If ISL is applicable, then the effective SSD at the applicator end can be obtained from the intercept with the distance axis.

In the event that ISL is not applicable close to the end of an applicator, further careful measurements may be needed to obtain specific stand off corrections for each applicator.

7. Acceptance and quality control

Many of the points discussed in Chapters 2–5 for megavoltage applications are applicable for kilovoltage systems, with some changes in detail where appropriate. The general approach and background are closely parallel to those presented in the preceding chapters. Thus, this section will be brief and will essentially deal only with those aspects that are specific to kilovoltage sets and that have not been covered already.

Acceptance and commissioning tests are often much less extensive than for megavoltage units, since published depth dose and other data are frequently used for the particular measured beam quality, and isodoses are often not required. However, this depends on the beam qualities and the clinical objectives, which may vary greatly from centre to centre. The performance of a kilovoltage set may differ significantly with the age and type of the equipment and will generally be less than that achieved with megavoltage units. Often the kilovoltage equipment in a centre is relatively old and, therefore, may not be equipped with certain safety features, e.g. a monitor chamber, and may be less reliable. These considerations must be borne in mind when evaluating suitable quality control programmes.

Some of the areas to be considered for kilovoltage units have been described in previous sections. These are:

(1) filter selection and position;

(2) kV/filtration interlock operation;

(3) measurement of first (and second) HVL as a quality specifier;

(4) measurement of output (dose rate or dose/monitor unit, depending on whether the set is timer or monitor controlled);

(5) verification of applicator (cone) defined SSD and the variation of dose with SSD;

(6) measurement of cone output ratios;

(7) measurement of in-air distributions;

(8) measurement of depth doses for each applicator.

All these, where necessary, must be investigated separately for each kV/filter combination to be used clinically.

Other aspects of the performance of kilovoltage sets that should be considered include the following.

1. Input-voltage stability, which is a common cause of performance problems.

2. Dose-rate stability for each kV/filter combination and for different beam directions. If problems are encountered, kilovoltage and tube current stability should be investigated.

3. The time for the high voltage to rise (or to step up) to maximum, or shutter timing if applicable, which can give rise to timer end effects. End effects can be either positive or negative.

4. Timer (or dose monitor) accuracy, reproducibility, linearity, and end-effect. The tests required will depend on the type of timer (or dose monitor). The reliability of electro-mechanical counters, in particular, may need to be checked regularly.

Table 6.1 Suggested quality control checks on kilovoltage equipment

Check	Frequency	Tolerance
Calibration constancy	Weekly/daily	±5%
Absolute calibration	Yearly	±3%
Timer/monitor		
Accuracy	Monthly	±2%
Linearity/end effect	Yearly	±1%
Dose-rate monitor	Six-monthly	±2%
Beam quality (HVL)	Yearly	±10%
Cone ratios	Yearly	±3%
Field distribution/coverage	Six-monthly	
Applicator distortion	Monthly	±2 mm
Light field/radiation field	Monthly	±2 mm
Collimation axis/radiation axis	Monthly	±2 mm
Timer termination	Daily	
Door interlocks	Daily	
Filter interlocks	Monthly	
Head leakage	Yearly	10 mGy hr^{-1} at 1 m
		300 mGy hr^{-1} at 5 cm[a]

[a]Leakage levels quoted for set operating at 50–500 kV with distances being 1 m from the focal spot and 5 cm from the surface of the tube housing respectively. For sets operating at up to 50 kV, the UK recommendation is 5 mGy hr^{-1} at 5 cm from the surface. Some countries have rather different recommendations.

5. The operation of meters, etc., in particular the dose rate meter that may be present on some sets and which can indicate whether there may be gross errors in kV, mA or filter during treatment. Changes of more than 5% should be investigated.

6. Tube ageing: this is indicated by HVL changes (beam hardening) with time due to target material deposits building up in the exit path of the X-ray beam. Frequent resetting of output factors due to mA variations may also be indicative of this. Once these effects become significant, a new tube is recommended.

7. Checks on the alignment of the applicator axis with its rotation axis, and their agreement with the radiation axis. This ensures that there is no shift of focal spot (due to tube insert shift or other reasons). For diaphragm-controlled sets, similar considerations apply to the alignment of the rotation axis and the radiation axis. The invariance of radiation-field edges, when the collimator is rotated, checks this alignment. Agreement between light field and radiation field is required to within 2 or 3mm. Diaphragm systems on kilovoltage units often have mirrors that are manually removable from the beam for treatment. Therefore, there is a need for interlock checks. Checks are also needed on the movements and positioning of the diaphragms themselves.

8. Applicators must be regularly checked for damage and distortion, where the cone meets the main cutout, where any side wall material may become detached, where any plastic end plate can be cracked or broken, and checked for any distortion of the cone direction and shape.

9. Filter and kV interlocks: interlocks and filter indication at the control panel must be checked regularly. The construction of filters, particularly multi-layer filters, and their condition and integrity must also be inspected. If no interlocks are present, special precautions must be built into operational procedures to ensure correct usage.

10. Other safety systems and interlocks: these include door interlocks; X-rays off controls; back-up timers; and monitors, which must have their function verified at an appropriate frequency.

11. Head leakage: this must be checked, to ensure compliance with national or international guidelines, paying particular attention to joins in shielding. These checks should be made when the equipment is new and after any removal and replacement of shielding.

Some suggested tests and frequencies for kilovoltage X-ray equipment are listed in Table 6.1. Such lists should only be viewed as a starting point and may need to be added to or increased in frequency, depending on design and behaviour of a particular machine. It may also be appropriate to reduce the frequency of some tests, where there is solid evidence to support this. Modification of tolerances may be considered to take into account the specific equipment and local practices, but generally should not be widened significantly. Some of these checks should be carried out for each applicator and/or for each kV/filter combination and some at different beam angles. Other checks can be simplified, for example, the alignment of the tube focus with the applicator axis of rotation only needs to be checked in one position and the same films can be used to check their leakage. The quality control programme can be planned so that a combination of these parameters may be used on a rolling basis so that over a reasonable time period a wide variety of conditions will have been checked.

8. References

British Institute of Radiology (1983). *Central axis depth dose data for use in radiotherapy. BJR*, Supplement 17. BIR, London.

British Institute of Radiology (1996). *Central axis depth dose data for use in radiotherapy. BJR*, Supplement 25. BIR, London.

Carlsson, C.A. (1993). Differences in reported backscatter factors for low energy X-rays: a literature study. *Phys. Med. Biol.*, **38**, 521–31.

Greening, J.R. and Wilson, C.W. (1951). The wavelength of X radiation at a depth in water irradiated by beams of X-rays. *Br. J. Radiol.*, **24**, 605–12.

Grosswendt, B. (1984). Backscatter factors for X-rays generated at voltages between 10 and 100 kV. *Phys. Med. Biol.*, **29**, 579–91.

Grosswendt, B. (1990). Dependence of the photon backscatter for water on source-to-phantom distance and irradiation field size. *Phys. Med. Biol.*, **35**, 1233–45; see also (1993) *Phys. Med. Biol.*, **38**, 305–10.

Harrison, R.M., Walker, C., and Aukett, R.J. (1990). Measurement of backscatter factors for low energy radiotherapy (0.1–2.0 mm) Al HVL) using thermoluminescence dosimetry. *Phys. Med. Biol.*, **35**, 1247–54 (and 1715–6).

Hubbell, J.H. (1982). Photon mass attenuation and energy-absorption coefficients from 1 keV to 20 MeV. *Int. J. Appl. Radiat. Isotop.*, **33**, 1269–90; see also Hubbell, J.H. (1999) Review of photon interaction cross section data in the medical and biological context. *Phys. Med. Biol.*, **44**, R1–22.

IPEMB (1996). Code of practice for the determination of absorbed dose for X-rays below 300 kV generating potential. *Phys. Med. Biol.*, **41**, 2605–25.

Institute of Physical Sciences in Medicine (1991). Report of the IPSM working party on low- and medium-energy X-ray dosimetry. *Phys. Med. Biol.*, **36**, 1027; *Br. J. Radiol.*, **64**, 836–41.

International Atomic Energy Agency (1987). *Absorbed dose determination in photon and electron beams*. IAEA Technical Report Series 277. IAEA, Vienna.

International Atomic Energy Agency (1993). Review of data and methods recommended in the international code of practice. In IAEA Technical Reports Series No. 277. *Absorbed dose determination in photon and electron beams working material*. IAEA, Vienna.

International Atomic Energy Agency (2000). *Absorbed dose determination in external beam radiotherapy based on absorbed-dose-to-water standards: an international code of practice for dosimetry*. IAEA Technical Report Series. IAEA, Vienna. (In press.)

International Commission on Radiation Units and Measurements (1970). *Radiation dosimetry: X-rays generated at 5 to 150 kV*. Report 17. ICRU, Washington, DC.

International Commission on Radiation Units and Measurements (1973). *Measurement of absorbed dose in a phantom irradiated by a single beam of X- or gamma-rays*. Report 23. ICRU, Washington, DC.

International Commission on Radiation Units and Measurements (1989). *Tissue substitutes in radiation dosimetry and measurement*. Report 44. ICRU, Washington, DC.

International Commission on Radiation Units and Measurements (1992). *Photon, electron, proton and neutron interaction data for body tissues*. Report 46 ICRU, Washington, DC.

Klevenhagen, S.C. (1982). The build-up of backscatter in the energy range 1 mm Al to 8 mm Al HVT. *Phys. Med. Biol.*, **27**, 1035–43.

Klevenhagen, S.C. (1989). Experimentally determined backscatter factors for X-rays generated at voltages between 16 and 140 kV. *Phys. Med. Biol.*, **34**, 1871–82.

Klevenhagen, S.C., D'Souza, D., and Bonnefoux, I. (1991). Complications in low-energy X-ray dosimetry caused by electron contamination. *Phys. Med. Biol.*, **36**, 1111–6.

Knight, R.T. (1992). *Backscatter factors for low- and medium-energy X-rays calculated by the Monte Carlo method*. Internal Report ICR-PHYS-1/93. Royal Marsden NHS Trust, Sutton.

Knight, R. and Nahum, A.E. (1994). Depth and field size dependence of ratios of mass energy absorption coefficients, water to air, for kV X-ray dosimetry. In *Proceedings Measurement assurance in dosimetry*. IAEA-SM-330/17, pp. 361–70. IAEA, Vienna.

Li, X.A., Ma, C-M., and Salhani, D. (1997). Measurement of percentage depth dose and lateral beam profiles for kilovoltage X-ray therapy beams. *Phys. Med. Biol.*, **42**, 2561–8.

Ma, C-M., Li, X.A., and Seuntjens J.P. (1999). Study of the dosimetry consistency for kilovoltage, X-ray beams. *Med. Phys.*, **25**, 2376–84.

Ma, C-M. and Seuntjens, J.P., (1999). Mass-energy absorption coefficients and backscatter factor ratios for kilovoltage X-ray beams. *Phys. Med. Biol.*, **44**, 131–43.

NCS (1997). *Dosimetry of low- and medium-energy X-rays*. Report 10 of the Netherlands Commission on Radiation dosimetry. NCS, Delft.

Nisbet, A., Aukett, R.J., Davison, A., Glendinning, A.G., Thwaites, D.I., and Bonnett, D.E. (1999). Kilovoltage X-ray dosimetry for radiotherapy. In *AAPM Symposium Proceedings No 11*, (ed. Ma, C.), AAPM, Maryland, (In press.)

Rosser, K.E. (1998). An alternative beam quality index for medium energy X-ray dosimetry, *Phys. Med. Biol.*, **43**, 587–98

Seuntjens, J., Thierens, H., van der Plaetsen, A., and Segaert, O. (1988). Determination of absorbed dose to water with ionisation chambers calibrated in free air for medium-energy X-rays. *Phys. Med. Biol.*, **33**, 1171–85.

Trout, E.D., Kelley, J.P., and Lucas, A.C. (1960). Determination of half value layer. *Am. J. Roentgenol.*, **84**, 729–40.

Chapter 7

Simulation and imaging for radiation therapy planning

J. Van Dyk and K. Mah

1. Introduction

The process of radiation therapy for malignant disease is complex and involves many steps, as is shown in the block diagram of Figure 7.1. It begins with patient diagnosis, contains a number of steps to patient treatment, and carries through with on-going follow-up. One crucial step in this process is the determination of the location and extent of disease relative to adjacent critical normal tissues. This can be done in a variety of ways, ranging from simple clinical examination to the use of complex imaging modalities, sometimes aided by contrast agents. Another step of the process is the selection of the necessary radiation beams to provide an adequate coverage of the tissues at risk, while minimizing the dose to healthy normal tissues. Before treatment is initiated, this treatment plan needs to be confirmed by an imaging procedure to ensure that the beams traverse the desired anatomical volume and correlate accurately with respect to critical structures.

Computerized tomography (CT) scanners, radiation therapy simulators, and CT simulators play a very important role in these components of the radiation therapy process. In addition, other imaging modalities are used primarily for tumour localization. The most important of these is magnetic resonance imaging (MRI), although single photon emission tomography (SPECT), positron emission tomography (PET), conventional nuclear medicine studies, and ultrasound imaging can provide important planning information for less common situations.

Simulators, CT scanners, and CT simulators can be used for localizing tumour extent and normal tissues. In addition, CT data may be needed for accurate dose calculations accounting for external contours and for variations in internal tissue densities. The simulator is used for the verification of the location of the treatment ports since it simulates the actual treatment geometries. Based on the approved simulated fields, reference marks are placed on the external skin surface of the patient and used for the daily treatment set-up. The CT-simulation process integrates all these functions.

The need for spatial accuracy in these stages of the planning process must be emphasized. Uncertainties in patient reference marks, as well as other uncertainties generated by the simulation or CT procedures, will be propagated throughout the entire treatment course. Therefore, it is important for the users of these devices to understand their limitations and capabilities and to develop strict quality assurance programmes, which regularly monitor their performance.

2. Definitions related to patient planning

The International Commission on Radiation Units and Measurements (ICRU), in an attempt to standardize radiation therapy terminology and dose specification procedures, has provided a number of definitions in ICRU Report 50 (ICRU 1993). These definitions are revisions and advancements over the definitions originally provided in ICRU Report 29 (ICRU 1978). The terminology pertinent to the planning process is summarized in this section with the aid of Figure 7.2.

2.1 Gross tumour volume (GTV)

Figure 7.2(a) illustrates a CT image with a tumour of the lung clearly indicated. The **gross tumour volume (GTV)** is the gross palpable or visible/demonstrable extent and location of malignant growth (ICRU 1993). Thus, what is clearly visible on the CT image of Figure 7.2a is the GTV. The GTV may consist of primary tumour, metastatic lymphadenopthy, or other metastases. No GTV will exist if the tumour mass has been excised. Because the determination of GTV may be dependent on the diagnostic modality (e.g. CT, ultra-

DIAGNOSIS
- tumour pathobiology
- staging

THERAPEUTIC DECISIONS
- cure/palliation
- treatment modalities

IMAGING FOR TREATMENT PLANNING
- CT, MR X-ray, SPECT, PET, other
- Image registration

TARGET VOLUME LOCALIZATION
- tumour/normal tissue definition
- image segmentation
- margins for microscopic spread and patient motion
- field shaping

FABRICATION OF TREATMENT AIDS
- compensators/bolus
- immobilization devices
- blocks/shields/MLC shaping

SIMULATION
- conventional simulation
  - beam design/placement
  - determination of external contours
- virtual simulation/beam display
  - patient marking
  - transfer of plan to marks on patient
- treatment verification
- confirmation of shields

TREATMENT PLANNING
- selection of technique
- computation of dose distribution
- optimization

TREATMENT
- verification of set-up/portal imaging
- verification of equipment performance
- dosimetry checks
- record keeping

PATIENT EVALUATION DURING TREATMENT
- treatment tolerance
- tumour response

PATIENT FOLLOW-UP
- tumour control
- normal tissue response

Figure 7.1 The various steps in the process of external beam radiation therapy. While all the steps are shown, not every patient will require each step, nor will the steps always be in the order indicated.

sound, mammography, palpation), the radiation oncologist should indicate which methods have been used for its determination.

The rationale for the definition of GTV is at least twofold (ICRU 1993). First, an adequate dose must be delivered to the entire GTV in order to obtain local

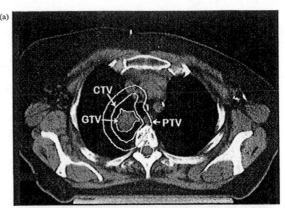

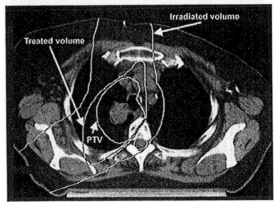

Figure 7.2 (a) A CT image of the mid-thorax showing a cancer of the lung. The obvious tumour mass is outlined as the GTV. The CTV and PTV are also shown. (b) The same CT image as in (a) showing the PTV, the treated volume and the irradiated volume. A two-field technique was used, with anterior and posterior oblique fields of 6 MV X-rays.

control. Second, its identification is necessary to allow for the recording of tumour response in relation to the delivered dose, the variation of dose across the GTV, and other relevant factors.

2.2 Clinical target volume (CTV)

Clinical experience has demonstrated that around the GTV, there is generally subclinical involvement. This could include individual malignant cells, small cell clusters, or microextensions that cannot be detected by staging or diagnostic procedures. The **clinical target volume (CTV)** is a tissue volume that contains a demonstrable GTV and/or subclinical microscopic malignant disease, which has to be eliminated. This volume thus has to be treated adequately in order to achieve the aim of therapy, cure or palliation (ICRU 1993).

The GTV combined with the surrounding volume of local subclinical involvement is usually designated by CTV I. When additional volumes of presumed subclinical spread, such as regional lymph nodes, are included, these are designated as CTV II, CTV III, etc. Figure 7.2a also shows a CTV around the GTV.

For external beam therapy, it is the CTV that has to be irradiated to a specified dose according to the prescribed fractionation scheme. When different doses are prescribed as occurs when a 'boost' is given, there is an implied CTV for each dose level. If there is a change of shape and/or location of the CTV during the course of a treatment, replanning of the patient may be required.

2.3   Planning target volume (PTV)

Ideally, the dose distribution is delivered exactly to the CTV. In practice, however, this is impossible due to:

(1) patient repositioning uncertainties from day-to-day;

(2) CTV movements within the patient as a result of breathing;

(3) changes in CTV shape as a result of issues such as bladder and rectum volume changes; and

(4) uncertainties associated with mechanical set-up, such as field size, gantry angle, collimator rotation, and couch rotation.

For these reasons, the **planning target volume (PTV)** is defined. The PTV is a geometrical concept, and it is defined to select appropriate beam sizes and beam arrangements, taking into consideration the net effect of all the possible geometrical variations, in order to ensure that the prescribed dose is actually absorbed in the CTV (ICRU 1993).

Conceptually, the dose distribution to the PTV has to be considered representative of the dose delivered to the CTV. The PTV is used for planning, prescription, specification, and reporting of dose. From this definition, it is clear that PTV is strictly a static, geometrical concept and is related to the beams through a fixed co-ordinate system. Indeed, it may surpass normal anatomical boundaries, such as unaffected bony structures, or even extend into air. The PTV is identical to the 'target volume' as defined in the older ICRU Report 29 (ICRU 1978). A typical PTV for lung cancer is shown in Figure 7.2a.

While Figure 7.2a shows the tumour and target volumes in a single two-dimensional plane, it needs to be emphasized that all tumour and target volumes contain a third dimension that is different from the one on the central plane. While in the past practical considerations often limited planning to a relatively few two-dimensional planes, the increased use of CT and MR scanners is providing the information in the third dimension much more readily.

2.4   Treated volume

Because of the geometric arrangement of radiation beams, the high dose region is usually larger than the

PTV. The **treated volume** is the volume enclosed by an isodose surface, selected and specified by the radiation oncologist as being appropriate to achieve the purpose of treatment (e.g. tumour eradication, palliation) (ICRU 1993). Sometimes the treated volume is nearly the same as the planning target volume, while at other times the treated volume is substantially larger, depending on the complexity and geometry of the radiation beams. Figure 7.2b illustrates the treated volume used to cover the PTV.

2.5   Irradiated volume

During normal treatment, radiation beams must traverse normal tissues in front of and/or behind the PTV. The **irradiated volume** is that tissue volume that receives a dose that is considered significant in relation to normal tissue tolerance (ICRU 1993). The significant absorbed dose level can be expressed in absolute dose or as a percentage (e.g. 50%) of the dose specified to the PTV. Figure 7.2b also illustrates the irradiated volume based on the two-field technique used to treat the PTV.

2.6   Organs at risk

Organs at risk are normal tissues whose radiation sensitivity may significantly influence treatment planning and/or prescribed dose (ICRU 1993). Again, possible movements of the organ at risk, as well as set-up uncertainties during the course of treatment, need to be considered. ICRU Report 50 (1993) divided organs at risk into three different classes:

1. **Class I organs**: radiation lesions are fatal or result in severe morbidity.

2. **Class II organs**: radiation lesions result in moderate to mild morbidity.

3. **Class III organs**: radiation lesions are mild, transient, and reversible, or result in no significant morbidity.

2.7   Absorbed dose distribution

Due to variations in dose delivery for different clinical sites, as well as different approaches that are evolving with three-dimensional (3-D) conformal radiation therapy (CRT), different concepts for dose prescription and recording are required. Generally, when planning a patient for treatment, an irradiation technique is developed that provides a maximum and uniform dose to the planning target volume and minimizes the dose to both the treated volume and the irradiated volume. However, in practice it is difficult to achieve the ideal dose distribution and some dose heterogeneity has to be accepted. ICRU (1993) recommends that this dose variation should be kept within +7% and −5% of the prescribed dose. Variation beyond these limits will need to be assessed on an individual basis by the radiation oncologist for acceptability. For palliative or subclinical disease, larger variations in dose delivery are often acceptable.

New imaging modalities and modern 3-D radiation therapy planning systems (RTPS) have the capability of handling the patient anatomy in full 3-D. Thus, it is important to generate anatomic data that will allow the extreme outlines of the GTV, CTV, PTV organs at risk, and tissue heterogeneities for dose calculations and external contours to be determined. The GTV, CTV, PTV, and organs at risk are required for beam placement and dose evaluation purposes, while the tissue heterogeneities and external contours are requirements for accurate dose calculations. In many instances, the organs at risk will have to be imaged in their entirety – even if the beam is only interacting with a fractional part of the organ. This is required because dose–volume histograms (Chapter 9, Section 1.3.3) are based on the fractional volume of the organ that is irradiated to a dose equal to or more than a particular dose.

For dose specification, ICRU has also defined various quantities:

1. **Maximum dose:** the maximum dose within the PTV, and the maximum dose at tissues outside the PTV A maximum dose volume is generally considered clinically meaningful if its minimum diameter exceeds 15 mm.

2. **Minimum dose:** the smallest dose in a defined volume. No volume limit is recommended for a minimum dose.

3. **Average dose:** the average of the dose values at the discrete dose-calculation points uniformly distributed in the volume in question.

4. **Median dose:** the central value of the doses at the discrete dose-calculation points uniformly distributed in the volume in question.

5. **Modal dose:** the dose that occurs most frequently at the discrete dose-calculation points uniformly distributed in the volume in question.

6. **Hot spots:** a hot spot represents a volume outside of the PTV, which receives a dose larger than 100% of the specified PTV dose. As for the maximum dose, the volume of a hot spot is considered clinically meaningful if its minimum diameter exceeds 15 mm.

2.7.1 The ICRU reference dose

The ICRU recommendations for dose reporting are based on the selection of a point within the PTV, which is referred to as the ICRU reference point. This point is to be selected according to the following criteria:

(1) the dose at the point should be clinically relevant and representative of the dose throughout the PTV;

(2) the point should be easy to define in a clear and unambiguous way;

(3) the point should be selected where the dose can be accurately determined;

(4) the point should be selected in a region where there is no steep dose gradient.

Thus, the ICRU reference point is firstly located at the centre, or in the central region, of the PTV, and secondly, on or near the central rays of the beams.

The dose at the ICRU reference point is the ICRU reference dose, and should always be reported. Variations in dose delivery to the PTV should also be recorded including at least minimum and maximum doses and possibly some of the other statistical dose values described above. In addition, dose–volume histograms or biologically weighted doses should be calculated as is appropriate and as might be required by clinical trials groups.

3. Methods of deriving patient-specific data

3.1 Patient positioning

One of the major uncertainties in dose delivery to the patient relates to the ability to set up the patient accurately and reproducibly from day to day. Therefore, it is important that, at the outset of the planning process, a comfortable and reproducible patient position is developed. The specific patient-positioning strategy will depend strongly on the volume to be irradiated. High-dose, small-volume techniques might require millimetre precision, whereas some large-volume techniques might allow a larger tolerance. Examples of the former are small-field eye treatments or stereotactic radiosurgery, and examples of the latter are whole abdominal fields and half- or total-body irradiation. Precise immobilization will help in reducing the margins required around the CTV to generate the PTV.

A number of techniques can be used to aid in reproducible patient positioning. These are summarized in Table 7.1 and are broadly divided into four categories:

(1) no immobilization;

(2) simple immobilization;

(3) complex immobilization;

(4) monitoring techniques.

Category (1) involves only patient-positioning aids, such as three-point laser set-ups, pillows, headrests, etc. For these set-up procedures, it is possible that the patient position might change during the actual beam-on time. Hence a review of patient set-up immediately after

Table 7.1 Patient positioning aids

No immobilization
   Head or neck rests
   Three-point laser set-up
   Upper-body elevator (breast technique)
   Indexed arm/hand poles
   Well-defined measurements (e.g. chin to sternal notch)
   Vacuum sandbags
   Foam cushions
   Specially constructed couch attachments
   Pillows
   Styrofoam shoulder wedges

Simple immobilization
   Tape chin or body straps
   Lateral head supports
   Bite blocks

Complex immobilization
   Casts, shells, moulds
   Expandable styrofoam
   Stereotactic head frame
   'Bunny wrapping' for children

Monitoring techniques
   Remote TV viewing
   TV monitoring with difference images comparing present set-up to initial set-up
   Port films
   Repeat simulator films
   Real-time electronic portal imaging

treatment will give some indication of its stability. Category (2) involves some restriction of movement and requires the patient's voluntary help. Category (3) involves individualized immobilization devices that restrict patient motion and ensure reproducible patient positioning. Category (4) includes techniques for monitoring patient positioning and reproducibility of set-up, and may or may not be used in conjunction with immobilization devices. However, the results of these monitoring techniques provide input information as to improvements that may be required in the immobilization techniques used. Television monitoring provides a means of detecting obvious changes in patient position. Real-time electronic portal imaging provides a means of observing patient positioning, although the resultant image gives a beam's eye perspective of the irradiated volume. Both of these techniques allow the radiographer (radiation therapist or radiation therapy technologist) to make positioning adjustments either before giving a full daily dose from all fields or by stopping the irradiation during treatment.

Several additional observations can be made regarding patient positioning.

1. If possible, the patient should be treated in one position only. Both internal anatomy and external contours can change dramatically if, for example, the patient is treated in both the supine and prone positions for anterior and posterior fields, respectively.

2. The treatment position may be constrained due to equipment limitations. For example, the limited aperture size of the CT scanner or the distance between the patient and the collimator assembly on the therapy machine as it rotates about the patient may constrain the arm positions. However, the patient-treatment position must be based on the procedures used during the planning process.

3. Clinical considerations may restrict patient positioning. Patient pain and discomfort or physical disabilities might result in very limited positioning.

4. Informing patients about the technical details of their treatment will allow them to aid in set-up and in remaining stationary during treatment.

5. Some special procedures will help the reproducibility of patient anatomy. Emptying the bladder in a consistent manner before treatment will provide more reproducible pelvic treatments. In some situations, especially for young children, analgesics and/or anaesthetics may be required.

6. Patient's clothes may interfere with the set-up.

7. Sliding the patient along a couch top may skew the skin marks. Careful attention should be given to ensure that the positioning procedure is performed reproducibly.

8. Simulation or CT scanning of patients on solid couch tops, while treating them on couch tops with stretchable 'tennis rackets' or Mylar windows, can result in discrepancies between the planned volume and the irradiated volume, as well as the delivered radiation dose.

9. The involvement of the same radiation therapy radiographer throughout the course of a patient's treatment can improve the reproducibility of daily set-ups and treatment. This familiarity can be extremely valuable, particularly for non-standard techniques.

10. Good record-keeping and the use of Polaroid pictures taken on simulation will help the radiographers reproduce the patient set-up.

11. The use of additional skin marks for field borders will aid in reproducing unusual treatment geometries, especially for positioning body extremities such as the arms or legs.

12. Under some circumstances, critical normal tissues may need to be moved out of the field or away from the field edge. Examples of this include rotation of the eye to spare the lens or testicle positioning to minimize gonadal dose. Occasionally, ovaries are moved surgically to locate them away from the irradiated volume.

3.2 *Measurement of external contours and internal anatomy*

The determination of accurate dose distributions and the corresponding delivery of the prescribed dose requires patient-specific information on body contours accompanied by external reference marks to align the incident radiation beams. Many methods of measuring external contours have been developed (Andrew and Aldrich 1982; Day and Harrison 1983; Sternick 1983), some of which are summarized in Table 7.2. These methods can range from the use of simple lead wire or mechanical pointers to more complex imaging techniques, such as ultrasound or CT scans. Patient positioning is also an important consideration for contour measurements, since the contours must reproduce the patient shape when in the treatment position.

While this report cannot recommend any particular contouring technique, the manual method that has probably been used most frequently is the lead wire or flexicurve, which is placed in position on the skin surface and bent to follow the patient's contour. Any reference

Table 7.2 Methods of patient contour determination

Mechanical
  Manual point measurement
    Single rods
    Multiple rods in one dimension
    Multiple rods in two dimensions
  Manual with lead wire or flexicurves
  Manual with mechanical coupling to recording on chart paper
  Manual with electronic coupling to display
  Automatic with mechanical coupling
  Use of acrylic or plaster cast

Optical
  Optical distance indicator on simulator or therapy unit
  Oblique viewing on television system; allows for digitization
  Stereophotographic
  Photogrammetry
  Moiré topography

Ultrasonic
  B-mode, similar to mechanical pointer
  Gives limited information on internal anatomy

Radiological
  Radiographs: either AP and lateral or oblique views
  CT scanning: gives detailed information on external contours and internal anatomy.

Magnetic resonance imaging
  Provides detailed information on external contours and internal anatomy; bone shows as low intensity; subject to geometric distortions

marks on the skin are marked on the wire. This is then carefully transferred to drawing paper and a direct tracing is made, including the reference marks. While this method is simple, it is prone to distortion in the wire's shape during transfer from the patient to the paper. To minimize this distortion, vertical and/or horizontal measurements can be taken between the contour reference marks and a fixed surface or point (e.g. couch top, isocentre) and these measurements can be transferred to the drawing paper. The relative distances provide a second check on the transferred contour.

A much more accurate technique involves the use of a mechanical pointer that is coupled to a device (pantograph) that traces onto drawing paper. As the pointer is traced along the patient's skin surface, the contour is directly transferred onto paper. This device is capable of providing very accurate contour measurements, although some difficulty may be encountered if contours are required around the couch side of the patient. A range-finder method can be used in conjunction with any isocentrically mounted simulator or therapy unit that has an optical distance indicator (ODI). The patient is positioned at the isocentre and ODI (range finder) readings are taken at various gantry angles. These data are then converted to distances from the isocentre and transferred to paper or to a computer to yield the patient contour. While this method is useful for relatively shallow contour gradients, as are found in the pelvic, abdominal, or thoracic regions, it does not produce accurate contours when the slopes change rapidly as is possible in the head and neck region.

Recent emphasis is on the derivation of three-dimensional information that can be entered digitally into the treatment-planning computer. While CT scanning is by far the most superior technique, since it provides information on target volume, internal densities, and external contours, it may not be cost-effective if only external contours are required for dose computations. The particular choice of device used for contour determination depends on whether the dose determination will be based on a single point, a two-dimensional plane, or a three-dimensional volume calculation. In general, an accuracy of 5 mm should be attained for contour measurements, although greater accuracy may be required for some special techniques such as 3-D CRT and stereotactic radiosurgery.

4. Simulators

4.1 *Role of treatment simulation*

The radiation therapy simulator is a diagnostic X-ray machine mounted on a rotating gantry that provides geometries identical with those found on megavoltage therapy machines. Simulators can be used in either a radiographic or a fluoroscopic mode to provide diagnostic quality images on a film or a television monitor, respectively. The simulator can be used at various stages during the planning or treatment process for the following purposes.

1. Tumour and normal tissue localization. The simulator might be used to determine the extent of tumour or the proximity of critical structures. To aid this process, radiographic contrast agents and medical procedures, such as cystoscopy, may be employed concurrently. At this stage decisions regarding beam arrangements are yet to be made.

2. Treatment simulation. Once a decision has been made regarding target volume and relevant normal tissue locations, a trial selection of numbers of beams, their directions, and their sizes can be made. These beams can be simulated using the radiographic or fluoroscopic systems and will mimic the real radiation therapy beams with respect to geometric divergence and volume of anatomy exposed. This simulation trial can then be modified to optimize the proposed treatment technique.

3. Treatment plan verification. It is possible that a treatment plan is developed without the use of step (1) and/or step (2), as might be done with CT planning. In this case, a radiographic confirmation of the plan might be made to ensure proper target-volume coverage and minimal normal-tissue coverage. This check is particularly relevant at off-axis locations, if the treatment plan is designed in two-dimensions only. Furthermore, the physical reference depths measured on the simulator must confirm the depths predicted by the treatment plan to ensure accurate dose delivery on the therapy machine.

4. Treatment monitoring. A review of the treatment procedure can be made at various stages during the treatment course. This might be done for a variety of reasons including:
    (a) a simple check of treatment reproducibility;
    (b) a concern about change of anatomy as a result of tumour shrinkage or patient weight-loss with a corresponding effect on beam location;
    (c) confirmation of boost fields or additional shielding part way through treatment.

4.2 *Specifications*

The typical radiation therapy simulator features a rotating gantry with a diagnostic X-ray tube at one end and an image intensifier coupled with a film cassette holder at the other. Figure 7.3 is a schematic diagram of a simulator with its various motions and components, including the patient support assembly (also known as the patient couch or table).

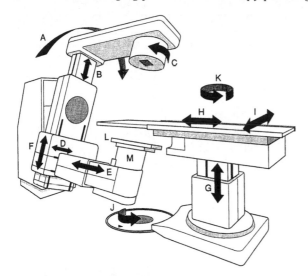

Figure 7.3 The basic components and motions of a radiation therapy simulator: A, gantry rotation; B, source–axis distance (SAD); C, collimator rotation; D, image intensifier (lateral); E, image intensifier (longitudinal); F, image intensifier (radial); G, patient table (vertical); H, patient table (longitudinal); I, patient table (lateral); J, patient table rotation about isocentre; K, patient table rotation about pedestal; L, film cassette; M, image intensifier. Motions not shown: (a) field size delineation; (b) radiation beam diaphragms; (c) source–tray distance.

seven major mechanical motions of a simulator are summarized in Figure 7.3 and include:

(1) gantry rotation;

(2) source–axis distance (SAD) motion in the radial direction;

(3) collimator rotation;

(4) image intensifier motion in the lateral, longitudinal, and radial directions;

(5) table translation in the vertical, longitudinal, and lateral directions;

(6) table rotations both about the isocentre and the pedestal;

(7) mechanical motions of the X-ray field collimators and treatment field delineator wires (see representative simulator radiograph in Figure 7.4).

For each motion, it is important to note its extent, speed, read-out, and accuracy in both the manual operator mode and the automated set-up mode, if available. Various authors (Connors *et al.* 1984; Doppke 1987) have published sample specification data for a number of commercially available simulators. The implementation of asymmetric diaphragms has resulted in additional controls and read-outs.

Controls for many of these mechanical parameters can be found both inside the simulator room and at the

Ideally, the therapy simulator should mimic all the mechanical features and geometric field arrangements of the radiation therapy treatment machines. This includes accessories for trays, such as shielding, which should be identical in size and distance from the source as they are on the therapy machine. Thus, to allow for variation from different manufacturers, the source–tray distance may have to be variable. Under some conditions, simulators can be more restrictive than therapy machines because of the bulky image intensifier. This is particularly true when simultaneous couch and gantry rotations are required.

The design specifications of a simulator can be divided into three broad topics:

(1) mechanical;

(2) X-ray source;

(3) image detection.

Each of these topics will be discussed in the following sections.

4.2.1 Mechanical specifications

Designed to mimic various radiation therapy machines based on different designs from different manufacturers, and requiring an image detection system, simulators are constructed with multiple motions and read-outs. The

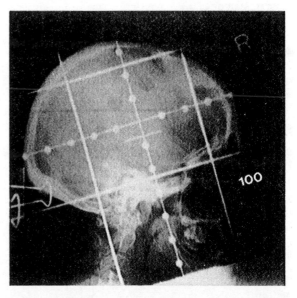

Figure 7.4 Simulator film of a lateral skull showing field-edge delineators, cross-hairs, and magnification graticule with beads projecting at 2-cm intervals at the isocentre. The patient is wearing a plastic cast. Included on the film are lead beads on the anterior surface of the cast for measurement purposes. On the posterior (left) side are clamps for immobilizing the plastic cast.

simulator control console. The latter allows for the remote control of these parameters, while the beam is on in the fluoroscopic mode. Most manufacturers now provide some kind of anticollision device in order to preclude patient–machine contact and to prevent collision between different components of the simulator. Many simulators also provide motion-enable buttons or bars for safety reasons. Motion read-outs need to be assessed for accuracy (or calibration), linearity, and point of origin. These should all be consistent with the treatment machines, particularly if they are computer-linked for record-and-verify systems or for dynamic therapy. It is also important to check for correctness of read-outs of field size at different SADs. Some simulators also have a graticule consisting of a series of radio-opaque dots or lines that project a constant spacing as defined at the isocentre or reference distance. These can be seen on Figure 7.4.

An additional consideration, in the context of mechanical specifications, is the ability to add ancillary devices to the simulator using the same geometrical constraints as would be found on radiation therapy machines. Most manufacturers now provide the ability to attach beam block tray assemblies at variable source–tray distances. However, for some simulators, these block tray assemblies do not rotate with the collimator, whereas on the therapy machines they do.

It should be recognized that some simulators are not able to support the full weight of a shielding tray with blocks, and thus some form of simulated blocking (using, for example, lead wire, lead rubber, or aluminium-coated Styrofoam) may be required. Some simulators also provide the ability to implement electron beam cones as attachments that can be used in the simulation process.

Table 7.3 is adapted from a previously published report (Brahme 1988) and provides the performance standards for the mechanical, radiation, and optical systems of a simulator. The tolerance defines the specification of the machine at the time of installation and its acceptance within the department. The Interna-

Table 7.3 Performance standards for mechanical, radiation, and optical systems of a radiation therapy simulator

Parameter	Tolerance level	Action level
Gantry rotation		
Radius of sphere of convergence	1.0 mm	2.0 mm
Delineator lines		
Perpendicularity (X-ray image)	90 $\pm 1°$	Four lengths of diagonals within 1.0 mm of each other
Agreement of field size on X-ray image with indication(s)	0.5 mm	1.0 mm $\leq 15 \times 15$ cm^2 2.0 mm $> 15 \times 15$ cm^2
X-ray and optical image congruence	1.5 mm	2.0 mm
Cross-hair intersection		
X-ray image wander	0.5 mm	1.0 mm
Optical image wander	0.5 mm	1.0 mm
X-ray and optical image coincidence	0.5 mm	1.0 mm
X-ray image shift with focal spot change	0.5 mm	0.5 mm
Central axes (intersection of diagonals)		
X-ray image wander	0.5 mm	1.0 mm
X-ray image coincidence with cross-hair intersection on X-ray image	0.5 mm	1.0 mm
X-ray image coincidence with central axis on optical image	1.0 mm	1.0 mm
X-ray image coincidence with cross-hair intersection on optical image	1.0 mm	1.0 mm
SAD variation		
Cross-hair intersection wander (X-ray image)	1.0 mm	1.0 mm
Accuracy of field at SAD (X-ray image) with indicator (if so equipped)	1.0 mm	Within 1.0 mm of (150 $\pm$ 1) (SAD/100)
Accuracy of SAD and SSD indicators	1.0 mm	1.0 mm digital 2.0 mm mechanical
Table movement		
Cross-hair intersection (X-ray wander) with vertical motion	1.0 mm	2.0 mm
Cross-hair intersection (X-ray image) wander with table rotation	2.0 mm	2.0 mm
Difference in vertical deflection with patient load relative to treatment table	2.0 mm	3.0 mm

All measurements except those requiring SAD or table height variation to be made at 100 cm. From Brahme (**1988**).

tional Electrotechnical Commission (IEC) and the British Institute of Radiology (BIR) (Bomford *et al.* 1989) have also proposed similar data.

4.2.2 X-ray source specifications

A major difference between conventional radiography and therapy simulation is the large distance between the focal spot and the image receptor. This is typically between 100 and 170 cm for simulators. This reduces the beam intensity and, depending on the location of the image detector, could result in increased scatter to the detector. Furthermore, simulation often involves a radiographic beam–patient geometry not normally used in conventional radiography, such as lateral or oblique views through large body thicknesses. Target-volume localization often involves longer fluoroscopy times. As a result, the tube and generator ratings need to be substantially greater than for conventional radiology. In the past, a three-phase generator capable of high radiographic outputs with minimal voltage regulation was considered desirable. However, the advent of high-frequency generators has led to a reduction of their size and to a total dynamic and instantaneous control of exposure factors. Thus high-frequency generators would now be preferred.

A further requirement is that the simulator produces an image on an X-ray film identical with that visualized during fluoroscopy. This will only be possible if the focal spots for the two imaging modes coincide. While a large focus–object distance allows for a larger focal spot size, image sharpness of fine field-defining wires (Figure 7.4) or sharp anatomic boundaries requires a small focal spot size.

McCullough and Earle (1979) have reviewed both the radiographic and fluoroscopic needs of a simulator. For radiographic procedures, an acceptable generator would provide 600 mA at 80 kV_p (three-phase). In considering fluoroscopic requirements and using several relevant clinical geometries, they concluded that the desirable X-ray generator should provide a minimum of 10 mA at 60–130 kV_p as independent variables on a continuous basis. Exposure reproducibility and linearity are important considerations for ensuring consistent quality of the radiographic images. Exposures should be reproducible to 5% and maximum deviations from linearity in microgray per milliampere-second ($\mu Gy\ mAs^{-1}$) should also be less than 5%.

4.2.3 Image detection specifications

Large-screen image intensifiers are required if large therapy beams are to be visualized in their entirety. However, it must be recognized that there may have to be a compromise between phosphor diameter and axial tube length if geometric constraints in some set-ups are to be

avoided. Generally, image intensifiers that are 30–35 cm (12–14 in) in diameter are found to be the most practical for therapy simulation.

Both the radiographic and fluoroscopic modes must provide high-quality images so that appropriate image resolution and contrast is maintained. Some simulators are equipped with automatic exposure controls for the radiographic mode and automatic brightness controls for the fluoroscopic mode. While these functions are useful for ease of settings on the controls, the adequacy of these functions must be thoroughly checked and maintained to ensure optimal image quality under relevant clinical conditions.

For the radiographic mode, an important consideration is the maximum film cassette size possible on the simulator. Many companies provide cassettes of dimensions $35 \times 35\ cm^2$ ($14 \times 14\ in^2$) maximum, although larger cassettes are often preferred since radiation therapy field sizes can be as large as $40 \times 40\ cm^2$ at the patient and therefore larger at the film. Cassettes and grids should be chosen to provide the largest films possible with the specifications that provide diagnostic images of the best possible quality.

Film processing is an integral part of image detection when using the radiographic mode and requires strict quality control to maintain optimum image quality. Radiation therapy simulation may require film processors capable of handling larger format films (i.e. greater than $35 \times 35\ cm^2$) and possibly low daily processor workloads.

4.2.4 Additional considerations

Design constraints

In general, the simulator geometries should mimic those on the radiation therapy machines. In practice, there are some situations that are impossible to simulate because of differences between the therapy unit and the simulator. One such constraint is the combined rotation of both the gantry and the treatment couch to yield an oblique beam with respect to the patient's longitudinal axis. While such oblique beams can be achieved on therapy machines that do not have beam stoppers, simulators are unable to simulate such set-ups because of the interference from large image intensifiers. This is not a problem for the virtual simulation process described later in Section 6.

Therapy machine heads are usually larger than simulator heads because of shielding requirements on megavoltage machines; therefore, the floor–isocentre height is usually lower on the simulator (typically 115–125 cm) than on the therapy machines (typically 120–130 cm). While a lower isocentre height is advantageous from a radiographer's perspective, it may cause severe constraints for some specific patient set-ups on the simulator. For example, some institutions treat cancer of the breast by positioning the patient on a special upper-body elevator that slopes the patient's superior–inferior chest contour to be almost horizontal. However, this elevation of the patient results in a substantial lowering of the couch top below the isocentre, since the treatment volume is located anteriorly in the patient. On some simulators with a low floor–isocentre distance, this set-up may not be possible because of the size of the intervening image intensifier.

Simulator couch

Ideally, the couch on the simulator should be identical with that on the therapy machine, although compatibility becomes difficult when treatment machines from different manufacturers are in use. However, the couch should be radiographically transparent throughout the region used for imaging. This precludes the use of bars or any metallic support that can be found on therapy machine couches. Most therapy couches have a 'tennis racket' or Mylar window to allow for skin sparing for upward-directed fields. Generally, simulator couch tops are hard and will not provide the same flex as therapy couch tops with thin windows. These differences can result in discrepancies in target-volume irradiations, typically by 0.5–1.0 cm, in comparison with the simulated geometry. For those simulator couch tops that offer 'tennis rackets' or Mylar windows, the area of the window should equal that on the treatment machine in order to achieve equivalent flex and adequate field coverage. The longitudinal flex of the couch due to patient weight should be minimal and comparable with that on the therapy unit. Ideally, the couch width should be identical with that on the therapy unit to ensure identical patient set-ups and to reduce the probability of machine head–couch collisions.

Optical positioning lights

Accurate patient positioning and beam alignment are crucial components of the simulation process. Once the appropriate beam locations have been determined, reference marks for the purpose of patient treatment are placed on the patient's skin surface. Generally, three optical systems aid in this process:

(1) field light with cross-hairs to show the radiation field outline and its centre on the skin surface;

(2) ODI, which is used to indicate the source–skin distance (SSD) or the SAD;

(3) laser-positioning lights to provide an optical indication of the position of the isocentre.

The first two are an integral component of all simulators, whereas the laser-positioning lights are wall- and ceiling-mounted and generally considered to be optional equipment by the simulator manufacturers (see Figure 7.5). Lasers A and B in Figure 7.5 identify the horizontal line through the isocentre perpendicular to the

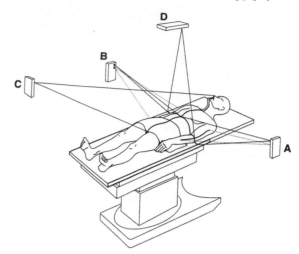

Figure 7.5 Schematic diagram of the laser lights as they are positioned on the simulator and therapy machines. A and B are lateral wall-lasers providing one vertical line and one horizontal line. C is a laser-mounted on the wall nearest the foot-end of the couch. D is the ceiling laser to provide a transverse line.

axis of rotation of the gantry and axis of the couch turntable. Laser C in Figure 7.5 is used to define the vertical plane containing the axis of gantry rotation. This plane is useful for initially positioning the patient on the couch to ensure that the longitudinal axis of the patient is coincident with the gantry axis of rotation. A fourth ceiling-mounted laser (laser D in Figure 7.5) provides a transverse line through the central ray. While this laser does not provide any light marks on the patient when the gantry is in the vertical position, it does provide an important check on patient positioning when the gantry is angled obliquely. With the gantry in the vertical position, the field light with cross-hairs is used to indicate the axis of the collimator and couch rotations.

An important component of commissioning and quality assurance protocols for simulator installations is to ensure that all the optical systems are aligned accurately. Patient reference marks are usually based on these light systems. The same alignment is used with similar optical systems on the radiation therapy machines. All these optical systems should be checked for consistency both at the isocentre and at other distances.

4.3 Selection criteria, purchase, and acceptance

The complexities of a modern simulator have made the selection process onerous and difficult. On the one hand, the simulator must be able to emulate all the megavoltage therapy equipment and techniques in a particular department. On the other hand, the simulator should provide the best possible diagnostic quality images in both the radiographic and fluoroscopic modes. The complexity of a modern simulator is reflected in its cost, which has become substantial (almost 65% of a single-beam low-energy linear accelerator, and about 50% of a dual-photon and multi-electron energy linear accelerator). Furthermore, various committees have recommended that every radiation therapy department should have at least one simulator (Bomford *et al.* 1989; ISCRO 1991). The actual number of simulators per department will be dependent on various factors, including number of radiation therapy courses, types of treatments (i.e. palliative versus radical), types and complexities of treatment techniques, average number of simulations per treatment course, the number of studies requiring contrast agents, and whether or not a CT-simulator is available. Most oncologists would recommend one simulator for every three to four megavoltage machines, although this number will be dependent on the various factors listed above.

Mechanical considerations are an important component of the selection process. The simulator should be able to reproduce techniques used routinely in the department including extended-distance, large irregular field techniques. Perhaps the latter, as would be required for routine 'upper-mantle' irradiation for Hodgkin's disease or large abdominal fields for cancer of the ovary, provide one of the greatest constraints on modern simulators. The large field sizes often do not fit on conventional films, and special films, cassettes, and holders may have to be developed. Thus, each department will have to assess its particular techniques to ensure that these can be simulated by the machine of choice.

McCullough and Earle (1979) have provided an excellent review of the factors to consider in the selection process. Selection considerations include the following:

(1) motions and read-outs;

(2) X-ray and image receptor systems;

(3) mechanical tolerances and limits;

(4) collision avoidance and other safety features;

(5) ease of use;

(6) ability to use with computers, record-and-verify systems, and oncology management systems of other manufacturers;

(7) warranty, service, and parts availability;

(8) options and extras;

(9) cost.

Several authors (Connors *et al.* 1984; Doppke 1987) have tabulated the technical specifications for a number of commercial radiation therapy simulators. Such a review is an essential component of the selection process, so that there is a clear understanding of the capabilities and limitations of each simulator currently available on the market. In addition to the technical specifications, installation requirements also need to be addressed, especially if the simulator requires a floor pit for its base. Some simulators require pits that are up to 33 cm deep and thus require a substantial floor depression if a raised floor with ramps is to be avoided. Other simulators are floor-mounted or require shallow depressions. The resulting side-pedestal design of some such simulators provides adequate patient-support stability, although patient access by the radiographer may be limited to one side only.

The comparison of motion read-out conventions of treatment units with that of the simulator is an important component of the selection process. Inconsistent read-outs can generate confusion and are a potential source of treatment error. Indeed, under some conditions, there may be an advantage in purchasing simulators and therapy machines from the same manufacturer, although this is not always a prerequisite. Ideally, all manufacturers should use the same convention, as has been proposed by the IEC, for example. Table-top size and the use of patient-repositioning devices should be very similar to those on the therapy machines.

The process of purchasing a new simulator should include the following considerations.

(1) Definition of the departmental requirements.

(2) Acquisition and comparison of the specifications of all commercial simulators.

(3) Review of these data and the elimination of any products that do not fit the departmental requirements; short-listing of the remaining machines.

(4) Site visits to see the top two or three machines. Site visits are best carried out at institutions that are using these machines clinically. The visiting team should preferably include a physicist, radiographer, and a radiation oncologist. If possible, the image quality should be tested as part of the visit.

(5) Call for tender. This should include a request for specifications and quotations on all optional items.

(6) Purchase. The purchase order should include a set of well-defined acceptance tests. If the manufacturer has defined these, the adequacy and completeness of the tests should be reviewed and revised as necessary since manufacturer's tests often constitute a minimum assessment. Various reports (Brahme 1988; Bomford *et al.* 1989; McCullough and Earle 1979) have provided a detailed set of tests that can be used as a guideline.

Before acceptance testing or clinical implementation, a radiation survey should be performed in areas around the simulator room to ensure the adequacy of the room's

YEAR: _____   UNIT: _____

MONTH: _____

NO.	TEST	FREQUENCY	M	T	W	T	F	M	T	W	T	F
	DATE:											
1	warning lights	daily										
2	door interlocks	daily										
3	emergency switches	daily										
4	dead-man switches	daily										
5	collision device	daily										
6	gantry angle	daily										
7	O.D.I.	daily										
8	laser lights	daily										
9	light/radiation field	daily										
10	light/numerical field	daily										
11	cross-hairs alignment	daily										
12	focus film distance measurement	daily										
13	image processor test	daily										
14	exposure reproducibility measurement	6 months										
15	exposure linearity measurement	6 months										
16	half value layer measurement	6 months										
17	peak kilovoltage measurement	6 months										
18	automatic exposure termination	6 months										
19	fluoroscopic resolution test	6 months										
20	fluoroscopic exposure rate control test	6 months										

Figure 7.6 An example QC form listing the tests and their corresponding frequency of performance.

shielding for the safety of staff, visitors, and patients. Standard protocols for radiation safety of diagnostic radiological equipment can be used (Lin *et al.* 1988).

4.4 Quality assurance

The simulator quality assurance (QA) programme includes a series of systematic tests to ensure that the simulator continues to perform according to a set of predefined standards. Since a simulator consists of three main subsystems, standards and tests should be defined to ensure the quality of each of these subsystems. These subsystems include the following:

(1) the mechanical system;

(2) the image-forming system;

(3) the image detection system of which the film processor is an important component.

A number of the quality control (QC) tests of the mechanical aspects of the simulator are similar to those described in Chapter 5 for linear accelerators.

Figure 7.6 gives an example of a series of safety and QC tests and their corresponding frequency of performance. The first five tests are basic safety tests. Tests 6–12 are QC tests of the mechanical system, including the various read-outs and light versus radiation field sizes. Tests 13–20 relate to the image forming and detection systems. While test results are usually classified as acceptable and unacceptable, some QC test results can be defined to be marginal.

An **acceptable** result is defined as follows:

(1) for a safety test, a test that is completely successful;

(2) for a QC test, a result that is within the stated tolerance.

A **marginal result**, for some tests, such as 6–12 that have tight tolerances, is a result beyond the stated tolerance but less than or equal to twice the stated tolerance. A marginal result occurring once does not require direct action; however, if it occurs repeatedly, corrective action is required.

An **unacceptable** result is defined as follows:

(1) for a safety test, a test which is not completed successfully;

(2) for QC tests, such as 6–12, a result that is beyond more than twice the stated tolerance;

(3) for QC tests, such as 13–20, a result that is beyond the stated tolerance.

Unacceptable results require immediate corrective action.

Figure 7.6 is a typical QC result sheet that contains a summary of the outcome of each QC test as it is performed. The procedure for each test is detailed in a simulator QA manual. Some of the tests require special QC equipment. For example, tests 6–12 require a mechanical level for testing the gantry angle, a special lucite jig with levelling screws positioned on the patient-support assembly for testing the ODI, the laser lights, the light field, and cross-hairs, and the light and radiation field coincidence (8–10). Some institutions will build their own QC equipment, although some of it can be purchased commercially. The X-ray image-forming and image-detection systems require the use of special equipment (Gray *et al.* 1983), such as a digital-dosimeter system, aluminium sheets for HVL measurements, a kV_p meter, a contrast resolution test tool, and a sensitometer and densitometer for assessing the image processor. It must be emphasized that Figure 7.6 is only an example of QC tests as performed on particular simulators. Other simulators may require some additional tests as they relate to the emergency hand pendant, automatic load and unload functions, and electron applicators. In this sense, every institution will need to assess and develop its own specific QC tests. While it is beyond the scope of this chapter to outline the details of each test, it is clear that a well-documented QA programme will provide a thorough understanding of the standard of operation of the radiation therapy simulator and its imaging systems.

4.5 Additional considerations

Computerization of radiation therapy equipment simplifies its operation from a user's perspective but provides another source of potential error since the software may not necessarily be free of faults. While it is the manufacturer's responsibility to provide fault-free programs, it is up to the user to confirm proper operation, calibration, and safety of computer-controlled systems. Some modern simulators have a computer as the actual control console of the unit. In addition to computerized controls, more radiation therapy units are being networked with record-and-verify systems, digital image-transfer systems, and departmental management systems. On accelerators, record-and-verify systems will not allow treatment to proceed until all the machine parameters are set to agree with the parameters stored in the computer. The source of the appropriate machine settings could be:

(1) a treatment plan that is either entered at the accelerator record-and-verify system on the first day of treatment or transferred directly from the treatment planning computer or CT-simulator; or

(2) data recorded at the simulator from the parameters derived from the simulation process.

In the latter case, the simulator record-and-verify station must be networked with the record-and-verify station on the accelerator, allowing direct transfer of each patient's prescription and machine-related data. While this process has several benefits in terms of efficiency and accuracy of data transfer and reproducibility of patient set-up, it must be recognized that it could lead to the possibility of reproducible errors if inaccurate data are stored in the computer. Extra precautions are required to test the integrity of the programs and to ensure the quality of data transfer.

5. CT scanners for therapy planning

5.1 Role of CT scanners

The easy availability of CT scanners in the late 1970s led to major improvements in the radiation therapy planning process. The cross-sectional images provided by these diagnostic imagers provide a wealth of anatomical data and are ideally suited for planning purposes. The application of CT scanning to radiation therapy lies in four major areas.

1. *Diagnosis.* As a diagnostic tool, the CT scanner provides qualitative information about irregularities within tissue structures, which can be assessed by the radiologist for the extent and stage of disease. This is information required by the radiation oncologist to decide on treatment modality, technique, and prescribed dose.

2. *Tumour and normal tissue localization.* With a diagnosis of malignant disease, the radiation oncologist needs detailed quantitative information about tumour extent and intervening or adjacent normal tissues. This allows for detailed decisions about field sizes and beam configurations in order to maximize tumour dose, while minimizing the dose to critical normal tissues. Because of its ability for low-contrast detection, CT provides much better soft tissue/tumour delineation than can be obtained with conventional simulation.

3. *Density data for dose calculations.* CT images consist of a matrix of relative attenuation coeffi-

cients. These CT numbers are easily converted to relative electron densities that are necessary for accurate dose calculations. Compton scattering is the predominant interaction process for megavoltage photons in tissue, and the probability of Compton interaction is directly proportional to electron density. Thus CT scans not only provide information on external contours and internal structures but, in addition, they provide detailed density information that can be used for dose calculations that account for tissue inhomogeneities. Both the spatial and density accuracy are provided by CT in a manner unparalleled by any other imaging modality.

4. *Treatment monitoring.* Follow-up CT images either during or after treatment afford a means of assessing tumour regression or recurrence, or normal tissue damage. This type of information is useful not only in clinical studies that provide statistical information on efficacy of treatment techniques but also for assessing follow-up therapies for individual patients. At times, boost field techniques are based on tumour regression data derived from CT images taken during treatment.

The clinical impact of CT on the therapy planning process is now well established (Goitein 1982; Brahme 1988). Various studies have indicated modifications in 30–80% of a selected number of conventional non-CT treatment plans because of the additional information provided by CT. Some 10–40% of all radiation therapy patients might benefit from CT scanning for therapy planning. Furthermore, a theoretical estimate indicates that the use of CT planning could improve the local control probability by 6% with an estimated 3.5% increase in 5-year survival rates (Goitein 1982). CT for therapy planning has been used for the majority of malignancies throughout the human body. Perhaps the greatest impact has been in pelvic, abdominal, and thoracic tumours, with the latter having the added impact of calculating doses that account for tissue inhomogeneities. In addition, CT has proved to be a tremendous aid for the treatment of small brain tumours by the use of stereotactic radiosurgery/radiation therapy.

In addition to improvements in conventional two-dimensional treatment planning, CT provides volumetric information well suited for more sophisticated 3-D treatment planning. Current practice is moving towards 3-D CRT. This includes the use of smaller planning target volumes that can be irradiated to higher doses, thus improving the likelihood of cure while maintaining normal tissue complications at similar or lower levels in comparison to conventional treatments (Fuks *et al.* 1991). This requires more sophisticated procedures for plan optimization possibly using dose–volume histograms (DVH) and inverse-planning techniques with the use of intensity-modulation radiation therapy (IMRT) (Carol 1995). True conformation therapy with complex shielding, moving fields, or multi-leaf collimators would not be possible without the 3-D information provided by CT. The ability to reconstruct images in any plane and to use volume-rendered display allow for an improved perspective of tumours and normal tissues and the corresponding dose distributions. This is discussed in more detail in Section 6 on CT simulators.

5.2 Practical considerations

While the benefits of CT scanning in the context of radiation therapy planning have been well demonstrated, its use must be accompanied by consideration of a number of related issues and concerns. Organizationally, many radiation therapy departments do not have easy access to CT scanners. Usually, these are housed in other departments, often within other institutions. Hence, organizational issues related to easy access to radiation therapy patients must be resolved between the two departments.

Once radiotherapy patient access is available, it needs to be emphasized strongly that the radiation therapy patient scanning procedures are distinctly different from conventional diagnostic procedures. Some practical issues that need special consideration for the therapy-planning process are listed in Table 7.4. As in the simulation process, patients must be positioned in identical positions to those that will be used on the therapy machines. Again, laser set-ups, as used on simulators and therapy machines, will greatly aid this process. Since diagnostic imaging is usually performed with curved couch tops, a flat insert is required to emulate the therapy machine couch top.

Table 7.4 Special considerations in CT scanning for therapy planning

Flat tabletop
Laser positioning lights
Patient positioning
   Supine/prone
   Arms in/arms out
Respiratory condition
Beam reference marks
Immobilization or treatment devices
Fillable organs
Patient size and circle of reconstruction
Accurate CT numbers
Slice thickness
Transmission scans
Contrast agents
Prostheses
Scan time

Supine versus prone set-ups or whether the arms are in or out of the image are also important considerations. Both these situations will alter external contours and the shapes and positions of the internal organs to the extent that the choice of one or other of such positions can dramatically influence the shape of the irradiation volume and the doses delivered to specific tissues. Whichever position is chosen, it should be maintained reproducibly. In cases where the patient is treated in both the supine and prone positions, the true dose delivered to individual tissue elements may become rather difficult to establish. To ensure proper patient positioning, it is very useful to have a radiation therapy radiographer, who is well acquainted with the details of the treatment procedures, participate in the CT scanning process.

Respiratory condition during the scanning process is an important consideration for accurate target-volume delineation and dose delivery, especially in the thoracic region. For diagnostic purposes full inspiration scans are preferred. These provide the greatest contrast for the lung region and keep the patient from moving. However, therapy patients are treated under normal respiration conditions. Hence, therapy-planning scans should also be taken under shallow breathing conditions, recognizing that such scans will be of somewhat reduced quality due to motion artefacts.

Reference marks are required on a CT image in order to relate the positions of the radiation beams to points on the external contours. Such reference marks can be produced by the use of small pieces of thin radio-opaque solder wire, strands of copper wire, or small catheters filled with dilute barium sulphate or hypaque contrast material. Under some conditions, when the position and shape of a radiation beam is known, the entire field, as located on the skin surface, can be confirmed on the images by the use of such radio-opaque markers.

Patient support or immobilization devices used for therapy should also be used during the scanning process, although the use of metallic screws or metal clips must be avoided since these can create serious artefacts or distortions in the images. Headrests, casts, or moulds should be made of low-density or tissue-equivalent materials. Sometimes tissue-equivalent bolus is used for improving the dose distribution required in the target volume. It is beneficial to confirm their tissue equivalence by scanning these materials while in the treatment position.

Certain organs within the body can change shape from hour to hour for physiological reasons. Gas in the intestines or bowel can show up on CT images as sizeable volumes at one time and not at all at another. Clearly, dose computations including such large volumes of gas will be substantially different in comparison with the absence of gas. Perhaps inhomogeneity corrections should be avoided under these conditions. However,

under other conditions, some control over organ volume may be possible. Hence, for pelvic treatments it may be useful to ask the patient to empty the bladder routinely prior to simulation, CT scanning, and treatment.

Diagnostically, the smallest possible circle of reconstruction is generally chosen to yield the best resolution of the internal anatomy. However, under some conditions this could truncate parts of the patient, making it difficult to calculate dose distributions, since the full external contour of the patient is not available. Generally, the smallest possible circle of reconstruction that still encompasses the entire patient over the entire volume that is scanned should be used. Furthermore, the scanner couch position should not be moved vertically during the scanning procedure, since spatial relationships become difficult to assess. This is particularly relevant for three-dimensional calculation or display. While this appears obvious in the context of therapy planning, this is generally not a constraint for diagnostic procedures.

CT number accuracy can be affected by a variety of conditions including:

(1) part of the patient being outside of the circle of reconstruction;
(2) beam-hardening effects due to bone, patient shape, immobilization devices, metallic surgical clips, metal prostheses, or contrast agents.

The latter should be avoided if CT images are to be used for dose inhomogeneity corrections since they can affect the resultant dose distributions.

Slice thickness generally can vary from 1 mm to 1 cm. It used to be that slice thicknesses of 1 cm were adequate for thoracic and pelvic scans. However, with the use of 3-D treatment planning and 3-D reconstructions including volume rendering, a smaller slice thickness and slice spacing is required to obtain adequate displays. Similarly, for head and neck treatments, slice thicknesses of less than 0.5 cm (0.2–0.3 cm) are preferred because of rapid changes in contours and tissue structures. Again, thinner slices are required for 3-D reconstructions, although the thinner images could have more noise unless a higher radiation dose is given to yield images with the same noise as the thicker images. Higher noise results in poorer low-contrast resolution. While radiation dose due to imaging is normally not an important consideration for patients who are undergoing high-dose radiation therapy, scanning many slices with high doses can place a severe heat load on the scanner X-ray tube, as well as reduce patient throughput. Furthermore, more slices will increase image storage requirements, image transfer times through the network, and staff time required to perform contouring and image segmentation. The couch interval will also have to be carefully selected and should be appropriately correlated to the slice thickness. Sometimes there are benefits to overlapping slices for better longitudinal resolution in reconstructed images.

Spiral CT scanners now provide a means of scanning the patient very rapidly. The patient is automatically moved through the scan plane, while the X-ray tube is rotating continuously around the patient. The advantage is that the high-speed scan generally involves minimal patient motion and, therefore, improved images that are ideally suited for 3-D reconstructions. One of the requirements for such scanners is a very high heat capacity X-ray tube due to the very high heat loading as a result of the X-ray tube being on continuously for multiple slices. Scan volumes could be as long as 40–120 cm for treatments such as those associated with lymphomas, cancer of the ovary or total CNS irradiation. The need for spiral CT has become even more important for CT-simulation (Section 6.2).

Transmission scans (also known as pilot or scout scans) are very useful for an initial survey of patient landmarks and for defining the first and last scan. However, transmission scans are geometrically not the same as simulator films for two reasons. Since the patient moves through the plane of a fan beam, the transmission scan does not contain any beam divergence in the longitudinal direction, while in the transverse plane the divergence is determined by the source–patient–detectors geometry, which generally will not be the same as the simulation or treatment geometry. Hence transmission scans are only useful for crude localization of patient structures and for the definition of upper and lower scan limits but should not be used for outlining radiation beams or for planning purposes.

Metallic prostheses used for bone replacement can generate enormous artefacts in images and may render the images useless. However, methods have been developed that mathematically remove the prosthesis from the image and reconstruct the image to provide reduced artefacts. These metal artefact reduction algorithms should be thoroughly assessed, particularly for geometric accuracy and accuracy of CT numbers, before this approach is used for therapy planning.

At times it may be desirable to image patients who have applicators inserted that are to be used in conjunction with brachytherapy sources. While such procedures may be useful for source localization and dose computations, the resultant images should be checked for geometric distortions if the applicators are made of metal.

In conventional CT-planning, once a patient has been scanned, the CT data need to be transferred to a treatment-planning computer. One approach is to enlarge hard copies of CT images and to enter the outlines of external contours and internal structures into the treatment-planning computer using a graphical digitizer.

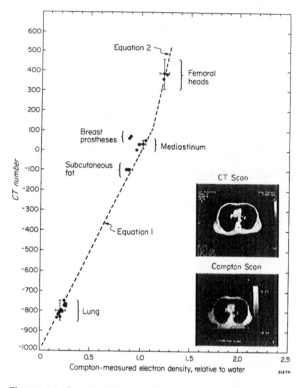

Figure 7.7 Graph of CT number versus relative electron density (from Gray *et al.* 1983).

For dose calculations, some assumptions will have to be made regarding the densities of the internal structures. However, it is preferable to enter the CT data directly into the treatment-planning computer. This requires:

(1) a treatment-planning computer system capable of handling CT data directly; and

(2) a proper CT handler to read the CT data for each particular scanner in use.

Furthermore, a calibration curve must be derived to convert CT numbers to electron densities for each scanner or even for different scan protocols using different kilovoltage settings from the same scanner. Often, these calibration curves are bilinear with one linear portion for soft tissue and another for bony structures. Figure 7.7 is an example of such data, which were derived by directly comparing the same tissue elements using a CT scanner and a Compton scanner to give electron densities directly (Battista and Bronskill 1981).

5.3 Specifications

CT scanners are routinely found in diagnostic-imaging departments and usually consist of an X-ray tube that

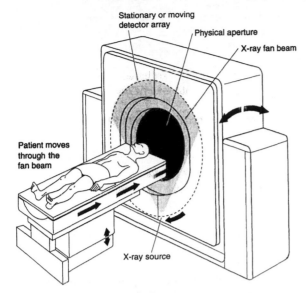

Figure 7.8 Schematic diagram of a CT scanner and its various mechanical motions.

rotates about a patient (Figure 7.8). Most modern scanners are third or fourth generation. In the third-generation scanner, both the X-ray tube and a group of detectors rotate about the patient, while the fourth-generation scanner has multiple fixed detectors in a circle and only the X-ray tube rotates. While some would argue that image quality for therapy planning need not be as stringent as for diagnostic use, others prefer the best diagnostic quality images for therapy planning. The issues to be considered for a scanner that is to be used specifically for radiation therapy planning are discussed below. They are broadly divided into four subsections:

(1) mechanical;
(2) imaging system;
(3) image analysis;
(4) organizational.

5.3.1 Mechanical

1. The scanner should have the largest physical aperture possible to aid patient set-up in the therapy mode. Even the largest aperture sizes (about 70-cm diameter at present, although one CT-simulator manufacturer has an aperture of 91.5 cm) can be restrictive for some patient set-ups. Hence even a small reduction in aperture size will create severe practical limitations on some patient set-ups.

2. By analogy with simulator and therapy machine set-ups, precise positioning lasers and patient-reference marks are required. Light localizers or lasers in the scan plane provide a further check on patient positioning.

3. All scanners are equipped with a concave couch top. Either the manufacturers or the institution will have to provide a flat insert to simulate therapy-couch tops. There should be the possibility of some adjustment in the couch vertical position while the patient is being positioned in the scanner aperture. This will aid patient set-up with the lateral lasers.

4. Because of the quantitative nature of therapy planning, accurate couch registration is essential. The accuracy should be better than 0.5 mm.

5.3.2 Imaging system

1. The scanner should be a state-of-the-art diagnostic imager.

2. The circle of reconstruction (field of view) of all present commercial scanners is smaller than the physical aperture size. To minimize a loss of information and the exclusion of the patient's external contour, the largest possible circle of reconstruction should be obtained (about 50-cm diameter at present).

3. Rapid scan capabilities with thin CT slices over large volumes are useful for three-dimensional treatment-planning purposes. As a result of rapid large-volume scanning, the CT scanner X-ray tube should have a high tube rating. Modern spiral CT scanners now provide such rapid scanning capabilities with high tube ratings.

4. The CT scanner should be capable of various reconstruction planes with sagittal and coronal reconstructions being the minimum. These reconstructed images should be transferable to the treatment-planning computer, or preferably the treatment-planning computer should be capable of performing such reconstructions.

5. The scanner should be capable of anterior–posterior (AP) and lateral transmission scans. This is useful for determining the location of the CT slices to be obtained for therapy planning.

5.3.3 Image analysis

1. Because the CT data may be used directly for dose calculations, the CT scanner should provide images with high CT number precision and accuracy (<2%).

2. The CT numbers should be readily convertible to electron densities. While a simple calibration of a series of known materials will yield an adequate conversion for megavoltage photon calculations, electron beam calculations could make use of atomic number data as well, since mass scattering powers

are proportional to atomic numbers. A dual-energy scanning technique with appropriate reconstruction algorithms is capable of providing both electron density and atomic number information. However, most commercial scanners available at present are not capable of providing this information. It is hoped that future research will make these conversions readily available.

3. Some scanners have a dynamic reference consisting of detectors that measure radiation that emanates from the X-ray tube just outside the circle of reconstruction. These reference measurements provide a means of dynamically calibrating the detectors for variation in X-ray output during each scan. However, if part of the patient is outside of the circle of reconstruction, this dynamic reference will be in error and the resultant images will have distortions and inaccurate CT numbers. Therefore, the scanner should have an option of turning off the dynamic reference, if parts of the patient are outside of the circle of reconstruction.

4. Good display and hard-copy capabilities are essential. Another desirable feature is good image analysis software capable of delineating regions of interest for CT number statistics, distance rulers, geometric zooms, image subtraction, and multiple-format viewing.

5. Appropriate beam-hardening correction is important if accurate CT numbers are to be provided. This can be done through the use of physical or software compensation. The use of a metal artefact reduction algorithm is useful, since cancer is generally a disease occurring within an older population with a higher frequency of metallic prostheses.

5.3.4 Organizational

1. While a simple transfer of CT data via magnetic tape to the treatment-planning computer is possible with most scanners, ideally the scanner and treatment-planning computers should be networked to allow for direct transfer of CT images.

2. The CT number data file format must be provided by the manufacturer either directly to the user or to the manufacturer of the treatment-planning computer so that programs can be developed to transfer the data on to the treatment-planning system. This is useful not only for dose computation procedures but also for those who wish to use the data directly for monitoring outcome of treatment.

3. The CT scanner should be capable of a large amount of data storage for extra large volumetric scans (e.g. sometimes 30 cm length with 0.5 cm spacing, i.e. 60 slices per patient).

The above considerations provide some guidelines for those involved with the use of CT scanning for therapy planning. It is clear that all the above specifications cannot be readily found in any one scanner. However, the users must compromise between their departmental priorities and the capabilities of the available scanners.

5.4 Selection criteria, purchase, and acceptance

The selection of a CT scanner is dependent on local needs and, specifically, whether the scanner is to be used for therapy planning only or whether it is to be shared with routine diagnostic use. The selection criteria for the latter may be different from the former. In either case, the purchasers must define their requirements and ensure that the selected CT scanner is capable of delivering their requests.

Once these requirements are established, the purchaser should produce a list of parameters for which manufacturers should provide general and technical details. While an exhaustive list is beyond the scope of this chapter, it should include some of the following information (Kelsey *et al.* 1980; Goitein 1982):

(1) scan performance (including scan speeds, circles of reconstruction, slice thickness, spatial resolution, noise, linearity, dose per scan and dose profile, table accuracy, scan repetition rate, reconstruction time, matrix size);

(2) system components (including tube specifications and cooling especially for spiral CT, detectors, computer system(s), hard-copy units such as laser camera, laser printers, display system(s), data storage);

(3) mechanical requirements (including gantry aperture, gantry tilt, patient table including vertical positioning constraints when moving into the aperture and physical stability, accessories for head scans, and patient alignment lights and their accuracy);

(4) ease of operation (including cold start time, type of computer display, interactive sequences, display and features associated with image manipulation, image magnification, quantitative measurements including distances and CT number statistics, cursors, grids, sagittal/coronal displays);

(5) options and extras (including metal artefact reduction algorithms, high speed or spiral scanning, special patient holders, networking, picture archive and communications system);

(6) special requirements for therapy planning discussed above;

(7) warranty, service, and training;

(8) installation requirements;

(9) cost.

By analogy with a simulator purchase, these data should be obtained from all manufacturers and summarized in tabular form. After reviewing the data, some models not meeting appropriate requirements should be eliminated and a remaining short-list prepared. Site visits should be organized, preferably to locations where these machines are in clinical service. The visiting team should consist of a physicist, a radiation therapy radiographer, a radiation oncologist, and a radiologist. If possible, various image parameters should be tested while on the site visit. After a call for tender, a final selection and purchase can be made. The purchase order should include a set of well-defined acceptance tests as well as agreements related to access to software and data file formats, if these are required for therapy-planning purposes. It should be emphasized that manufacturers are quick to make promises before a sale but slow to release information afterwards. Hence, clear legal documents are required to avoid disappointment to the purchasers.

5.5 *Quality assurance*

CT scanner QA procedures are well established, especially as they relate to diagnostic use (Dick Loo 1991). While most therapy-planning requirements will be incorporated in these diagnostic QC tests, some additional tests should be performed to ensure the integrity of the CT-planning process. These tests relate to patient-positioning accuracy, including reference lasers and accuracy of couch positioning, image geometric accuracy, and accuracy in CT numbers and their conversion to electron densities.

The QC of both the geometric image accuracy and the accuracy of the CT numbers and their conversion to electron densities can be carried out using a single phantom. A circular water or water-equivalent phantom of known diameter and containing a number of circular inserts with known physical properties, including electron densities, can be used for this purpose. By scanning this phantom, entering the data into the treatment-planning computer, and plotting the external contour, a test exists to evaluate not only the geometrical accuracy of the CT image but also its transfer to the treatment-planning computer, the automatic contouring techniques, and the integrity of the output device. The diameter of the external contour from the output device should agree to within 2 mm of the physical diameter of the phantom.

The phantom inserts will initially be used to generate the CT number to electron density relationship as used by the treatment-planning computer, and can then be used routinely as a means of assessing the reproducibility of these electron densities as derived from the CT scanner. The geometric accuracy and the electron density tests should be carried out every 3–6 months or whenever there is a change of software in either the CT scanner or the treatment-planning computer.

Another means of ensuring the accuracy of conversion of CT number to electron density for every scan is to use inserts of different materials under the flat couch top used for planning scans. Rods of two or three materials ranging from low density (e.g. wood or cork) to tissue-equivalent densities (e.g. polystyrene or lucite) to bone-equivalent materials could be used for this purpose. A quick check of the CT numbers for these materials for every patient will ensure the quality of the CT data.

By analogy with simulators, a radiation survey should be performed in the areas around the CT-scanner room to ensure the adequacy of shielding in all the walls.

6. CT simulators

6.1 *Role of CT simulators*

Over the last decade, the advent of high-dose 3-D CRT has brought about the development of CT simulators (Nishidai *et al.* 1990; Sherouse and Chaney 1991; Jani 1993; Coia *et al.* 1995). A CT simulator is a standard diagnostic CT scanner with additional software that provides beam edge display, beam's eye view (BEV) display, 3-D images, and high quality digitally-reconstructed radiographs (DRRs). A DRR is a ray-line reconstruction through a 3-D volumetric CT data set, which generates the equivalent of a conventional transmission radiograph using a virtual source and the geometry of the planned radiation therapy beam (Goitein *et al.* 1983; Sherouse *et al.* 1990; Rosenman *et al.* 1991). Target volumes and critical structures can be outlined on the CT axial images and the CT-simulator software integrates these targets and structures with therapy beam geometries to perform 'virtual' simulation in 3-D. Users may display these beams in any plane or in any BEV. Ideally, CT simulation can unify the tasks of CT imaging for 3-D target and normal tissue localization, treatment field design, dose calculations, patient marking, and verification simulation into one physical location. The major components of a state-of-the-art CT simulator are illustrated in Figure 7.9 and include:

(1) a CT scanner and couch;

(2) a CT computer console;

(3) one or more networked 3-D image and virtual simulation workstations;

(4) a laser-marking system;

(5) a laser hardcopy device.

The integration of dose computations into commercially available systems is currently under development,

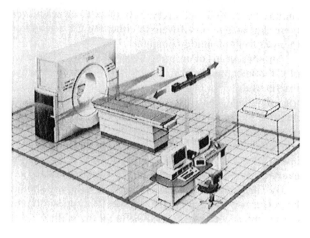

Figure 7.9 Layout of a typical CT-simulator suite. The major components include a CT scanner and couch, a CT computer console, a virtual simulation workstation, a (movable) laser marking system, and hardcopy devices. (Courtesy of Picker International, Cleveland, Ohio.)

although target volumes and beam geometries developed by virtual simulation may be exported to some external treatment-planning computer systems.

The CT simulator is capable of performing almost all the functions of both a conventional simulator and a conventional CT scanner as described in Sections 4.1 and 5.1, respectively. Additional capabilities of a CT simulator include:

Three-dimensional target and normal-tissue visualization

Since it comprises a digital database, the CT volumetric data can be manipulated using any of the display tools, post-processing tools and image formats that, up till now, have been exclusively in the domain of diagnostic imaging. Not only can radiation oncologists view anatomy from new perspectives quickly and accurately, but also tissues of interest can be highlighted amid the wealth of 3-D data available. These tools can better help to define GTV, CTV, or PTV.

Standard display tools consist of window/level adjustments, brightness/contrast adjustments as well as zoom, pan, and cine functions. Contoured regions of interest can be displayed in wire frame, outline, or colour-wash mode, and selectively turned on or off to enhance the viewer's perspective. It is even possible, if the user wishes, to change CT numbers in the images. This might be useful for dose calculations, especially if the images contain artefacts as might be generated by metallic prostheses. Changing the CT number on any structure that is contoured to −1000 (air equivalent), enables the user in essence to 'remove' the structure from

the 'virtual' patient and helps to improve the image quality of the DRR (i.e. fewer obstructing tissues so that the signal of the tissues of interest is improved). Not only can structures be manipulated in this fashion, the user can define a volume of interest such that a portion of the patient is eliminated. The subsequent 'thin slice' DRR will have excellent image quality in the specific regions of interest. For example, if one defines the volume of interest to be only the posterior half of the patient in the abdominal region (i.e. cut away in the coronal plane), then one will see the kidneys quite clearly on a PA DRR without having to outline the structure (i.e. all the anterior structures have been eliminated from the DRR reconstruction process).

The CT data base may be displayed in various image formats providing new perspectives to the planning process, as well as non-axial contours for dose computational purposes. The 3-D imaging and virtual simulation workstations can generate multiple planar reformatted (MPR) images (in axial, coronal, sagittal, or any arbitrary plane), 3-D images (with volume rendering and segmentation options), and DRRs. Tissues previously delineated can be displayed on each format. Example formats of a sagittal MPR, a coronal MPR, a 3-D image, and a DRR are shown in Figs. 7.10a–d, respectively.

Not all soft or malignant tissues are readily imaged with CT. In these cases, magnetic resonance imaging (MRI), single photon emission CT (SPECT), and positron emission tomography (PET) may provide complimentary data to enhance the 3-D CT-planning process through the use of multi-modality image registration techniques (see Figure 7.11). This will be discussed further in Section 7.4.

Enhanced planning capabilities through the use of virtual simulation

Although the value of the high-resolution data provided by CT to tissue localization has long been recognized, its potential advantage in the planning process had not been fully realized until the evolution of virtual simulation. Using computer software, virtual simulation is able to simulate any radiation therapy beam geometry directly onto the CT data, eliminating the need for conventional simulation as well as its associated transfer errors. Clinically, the ability to view all beams simultaneously, in any orientation, overlaid with accurate anatomic data of critical structures can increase field placement and shielding accuracy (Goitein *et al.* 1983). Organizationally, virtual simulation can help improve resource utilization in the planning process for certain types of techniques.

One of the greatest assets of CT simulation is the ability to see soft tissues projected in any BEV on a standard radiograph-like projection, the DRR. This is valuable not only for new conformal techniques but can have a significant impact on the accuracy of conventional

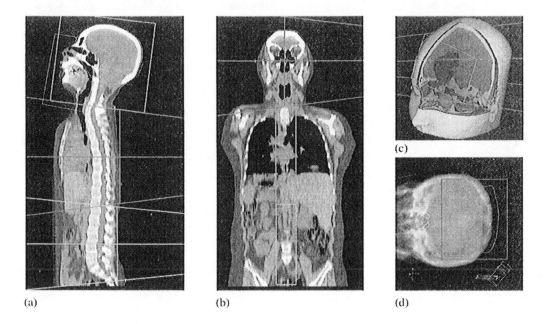

(a)   (b)   (d)

Figure 7.10 Various image formats available for localization and virtual simulation. (a) A sagittal, mid-line multiple plane reconstructed (MPR) image displaying a lateral cranial field and two posterior spinal fields. (b) A coronal, mid-line MPR displaying the same fields as in (a). (c) A 3-D image of the head with regions 'cut away' to display internal tissues of interest. (d) A digitally-reconstructed radiograph (DRR) of an anterior, obliquely-oriented vertex field. The projection of the planning target volume and field are graphically overlaid. See also colour plate section.

techniques. For the latter, inaccuracies associated with a clinician's ability to mentally translate geometric information from diagnostic scans to treatment portals are eliminated. Shielding can be designed with greater accuracy by using a visual of individualized critical structures, without the need for referencing to bony landmarks, average anatomy data, or the use of injected dyes such as those used for kidney localization.

The planning of multiple-field techniques can be simplified and expedited with virtual simulation. Unlike conventional simulators, virtual simulators can display all fields simultaneously in any plane and hence junctions can be matched anatomically for individual patients. An example of the multiple fields of craniospinal irradiation can be seen in Figure 7.10a and b and in Mah *et al.* (1998). Interactive selection of gantry, collimator, and table rotations, SSD/SAD, and field sizes allow the user to match beams accurately and quickly. The viewing of multiple-image planes can be used to determine which volume of tissues may be irradiated in the exit portion of beams.

Without the hindrance of a bulky image intensifier, virtual simulators can be used to design beams with all the combinations of gantry and table angles that are possible on the treatment machine. One prime example is

the simulation of oblique vertex beams for brain and base of skull lesions (Figure 7.10d). In these cases, CT simulation does two things. First, it maps the exact location and shape of these soft tissue lesions in a BEV. Second, it can simulate beams oriented at various angles through the vertex. Sometimes this is the optimal configuration in terms of the dose-volume profiles for both target and critical normal tissues.

DRRs are digital radiographs representing the equivalent of conventional simulator films. DRRs can be further processed to generate images similar to electronic portal images from high energy therapy machines. Electronic portal images, by nature of their design, come in a digital format. Radiographs can also be converted to digital format by appropriate scanners. In both instances, the resultant images can be compared directly, either visibly or digitally, with the corresponding DRR. Digital comparisons provide a means of quantitative assessment that allows for easier, less subjective and more accurate field placement corrections then is generally possible when we do this by eye as is conventionally done when comparing simulator and port films. Automated field set-up corrections from digital images are still in a state of infancy and will require a substantial amount of technological development before this becomes routine clinical practice.

The disadvantages of CT simulation are few but not negligible. The physical diameter of the CT bore and restricted couch ranges may limit patient-positioning options or the use of some large accessories. Observation of dynamic motions in relation to treatment portals is not currently possible with CT simulation. Planning techniques, in which respiratory or cardiac motion must be observed in real-time, must be done with conventional simulators.

6.2 Practical considerations

The practical issues and concerns previously described for conventional CT scanning in Section 5.2 are pertinent for CT simulators. However, additional considerations will arise from the intended use of the CT simulator. These include markedly different effects on resource utilization, cost-effectiveness, staff productivity, and patient time. Clearly, there will a substantial variation with institution and technique.

In the simplest approach, a patient could be scanned in the treatment position using arbitrary reference marks, have virtual simulation performed with or without contours at a later time, and have the isocentre of the planned treatment fields set up as shifts from the reference marks. In these cases, the ability to perform virtual simulation reduces both the number and length of the patient's appointments for the planning process. The conventional CT-planning process in which a pre-CT simulation, CT scanning, and plan verification simulation are required with the patient's presence, can be replaced by a single CT-simulation session. Furthermore, fast spiral scanning technology and the elimination of waiting periods for film development, staff consultation, and multiple field set-ups can lead to significant time reductions. This is particularly advantageous for both patient and staff when planning paediatric or difficult patients who cannot be immobilized for long periods of time without undue distress.

Alternatively, a CT-simulation session can encompass all facets of planning while the patient remains on the scanner couch for the duration. This could include the fabrication and registration of immobilization devices, CT data acquisition, target and normal tissue localization, virtual simulation of treatment apertures, generation of dose distributions, marking the patient with the planned fields, and production of images for treatment verification (DRRs). This approach is generally more resource intensive requiring a radiation oncologist, a dosimetrist, a radiographer, a medical physicist, and, possibly, a diagnostic radiologist to be present during the CT-simulation session. Depending on the complexity of the plan, the session will generally exceed 30 minutes and a further verification simulation on a conventional simulator may be required.

To minimize the time a patient must remain immobilized, fast CT-scan acquisition and networked computers are essential in CT simulation. The production of high-quality DRRs may require 50–200 axial images, depending on the anatomic site. To this end, fast spiral CT-scanning technology can offer numerous advantages over conventional axial acquisitions. Spiral acquisition can:

(1) significantly reduce total acquisition time (typically 10 minutes for spiral acquisition and reconstruction of 60 images compared to 20 minutes for axial mode);

(2) consequently, minimize gross patient motion, which can lead to misregistration in the volumetric data;

(3) permit the reconstruction of overlapping images without additional radiation exposure in an attempt to further improve longitudinal resolution in the DRRs (Brink and Davros 1995).

To handle the large volume of data that must be transferred quickly, a Fast Ethernet or fibre optic FDDI (fibre distributed data interface) network topology must be reliably available. Not only is speed required in the transfer from the CT console to the virtual simulation workstation, but also between multiple workstations in centres with such configurations. In addition, the simultaneous transfer of images to the virtual simulation workstation as they are reconstructed on the CT console allows target-volume delineation to commence prior to the completion of the CT study.

6.3 Specifications

6.3.1 CT Scanner

In this section, specific issues related to the use of a CT scanner for the purpose of CT simulation are described. These represent issues in addition to those described in Section 5.3 for conventional CT and are broadly divided into:

(1) mechanical;

(2) imaging system;

(3) image storage and networking.

Mechanical

1. The scanner should be capable of helical or spiral scanning mode with a wide range of pitches. A slip-ring gantry in which the X-ray tube, transformers, generator, and detectors are all mounted on the rotating portion of the gantry, enables the continuous rotation required for helical/spiral acquisitions. The pitch is defined as the table increment per gantry rotation divided by the X-ray collimation. By increasing the pitch, the longitudinal coverage of

the patient can be increased for the same tube loading. The selection of pitch, X-ray collimation (or slice thickness), and reconstruction interval will affect the longitudinal resolution of the CT data base and subsequent DRRs (Wang and Vannier 1994). For radiation therapy planning, a pitch of 1–2 is generally sufficient.

2. To transfer a virtual-simulated isocentre or field from the workstation to the patient, a laser-marking system should be available in the CT-simulator suite. Whether the marking system provides a three-point set-up or outlines the field shape on the patient's skin (Ragan *et al.* 1993), its accuracy should be 1 mm.

3. Although previously stated, the importance of accurate couch registration should be re-emphasized, particularly in the context of 3-D volumetric data manipulation and DRR production. With increasing flexibility in varying scan parameters during a single patient CT study, the couch index provides the geometric basis for coalescing images along the longitudinal axis in all 3-D image formats. Therefore, the couch incrementation accuracy should be better than 0.5 mm for maximum load.

Imaging system

1. Spiral scanning of large volumes and thin sections for 3-D treatment planning, significantly challenges the X-ray generators, tube, and anode cooling system compared to conventional scanning. The range in heat capacity for commercially available tubes for spiral CT is 2.0–5.2 million heat units, with anode cooling rates of up to 0.9 million heat units/minute.

2. To support fast, high-quality image acquisition, while minimizing production of X-rays, detectors for spiral scanning must have high X-ray efficiency. Solid state and xenon-filled ionization chambers appear to be the detectors of choice for the commercially available spiral scanners. The state-of-the-art CT scanner typically has 4800 detectors.

3. The scanner software should provide efficient and flexible tools for planning multiple spiral acquisitions on the transmission scans. Variable slice collimation, reconstruction interval, and site-specific algorithms are essential for both optimal image quality and DRR production and provide flexibility for image storage considerations.

Image storage and networking

1. Image format standards have evolved such that most manufacturers are now providing DICOM compatible formats. DICOM is the acronym for 'Digital Imaging and Communications in Medicine' and is a standard developed through a committee set up by NEMA (National Electrical Manufacturers Association) and the American College of Radiology (ACR). To transfer data in a radiation therapy department, including CT images, volumetric structures, and isodose distributions, DICOM-RT has recently become available. This will not only aid the transfer of data within individual departments and computer systems but will also allow for easy transfer of data from one department to another or from a department to a collaborative clinical trials group.

2. Disk storage requirements on a CT computer differ for axial and spiral scanners. Although image sizes are identical, spiral studies contain a higher average number of images (typically 50–200 images) and hence require greater image storage space per study. In addition, 300–500 megabytes are required to maintain the raw data sets from multiple acquisitions per study required for reconstruction. In contrast, axial scanning requires only 32–64 megabytes for the raw data. A typical CT console should contain at least 2 gigabytes for compressed image storage.

3. The archival system on the CT console should be efficient and reliable, since storage on the console may be typically only a few weeks for a busy centre.

4. Networking is essential for an efficient CT-simulation program. If the intent is to plan and mark the patient during the CT-simulation session, simultaneous and fast network transfer between the CT console and the virtual simulation workstation during the reconstruction process is essential to minimize patient motion between scanning and field marking.

6.3.2 3-D Imaging/virtual simulation workstation

Tools for tissue localization

The accuracy, ease, and speed with which structures can be localized and drawn are key factors for a successful CRT and CT-simulation program. Presently, the contouring of all relevant structures is considered to be the most labour intensive aspect of planning 3-D CRT. Software tools to expedite this process are essential. User 'unfriendly' software and the time required to outline the critical structures may hinder the potential use of CT simulation. Flexibility may be the key to user satisfaction. With commercially available software, the localization of structures is performed on high-resolution 2-D axial images.

1. The modalities by which outlines can be entered include keyboard, mouse, trackball, light pens, and others. Users will often have individual preferences, although response time, sensitivity adjustment, and accuracy should be considered as priorities.

(a) 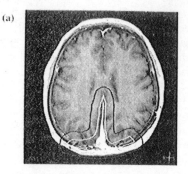 (b) 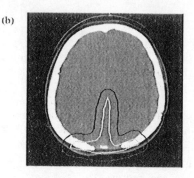 (c)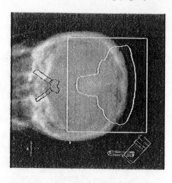

Figure 7.11 Registration of (a) magnetic resonance image (MRI) with (b) a planning, axial CT image. The clinical target volume (CTV) (white outline) may be localized on the MRI and simultaneously displayed on the registered CT data set. Software tools to produce automatic uniform or non-uniform margins can help produce planning target volumes (black outline) quickly and accurately. (c) The planning target volume (PTV) can then be graphically overlaid onto the DRR in a beam's eye view.

2. Manual localization options should include point and click (e.g. rubber band) and continuous modes. Interpolation between slices and the ability to copy an outline to subsequent images can aid in this process.

3. Semi-automatic or automatic localization options should be available to outline normal structures demonstrating high contrast with adjacent tissues. Skin, lungs, spinal cord, and bones are examples of such tissues.

4. The ability to automatically add uniform or non-uniform margins around localized volumes will aid those individuals wishing to implement the concepts of ICRU Report 50 (1993) (e.g. see Figure 7.11).

5. Editing functions, such as erase, stretch, translate, scale, and rotate, as well as editing of CT numbers, should be applicable to single slice outlines or to entire structures.

6. Measuring functions should include rulers, statistics, voxel values, and CT histograms.

Virtual simulation

1. The virtual simulation process includes the determination of an isocentre or reference point that has been or remains to be marked on the patient. The depth to the isocentre should be accurate to within 1 mm, whether it be calculated automatically or determined with a measuring tool.

2. The tolerance levels listed in Table 7.3 for conventional simulators are applicable to virtual simulation for field size (in asymmetric or symmetric modes), SAD/SSD, and gantry, collimator, and table angles.

3. For DRRs to be clinically accepted, the longitudinal resolution must be adequate and the computation time 'nearly' interactive. These two factors are clearly in opposition. The former requires more

images with small reconstruction intervals, while the latter increases with an increased number of images. At least one commercially available system makes use of special rendering hardware to produce a coarse DRR within a second and a full resolution image in less than 20 seconds. These images and computation times include the projection of all delineated structures as well as any user-designed shields.

Image display capabilities

1. Whole or parts of the CT volumetric data set should be displayed in various image formats and planes. Figure 7.12 shows a typical screen display of virtual simulation and DRR images. In addition to the conventional axial view, multi-planar reconstructed images in sagittal, coronal, and other user-defined planes are invaluable for planning many techniques. These views help planners assess the volumes and types of structures, which are encompassed within the planned beams. They can provide external contours in non-conventional planes for use in external dose-computation systems. True 3-D images displaying beam geometries can be useful, particularly if volume rendering and segmentation capabilities are provided. A virtual light field of the planned beam onto the skin is included on the 3-D images of some commercially available systems.

2. Beam and anatomic data may be displayed using various perspectives, the most useful of which is the BEV and the DRR. These should include the display of shielding. Observer-eye view and room-eye view displays are other options (Martin 1995).

3. The workstation should provide the flexibility to change monitor display, file save, and hardcopy configurations. Users should be able to zoom any

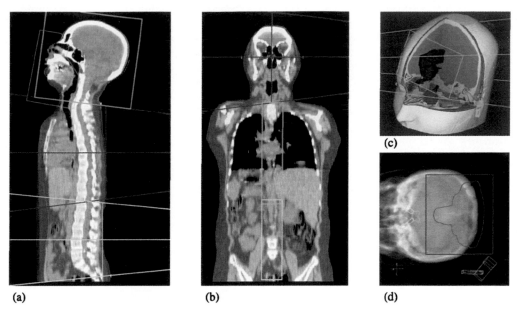

Figure 7.10 Various image formats available for localization and virtual simulation. (a) A sagittal, mid-line multiple plane reconstructed (MPR) image displaying a lateral cranial field and two posterior spinal fields. (b) A coronal, mid-line MPR displaying the same fields as in (a). (c) A 3-D image of the head with regions 'cut away' to display internal tissues of interest. (d) A digitally-reconstructed radiograph (DRR) of an anterior, obliquely-oriented vertex field. The projection of the planning target volume and field are graphically overlaid.

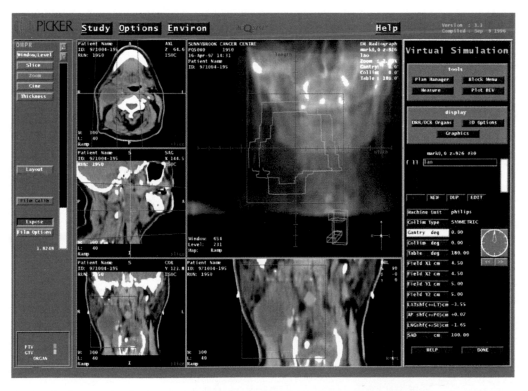

Figure 7.12 A typical screen display for virtual simulation. MPR images in the axial, sagittal, coronal, and isocentric plane orthogonal to the beam axis are shown in the small viewports. An anteroposterior DRR of a beam in the neck region is displayed in the larger viewports. Appropriate beam edges and axes may be displayed on each image. Various display manipulation functions are located in the left panel. Simulation functions include gantry, collimator, table, field size, and location manipulations along with tissue display options are located in the right panel.

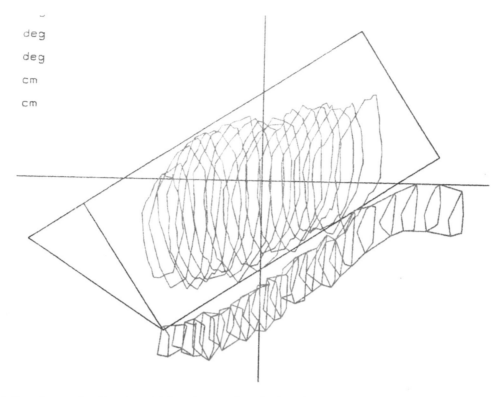

deg

deg

cm

cm

Figure 9.3 Beam's eye view for a target lying close to the spinal cord.

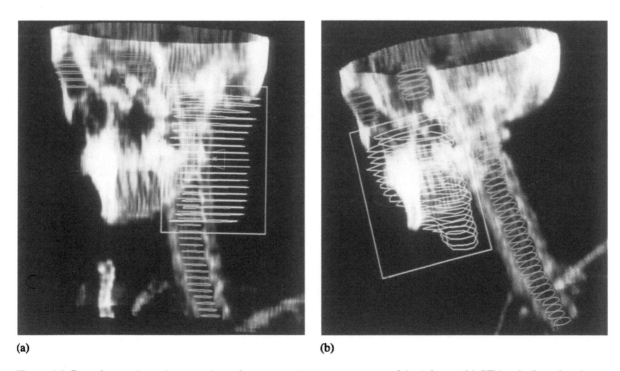

(a)   (b)

Figure 9.8 Beam's eye view of non-coplanar beams used to treat a tumour of the left parotid. PTV, spinal cord and eyes are outlined (a) anterior oblique beam, (b) posterior-superior oblique beam.

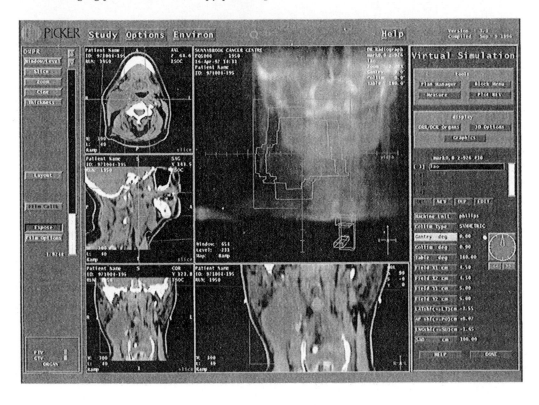

Figure 7.12 A typical screen display for virtual simulation. MPR images in the axial, sagittal, coronal, and isocentric plane orthogonal to the beam axis are shown in the small viewports. An anteroposterior DRR of a beam in the neck region is displayed in the larger viewports. Appropriate beam edges and axes may be displayed on each image. Various display manipulation functions are located in the left panel. Simulation functions including gantry, collimator, table, field size, and location manipulations along with tissue display options are located in the right panel. See also colour plate section.

one selected image type as a full screen display or save, as well as to view multiple-image types simultaneously.

Image storage and networking

1. *Disk space*. The large amount of memory, processing capability and storage needs of a virtual simulation workstation are considerable even when compared to those for the CT console. The storage needs on a virtual simulation station include storage for the CT study, contour data, patient information, planned beam data, and DRRs. The latter require typically 0.5 megabyte each. It has been estimated that a virtual simulation workstation would require at least 7 gigabyte of local storage space to accommodate a workload of eight patients per day for 28 days, assuming each patient had 70 CT images and 4 DRRs (Martin 1995).

2. *Archival systems*. The archival system on the virtual simulation workstation should be efficient, reliable, and automatic. It is essential to archive the contoured data-set as well as the configuration of all planned beams, since they represent a significant proportion of staff time and effort. To be highly efficient, the ideal system should archive automatically in the background, each time a change to either a contour or plan is saved. This is particularly important in large centres where numerous staff may access any one patient file during the course of planning.

3. *Networking*. In addition to transfers between the CT console and the virtual simulation workstations, fast network transfers to additional virtual simulation workstations, external dose-calculation computers, picture archive and communication systems (PACS), electronic portal imaging devices (EPID), and other in-house computer systems may be required. The

Table 7.5 Acceptance testing of the major components of a CT simulator

Component	Acceptance test	Tolerance
Transfer of CT data	Speed, data integrity after transfer and any format conversion	
External laser system	Orthogonality or accuracy	± 1 mm
	Alignment of lasers with CT image plane	± 1 mm
Anatomic data	Geometric accuracy of image planes	Error $\leq$ 1 pixel
	Geometric accuracy in all image formats	Error $\leq$ 1 pixel
Image use	Window/levelling, zoom	
Localization	Contour verification	Error $\leq$ 1 pixel
	Semi- and automatic contouring options	Error $\leq$ 1 pixel
	Isocentre calculation	*
	Area and volume statistics	
	Automatic margin placement	*
Virtual simulation parameters	Gantry rotation	$< 1°$ over $90°$ interval
(to be checked in all image	Collimator rotation	$< 1°$ over $90°$ interval
formats and principle planes)	Table rotation	$< 1°$ over $90°$ interval
	Field size	*
	Isocentre	*
	SSD/SAD	*
	Magnification	$\leq 1\%$ over total range
	Combinations of all above	Combined tolerances of individual tests
DRRs	Ray tracing	Angular divergence $< 1°$
	Spatial linearity	Error $\leq$ 1.0 mm over 10 cm
Contour verification on DRRs	Contour divergence	Error $\leq 1°$ for all field sizes at all clinical SSDs
	Spatial linearity	Error $\leq$ 1.0 mm over 10 cm
	Accuracy of translation from axial planes	
	Consistency between display modes	
Hardcopy output	Data integrity	

* $\leq$ 1/2 slice thickness in scan axis or 1 pixel in transaxial axis

large volume of data transferred may require a dedicated segment of the local area network to minimize traffic delays.

6.4 Acceptance and implementation of virtual simulation

The CT-scanner component of a virtual simulation package can be accepted and implemented as described in Section 5.4. All facets of the planning process of the virtual simulation program need to be verified using a comprehensive set of tests. Minimum standards can be adopted from conventional simulator and CT-planning practice. The major areas of consideration are listed in Table 7.5. Sections of this table have been adapted from McGee and Das (1995).

6.5 Quality assurance

The QA procedures for the CT-scanner component of CT simulators were described in Section 5.5. Further testing of accurate image reconstructions should be done for spiral acquisitions. In addition to these, the laser-marking system of CT simulators should be tested on a daily

basis. For a three-point system, tests should be performed to assess orthogonality of the lasers, its distance from the scan plane along the scan axis, and the linearity of any moving laser. The accuracy of isocentre localization by the lasers should be tested in conjunction with the virtual simulation software. Whether the marking system outlines three points or the entire beam aperture, the test should be designed to mimic the clinical procedures. A simple procedure could involve scanning a phantom with markers fixed to various locations, placing the 'isocentre' on a marker by virtual simulation, moving the couch and lasers to the programmed positions, and verifying that the marker is illuminated by all lasers.

The hardware and software components of the virtual simulation workstation should be thoroughly tested at the time of initial acceptance and again any time a component is upgraded or a new function installed. Essential components such as gantry, collimator, and table rotations, field size, isocentre location, SSD/SAD, beam divergence, contour accuracy in all projections, magnification, and DRR projection accuracy should be thoroughly checked. QA phantoms specifically designed for virtual simulation need to be developed to make these

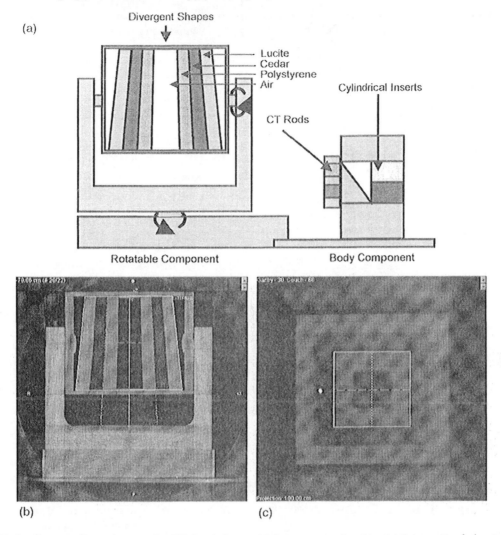

(a)

Divergent Shapes

Lucite
Cedar
Polystyrene
Air

Cylindrical Inserts

CT Rods

Rotatable Component

Body Component

(b)

(c)

Figure 7.13 Quality assurance phantom for CT simulation and 3-D treatment planning. (a) Schematic of phantom design showing two components: (1) a 'rotatable component' with the rotations representing gantry and couch rotations and the divergent cones representing different divergent beam sizes; (2) a 'body component' with different volume inserts to assess volumes and dose–volume histograms. The latter also contains a number of different materials for assessing consistency in CT number to electron density conversions. (b) CT images of the phantom with zero degree gantry and couch rotations. Also shown are the beam edges of a 10 × 10 cm^2 field showing good agreement with the edges of the different densities in the phantom. (c) A DRR with superimposed 10 × 10 cm^2 field again showing good agreement.

checks practical on a routine basis. An example of such a phantom and the corresponding beam display assessment is shown in Figure 7.13 (Craig *et al.* 1999).

7.   Specialized imaging procedures

7.1   *Magnetic resonance imaging*

Magnetic resonance imaging (MRI) continues to show improvement as an imaging modality for the assessment

of malignant disease, particularly for sites such as the central nervous system, brain, head and neck, prostate, and lymph nodes. MRI is very useful for defining tumour localization, as well as following tumour response after treatment. MRI also provides unrestricted multiplanar and volumetric imaging, as well as physiological and biochemical information with magnetic resonance (MR) spectroscopy and angiography. However, MR images are subject to geometric distortion and MR parameters are not directly translatable to relative electron densities. Thus, MR is a useful tool for providing additional information to the therapy-planning process, especially for 3-D considerations, although it is not capable of replacing CT scanning. As such, these are complementary tools. A recent review article provides an excellent summary of the use of MRI in radiation therapy planning (Khoo *et al.* 1997). Some of the following is based on this article.

7.1.1 Principles of MRI

Briefly, an MR scanner consists of a large external magnetic field with superimposed radiofrequency pulses. The MR process consists of the measurement of the radiofrequency radiation resulting from transitions between nuclear spin states of hydrogen atoms (protons). While CT is dependent on X-ray attenuation that is a function of electron density and atomic number of the tissues, the relative pixel values in MRI are a function of tissue relaxation times and proton densities. For MRI, a major source of pixel value variation is due to the difference in relaxation times between different tissue types.

Spin–lattice (T1) and spin–spin (T2) relaxation times are the two parameters that are often used to characterize the MR signal and MR contrast. MR images are derived from signals acquired by using particular pulse sequences and magnetic field gradients. The resulting images are dependent on the relative timing of the applied pulses, gradients, and signal acquisition. MRI has no standard imaging sequence; however, resulting images are often weighted according to a specific relaxation time such as T1- or T2-weighted images. Thus, MRI has a tremendous variation in terms of imaging parameters and pixel intensities with settings often being adjusted on an empirical basis.

7.1.2 MRI for radiation therapy planning

MRI has a much superior ability to assess soft-tissue variations in comparison to CT. Varying the image sequence parameters provides tremendous soft-tissue contrast. This is very useful for evaluating the extent of malignancies, especially those that are adjacent to or infiltrating muscle. MRI has been shown to be superior to CT in the staging of soft-tissue and pelvic tumours. It is also sensitive to assessing bone marrow disease and bony metastases. It is the imaging modality of choice for brain, spinal cord, some head and neck tumours and, in combination with contrast agents, it has further scope in oncology especially within the central nervous system (Lattanzi *et al.* 1997).

One feature of MRI that is in contrast to CT is that bone appears with very low signal intensity. This provides the advantage of clearer definition of lesions near bony structures, including the posterior fossa, the brainstem, and the spinal cord. The disadvantages relate

to radiation dosimetry and image correlation problems when trying to compare MR to CT.

A major feature of MRI that is particularly suited to 3-D conformal radiation therapy is the ability to determine images with equivalent characteristics in any plane in 3-D. However, MRI still has some substantial limitations for radiation therapy planning in comparison to CT (Henkelman *et al.* 1984). These include:

(1) the lack of electron density information, which is essential for radiation dosage calculations;

(2) the absence of MR signals from cortical bone;

(3) the presence of image distortions;

(4) tumour boundaries can be obscured by peripheral edema;

(5) the lack of availability of adequate computer software to integrate and manipulate MR images in radiation therapy planning systems.

The correction of distortions requires constant imaging conditions between patient and phantom studies. Care has to be taken to avoid imaging patients with magnetic materials or pacemakers, as these could create substantial image or clinical concerns. Furthermore, external ferromagnetic objects must be avoided and kept out of the MRI room to avoid accidents with mobile objects in these strong magnetic fields or to avoid image distortions. Thus rigorous QA is essential to prevent any untoward misadventures. As for CT, accurate immobilization and positioning with appropriate reference marks are essential for therapy planning and image correlation. Again immobilization devices need to avoid metallic substances. MRI-scanner tunnels are generally even more constrained than CT scanners. Scan times should be limited to minimize motion artefacts. Unfortunately, organizational issues often make MR scanning, specifically for therapy planning, very difficult. Difficulties include:

(1) MRI scans are generally performed for diagnostic reasons before the patient enters a radiation therapy department and, thus, are not done for planning purposes;

(2) head immobilization devices do not fit in the MR imager because the MR radiologists want head patients in very small head coils;

(3) MR imagers use curved couches.

For these reasons, appropriate image correlation software is crucial to correlating target volume image information on MR and CT.

In summary, MRI has considerable potential for therapy planning, although it will usually need to be used in conjunction with CT. MR-image distortions remain a concern and reliable methods of distortion correction remain to be developed. Furthermore, precise methods of image segmentation (organ/structure outlining), correlation, and registration are required so that MR could be used alone or with CT for radiation therapy planning.

7.2 Simulator with CT mode

Some researchers (Kotre *et al.* 1984; Redpath and Wright 1985) and manufacturers have developed techniques whereby the imaging device on the simulator can be used to record transmitted beam intensities as the simulator gantry rotates. The resultant reconstructed images are analogous to conventional CT images. The advantages of such a device are two fold. First, the cost is low and, therefore, these can be considered as inexpensive CT scanners. Second, the geometry of the simulation is more representative of the therapy machine geometry; hence, patient set-ups produced by such a simulator with a CT mode are not as constrained as they are with conventional CT scanners with their limited aperture sizes. However, there are several concerns with the use of these devices. First, the images are of a slightly poorer quality compared to modern CT scanners. Hence, interpretations should be regarded with caution. Second, simulators with a CT option acquire images slowly compared to CT scanners, requiring about one minute per revolution. This can increase the probability of motion artifacts both within and between the slices. Certainly these scans should not be used for tumour localization. Third, it is difficult to obtain a full set of CT images, making it difficult to use these data for 3-D reconstructions.

The greatest advantage of these devices is that they are capable of providing both external contours and information on gross internal structures such as lungs, bones, chest wall thicknesses, etc. While modern simulators with a CT mode provide reasonably good CT number data, older versions did not provide accurate CT numbers and thus, for tissue inhomogeneity corrections, assumptions had to be made about tissue density (Van Dyk *et al.* 1982). It must be emphasized that a CT mode on a simulator will not replace the diagnostic use of conventional CT, nor will it allow for detailed tumour localization or follow-up studies. As such, it remains an additional procedure to the rest of the therapy-planning process with the convenience of obtaining some relatively crude CT images during the simulation process, primarily for the derivation of internal and external contours.

7.3 Other imaging procedures

Improvements in imaging technology continue to enhance the ability of the diagnostic radiologist and the radiation oncologist to diagnose, stage, and evaluate the response of malignant disease. The role of various imaging modalities, such as CT, magnetic resonance, radionuclide, ultrasound, and others, will continue to increase (Glatstein *et al.* 1985; Photon Treatment Planning Collaborative Working Groups 1991). Ideally, the treatment-planning system would allow for a direct correlation of these various imaging modalities. Some imaging modalities that have been used as part of the planning process are outlined briefly below. In the future, we can expect to see them used more frequently as they become more readily available and computer software allows for easier image correlation.

7.3.1 Radionuclide scanning

Radionuclide scans are extremely useful for demonstrating tumour uptake and the spread of metastatic disease. Furthermore, lymphoscintigraphy has been demonstrated to be useful for the localization of internal mammary lymph nodes. As for MRI, these nuclear medicine procedures provide additional information that is useful for the therapy-planning process and the delineation of target volumes.

7.3.2 Ultrasound scanning

Ultrasound, in the context of radiation oncology, can be used as a means of deriving patient contours, as well as some limited information on internal structures, such as chest-wall thicknesses, and the localization of specific tumours or normal tissues, such as bladder, rectum, and kidneys. Recent applications include ocular melanomas and retinoblastomas where tumours can be localized with respect to radioactive plaques and the location of the lens can be accurately determined for dose-determination purposes. Transrectal ultrasound is now being used for assessing tumour extent and localization for prostate cancer. Indeed, it is proposed that 3-D ultrasound could be used as a means of localizing the prostate disease on a daily basis and to arrange the radiation beams as to the actual location of the prostate rather than using surface landmarks. This approach could be a tremendous aid to the application of 3-D conformal radiation therapy.

7.4 Image correlation

Modern radiation therapy equipment utilizes a number of imaging modalities for diagnosis, tumour localization, simulation, and port verification. Many of these have been discussed in this chapter, although very few institutions are making full use of all these applications. One of the greatest challenges that faces the medical-physics community is the ability to combine some or all of these imaging modalities, so that the data can be intercompared accurately in the planning and verification stages. In doing so, unique information from each modality can be coalesced to provide maximum input for therapy-planning purposes. Ideally, since all these imaging modalities can provide digital information, this intercomparison can be performed through computer technology (Kessler *et al.* 1991). However, such image correlation is complicated by a number of factors including:

(1) patient positioning;

(2) pixel or voxel size;

(3) image distortions as can occur in MRI;

(4) different anatomy as observed by different imaging modalities (e.g. CT, MRI, nuclear medicine);

(5) differences in spatial resolution.

Initial correlation can be made by a visual inter-comparison of various images. Computer correlation is aided by the use of fiducial markers on the patient or by matching surfaces derived from known anatomical structures, such as bony landmarks. However, considerable research is still required to make computerized image correlation a practical reality.

8. Summary and conclusions

The treatment of malignant disease using megavoltage radiation requires sophisticated technology for the diagnosis of the disease and for the localization of the tumour and critical normal tissues. An important component of the therapy-planning process is the determination of appropriate fields with necessary shielding in order to maximize the dose to the tumour and to minimize the dose to normal tissues. A review of clinical data has shown that departments not using treatment simulators as a part of the planning process yield substantially worse clinical results compared with those that do (Hanks *et al.* 1985). More recently, CT scanners have proved to be an essential tool not only for diagnosis and localization but also for deriving tissue densities essential for accurate dose calculations. It is now well recognized that radical radiation therapy requires a dose delivery accuracy of better than 5%. This is important for individual patients, as well as for deriving interpretable results from clinical trials. Without the use of therapy simulators, CT scanners, or the combination in the form of CT simulators, this accuracy in dose delivery would not be possible.

9. References

Andrew, J.W. and Aldrich, J.E. (1982). A microcomputer-based system for radiotherapy beam compensator design and patient contour plotting. *Med. Phys.*, **9**, 279–83.

Battista, J.J. and Bronskill, M.J. (1981). Compton scatter imaging of transverse sections: an overall appraisal and evaluation for treatment planning. *Phys. Med. Biol.*, **26**, 81–99.

Bomford, C.K., Dawes, P.J., Lillicrap, S.C., and Young, J. (1989). *Treatment simulators*. BIR Supplement 23. British Institute of Radiology, London.

Brahme, A. (ed.) (1988). Accuracy requirements and quality assurance of external beam therapy with photons and electrons. *Acta Oncol.*, Supplement 1.

Brink, J.A. and Davros, W.J. (1995). Helical/spiral CT: technical principles. In *Helical/spiral CT a practical approach* (ed. R.K. Zeman, J.A. Brink, and P. Costello). McGraw–Hill Inc., New York.

Carol, M.E. (1995) Beam intensity modulation conformal radiotherapy. International symposium proceedings. In *3D radiation treatment planning and conformal therapy*, pp. 435–45. Medical Physics Publishing. Madison, WI.

Coia, L.W., Schultheiss, T.E., and Hanks, G.E. (ed.) (1995). *A practical guide to CT simulation*. Advanced Medical Publishing, Madison, W.I.

Connors, S.G., Battista, J.J., and Bertin, R.J. (1984). On technical specifications of radiotherapy simulators. *Med. Phys.*, **11**, 341–3.

Craig, T., Brochu, D., and Van Dyk, J. (1999). A quality assurance phantom for three-dimensional radiation treatment planning. *Int. J. Radiat. Oncol. Biol. Phys.*, **44**, 955–66.

Day, M.J. and Harrison, R.M. (1983). Cross sectional information and treatment simulation. In *Radiation therapy planning* (ed. N.J. Bleehen, E. Glatstein, and J. Haybittle), pp. 87–138. Marcel Dekker, New York.

Dick Loo, L.N. (1991). CT acceptance testing. In *Specification, acceptance testing and quality control of diagnostic X-ray imaging equipment* (Proc. AAPM Summer School 1991) (ed. J.A. Seibert, G.T. Barnes, and R.G. Gould), pp. 1042–66. American Institute of Physics, New York.

Doppke, K.P. (1987). X-ray simulator developments and evaluation for radiation therapy. In *Radiation oncology physics – 1986* (ed. J.G. Kereiakes, E.R. Elson, and C.G. Born), pp. 429–41. American Institute of Physics, New York.

Fuks, Z., Leibel, S.A., Kutcher, G.J., Mohan, R., and Ling, C.C. (1991). Three-dimensional conformal treatment: A new frontier in radiation therapy. In *Important advances in oncology* (ed. V.T. DeVita, S. Hellman, and S.A. Rosenberg), pp. 155–72. Lippincot, Philadelphia.

Glatstein, E., Lichter, A.S., Fraass, B.A., Kelly, B.A., and van de Geijn, J. (1985). The imaging revolution and radiation oncology: use of CT, ultrasound, and NMR for localization, treatment planning and treatment delivery. *Int. J. Radiat. Oncol. Biol. Phys.*, **11**, 299–314.

Goitein, M. (1982). Applications of computed tomography in radiotherapy treatment planning. In *Progress in medical radiation physics*, Vol. 1 (ed. C.G. Orton), pp. 195–293. Plenum Press, New York.

Goitein, M., Abrams, M., Rowell, E., Pollari, H., and Wiles, J. (1983). Multi-dimensional treatment planning: II beam's eye-view, back projection, and projection through CT sections. *Int. J. Radiat. Oncol. Biol. Phys.*, **9** 789–97.

Gray, J.E., Winkler, N.T., Stears, J., and Frank, E.D. (1983). *Quality control in diagnostic imaging*. University Park Press, Baltimore, MD.

Hanks, G.E., Diamond, J.J., and Kramer, S. (1985). The need for complex technology in radiation oncology. *Cancer*, **55**, 2198–201.

Henkelman, R.M., Poon, P.Y., and Bronskill, M.J. (1984). Is magnetic resonance useful for planning of radiotherapy? In *Proceedings eighth international conference of computers in radiation therapy* (ed. J.R. Cunningham, D. Ragan, and J. Van Dyk), pp. 181–5. IEEE Computer Society, Silver Spring, MD.

International Commission on Radiation Units and Measurements (1978) *Dose specification of reporting external beam therapy with photons and electrons.* Report 29. ICRU, Washington, DC.

International Commission on Radiation Units and Measurements (1993). *Prescribing, recording, and reporting photon beam therapy.* Report 50. ICRU, Washington, DC.

Inter-Society Council for Radiation Oncology (1991). *Radiation oncology in integrated cancer management.* National Institutes of Health, Washington, DC.

Jani, S.K. (ed.) (1993). *CT-simulation for radiotherapy.* Medical Physics Publishing, Madison, WI.

Kelsey, C.A., Berardo, P.A., Smith, A.R., and Kligerman, M.M. (1980). CT scanner selection and specification for radiation therapy. *Med Phys.*, **7**, 555–8.

Kessler, M.L., Pitluck, S., Petti, P., and Castro, J.R. (1991). Integration of multimodality imaging data for radiotherapy treatment planning. *Int. J. Radiat. Oncol. Biol. Phys.*, **21**, 1653–67.

Khoo, V.S., Dearnaley, D.P., Finnigan, D.J., Padhani, A., Tanner, S.F., and Leach, M.O. (1997). Magnetic resonance imaging (MRI): considerations and applications in radiotherapy treatment planning. *Radioth. Oncol.*, **42**, 1–15.

Kotre, C.J., Harrison, R.M., and Ross, W.M. (1984). A simulator-based CT system for radiotherapy treatment planning. *Br. J. Radiol.* **57**, 631–5.

Lattanzi, J.P., Fein, D.A., McNeeley, S.W., Shaer, A.H., Movsas, B, and Hanks, G.E. (1997). Computed tomography-magnetic resonance image fusion: a clinical evaluation of an innovative approach for improved tumor localization in primary central nervous system lesions. *Radiat. Oncol. Investig.*, **5**, 195–205.

Lin, P.P., Strauss, K.J., Conway, B.J., *et al.* (1988). *Protocols for radiation safety of diagnostic radiological equipment.* AAPM Report 25. American Institute of Physics, New York.

Mah, K., Danjoux, C.E., Manship, S., Makhani, N., Cardoso, M., and Sixel, K.E. (1998). CT-simulation of craniospinal fields in paediatric patients: improved treatment accuracy and patient comfort. *Int. J. Radiat. Oncol. Biol. Phys.*, **41**, 997–1003.

Martin, E.E. (1995). CT simulation hardware. In *A practical guide to CT simulation* (ed. L.W. Coia, T.E. Schultheiss, and G.E. Hanks), pp. 51–9. Advanced Medical Publishing, Madison, WI.

McCullough, E.C. and Earle, J.D. (1979). The selection, acceptance testing, and quality control of radiotherapy treatment simulators. *Radiol.* **131**, 221–230.

McGee, K.P. and Das, I.J. (1995) Commissioning, acceptance testing, and quality assurance of a CT simulator. In *A practical guide to CT simulation* (ed. L.W. Coia, T.E. Schultheiss, and G.E. Hanks), pp. 5–23. Advanced Medical Publishing, Madison, WI.

Nishidai, T., Nagata, Y., Takahashi, M., Abe, M., Yamaoka, N., Ishihara, H. *et al.* (1990). CT simulator: a new 3-D planning and simulation system for radiotherapy: part 1. Description of system. *Int. J. Radiat. Oncol. Biol. Phys.*, **18**, 499–504.

Photon Treatment Planning Collaborative Working Groups (1991). State-of-the-art of external photon beam radiation treatment planning. *Int. J. Radiat. Oncol. Biol. Phys.*, **21**, 9–23.

Ragan, D.P., He, T., Mesina, C.F., and Ratanatharathorn, V. (1993). CT-based simulation with laser patient marking. *Med. Phys.*, **20**, 379–80.

Redpath, A.T. and Wright, D.H. (1985). The use of an image processing system in radiotherapy simulation. *Br. J. Radiol.*, **58**, 1081–9.

Rosenman, J., Sailer, S.L., Sherouse, G.W., Chaney, E.L., and Tepper, J.E. (1991). Virtual simulation: initial clinical results. *Int. J. Radiat. Oncol. Biol. Phys.*, **20**, 843–51.

Sherouse, G.W. and Chaney, E.L. (1991). The portable virtual simulator. *Int. J. Radiat. Oncol. Biol. Phys.*, **21**, 475–82.

Sherouse, G.W., Novins, K.L., and Chaney, E.L. (1990). Computation of digitally reconstructed radiographs for use in radiotherapy treatment design. *Int. J. Radiat. Oncol. Biol. Phys.*, **18**, 651–8.

Sternick, E.S. (1983). Special contouring techniques. In *Advances in radiation therapy treatment planning* (ed. H.E. Wright and A.L. Boyer), pp. 138–48. American Institute of Physics, New York.

Van Dyk, J., Keane, T.J., and Rider, W.D. (1982). Lung density as measured by computerized tomography: implications for radiotherapy. *Int. J. Radiat. Oncol. Biol. Phys.*, **8**, 1363–72.

Wang, G. and Vannier, M.W. (1994). Longitudinal resolution in volumetric X-ray computerized tomography – analytical comparison between conventional and helical computerized tomography. *Med. Phys.*, **21**, 429–33.

Chapter 8

Treatment planning for external beam therapy: principles and basic techniques

A.T. Redpath and J.R. Williams

1. Introduction

Treatment planning is the process whereby the therapeutic strategy of the radiation oncologist is realized as a set of treatment instructions together with a physical description of the distribution of dose in the patient. The aims of treatment planning can be summarized as follows:

1. To localize the tumour volume in the patient and to define the target volume for treatment.

2. To measure the outline of the patient and to place within it the target volume and other anatomical structures, which may affect the dose distribution or for which dose constraints may be necessary.

3. To determine the optimum treatment configuration required to irradiate the target volume to the specified dose within particular clinical constraints.

4. To calculate the resultant dose distribution in the patient.

5. To prepare an unambiguous set of treatment instructions for the radiographers.

The first two of these aims have been discussed in detail in Chapter 7. Other basic aspects of treatment planning are considered in this chapter in respect of photon beam therapy. More complex aspects of external beam photon therapy are considered in Chapter 9. Although many of the general points relating to photon therapy apply to external beam electron treatment, treatment planning aspects specific to this modality will be considered separately in Chapter 10.

Requirements for accuracy and prescription in the dose to be delivered to the tumour were discussed in Chapter 1. In treatment planning, consideration must not only be given to the accuracy and precision of dose to a specified point or points, but also to the geometric tolerance of dose delivery. It has been estimated that there is a ±4 mm positional error in treatment and this should be taken into account when the target volume is defined.

Optimization of radiotherapy may be constrained by several factors. There are physical factors, such as the fundamental nature of the radiations used and the limitations of treatment equipment. Resources may be limited, which may make it necessary to compromise the treatment given. There are also clinical factors, which may make it inappropriate to give the most sophisticated treatment when the patient will not gain any significant benefit.

Dose distributions are calculated to provide the clinician with a physical description of the treatment prescribed and to provide a record of that treatment. Formerly, all treatment plans were produced laboriously by hand. This compromises accuracy, but more importantly hand planning limits the opportunity for optimization of the dose distribution and limits the degree of sophistication to which patients may be treated. Computer systems are now almost universally used for radiotherapy planning and this has been made possible by the decreasing cost of hardware and the expanding market in software, much of it developed by physicists working in the clinical environment.

The final product of treatment planning is the treatment card or prescription sheet. This provides a set of instructions for the radiographer enabling the treatment to be delivered as described by the dose distribution. The instructions must be both unambiguous and accurate. Accuracy has to be assured by a series of checks through the whole planning process, and these should form a part of a fully documented quality assurance system (see Chapter 14).

The definition of terms recommended by the ICRU will be used in this chapter (ICRU 1993). These definitions have already been summarized in Chapter 7, Section 2. It is assumed that field sizes are defined as the width of the 50% isodose at the isocentric distance, which is the definition recommended by the ICRU.

In this chapter reference will be made to the planning target volume (PTV) and care is needed to ensure the exact definition of this term. The tumour mass that is to be irradiated, known as the gross tumour volume (GTV), is surrounded by a region of subclinical tumour infiltration. The GTV plus this surrounding region is known as the clinical target volume (CTV). A further allowance must be made for possible errors in localization, for potential positional errors in the daily set-up of the patient, including the tolerances on machine performance, and for patient movement, e.g. those movements caused by breathing. The margin allowed depends, amongst other factors, on local protocols, tumour size, and site. For example, for a tumour close to the spinal cord, a smaller margin may be allowed in order to ensure that the treatment is delivered safely. Typically, the margin surrounding the tumour volume is in the range 5–15 mm. The total volume defined in this way is the planning target volume. The specification of these volumes are described in more detail in Chapter 9.

2. General principles and planning techniques

2.1 Single fields

Single-field treatment is a term applied to those situations in which the irradiated volume does not overlap any other volume treated concurrently. In photon therapy, treatments with a single field are generally used only for palliative purposes, a typical example being the irradiation of the spine to relieve pain in patients who have spinal metastases. In general, it is only with low-energy X-rays (below 150 kV) that single photon beams are used curatively. This modality is described in Chapter 6.

Methods of calculation of the dose for single fields and other planning considerations for these treatments are described below. These details may also be applied with other treatment configurations.

2.1.1 Calculation

The dose distribution in a central plane of a single-field irradiation can be described by an isodose chart. A typical dose distribution is shown for a 6 MV X-ray beam in Figure 8.1a. An isodose is a line of equal dose. The dose represented by the line is expressed as a percentage of the dose on the central axis at the depth of dose maximum. By convention the single-field isodose curves are plotted at 10% intervals and are presented on a 1 : 1 scale. This dose distribution represents a full description of the treatment in a single plane, provided that the section of the surface through which the patient

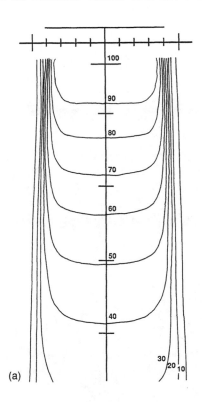

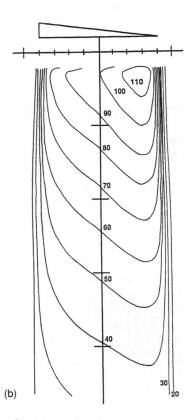

Figure 8.1 Isodose distributions for a 6 MV X-ray beam with an 8 × 8 cm² field size: (a) is for an open field; and (b) is for a field with a 45° wedge.

is treated is flat and perpendicular to the central axis of the beam, and that the tissue within the volume irradiated is homogeneous and equivalent to water in its attenuating properties.

Single-field treatments are normally prescribed in terms of the dose to be given to a point at a specified depth on the central axis of the beam, and the dose distribution is not required. Two data charts are required for the calculation of the monitor units on a linear accelerator, or of the time to be set on a cobalt unit, in order to deliver the prescribed dose to the target. These are an output chart and, if the dose is prescribed to a depth other than the dose maximum, a depth–dose table.

The data in the two charts are normally tabulated for square fields. If the field is rectangular, an equivalent square field size that would have the same output and depth–dose characteristics is used. This is not simply equal to the square root of the field area, as the effect of scatter at the central axis of the beam is not simply dependent on field area. It also depends on the distance that the scattered photons have to travel in order to reach the central axis. There are standard tables for calculating the equivalent square of rectangular fields, such as given in *BJR* Supplement 25 (BIR 1996). It has been shown that these data can be adequately represented by the following relationship:

$$s = \frac{2ab}{(a+b)}$$

where s is the side of the equivalent square, and a and b are the sides of the rectangular field. This is an empirical relationship, which should be used with caution for those fields with equivalent square sides greater than 20 cm or with elongation factors greater than 2. A full discussion on its limitations is given in BIR (1996). Table 8.1 is an example of an output chart for a 6 MV linear accelerator. The data are given in terms of the number of monitor units required to give a dose of 100 cGy to the dose maximum. Table 8.2 is a typical depth–dose chart. It should be noted that both of these charts are for a specified source–skin distance (SSD) of 100 cm. The

Table 8.1 Sample output chart for a 6 MV X-ray beam giving the required number of monitor units to deliver a dose of 100 cGy to the position of the dose maximum on the central axis at 100 cm SSD

Field size (cm²)	Output mu/100 cGy
6 × 6	104.3
8 × 8	102.0
10 × 10	100.0
12 × 12	98.5
15 × 15	96.7
20 × 20	94.8

Table 8.2 Sample depth–dose chart for a 6 MV X-ray beam for a treatment distance of 100 cm SSD

Depth (cm)	Field size (cm²)					
	6 × 6	8 × 8	10 × 10	12 × 12	15 × 15	20 × 20
1.5	100.0	100.0	100.0	100.0	100.0	100.0
2.0	98.1	98.2	98.3	98.4	98.5	98.5
4.0	89.3	89.8	90.2	90.4	90.7	91.0
6.0	80.6	81.8	82.6	83.2	83.9	84.6
8.0	71.6	72.9	74.0	74.7	75.5	76.5
10.0	63.7	65.1	66.2	67.0	68.0	69.2
12.0	56.7	58.1	59.3	60.2	61.3	62.7
14.0	50.4	51.9	53.1	54.1	55.3	56.7
16.0	44.9	46.4	47.6	48.6	49.8	51.3
18.0	39.9	41.4	42.6	43.7	44.9	46.5
20.0	35.5	37.0	38.2	39.2	40.5	42.1

Table 8.3 An example of the calculation of the required daily monitor units for a single-field treatment

Prescribed dose	1500 cGy
Number of fractions	5
Target depth	6 cm
Field size	12 × 7 cm²
SSD	100 cm
Equivalent square	8.8 cm
Per cent depth dose	82.1%
Output factor	101.2 mu/100 cGy

Daily monitor units = (1500/5) × (101.2/100) × (100/82.1)
= 370 mu

Output and depth–dose data have been interpolated from Tables 8.1 and 8.2.

data in the tables are presented for a limited number of field sizes and depths. For manual calculations, more extensive data-sets should be provided to minimize the need for interpolation and to ensure that linear interpolation between the data points provides adequate accuracy.

An example of a single field calculation for a prescription to a specified depth is shown in Table 8.3.

2.1.2 Use of shielding blocks

This simple type of calculation is sufficient for most single-field treatments. However, if a shielding block is used to protect a sensitive structure in part of the field, some modification is required. The equivalent square field size is changed resulting in an alteration to both output and depth dose. The method of calculation is to subtract the projected area of the block at the treatment distance from the square of the equivalent field size and to take the square root of this difference. If a corner of the beam in the example in Table 8.3 was blocked in the form of a triangle with two sides of 4 cm, the equivalent square of the resultant field would be 8.4 cm. This is a reasonable approximation, provided that the area blocked is at the edge of the beam and the area blocked is less than about 15% of the total area of the beam. For a more accurate method of calculating blocked beams see Section 7.1.

Shielding blocks are normally positioned on a tray attached to the treatment head. The tray attenuates the beam and, therefore, the output has to be corrected by a tray factor. This factor may vary sufficiently with field size for that to have to be taken into account. Care should be taken to specify the appropriate factor if there is more than one tray available on the set. It should be noted that the use of the shielding tray and blocks can increase the surface dose to the patient due to electrons generated in them by photon interactions.

2.1.3 Non-standard treatment distance

For most single-field treatments, a standard SSD is used and this is normally the distance from the radiation source to the isocentre of the treatment unit. Non-standard distances may be used in certain circumstances, the most common being when the field size needed is larger than can be obtained at the standard SSD and so an extended SSD is required. This is unusual for single-field irradiation. Alternatively, shortened SSDs may be used in order to increase the dose rate and, therefore, to decrease treatment time. This is most likely to occur on a cobalt unit. Altering SSD causes a change in output factor and, to a lesser extent, in the depth dose. The variation in output factor with SSD can be assumed to depend on the inverse square law (ISL), provided that the deviation from the standard SSD is not large (less than about 10 cm). The correction to be applied to the output factor is:

$$\left(\frac{f + d_{max}}{f_0 + d_{max}}\right)^2$$

where f is the treatment distance, f_0 is the nominal SSD and d_{max} is the depth of dose maximum. This relationship should be treated with caution for cobalt units, for which the source height may be several centimetres so that the effective SSD may be greater than the distance from its front surface. ISL corrections should be confirmed by measurement.

The ISL correction above is a multiplicative factor in the case of the data presented in Table 8.1. However, if the data are presented as dose per minute, as is the case for cobalt units, the output should be divided by this factor. If treatments are regularly given at non-standard treatment distances, it is good practice to prepare output charts based on measurements for a range of SSDs, which encompass the values used for treatment. The SSD intervals should be sufficiently close to permit accurate linear interpolation.

The variation of dose with depth depends on both the attenuating properties of tissue and on the ISL. To convert a depth–dose value to an alternate SSD it is necessary to correct the measured data to infinite SSD, i.e. by removing the inverse square component, and then converting to the SSD of treatment. For a point at a depth d in a beam with its dose maximum at d_{max}, the form of the correction to the depth dose measured at an SSD of f_0 is:

$$\left(\frac{f_0 + d}{f_0 + d_{max}}\right)^2 \left(\frac{f + d_{max}}{f + d}\right)^2$$

where f is the treatment distance. The net effect is that per cent depth dose increases with SSD. The correction should be applied to the depth–dose data at f_0 for the field size to be used at the non-standard treatment distance, f. This is because the scatter component of the central axis depth–dose curve depends on the field size at the depth of dose maximum and not on the collimator setting.

In changing from an SSD of 100 cm to one of 90 cm, this correction affects the depth dose at a depth of 5 cm by just under 1%, but it should not be ignored in these calculations. The correction is an approximation based on the ISL and is only valid for the primary component of the radiation beams. If regular use is made of SSDs, which differ for more than 10 cm from the SSD used for measurement, alternative data should be measured.

2.1.4 Adjacent treatment volumes

A single field may be treated that is adjacent to a volume that has either been irradiated previously or that is to be treated concurrently. A common example of the latter situation is in the treatment of breast cancer. For this treatment the supraclavicular region may be irradiated using a single anterior field and this is matched to a two-field irradiation of the breast. This special case will be discussed in Section 6.4.

For the general situation when two areas of single-field treatment are adjacent to each other, account must be taken of beam divergence. If the two field edges are matched at the skin, the dose at any depth below the skin will be significantly increased in the region of overlap in comparison with the dose elsewhere at the same depth. If the beam edges at the surface are separated by a distance that is sufficient to cause an exact match at the depth of dose specification, there will then be underdosing at more superficial depths. This is shown in Figure 8.2a. Better matching can be achieved if the two adjacent beams can be angled as shown in the Figure 8.2b so that their edges are parallel. This minimizes the discontinuity in dose and produces optimum matching at all depths. It is assumed in this discussion that the beam edge corresponds to the 50% dose level.

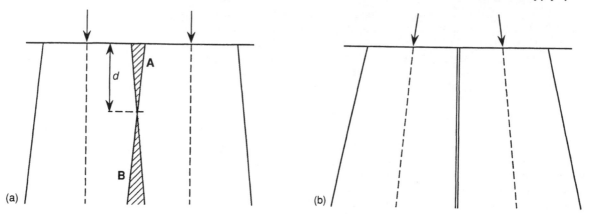

Figure 8.2 The effect of using two single adjacent beams: (a) represents beams with parallel central rays matched at depth *d* leading to underdosing in the hatched area, A, and overdosing in the area B; and (b) has precise matching at the beam edge at all depths with the central rays angled outwards at the angle of beam divergence.

When beams are matched in this way it should be noted that the effective divergence on the opposite side of the beams is doubled. This may need to be considered if irradiation of sensitive structures is to be avoided. Also it becomes more difficult to add a third field.

Beam matching inevitably causes some discontinuity in dose, even if the set-up is perfect. When two fields are treated concurrently, a daily variation in the position of the junction between the two fields may help to minimize systematically occurring discontinuities. It is also necessary to consider the possible discrepancies between the light field and X-ray beam. Quality control tests permit a discrepancy of 2 mm at the beam edge (Chapter 5, Section 12.1.9). For critical applications, this difference should be noted for the two beam edges to be matched and the position of the light beam edge on the skin adjusted accordingly.

If a single field has to be matched to a volume that has been irradiated by two or more fields, then a smaller angular change in the central axis needs to be made. In multiple-field treatments, it can be assumed that the isodoses at the edge of the volume lie in a plane parallel to the plane containing the central axes of the beams. In the case of the opposed beams, the match plane is parallel to the edge of the beam to be matched. The single field then has to be angled so that its edge is parallel to this plane. The position of the beam should be such that its edge coincides with the edge of the other beams at the depth of the target volume.

Improved field matching may be achieved using asymmetric jaws if that option is available on the linear accelerator's collimator system. This will be discussed in more detail in Section 7.3 and Chapter 9, Section 2.3.

2.2 Opposed coaxial fields

Two opposed coaxial beams can be used to irradiate volumes of tissue in which the tumour cannot be accurately defined or because the intention is to give a relatively low dose for palliation. Many tumour sites may be irradiated in this way, and the type of treatment is commonly referred to as a parallel pair or parallel opposed irradiation.

2.2.1 Opposed field dose calculation

Figure 8.3 shows a typical isodose distribution that results from opposed coaxial fields. Certain features should be noted. It can be seen that the dose to the subcutaneous region at the depth of dose maximum is greater than the dose at the central point. In this example, for an 18-cm thick section treated in a 6 MV X-ray beam, the difference is about 4%. The difference depends on the beam quality and the separation between the skin entry points. For higher energies and/or smaller separations the central dose may be greater than the subcutaneous dose. However, even for this situation the relatively high subcutaneous dose provides a constraint on the dose that can be delivered at the mid-point of the patient. It may also be seen that the isodose curves show that the dose profile at the mid-line is less uniform than at the surface due to the effects of scatter. In addition, the penumbra width increases with depth.

Presentation of full isodose data for parallel-pair treatments is not the usual practice. In general, these treatments are prescribed in terms of the dose to the mid-point of the target volume. In addition, the dose at the depth of dose maximum below the skin is usually

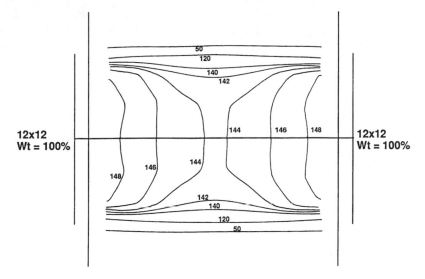

Figure 8.3 Opposed coaxial field irradiation for 6 MV X-rays with separation of the entry points equal to 18 cm and for a 12 × 12 cm² field size.

calculated. When calculating this dose it is necessary to look up the depth dose on the exit side of the beam at a depth that is equal to the total separation minus the depth of build-up. The method of calculation may be demonstrated by an example as shown in Table 8.4.

2.2.2 Isocentric opposed fields

The example shown in Table 8.4 is for a treatment at a fixed SSD. In many centres there is a preference for performing these treatments isocentrically. Isocentric irradiation involves positioning the patient so that the centre of the target volume is coincident with the centre of rotation of the treatment unit. When the first beam has

Table 8.4 Sample dose calculation for opposed coaxial fields using a 6 MV X-ray beam

Prescribed dose	3000 cGy
Number of fractions	10
Field size	14 × 8 cm²
SSD	100 cm
Separation	18 cm
Equivalent square	10.2 cm
Central depth dose	70.2 × 2 = 140.4%
Maximum % dose	100 + 46.5 = 146.5%
Output	99.8 mu/100 cGy

Daily monitor units = (3000/10) × (99.8/100) × (100/140.4)
= 213 mu

Maximum dose = 3000 × (146.5/140.4) = 3130 cGy

Output and depth dose data have been interpolated from Tables 8.1 and 8.2.

been set up and treated it is then only necessary to rotate the gantry through 180° before treating the second field. This has the advantage of minimizing set-up time for the second field and thus the overall treatment time. In addition, for opposed fields the effect of errors in setting up the treatment distance is minimized. Since treatment is carried out at a non-standard SSD, the output and depth–dose charts cannot be used directly and corrections should be made as indicated previously. For depth doses it is preferable to prepare tables of data at a distance 10 cm less than the distance to the isocentre, normally 90 cm. This corresponds to a typical mid-point depth of 10 cm and can be used over the typical range of clinical separations without a significant loss in accuracy. Separations of 12–24 cm would produce an error of 0.5% or less. Output charts should be available that cover a range of SSDs, if these treatments are planned manually, although computerized calculation is generally more reliable.

An alternative method to that described here for the calculation of the dose to the isocentre is to use the tissue maximum ratio (TMR) method (Chapter 4, Section 4.3). The advantage of this parameter is that it is independent of SSD, so that a single table of TMRs as a function of field size at the isocentre s and of depth d is required. The number of monitor units (mu) for a dose D at the isocentre is given by:

$$mu = \frac{D}{\text{TMR}(d, s)\text{OF}(s)}$$

where OF(s) is the output factor for field size s, in terms of dose per monitor unit, at the source–axis distance (SAD) and at the depth of maximum dose.

2.2.3 Beam weighting

The weight of a treatment beam is the relative contribution of that beam to the treatment plan. For treatments at fixed SSDs, the weight represents a multiplying factor for the dose at the depth of dose maximum, usually expressed as a percentage. In the example of the opposed fields in Figure 8.3, the weight of each field is 100%. For isocentric treatments, the definition of the field weight varies for different centres. The weight is defined as either the relative contribution to the dose at the isocentre or the relative contribution at the depth of dose maximum. In this chapter the latter definition of weight is used.

In certain clinical situations, coaxial opposed beams may be treated with unequal weights. This arrangement may be preferred when the target volume is not central in the patient's cross-section or when one of the fields is directed through a particularly radiosensitive structure, such as the spinal cord. A single-field treatment could result in an excessive dose to the subcutaneous region and an unacceptable degree of dose heterogeneity over the target volume. Equally weighted coaxial opposed beams could result in an unacceptably high dose outside the target volume. Figure 8.4 gives an example of an isodose distribution for unequally weighted beams for which the field weights are 100% and 50%. The dose would normally be specified in terms of the dose to the centre of the target volume and further calculations would be required for the maximum subcutaneous dose. In addition the dose to other sensitive regions may be required.

2.3 Factors affecting dose distributions

There are a number of factors that can modify the dose distribution of a single field from that shown in Figure 8.1a. Dose distributions are measured with the central axis of the beam perpendicular to the surface of a water-filled phantom. The phantom should be large enough to provide at least 5 cm of water outside the geometric edge of the beam at all depths, which are measured and 5 cm beyond the maximum depth of measurement. This ensures full scatter conditions. The measurement conditions do not correspond to the majority of clinical situations.

Normally the surface of the patient is not flat and the SSD varies over the area of the field. Corrections have to be made for the resultant excess or missing tissue. Compensation for surface obliquity may be made in special cases by using custom-made compensator devices. This is discussed in more detail in Section 7.2. For the general case in which the beam is at an angle to a surface, a wedge filter may be used as a compensating device. Wedge fields have isodose distributions as shown in Figure 8.1b. The raised dose at the thinner end of the wedge compensates for the excess tissue in the non-flat surface.

Isodose distributions are affected by tissue inhomogeneities within the patient's cross-section. For megavoltage photon beams, the predominant interaction process is the Compton effect and, therefore, the mass attenuation coefficient does not depend significantly on the elemental composition of the tissues. The principal factor affecting attenuation is the electron density, which is closely related to the physical density. In practice, most tissue heterogeneities are ignored, either because the density differences are small or, as in the case of bone, the thicknesses are sufficiently small for there to be little effect on the dose distribution. The exception to this general rule is for treatments that include lung. This has a

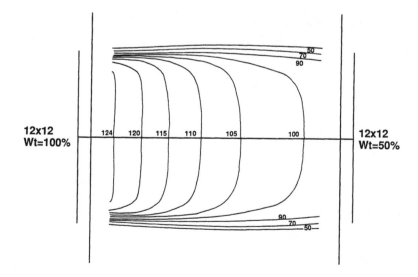

Figure 8.4 Opposed coaxial field irradiation with unequal beam weights.

density that is approximately 25% of that of water and it is large enough to increase the dose to the target volume by up to 20% in certain clinical situations.

There are a number of clinical situations in which a part of the radiation beam is not intercepted by the patient's body. This may occur when a relatively superficial target volume is irradiated and the cross-section of the patient varies significantly over the length of the treatment fields. Examples are the irradiation of the breast, and treatments in the head and neck region. The missing tissue in the treatment field causes a reduction in scatter and, therefore, in dose; correction for this effect requires sophisticated dose-calculation methods. Methods of correcting for surface obliquity and for tissue inhomogeneity are described in Section 3 and in more detail in Chapter 9.

2.4 Multiple fields

Single-field and coaxially opposed field irradiations are mainly used for palliative treatments for which the dose to the target volume is relatively low. Curative treatments generally require a higher dose and these simple treatment techniques are unsatisfactory because the dose to the tissues overlying the target volume would be excessive and could cause unacceptable early and late radiation effects. In these circumstances three or more fields are used, although there are some high-dose treatments, particularly within the head and neck region, which may only require two fields because the depth of the target volume is relatively small. For multiple-field and for non-opposed two-field treatments, the dose distribution in the target volume and in the surrounding tissue is less predictable than for the treatment methods previously described. Optimization of the treatment is required to ensure that a uniform dose is delivered to the target volume and that the dose to the surrounding tissues is as low as possible and within specified constraints. This requires the calculation of a full dose distribution.

Treatment planning is concerned with the selection of the parameters required to produce the optimum dose distribution within the patient. The parameters that may be selected in the planning process are number of fields, orientation of fields, field sizes, wedges, and weights. In this section these different parameters are considered with illustrations for one treatment site.

2.4.1 Field arrangement

The field arrangement, i.e. the number and orientation of the fields, determines the basic treatment technique. Most treatments are carried out in accordance to protocols that have been adopted in the radiotherapy centre for each treatment site and disease stage. The technique is specified not only on the basis of the physical dose distribution, but also on clinical constraints. In general,

the number of fields required is fewer for high energy beams and for smaller depths. For most sites, two to four fields are specified. The orientation of the treatment fields is chosen to provide a uniform dose distribution and to avoid irradiation of sensitive structures. Generally, the most even dose distribution is achieved if the beam directions are chosen to be spaced uniformly around the patient. However, this is not necessary for the achievement of uniform target dose if wedges are used as discussed below.

2.4.2 Field dimensions

In this section, the determination of the field dimensions to cover the planning target volume will be described. The planning target volume includes not only the tumour and its subclinical spread, but also the margins that have been added to allow for uncertainties in localization, movement, and treatment set-up (see Section 1). The planned isodose distribution should encompass this volume with a minimum dose, which is typically specified as 90% of the central dose. To achieve this the field dimension must be greater than the volume size. The extra margin depends on the distance in the penumbra of each field, between the points corresponding to 50 and 90% of the central axis dose at the depth of the centre of the target (typically 5–10 mm for deep-seated tumours) and on the geometry of the field arrangement.

Figure 8.5 illustrates a four-field treatment technique. Point A is at the edge of the planning target volume. From fields III and IV it receives a dose that is approximately equal to the dose contributed by those fields to the isocentre. The contribution from fields I and II will depend on the field width. If a minimum target dose of 90% is specified, the contribution to point A from fields I and II need not be as high as 90% because of the

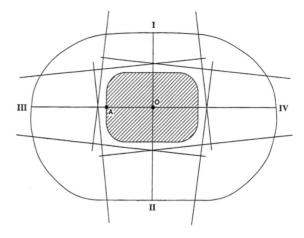

Figure 8.5 Four-field treatment technique showing the geometric edges of the beams.

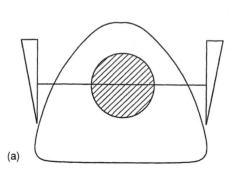
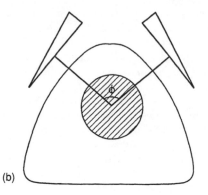

(a)   (b)

Figure 8.6 The two applications of wedge filters: (a) to compensate for missing or excess tissue; and (b) to correct for the non-uniformity of the dose distribution for irradiations in which the fields are not equally spaced about the patient's cross-section. ϕ is the hinge angle between the two fields.

contribution of the other two fields. For this situation, the field width would not need to be more than about 1 cm greater than the size of the planning target volume. If this volume were treated by opposed fields (I and II) only, and the minimum dose is specified to be not less than 90%, then the field width would have to be increased further due to the lack of contribution from the lateral portals. The difference between field size and target width would need to be approximately double what is required for the four-field plan. For most multiple-field plans, a smaller additional size is required if the fields are positioned uniformly around the patient. However, for the determination of field length, the size has to be increased to the same extent as would be required for opposed coaxial fields.

For non-isocentric treatments, the field size at the surface may be calculated from the required size at the centre of the target volume by a simple linear correction depending on SSD and depth of the centre.

Treatment planning practices and protocols are not standardized and care is required when comparing plans from different centres. In many centres it is not the planning target area that is drawn into the patient's outline or delineated on the CT slices, it is the target area without any margin for the physical uncertainty in treatment delivery. Local protocols should require that field sizes are chosen, so that the minimum dose to this volume is greater than 90% to allow for these physical uncertainties. This illustrates that care is needed in the use of the term 'minimum dose' because it depends on the exact delineation of the target area.

In those centres in which the volume is determined by conventional simulation, the field sizes for each beam may be specified by the radiotherapist at the time of simulation. Protocols may then be required to ensure that the target area that is derived from field size accurately represents the intended treatment.

2.4.3 Wedges

Wedges are used to provide a non-flat dose distribution across the beam as shown in Figure 8.1b. Wedges may be used for two purposes: to compensate for surface obliquity, as discussed previously, and to facilitate treatment techniques in which the beams are not uniformly spaced around the patient by correcting the non-uniformity in dose within the target volume that would otherwise result. The two uses of wedges are illustrated in Figure 8.6.

The IEC definition of wedge angle is assumed, i.e. the angle of the isodose curve to a plane at right angles to the central axis at a depth of 10 cm. Selection of the optimum wedge angle for two-field treatments shown in Figure 8.6 will now be considered. When the wedge is used as a compensator (Figure 8.6a) the angle required is between 50 and 75% of the angle of the surface obliquity depending on the depth of interest and the beam energy. For the type of treatment shown in Figure 8.6b the wedge angle is calculated from the angle between the beams, which is commonly referred to as the hinge angle (ϕ):

$$\text{wedge angle} = 90 - \phi/2.$$

In some treatments two wedges may be combined. An example is when the wedge is used to compensate for surface obliquity in both dimensions. Treatment is carried out alternately with a steeper wedge pointing laterally as shown in Figure 8.6b for half the total number of fractions and in the patient's longitudinal dimension for the other half. Another example is the situation in which an intermediate wedge angle is required to optimize the dose distribution. In these situations the effective wedge angle θ_0 of the combined fields is not the average angle of the two wedges, but is derived from the weighted averages of the tangents of the two angles:

$$\tan \theta_0 = \frac{w_1 \tan \theta_1 + w_2 \tan \theta_2}{w_1 + w_2}$$

in which w_1 and w_2 are the relative contributions to the dose at the depth of dose maximum for the two fields with wedges at angles θ_1 and θ_2 respectively.

A particular example of the combination of differently wedged fields through a single portal is the use of a motorized wedge. In this system the treatment unit has a single wedge, typically 60°, which is combined with an open field to produce any wedge angle up to 60°. This has the advantage of reducing set-up time. Also, because the radiographer does not have to handle the wedge, there is a reduction in the risk of injury to the patient and, in the case of high-energy accelerators, there is a reduction dose to the radiographer due to activation.

Using the equation above it can be seen that if equal weighting, i.e. equal dose, is given with and without a 60° wedge, the effective wedge angle is given by:

$$\tan \theta_0 = \frac{\tan 60}{2}$$

i.e. $\theta_0 = 41°$. This may be compared with an average angle of 30°. It is estimated that the equation produces a maximum error in θ_0 of about 3° at large field sizes.

2.4.4　Beam weighting

The second method for achieving uniformity in the target volume is to adjust the contribution from each beam, i.e. the beam weight. Beam weighting for coaxially opposed fields was discussed in Section 2.2.3. The use of beam weights to achieve a uniform dose over the target volume will be illustrated by an example.

Figure 8.7 shows a three-field treatment technique. The dose to five points within the target volume is to be

Table 8.5 Depth–dose data for the field arrangement in Figure 8.7

Point	I	II	III
A	70	48	44
B	58	62	40
C	52	56	50
D	58	42	56
O	60	52	48

balanced by altering the relative weights of the three fields. Table 8.5 shows the depth doses for five points from each of the fields. The procedure is as follows.

1. Make sure that the dose to B and D from field I are (approximately) equal. If not use a wedge on this field to make them equal.

2. Determine the weights w_2 and w_3 for fields II and III, such that the doses to B and D from these fields are equal:
   dose to B $= 62w_2 + 40w_3$
   dose to D $= 42w_2 + 56w_3$
   therefore $20w_2 = 16w_3$
   and if $w_2 = 1.00$, $w_3 = 1.25$.

3. Determine the weight for field I so that the total dose to points A and C are equal:
   dose to A $= 70w_1 + 48w_2 + 44w_3$
   dose to C $= 52w_1 + 56w_2 + 50w_3$
   therefore $18w_1 = 8w_2 + 6w_3$
   $w_1 = 0.86$.

4. Use these weights to calculate the doses to each point:
   dose to A $= 163$
   dose to B $= 162$
   dose to C $= 163$
   dose to D $= 162$
   dose to O $= 164$.

2.4.5　Dose calculation

Dose calculation for multiple fields involves the summation of the dose distributions of the individual fields. The total relative dose D_p at a point P for an irradiation with n fields is given by:

$$D_P = \sum_{i=1}^{n} w_i DD_{i,p}$$

where $DD_{i,p}$ is the depth dose at point P from the ith field and w_i is the weight for that field. In hand planning for fields with equal weights, this is achieved by overlaying the isodose distributions for two fields. The point of intersection of two curves represents the point at which the per cent dose equals the sum of the two isodoses. Identification of intersection points that add up to a

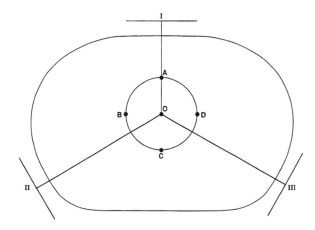

Figure 8.7 A three-field technique in which the doses to points A, B, C, D, and O are to be balanced by adjusting beam weights.

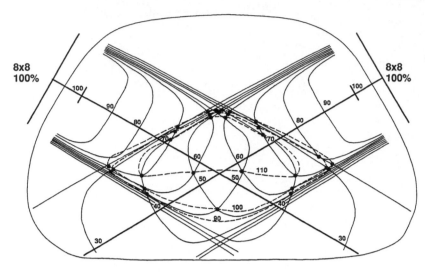

Figure 8.8 An example of hand planning in which the isodose curves for two fields (solid lines) are summed by drawing between the isodose crossing-points (solid circles) to give the summed isodose curves (broken lines).

particular value enables a summed isodose curve to be interpolated from the two contributing fields. In this way a full isodose distribution from the two fields may be constructed as shown in Figure 8.8. A third field may then be added by overlaying its isodose distribution with that calculated from the first two fields. The resultant distribution can be determined by consideration of the intersection points of the two distributions. This is a lengthy and tedious process in which the precision of calculation can be severely compromised.

A second method of hand planning is to calculate doses on a matrix of points within the patient's cross-section. Overlaying the isodose curves over the calculation matrix allows the dose at each point to be evaluated. Summing the dose for all fields leads to the full dose matrix from which the isodose distribution may be interpolated. For hand planning, the total number of dose points required to calculate a full isodose distribution is prohibitive and the quicker graphical method is preferred. However, for computer planning, a sufficiently large matrix of points may be used to enable sufficient spatial accuracy to be achieved. Computer planning is described in Section 5.

2.4.6 Example of multiple-field planning

To illustrate the general points discussed in the preceding paragraphs, the dose optimization and calculation for one treatment site will be discussed. The site chosen is the bladder and the outline and target area are shown in Figure 8.9a. The target area does not include any margin for the physical uncertainties in treatment delivery. This tumour is centred on the mid-line of the patient and is

anterior of the mid-point. Critical normal tissues for this site are the rectum and the subcutaneous tissues. In addition, the radiotherapist may wish to restrict the dose to the femoral heads and necks that may be within the irradiated cross-section at the lower end of the fields.

Quite often these patients are treated prone, which has the advantage in obese patients of flattening the anterior surface and thus preventing dose inhomogeneities in the longitudinal direction.

Due to the symmetry of the target volume, outline, and critical tissues about the mid-line of the patient, a field arrangement with left–right symmetry is selected. It will be seen that three fields are sufficient to produce a satisfactory dose distribution for 10 MV X-rays, as used in this example. An anterior field is always selected as one of the three fields because this has the shortest distance from the entry point to the centre of the target volume.

The dose distributions in the figure are all for isocentric treatments. The isodoses have been normalized to an average target dose of 100%.

1. The first dose distribution (Figure 8.9b) has an anterior field with two posterior obliques at 120°. This gives an equal angle between each of the three beams. In this example, wedges have not been used. The beam weights of the oblique fields (62%) are greater than for the anterior field (49%).

2. Figure 8.9c is a variation on the first plan. Wedges (10°) have been used on the oblique fields to allow the weights of these beams to be reduced. The oblique-beam weights are 55% with an anterior beam weight of 57%.

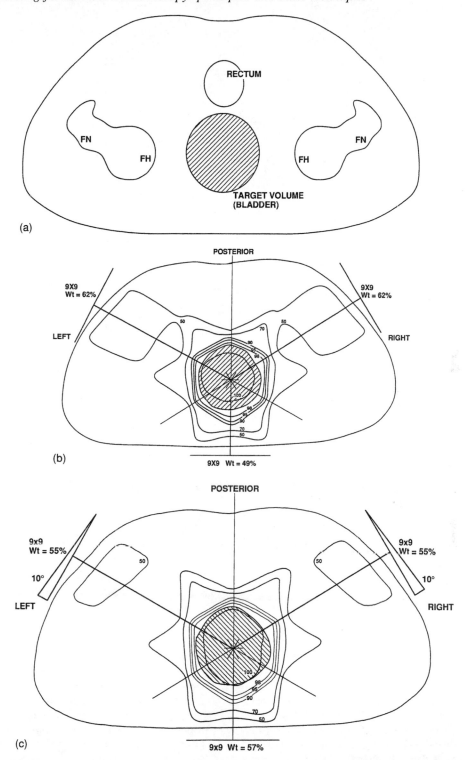

Figure 8.9 Alternative treatment plans for a bladder tumour: (a) patient outline in the prone position showing the position of the target volume and the critical normal tissues: rectum, femoral heads (FH), and femoral necks (FN); (b) patient treated with an anterior field and two unwedged posterior obliques; (c) same as (b) but with wedges on the oblique fields; (d) treatment with wedged lateral fields; (e) treatment with patient supine and using two anterior obliques at 60° to the anterior field.

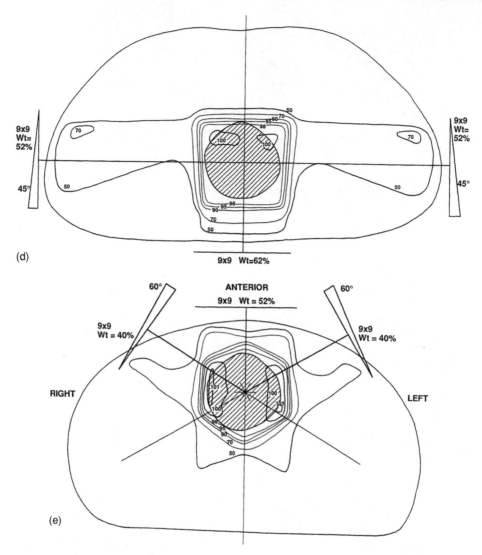

Figure 8.9 (*continued*)

3. Figure 8.9d shows a dose distribution when two lateral fields are used with the anterior beam. In this example the wedges on the lateral beams are used both to compensate for oblique incidence of these beams and to offset the dose gradient from the anterior beam. Steeper wedge angles are required then for the previous plan (45°). It may be noted that the dose in the subcutaneous region is increased for the lateral fields due to the exit contribution, and that the dose in the region of the femoral necks is also increased.

4. Figure 8.9e shows a distribution for a technique using an anterior field with two anterior obliques. With this arrangement the patient has to be treated supine because it would be difficult otherwise to treat all three portals without obstruction from the couch top. In this technique steeper wedge angles (60°) are required than for the previous example because all three beams are directed from the anterior half of the patient. The advantage of this technique is that the distance from the skin entry point to the tumour is minimized. Because opposed fields are not used, as in the second technique, the dose at the skin is reduced. However, this is offset because of the need to use a steep wedge. Reduction of the hinge angle is not practical because it would increase the overlap of fields close to the anterior surface.

This series of plans has been selected to demonstrate that equally satisfactory, homogeneous dose distributions over the target volume can be achieved using a number of different field arrangements. The critical factor involved in the choice of technique is the dose to tissue outside the target. For this routine type of therapy, treatment protocols are based on the clinical judgement of the therapist and assessment of the patterns of morbidity observed following treatment.

The most common field arrangement for treatment of the bladder is that shown in Figure 8.9b and c, although in many centres the patient is treated supine. The choice of whether to use a wedge or not and the calculation of beam weights are part of the physical optimization process. They will depend on the size of patient, the position and size of the target volume, and the energy of the treatment beam.

3. Dose calculation within the patient

In the previous section, the calculation of the dose at a point has assumed that the radiation beam has been normally incident on a unit density medium. In practice, a patient differs from this homogeneous situation both in shape and composition, and these differences must be taken into account when calculating the depth dose. The methods used vary considerably in their complexity. Some may be evaluated manually, but the majority of algorithms are sufficiently complex to require computer processing, and these in general will produce much higher accuracy. The algorithms are described in Chapter 9.

Only manual methods of correction are described in this Chapter but they provide a useful introduction to the more complex algorithms used for computer planning. Some of these manual methods may be used in the simpler computer algorithms. In addition, for certain non-standard planning situations, it is helpful to be able to calculate the dose at a limited number of points directly from isodose curves.

The more complex algorithms deal with body shape and body composition in a similar manner; for example, oblique incidence can be considered as a zero-density inhomogeneity present on the skin surface. However, manual methods deal with these two problems separately.

3.1 Correction methods for patient shape

3.1.1 Effective SSD/isodose shift

This method is illustrated by reference to Figure 8.10, where the patient's surface is represented by S. If the surface had been at S', then the primary component of the dose to p' would be unaltered. There will be small changes to the scattered dose to p', but this is ignored as

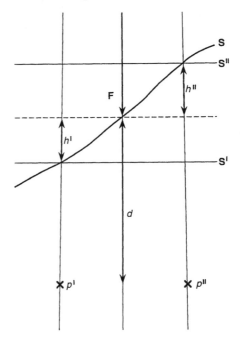

Figure 8.10 Calculation of the effect of surface obliquity for a beam at SSD = F incident on the surface S.

is the change in per cent depth dose with change in SSD from F to F + h'. The dose to p' can be found by sliding the isodose chart away from the source by a distance h' and reading off the new value. This accounts for the change in attenuation to p' but introduces an inverse square law (ISL) error because the distance of p' from the source has not changed. This must be removed and this is done by multiplying the depth dose by:

$$\frac{(F + d_{max})^2}{(F + h' + d_{max})^2}$$

where d_{max} is the depth of maximum absorbed dose (and is often omitted from the expression). In a similar manner, the dose to p'' can be found by sliding the isodose chart towards the source by a distance h'', reading off the depth dose at p'', and multiplying by:

$$\frac{(F + d_{max})^2}{(F - h'' + d_{max})^2}.$$

In this method, sliding the isodose chart by the full amount h of the excess or lack of tissue overestimates the correction required, and the use of the ISL factor reduces this overestimate to give an approximately correct result. If the isodose chart was moved a distance less than h, then the correct result would be obtained without having to multiply by the ISL factor. This is the basis of the isodose shift method. The fraction of h through which the isodose chart has to be shifted varies with energy as shown in

Table 8.6 Isodose shift as a function of radiation energy

Radiation energy	Fraction of h for isodose shift
Up to 1 MV	0.8
1–5 MV	0.7
5–15 MV	0.6
15–30 MV	0.5
Over 30 MV	0.4

Table 8.6. For manual planning, the isodose shift is the most commonly used method for correcting for patient shape as it can be implemented by the use of isodose charts only and requires no arithmetic calculation.

3.1.2   Effective attenuation coefficient

In this method, a correction factor is determined for the excess or lack of tissue h' along a fan-line to a calculation point such as p′ in Figure 8.10. The depth dose at p′ is determined as for normal incidence and is multiplied by the correction factor evaluated from $\exp(-\mu h)$, where μ is the effective linear attenuation coefficient of tissue. Values of μ are obtained from depth–dose curves by removing the effect of the ISL or from tables of TARs, and will vary with beam area. For ease of use, correction factors are generally supplied in graphical from, as shown in Figure 8.11 for a 4 MV X-ray beam. This gives factors for excess or lack of tissue equivalent material including the variation with beam area.

3.1.3   Tissue–air ratio method

This is essentially an application of the previous method, but as well as taking into account the beam size it also accounts for the depth of the point. Again with reference

to Figure 8.10, a correction factor C_F for point p′ can be obtained from the ratio of TARs for the depths $d - h'$ and d corresponding to the lack of tissue and to normal incidence respectively:

$$C_F = \frac{\mathrm{TAR}(d - h', r)}{\mathrm{TAR}(d, r)}$$

where r is the effective beam radius for the dimensions of the field. TARs are defined in BIR (1996) and in Chapter 4, Section 4.3.

3.2   Correction methods for patient composition

The presence of tissues of composition different from that of water affect the dose distribution in two ways. First, there will be a change in the primary component of dose to a point due to a change in attenuation; and second, the dose due to scattered radiation will be influenced by the presence of any nearby inhomogeneity. This latter effect becomes less important the further the distance from the inhomogeneity, and is smaller for high-energy beams. These reasons, together with the fact that correcting for changes in scatter dose is complicated, mean that manual methods only attempt to correct for the changes in the primary component of dose.

At high energies, the magnitude of the shielding effect due to bone is not affected by its atomic number and is due only to its increased density. It is unusual to apply a correction for bone in manual planning owing to the small amounts of bone involved, and corrections are only made for the presence of lung tissue.

3.2.1   Use of correction factors

The simplest method of correcting for the presence of lung tissue is to apply correction factors such as those

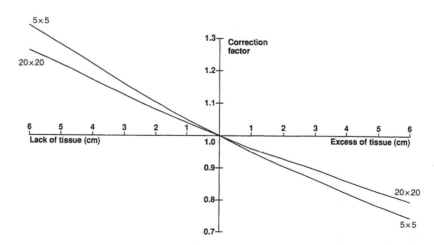

Figure 8.11 Correction factors for missing or excess tissue for 4 MV X-rays using the effective attenuation coefficient method.

Table 8.7 Corrections to depth dose necessary after transmission through lung tissue

Energy	% increase in dose per cm of lung tissue traversed
^{60}Co	+3
4 MV	+2.5
10 MV	+2
20 MV	+1.5

given in Table 8.7. The depth dose is increased by the percentage shown for every centimetre of lung traversed according to the energy of the radiation used. For example, if the depth dose to a point is 60% in unit density material, then at 4 MV the depth dose to the same point with 10 cm of lung tissue above the point will be increased by $10 \times 2.5 = 25\%$, i.e. the depth dose would increase to $60 \times 1.25 = 75\%$.

3.2.2 Effective-depth method

All manual methods require the determination of the unit density equivalent thickness of material between the entrance surface and the point of calculation, usually known as the effective depth. This is the thickness of unit density material that would attenuate the beam by the same amount as the body composition along a fan-line to the point. This can be demonstrated by Figure 8.12, where the depth dose to point P at a depth $d = 15$ cm beneath the surface is required. This distance is made up of 2 cm of unit density material followed by 8 cm of lung of assumed density 0.3, and a further 5 cm of unit density material. The effective depth d_{eff} of unit density material is $2 + (8 \times 0.3) + 5 = 9.4$ cm. The depth dose to P can then be evaluated by interpolating from the appropriate isodose chart at a depth of 9.4 cm instead of 15 cm. However, as in the effective SSD method for correcting for patient shape, the distance of P from the radiation source has not changed and although the above corrects for attenuation it introduces an ISL error that has to be removed. The depth dose to P must therefore be corrected by multiplying by an ISL factor:

$$\frac{(F + d_{eff})^2}{(F + d)^2}.$$

3.2.3 Effective-attenuation method

This method operates in a similar manner to that used to correct for patient shape. Correction factors are determined from $\exp[-\mu(d - d_{eff})]$, where again d is the true depth and d_{eff} is the effective or water-equivalent depth. In the example in Figure 8.12, $d - d_{eff}$ is the lack of tissue-equivalent material to the dose calculation point

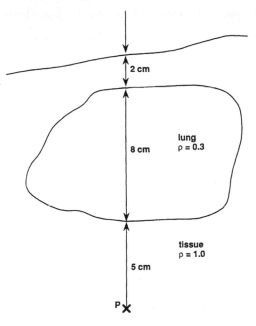

Figure 8.12 Lung correction for a point P in unit density tissue behind lung with density 0.3.

and, as an example, a correction factor can be read from Figure 8.11 for a 4 MV beam.

3.2.4 Tissue–air ratio method

This method again applies a correction factor C_F by using the ratio of two TARs:

$$C_F = \frac{TAR(d_{eff}, r)}{TAR(d, r)}$$

where again d is the true depth, d_{eff} is the water-equivalent depth, and r is the effective beam radius for the beam used. This method takes account of the beam size and the depth of the point of calculation. It does not take account of the position of the calculation point with respect to the inhomogeneity or of the lateral extent of the inhomogeneity. However, it is accepted as the most accurate of the manual methods.

4. Optimization

Optimization of external beam treatment planning can be defined as the determination of the various beam parameters that will produce a dose distribution such that the target volume will receive the required lethal radiation dose without producing any patient morbidity.

4.1 Specification of the planning problem

The treatment-planning process can be considered in two parts, the first of which is the clinical optimization. The radiotherapist will assess the site and extent of the tumour by a number of different means, including surgical and pathology reports, physical examination, and a range of imaging modalities. If radiotherapy is the chosen method of treatment, this initial assessment will lead to a clinical decision regarding the optimum technique to be used including modality, radiation energy and, usually, the field arrangement. The therapist will also decide on the most appropriate method for the accurate localization of the target volume, normally by CT scanning or conventional simulation.

The sequence of steps in this part of the radiotherapy process varies from centre to centre and, to a certain extent, with tumour site. In some centres the target volume is defined at simulation, and the choice of field size is part of the physical planning process. Elsewhere field size may be selected in the simulation process.

Following simulation, the therapist selects the target dose and fractionation scheme. The critical dose to vulnerable structures must also be considered so that any dose constraints can be fed into the physical planning process.

The second part of the planning process is to produce a treatment plan, and this is often referred to as physical optimization. If the direction and size of the beams have been established, then it consists of determining beam weights and wedges, such that the resulting dose distribution will best match that required from clinical assessment.

This text is only concerned with physical optimization and any method that attempts this must incorporate criteria that define the ideal dose distribution. These have been expressed in detail by Hope *et al.* (1967) who formulated the following six criteria.

1. The dose gradient across the tumour should be minimized.

2. The tumour dose relative to the largest incident dose should be maximized.

3. Integral dose should be minimized.

4. The shape of the high dose volume should be matched to that of the chosen target volume.

5. The dose to particular vulnerable regions should be minimized.

6. A higher than normal dose to regions of possible direct extension or lymphatic spread should be allowed.

It is unlikely that all these criteria will be considered or incorporated into an optimization procedure, and for that reason they can be summarized as follows:

1. a uniform dose distribution across the target volume (a simple example of optimization based on dose uniformity was given in Section 2.4.4);

2. Minimal dose to vulnerable regions.

4.2 Visual optimization

It is now normal for treatment-planning systems to present treatment plans visually on a graphics terminal. The operator can observe the effects of varying any of the beam parameters, and interactively arrive at what they consider to be an acceptable dose distribution. This is subjective and relies on the ability of the operator to judge the results correctly and consistently without any figure of merit to assist in the assessment of the quality of the plan. The final dose distribution achieved is unlikely to be optimal as the full effect of varying all the beam parameters cannot be investigated because of the time involved.

It is often argued that visual optimization is all that should be used, as any form of computer judgement using mathematical methods to produce optimum dose distributions removes the planning skills from the operator. However, using such methods to determine, for example, the optimum beam weights required to obtain a uniform target dose, can be instructive and relieve the operator of a tedious process. However, if such techniques are to be used successfully and routinely, not only must they provide the correct result but they must be readily available in existing planning software and their operation must be fast and efficient with the minimum amount of operator interaction.

There are two main methods of approach to physical optimization. One is to use exhaustive search techniques based on score functions; the other is to use mathematical optimization techniques. Physical optimization methods are incorporated in some planning systems, and an outline of the techniques will be summarized here.

4.3 Score functions

Score functions have been introduced based on the six criteria of judgement listed in Section 4.1 (Hope *et al.* 1967). A figure of merit for a plan can be calculated based on the degree to which the plan satisfies these conditions. An exhaustive search to find the best figure of merit is made for a large number of plans in which the treatment parameters vary over a preselected range.

In general, exhaustive search techniques can only provide the optimum value of a function that has discrete values, and if the function has many allowed values then the computational time can be prohibitive. Neither can the technique guarantee to provide the global solution to the planning problem, it is more likely to provide a solution that is an approximation to a local minimum.

The technique can be best described as a process that provides an improvement to some starting solution.

4.4 Mathematical optimization

Mathematical programming techniques provide the optimum value of a continuous function but can only guarantee to provide this if the function is unimodal. This is true of beam weight and wedge selection, and successful use has been made of mathematical programming to determine these parameters. The solution obtained is the optimum for the manner in which the problem is formulated.

Linear programming is a technique in which the minimum or maximum value of a linear function is found when the variables of the problem (or a linear combination of the variables) are constrained within set boundaries. The criteria are formulated as a set of linear equations, one of which is selected as an objective function. The problem is the choice of an objective function that is linear and that describes the quality of the treatment plan. A clinically meaningful parameter is the maximum difference between the mean target dose and the dose to any one of a number of preselected points within the target region (Redpath *et al.* 1976). This parameter represents the dose variations over the target.

There is sufficient evidence to support the uniformity of target dose as the criterion to be used as the objective function, and this can be expressed by the variance of the doses to preselected points within the target. Quadratic programming is similar to linear programming except that it will optimize the value of a second-order function, such as variance, subject to linear constraints. The dose to any point can be stated as a linear function and, therefore, a constraint can be used to keep this below a certain value. This technique has been used successfully in a treatment-planning system (Redpath *et al.* 1977). Similarly, use has been made of least squares optimization methods (McDonald and Rubin 1977; Starkschall 1984).

5. Computer planning

5.1 Hardware requirements

The first noted use of computers in external beam treatment planning was in 1955 (Tsien 1955), and since then their use in radiotherapy has followed closely the development of computer hardware. Initially, remote batch systems were used and eventually these were replaced by remote teletypes linked by modems to large time-sharing computers. In the 1970s, small minicomputer systems with visual displays produced a dramatic improvement in operator interaction and set the scene for the use of modern computer hardware. Present planning

systems use a wide variety of computer hardware but are tending to standardize on high-speed workstations using colour graphics displays.

The recent development in computer-processing speed is staggering, and at the same time the cost of computer memory has decreased, so that workstations with 256 megabytes of 32-bit memory are readily affordable. Hard discs are inexpensive, with multiple gigabyte capacity readily available for use as fast access store. Back-up storage tends now to be by digital magnetic tape or optical disc, and it may be necessary to have use of these in order to transfer CT or MRI images into the planning system if a fast network connection is not available.

Workstations now use large colour monitors with at least 1280×1024 resolution capable of providing the simultaneous display of 256 colours with 8-bit intensity resolution on each of the three primary colours. The use of a window environment allows both the display of images and text on the same monitor, and the display of multiple images. Many manufacturers can provide three-dimensional graphics packages as standard.

All planning systems require a digitizer for contour input and a printer/plotter for hardcopy, and these are usually linked by serial lines to the planning computer. Several types of digitizer are available based on different operating principles, e.g. magnetostrictive, inductive, or sonic. The latter should be avoided as it is sensitive to ambient conditions. It is usual for the planning system to have both a printer and a plotter, so that these functions can be separated. A large variety of plotters are available; however, the use of colour is desirable, and the simplest method is to use a multipen flatbed plotter, which will produce a coloured isodose line output within a few minutes. Colour printers are available that can produce life-sized outputs including grey-scale images of CT scans with isodose distributions superimposed in colour.

One of the main advantages of using the workstation approach is that it can be linked with a local network, such as Ethernet, allowing data collection and transfer from other areas of the department. It is straightforward to add another workstation as a second planning station, while sharing the peripherals already available on the network, including the storage media.

5.2 Beam data input and storage

All treatment-planning systems require the input of data specifying the wide variety of treatment beams to be used on the available machines. The data required depend on the type of beam model that is used, while the method of entry can vary considerably. Originally, the only method available was to type the data into the computer, an onerous task as it was supplementary to the acquisition of the data. The advent of beam data acquisition systems (BDAS), controlled by the planning computer, revolutionized the task and allowed data to be fed directly into the planning computer in the form required. More recently, BDAS have used their own processor and data transfer to the planning system has been done off-line. The digitizer on the planning computer has been used to enter beam profiles and central axis plots. Finally, another method that has been used is to create the necessary data by a beam-generation program working from a limited amount of data collected from the treatment machine.

The amount of data required depends on the beam model that is used by the planning system. In general, three methods of data storage have been used; mass storage, mathematical approximation, and separation into primary and secondary components.

5.2.1 Mass storage

This method requires the radiation dose distribution for a large number of radiation beams to be sampled at many points, and the values stored in a data file. The spatial resolution of the points is such that linear interpolation can be used to determine the depth dose from neighbouring points in a look-up table. It is not necessary to store data for every field size to be used, as interpolation from a discrete set is straightforward. However, a similar data-set has to be stored for every wedge on the treatment machine.

The most common model used is the fan-shaped grid, as shown in Figure 8.13. This approach has the advantage that the off–axis ratio (the ratio of the dose on a fan line to the dose at the same depth on the central axis) does not vary greatly along a fan line, thereby assisting linear interpolation both with position and field dimensions. Off–axis ratios are stored for a number of beam profiles (usually between 3 and 5) at selected depths, together with central axis data for the beam. The advantage of this method is that the computational time is fast; the drawback is that a substantial amount of work is required to measure and ensure the integrity of the data. Creation of the data-set by a beam generation program should be considered.

5.2.2 Mathematical approximation

A mathematical representation of the data can be employed as a means of data reduction. This is an empirical approach, where the dose at a point is determined from the evaluation of a mathematical function. A wide variety of functions have been used (Redpath and Wright 1981), and because of their complexity the calculation time per field is slow compared to table look up from the mass storage of data. In general, the mathematical representation is considered in two parts, where the dose is computed form the product of a central axis value and an off–axis

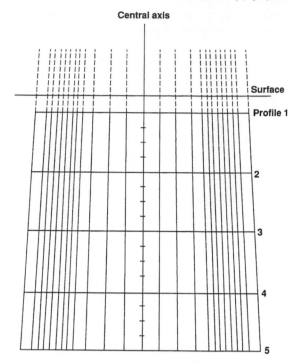

Figure 8.13 Fan-line grid for the mass storage of beam data. Data are stored at the crossing-points of the profiles and the fan lines and at the points marked on the central axis. Profile 1 is at the depth of dose maximum.

ratio. Each term is considered separately and approximately by a suitable analytical expression.

The method has several drawbacks. It is a difficult and time-consuming process to obtain the required accuracy when using curve-fitting techniques to model a wide range of data, and the process has to be repeated should any change occur in the data. Care must be taken not to use field sizes outside the range over which the mathematical approximation took place.

5.2.3 Separation into primary and scattered components of dose

The absorbed dose at any point in an irradiated medium can be split into a primary and a scattered component, each behaving in a different manner. In this approach, the two components are determined separately and added together to give the total dose.

The variation of the primary dose throughout a tissue-equivalent material is well known. The variation with distance from the source can be allowed for by the inverse square law. The variation across the beam can be calculated for ^{60}Co sources, or measured for linear accelerators. Attenuation of the primary in tissue-equivalent material, can be found from zero-area TARs.

Scattered dose arises from radiation scattered by the whole of the irradiated medium and it is not possible to calculate this from physical principles in the same way as it is for primary dose. Meredith and Neary (1944) introduced the concept of scatter functions, which they derived from a table of depth–dose data by subtracting out the primary component. From this idea, Cunningham (1972) proposed the use of scatter–air ratios (SARs), derived in an identical manner, except that TARs are used instead of depth–dose values, and hence are independent of SSD. Cunningham also proposed the use of differential SARs, which he calculated by differentiating the variation of SAR with beam radius. They represent the contribution to the SAR at a point from annular rings of a predetermined width at any distance from the point.

Differential SARs can be used to determine the scatter contribution of dose to a point by means of a method developed by Clarkson (1941), which is known as the sector integration method. This is shown in Figure 8.14, where radii are drawn from any point inside the field at 10 intervals, so that the field may be represented by 36 sectors. Each sector is divided into 1-cm lengths and the scatter contribution to any point P from a region such as S can be found by interpolation from a table of differential SARs. Allowance can be made for the fact that the scatter originating from any point, such as S, is proportional to the primary at S and, therefore, the method can deal with wedged fields.

This approach requires the storage of a small amount of physical data for any machine, namely in-air beam profiles, zero-area TARs and differential SARs. The method can also be used in a beam generating program to produce data for mass storage.

5.3 Patient data input and storage

In principle, the most accurate method of obtaining patient data is the use of CT scanning or simulator CT. This provides both the external outline and internal structure. These methods have become increasingly common and they will be discussed in Chapter 9.

A wide variety of other methods exist for obtaining the external contour of the patient, for example, the use of lead strips, pantographs or optical methods using lasers, and video cameras. The positions of internal structures are usually determined from orthogonal X-rays, possibly with the use of diagnostic CT images. Those outlines are entered by the use of a digitizer tablet and stored in the computer. The method used to represent the contours is the same regardless of the method by which they were obtained. It is generally accepted that an accuracy of 3 mm is sufficient for digital representation of the contours, and this is easily achieved by a polygon approximation using vectors 3 mm in length in a Cartesian co-ordinate system.

5.4 Calculation of dose distributions

The following discussion refers to dose calculation in two dimensions. A matrix of points at which depth–dose values are to be calculated is specified with respect to the external contour of the patient. It is usual for the spatial resolution of the points to be the same in both dimensions and the number of points used should be sufficient to give acceptable dose estimates when linear interpolation is used. The use of 1000 calculation points will give approximately 10 mm spacing in a large pelvis and 3 mm in the head or neck region. Thus a constant

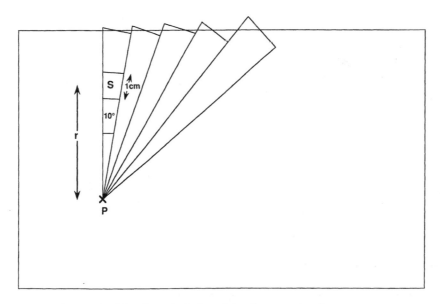

Figure 8.14 Sector integration method for the calculation of the dose at point P.

number of points will give a better resolution in the regions of the body where higher accuracy is required. Speed of calculation has often meant that the number of calculation points has been kept as small as possible and it is not uncommon for 1000 points to be used for the visual display of dose distributions. Speed of calculation is directly proportional to the number of calculation points, and also depends strongly on the beam calculation algorithm used. In the calculation of the dose distribution for visual display, the overall plan calculation time should be kept as small as possible for interactive planning. The number of calculation points is usually increased many times for hardcopy (to at least 6000), where speed of calculation is not important compared to accuracy. The higher resolution in the hardcopy can often result in the appearance of dose values higher than those seen in the visual display. The matrix points should be sufficiently close, so that the position of isodose lines as determined by contouring routines using linear interpolation will result in no significant loss in accuracy.

Each beam has a separate Cartesian co-ordinate system centred on the beam entry point. The co-ordinates of any dose calculation point, with respect to a beam co-ordinate system, can be found by a rotation and translation of the co-ordinates of the point. The dose distribution resulting from each beam in turn is calculated, multiplied by the beam-weighting factor and added into the patient–dose matrix. An alternative method is to have separate dose matrices for each beam and for the patient. It is then necessary to 'map' the dose distribution for a beam onto the patient–dose matrix by interpolation, and this can lead to large errors close to the external patient contour.

In the display of the dose distribution it is usual to alter the beam weighting, so that some normalization process occurs. For example, one of the following may be normalized to 100%:

(1) the mean target dose;

(2) the maximum dose in the plan;

(3) the isocentre, or the point of intersection of the central axes of the beams;

(4) the given dose on a specific beam.

The first three of these allow the dose at any point in the plan to be easily visualized as a percentage of the prescribed dose, whilst the third is the point at which the dose should be prescribed, or at least recorded, as stated in ICRU 50 (ICRU 1993).

6. Standard-treatment planning

In this section, planning of certain standard treatments will be considered. This is not intended as a complete list of all treatment sites; rather, examples have been selected to illustrate the physical aspects of treatment planning. A more complete description of the clinical problems can be found elsewhere (Bleehan *et al.* 1983; Dobbs *et al.* 1992). Following the normal convention, patient cross-sections are presented in the following examples under the assumption that they are viewed from the feet.

6.1   Pelvis

For a number of more advanced cancers in the pelvic region, it is common practice to treat not only the site of the primary disease, but also the lymphatic system to eliminate metastatic spread. The volume of tissue to be irradiated is large, typically 2000 cm^3, and it may be irradiated in conjunction with a booster dose to the primary tumour lying within it. Primary sites include the bladder (see Section 2.4.6), the cervix, for which the primary site may be treated by brachytherapy, and the rectum, commonly for recurrent or residual disease following surgery. Localization of the target volume may be done using CT or standard simulation based on anatomical markers. Figure 8.15 shows the target volume with the dose distribution for a three-field technique using a 16 MV beam. Although this is a very large volume, three fields produce a satisfactorily uniform dose distribution provided that the beam energy is sufficiently high (approximately 8 MV or greater). Balancing the dose distribution within the target volume is achieved through the appropriate selection of beam weights and wedge angles. These are chosen approximately to balance the subcutaneous doses for the anterior and lateral beams. It should be noted that, in order to reduce the maximum dose under the lateral fields, it is necessary to increase the wedge angle. At first sight this may seem paradoxical because the hot-spot dose under a wedge increases with wedge angle. However, an increase in angle is accompanied by a decrease in beam weight relative to the anterior field, in order to produce a uniform dose distribution in the target volume. Thus, the lateral skin dose is reduced at the cost of an increased anterior skin dose.

This example is for bladder cancer for which the dose to the rectum is kept to a minimum. Using a fourth, posterior field, would increase the rectal dose. If a four-field technique has to be used due to the non-availability of a high-energy accelerator, the weighting of the posterior field should be reduced to approximately 50% of the anterior field. In addition, the lateral fields should be wedged in order to compensate for the resultant non-uniformity in the AP direction but with a smaller wedge angle compared to the three field arrangement shown in Figure 8.15.

6.2   Oesophagus

Oesophagus tumours are not commonly treated by radical radiotherapy because of the relatively poor

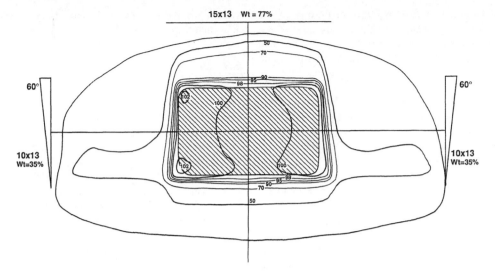

Figure 8.15 Treatment plan for the whole pelvis using 16 MV X-rays.

prognosis and ineffectiveness in their management by radiotherapy. However, tumours are sometimes treated for symptomatic relief and, in certain protocols, to relatively high doses requiring multiple field irradiation to avoid an excessive dose to the spinal cord. For these treatments the target volume generally has a relatively small cross-section (about 6–8 cm in diameter) but problems arise because of its length (up to 16 cm).

Localization of the target volume may be carried out on the simulator with the patient swallowing a barium contrast agent; alternatively, the CT scanner may be used. This is particularly valuable for the outlining of lung and for obtaining the position of the spinal cord.

Figure 8.16 shows a three-field plan for a 6 MV linear accelerator. The beams are positioned at equal angles round the patient and wedges are used to compensate of the different thickness of overlying lung tissue. This arrangement of fields has been selected to avoid irradiation of the cord (only the anterior field irradiates the cord directly) and to minimize the dose to the lung. A lower cord dose could be achieved using lateral fields, but this would be at the cost of increased lung dose.

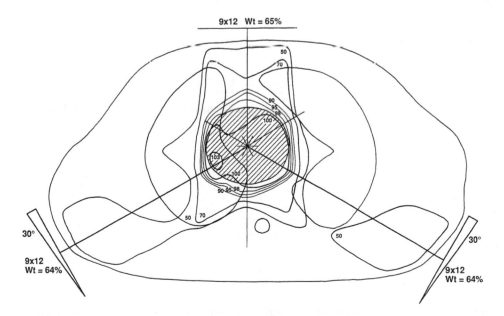

Figure 8.16 Treatment plan for an oesophageal tumour using 6 MV X-rays.

It should be recognized that this distribution only applies to the central plane of treatment. Because of the length of the treatment volume, it may seriously misrepresent the distribution in parallel planes. The upper and middle oesophagus is centrally placed but it follows the curvature of the spinal cord. This may require an increase in the irradiated cross-section, so that the target volume is included completely within the irradiated volume. However, this increased volume may include the spinal cord at one of its ends and may require beam blocks in the corner of the fields. Their position may best be obtained from the beams eye-view facility, if it is available in the planning software. Alternatively, simulator films may be used, although these may be difficult to interpret for oblique views. The lower oesophagus also runs from right to left within the patient.

If the target volume is at an angle to the rotation axis of the treatment unit, it may be necessary to rotate the diaphragm. The angle of rotation to be applied (δ) is given by $\tan(\delta) = \tan(\alpha) \sin(\theta) + \tan(\beta) \cos(\theta)$ in which α and β are the angles of the target volume to the rotation axis in the lateral and AP views respectively and θ is the angle of the treatment field (Casebow 1976).

An additional factor affecting the dose distribution along its length is the changing outline of the patient and the changing cross-section of the lungs. This is particularly significant when the upper oesophagus is treated. Multi-slice and 3-D planning are considered in more detail in Chapter 9.

6.3 Bronchus

Radiotherapy for bronchial cancer is generally only given for symptomatic relief using coaxially opposed fields. However, in a few cases radical treatment may be prescribed. For accurate treatment planning, CT outlines should be used, in particular to provide accurate localization of the lung. Radical treatments would normally only be given for unilateral disease, so that the lesion is non-central. It is important clinically to minimize the dose to the contralateral lung because of its relatively high radiosensitivity. Figure 8.17 shows a typical dose distribution using three fields. It should be noted that the anterior and the posterior oblique fields are symmetrically positioned either side of the anterior oblique field. The standard angle for the posterior oblique field is 120° but this may be changed depending on the position of the spinal cord relative to the target volume. Typically, 45° wedges are used but these may be changed depending on the precise geometry of the lung. The wedge for the anterior field is in part used to compensate for the changing overlying thickness of lung. It can be seen in this example that most of the left lung is receiving a dose that is less than 50% of the target dose.

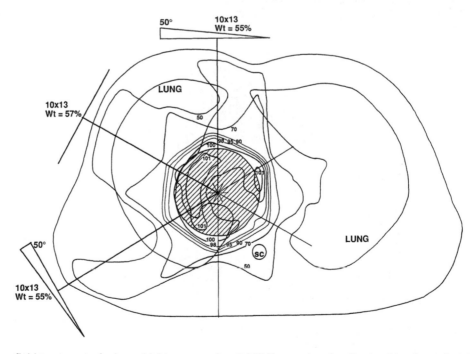

Figure 8.17 Three-field treatment of a bronchial tumour using 6 MV X-rays showing the target volume (hatched area) and the position of the spinal cord (SC).

As in the previous example, care must be taken to ensure that the spinal cord is not receiving an unacceptably high dose in the slices parallel to this central slice.

6.4 Breast

Post-operative irradiation of the breast is commonly prescribed for the elimination of residual tumour. This is frequently accompanied by the irradiation of the lymph nodes in the supraclavicular region and by a boost irradiation to the site from which the tumour was excised. The boost irradiation is normally given by electrons or using brachytherapy with, for example, iridium wire (Chapter 12).

Irradiation of the whole breast is normally carried out using coaxially opposed beams or with two beams at a shallow angle to each other. The lymph nodes are irradiated by a single straight-on field. This relatively simple irradiation geometry belies what is one of the more technically difficult sites for radiotherapy. The problems can be summarized as follows.

1. The cross-section of the breast varies over the length of the target volume.

2. The cross-section of the breast may vary over the time period of the treatment.

3. The sternum slopes when the patient lies flat requiring her either to be propped up in a position that may be difficult to reproduce or requiring a complex angulation technique.

4. The chest wall is curved and the depth of the lung below the breast tissue is small (approximately 2 cm), making it difficult to avoid irradiation of the lung.

5. A good match must be achieved at the border between the breast fields and the supraclavicular field over a width of approximately 20 cm. This is particularly important for this group of patients amongst whom there will be a high proportion of long-term survivors. Other borders may need to be considered if further fields are added.

Many different techniques for breast irradiation have been described in the literature. Techniques have been devised to produce an exact geometric match between the tangential fields for the irradiation of the breast and the supraclavicular field, which is generally angled outwards to avoid irradiation of the spinal cord. Matching may be achieved by means of blocks (or asymmetric jaws), or by angulation of the collimator and couch or by a combination of these (Lagendijk and Hofman 1992; Marshall 1993; Klein *et al.* 1994).

The dose distribution shown in Figure 8.18 is for the irradiation of the breast for which the isocentre is set at a point marked on the skin. The gantry angles are selected

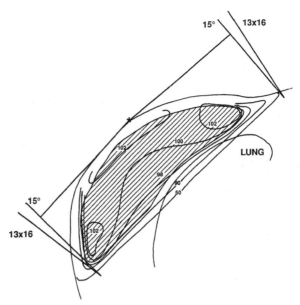

Figure 8.18 An isocentric technique for treatment of the breast with 4 MV X-rays.

such that the posterior margins of the two fields are coincident to minimize the dose to the lung.

6.5 Larynx

Figure 8.19 shows a fixed SSD treatment plan for an early stage carcinoma of the larynx. It is an example of coaxially opposed fields used for a radical treatment, which is possible in this site because of the narrow separation of the neck. Wedges are used to compensate for surface obliquity, with the surface angle being approximately 45°. The optimum wedge angle should be approximately two-thirds of this (see Section 2.4.3) and a 35° wedge has been used to produce a satisfactory distribution.

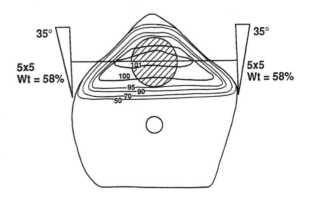

Figure 8.19 Treatment plan for the larynx using 4 MV X-rays.

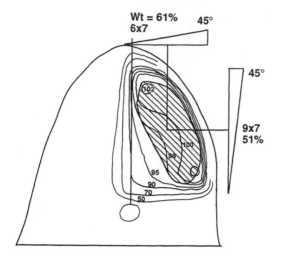

Figure 8.20 Treatment plan for a tumour of the floor of mouth using 4 MV X-rays.

6.6   Floor of mouth

Figure 8.20 shows a treatment plan for an advanced tumour originating in the floor of the mouth. As in the previous example, relatively superficial tumours in the head and neck region can be treated satisfactorily using a lower energy beam, in this case 4 MV. The minimum depth of the target volume is about 10 mm. If a higher energy beam were used it would be necessary to add bolus to the surface to provide full build-up and the outline should be modified accordingly. In this example, the required wedge angle calculated from the hinge angle (Section 2.4.3) is 45°. Steeper wedges might have been required to compensate for surface obliquity but the shallow depth of treatment increases the effective wedge angle.

As in many sites in the head and neck region, a more homogeneous dose distribution could be achieved if a third field were added, in this case through a right lateral portal. However, in this region, in which high target doses are given, irradiation of the normal tissues causes acute discomfort to the patient. Therefore, irradiation of areas outside the target volume should be avoided as much as possible and two-field techniques with the minimum target depth are almost always preferred.

6.7   Maxillary antrum

The last example in this series of treatment sites is the maxillary antrum. This provides particular problems for the planner because the target volume may be large and it

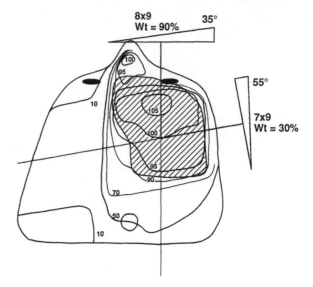

Figure 8.21 Treatment plan for the maxillary antrum using 4 MV X-rays. The positions of the brain stem and the lenses of the eyes are shown.

is close to the eyes and brain stem to which strict dose constraints apply.

Figure 8.21 shows a typical example of a tumour of the maxillary antrum. The ipsilateral eye is at the upper end of the target volume and in more advanced cases may not be spared because it is infiltrated by tumour. In less advanced disease, the therapist may choose to shield it using a block in the corner of the anterior field. The contralateral eye should be spared to avoid cataract formation as it has a relatively low dose threshold and the dose to the lens is normally constrained to about 10% of the target dose. This cannot be achieved without compromising the dose homogeneity within the target volume. The field arrangement chosen is unusual because one of the fields does not completely cover the whole target. In this example, the width of the lateral field is 7 cm, whereas the size of the target perpendicular to this field is 8 cm. In order to avoid gross dose inhomogeneity, the weight of this field is reduced considerably, in this case to one-third of the weight of the anterior field. This reduction in weight requires the wedge angle to be the maximum available. It can be seen that the consequence of this compromise in technique is that the dose in the target volume ranges from 90 to 107% which is very much worse than has been shown for the other distributions in this section. The lens of the right eye is close to the edge of both fields and is, therefore, in a region of a high-dose gradient. Precision of both planning and of treatment is, therefore, essential to ensure that it is not receiving an excessive dose. Direct measurements of eye dose should always be made for this particular treatment site to ensure that the calculated dose is correct (see Chapter 11, Section 2.5.5).

7. Treatment with non-standard fields

7.1 Irregular field calculations

Irregular shaped fields have always been used in radiotherapy. The simplest example of these is the insertion of a shielding block into the corner or edge of a field for the reduction of the dose to vulnerable structures, and in the majority of such cases it is sufficient to account for the change in beam area in the calculation of output and depth dose (Section 2.1.2). However, there are many other examples where the errors resulting from that assumption are not acceptable. The most common of these is the use of shielding blocks on a shadow tray to produce large irregular shaped fields in, for example, the treatment of Hodgkin's disease or lymphomas. In these, the use of equivalent beam area will result in the overestimate of both the output and depth dose at the centre of the field. More recently, multi-leaf collimators have provided an increase in the use of irregular stationary fields planned to conform to the shape of the target volume (see Chapter 9, Section 2.5).

The most commonly used method for calculation is based on the principle of separating the primary and scattered components of dose (Cunningham *et al.* 1972). Primary dose can be calculated from experimental measurements of the dose distribution in air over the beam portal or from a model of the geometry of the head of the treatment machine including the position and shape of the radiation source. The scattered component of dose can be calculated using a table of differential SARs in conjunction with the Clarkson sector integration method as described in Chapter 9, Section 1.5.4. Correction for patient–surface curvature requires a knowledge of its shape over the full beam portal if a full dose distribution is to be produced, and for this reason dose calculations have been performed one point at a time with the SSD input for each individual point. Correction for inhomogeneities is much more difficult and has been approximated by using an effective SSD for the calculations.

More recently, pencil beam algorithms (see Chapter 9, Section 1.5.5) have been used. The technique used is to integrate the pencil beams simulating the field over the beam portal, which means that the shape of the portal is irrelevant to the operation of the algorithm. Convolution methods will also deal with irregular shaped fields.

7.2 Compensators

The use of wedge filters to compensate for surface obliquity was discussed in Section 2.3. Generally, wedges provide adequate compensation if the surface inhomogeneity varies monotonically along one of the field dimensions. It may also be possible to use a combination of wedge directions if the surface obliquity is along both field axes. However, there are situations, as shown in Figure 8.22, for which standard wedges cannot help because of a significant tissue excess (or deficit) on both sides of the central axis. Particular clinical applications are in the head and neck region and for mantle fields. In these cases a more complex compensating filter may be required.

The simplest form of compensation is to use a tissue-equivalent material in contact with the skin over the full area of the field. This is built up to provide a flat surface perpendicular to the central axis. However, this brings the dose maximum towards the skin surface and for most curative treatments would be clinically unacceptable. An alternative is to use a tissue-equivalent filter of the same thickness, which is positioned on the accessory tray with its other dimensions reduced to compensate for the divergence of the beam. This restores much of the skin sparing but is more time consuming to produce for the individual patient and treatment field. Because tissue-equivalent filters need to be fairly thick, a higher density material is usually chosen.

The first stage in making a compensator is to measure the topography of the surface through which the field is directed. Many different ways of measuring these data have been described. Most have employed some form of pointer system either to measure distances directly on the patient's skin, from a plaster cast of the patient or the treatment shell. Commonly a grid pattern is projected on to the surface and the distance to each grid point measured. A system in which the pointer is pivoted at the simulated position of the source is the most convenient for this. Alternatively a multi-pointer system may be

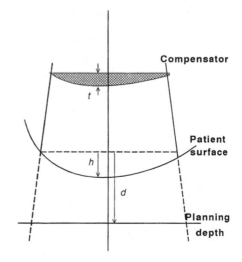

Figure 8.22 The use of a compensator to correct for surface non-uniformity.

used incorporating a jig to hold the pointers so that they diverge in an identical manner to the radiation beam. There are commercial systems that use pantographic devices to drive a milling machine to make an expanded polystyrene mould whilst the pointer traces over the patient's skin (Henderson *et al.* 1987). More recently, optical systems have become commercially available that analyse the digitized video signal from camera views of lasers projected onto the skin. The digitized data may also be used to control a milling machine. Other systems have made use of moiré fringe patterns. Alternatively the surface data may be obtained from CT scans.

There are three main types of compensator.

1. A grid-blocking system in which the compensator is made up of blocks of aluminium or brass from a range of standard thicknesses with each block having a fixed area, generally 1×1 cm^2 projected to the isocentre.

2. A contour system in which the compensator is built up from sheets of a standard thickness of lead (generally 0.5–1 mm). The lead sheet is cut to fit lines of equal tissue deficit interpolated from the surface measurements. When using this method care must be taken to ensure that the lead is of a uniform thickness(Aldrich and Andrew 1992).

3. A system using a machined compensator in which the surface of the block does not have any steps. These blocks are generally made by machining out the required shape in a polystyrene mould into which low melting point alloy (Lipowitz metal) may be poured. Commercial systems which use this technique are available.

The thickness t of material to be used in the construction of the compensator can be calculated from:

$$\exp(-\mu_{eff}t) = \frac{\text{TAR}(d, s)}{\text{TAR}(d - h, s)}$$

in which TAR(d,s) is the TAR at depth d for a field with equivalent square s; h is the tissue deficit (see Figure 8.22) and μ_{eff} is the effective linear attenuation coefficient of the material.

For lead, μ_{eff} values in the range 0.7–0.82 cm^{-1} have been reported. Some variation is due to filter thickness, distance from the skin and field size (Boyer, 1982). At higher energies, measurements of μ_{eff} should be made for the particular set-up to be used. An alternative method of calculating the thickness of material is to use a compensation ratio defined as the ratio of tissue to compensator thickness (Henderson *et al.* 1987).

Compensators can only achieve dose uniformity at a single depth. On other planes, the dose heterogeneity may by up to about 10% depending on the energy, field size, and the distance from the planning plane. If there are tissue inhomogeneities in the field, the compensator thickness may need to be modified. It should be noted that the presence of the compensator can increase the dose close to the skin owing to secondary electrons.

7.3 Asymmetric collimators

Asymmetric collimators are now standard equipment on the majority of currently available linear accelerators. In theory, asymmetric collimators allow the irradiation of any rectangular area within the maximum field size available on a linear accelerator. In practice, the movement of any one collimator blade is usually restricted to 10 cm beyond the central axis of the accelerator. Some of the clinical advantages to be gained from the use of asymmetric collimators are as follows.

1. Field matching: by moving one collimator blade to the central axis of the beam, that is used as a 'half-beam block', beam divergence at one edge of the field is eliminated. Matching to a similar field without beam overlap is greatly simplified, as there is no need to match the diverging edges of fields by gantry rotation.

2. Reduction in treatment volume: in treatment of Hodgkin's disease it may be desirable to cone down the treatment volume after a certain dose in order to limit the dose to the supraclavicular region. In other treatments it is often necessary to ensure that the spinal cord is out of the treatment volume, again after a certain dose has been given. These changes in treatment volume can be achieved simply by changing the position of one or more of the collimator blades without having to change the treatment set-up or make any major change to the dosimetry calculation.

3. Asymmetric collimators are particularly useful in enabling non-coplanar techniques to be set up with a common isocentre. An example of this is the use of 'half-blocked' fields in the treatment of carcinoma of the breast, where the isocentre can be set on the plane joining the tangential glancing fields to the anterior supraclavicular field. A further and similar example is in the treatment of nasopharyngeal cancer.

Dose calculation with asymmetric jaws can be a problem especially if the central axis of the beam is blocked. This is considered in the following section.

7.4 Monitor unit calculations

Output factors express the relationship between dose and machine units (or time) for different field settings at a specified treatment distance and depth. They have traditionally been measured at the depth of maximum absorbed dose on the central axis (d_{max}) relative to the value for a standard field size (generally 10×10 cm^2, see Chapter 4), and link other field size values directly to the absolute calibration of the treatment beam. Such output factors will be used with depth doses that are also normalized to d_{max} with beam modifier factors (e.g. blocking trays and wedges), also specified at d_{max}. With the almost universal adoption of isocentric techniques, an alternative method is to measure, store, and use factors at some other stated reference depth, e.g. 10 cm. This makes their use consistent with that of tissue–phantom ratio (TPR), also normalized at the same reference depth, and other factors should also be specified at this depth. However, many centres still utilize d_{max} referenced quantities for isocentric irradiation and this may necessitate careful conversions taking into account the appropriate field sizes both at the surface and at the isocentre distance, including inverse square law correction depending on how the data are stored.

Some recent recommendations (e.g. ESTRO 1997; NCS 1998) opt for all such quantities, measurements, and calculations to be referenced to 10 cm depth to minimize the problems of changing depth from d_{max} and from contaminant electron effects. However, it must be noted that changing from one system to another must be carried out with care and with full consultation with all groups involved in planning, including radiation oncologists and radiographers.

Simpler methods of tabulating output factors express the values against square field sizes or field area and interpolate intermediate or effective field sizes for rectangular or blocked fields from these values. This may be adequate to within acceptable accuracy for fields that do not differ substantially from regular settings. However, in situations where collimator settings and irradiated area differ significantly from one another or from a regular setting, it is more appropriate to separate collimator and phantom scatter effects and calculate the two components separately. Such situations may include, for example, when there is significant blocking (including multileaf collimation), the use of asymmetric collimators, or where exchange effects are significant for different collimator settings for the same field size (see Chapter 4). In this case, instead of using:

$$MU = \frac{\text{Dose required}}{D/MU(\text{ref}) \cdot OF}$$

the in-phantom output factor OF can be split into the product of the two components:

$$OF = S_{c,p} = S_c \cdot S_p$$

where S_c is the collimator scatter factor (or in-air output factor), dependent only on the collimator setting, and S_p is the phantom scatter factor, dependent only on the irradiated area. The appropriate values can be chosen to suit the irradiation situation. These can be measured at fixed FSD or isocentric conditions and their exact values and use will depend on the systems implemented in a given department. Chapter 4 discusses the measurement of appropriate data-sets at d_{max}, requiring the use of build-up caps, and also draws attention to the fact that measurements for other reference depths may be made using mini-phantoms. It may be noted that S_p values measured at d_{max} are normalized peak scatter factors (NPSF). Recent recommendations (ESTRO 1997; NCS 1998), which opt for all parameters to be specified and referenced to 10 cm depth recommend the in-air values to be measured in a mini-phantom.

8. Quality assurance

A general quality assurance programme in radiotherapy is essential and is discussed in Chapter 14. In treatment planning, this programme must ensure that adequate quality control (QC) procedures are applied to the treatment-planning system, as well as to the individual patient's plan.

8.1 QC of the treatment-planning system

Errors occurring in the treatment-planning system can affect a large number of patients. It is not possible in this text to detail all the tests required and only a brief outline will be given. The reader is referred for more detail to ICRU Report 42 (ICRU 1987) and to IPEMB (1996), IPEM (1999), and Starkschall and Horton (1991).

Necessary checks fall into two groups: those required at the time of commissioning the system; and those necessary for routine quality assurance on a daily, weekly, or monthly basis. It has been widely accepted that computer-calculated dose distributions are sufficiently accurate if the calculation is correct to within 2% or 2 mm in the calculation of the position of an isodose line, whichever is the greater. Thus, 2% would be the necessary accuracy in the centre of a field, whereas 2 mm would apply in the penumbral region. This accuracy requires a strict quality assurance programme.

The following is a list of QC checks that is not meant to be comprehensive and is probably the minimum that needs to be performed. The software checks only deal with external beam treatment planning.

8.1.1 Commissioning

1. Hardware tests:
   (a) correct performance of the processor, its memory, and any associated accelerators or array processors by the use of manufacturer's test software;
   (b) both digitizer and plotter accuracy by tracing in various outlines and comparing input to output;

(c) the performance of any interactive devices such as light pens and tracker balls;

(d) the linearity of graphic displays;

(e) the reliability of CT image transfer.

2. Software tests:

(a) the ability to deal with the changes in depth dose and machine output with SSD, beam area, etc.;

(b) the accuracy of the beam algorithm in a variety of situations; e.g. normal incidence in a homogeneous medium, surface obliquity, heterogeneous media, and calculations in off-axis planes;

(c) the ability to produce isodose charts to the required accuracy including interpolation from stored data;

(d) the ability to deal with beam modifiers such as wedges, blocks, asymmetric jaws, and compensators;

(e) the overall integrity of the stored data set compared to measured data;

(f) the relationship between electron density used for planning and CT number.

The above tests should be repeated for major hardware or software changes.

8.1.2 Routine checks

1. Daily:

(a) trace in, calculate, and plot out a plan – use a set of five plans covering a variety of treatment situations and beam parameters, and use a different plan each day of the week;

(b) check consistency of the isodose distribution (no planning is necessary);

(c) check output against input for patient contour accuracy.

2. Weekly:

(a) check the performance of the processor hardware using manufacturer's test software (many computers now test memory performance on boot-up);

(b) check the machine data set (this is best done by checking the data used against a master copy stored on archive media).

3. Monthly:

(a) check the transfer of CT image data to the planning system.

8.2 QC of the patient's plan

Errors in any treatment plan can seriously jeopardize the outcome for the individual patient. Planning requires a number of actions to be taken based on several individual items of information that are passed between different groups of staff. Therefore, the potential for error is high. The following general points may be made.

1. Any measurement from the patient that is to be used in the treatment calculation, for example, separation of field entry points or of treatment beam parameter, should be checked by a second person.

2. Treatment plan calculation should not be started until all the necessary data have been collected and checked for consistency. Standard forms for transferring such information are recommended; these should include a full description by the radiotherapist of the treatment required.

3. Following calculation of the plan, a full check should be made by a second person who is qualified to prepare the original plan. This should include a check of all the parameters entered in the treatment-planning system.

4. Following the final prescription by the radiotherapist and the completion of the treatment sheet, a second person should check that all data have been correctly transcribed and that the monitor settings have been correctly calculated.

5. There should be weekly checks of the treatment card to ensure that the treatment is proceeding as prescribed. For an isocentric treatment the SSD of each field should be remeasured to check for changes in patient outline.

The individuals carrying out the checks should sign the plan or treatment sheet to indicate that these checks have been completed.

As an additional check on the whole planning process, it is useful to have available an independent computer system to calculate the dose at a point, usually the isocentre, using the parameters that are written on the treatment sheet and measurements of SSD taken at the time of the patient's first treatment (Williams *et al.* 1991). Any discrepancy in excess of 2–5% should be investigated; the tolerance value depends on the type of treatment. For example, for treatments involving inhomogeneities, irregular field shapes, or in which there may be a relatively large daily variation in SSD, such as breast irradiation, a higher tolerance may need to be allowed.

It is essential that these QC procedures form part of a well-documented quality system. For example, there should be a clear protocol stating those circumstances when a patient may be treated before the checks described above have been completed.

9. References

Aldrich, J.E. and Andrew, J.W. (1992). Self-adhesive lead for compensator production and radiation shielding. *Med. Phys.*, **19**, 361–5.

Bleehan, N.M., Glatstein, E., and Haybittle, J.L. (ed.) (1983). *Radiation therapy planning*. Marcel Dekker, New York.

Boyer, A.L. (1982). Compensating filters for high energy X-rays. *Med. Phys.*, **9**, 429–33.

British Institute of Radiology (1996). *Central axis depth dose data for use in radiotherapy. Br. J. Radiol., Supplement 25.* BIR, London.

Casebow, M.P. (1976). The angulation of radiotherapy machines in the treatment of inclined lesions. *Br. J. Radiol.*, **49**, 278–80.

Clarkson, J.R. (1941). A note on depth dose in fields of irregular shape. *Br. J. Radiol.*, **14**, 265–8.

Cunningham, J.R. (1972). Scatter-air ratios. *Phys. Med. Biol.*, **17**, 42–51.

Cunningham, J.R., Shrivastava, P.N., and Wilkinson, J.M. (1972). Program IRREG – calculation of dose from irregularly shaped radiation beams. *Comp. Prog. Biomed.*, **2**, 192–99.

Dobbs, J., Barrett, A., and Ash, D. (1992) *Practical radiotherapy planning*, (2nd edition). Edward Arnold, London.

ESTRO (1997). *Monitor unit calculation for high-energy photon beams. ESTRO Booklet 3.* ESTRO/Garant, Leuven.

Henderson, S.D., Purdy, J.A., Gerber, R.L., and Mestman, S.J. (1987). Dosimetry considerations for a Lipowitz metal tissue compensator system. *Int. J. Radiat. Onc. Biol. Phys.*, **13**, 1107–12.

Hope, C.S., Laurie, J., Orr, J.S., and Halnan, K.E. (1967). Optimization of X-ray treatment planning by computer judgement. *Phys. Med. Biol.*, **12**, 531–42.

Institute of Physics and Engineering in Medicine (1999). *Physics aspects of quality control in radiotherapy. IPEM Report 81.* IPEM, York.

Institution of Physics and Engineering in Medicine and Biology (1996). *A guide to commissioning and quality control of treatment planning systems. IPEMB Report 68.* IPEMB, York.

International Commission on Radiation Units and Measurements (1987) *Use of computers in external beam radiotherapy procedures with high-energy photons and electrons. Report 42.* ICRU, Bethesda.

International Commission on Radiation Units and Measurements (1993). *Prescribing, recording and reporting photon beam therapy. Report 50.* ICRU, Bethesda.

Klein, E.E., Taylor, M., Michaletz-Lorenz, M., Zoeller, D., and Umfleet, W. (1994). A mono-isocentric technique for breast and regional nodal therapy using dual asymmetric jaws. *Int. J. Radiat. Oncol. Biol. Phys.*, **28**, 753–60.

Lagendijk, J.J.W. and Hofman, P. (1992). A standardized multifield irradiation technique for breast tumours using asymmetrical collimators and beam angulation. *Br. J. Radiol.*, **65**, 56–62.

Marshall, M.G. (1993). Three-field isocentric breast irradiation using asymmetric jaws and a tilt board. *Radioth. Oncol.*, **28**, 228–32.

McDonald, S.C. and Rubin, P. (1977) Optimization of external beam radiation therapy. *Int. J. Radiat. Oncol. Biol. Phys.*, **2**, 307–17.

Meredith, W.J. and Neary, G.J. (1944). The production of isodose curves and the calculation of energy absorption from standard depth dose data. *Br. J. Radiol.*, **17**, 75–82.

Nederlandse Commissie voor Stralingsdosimetrie (1998). *Determination and use of scatter correction factors of megavoltage photon beams. NCS Report 12.* NCS, Delft.

Redpath, A.T. and Wright, D.H. (1981). Beam modelling techniques for computerized therapy planning. In *Treatment planning for external beam therapy with neutrons* (ed. G. Burger), pp. 54–9. Urban & Schwarzenberg, Munich.

Redpath, A.T., Vickery, B.L., and Wright, D.H. (1976). A new technique for radiotherapy planning using quadratic programming. *Phys. Med. Biol.*, **21**, 781.

Redpath, A.T., Vickery, B.L., and Duncan, W. (1977). A comprehensive radiotherapy planning system implemented in Fortran on a small interactive computer. *Br. J. Radiol.*, **50**, 51.

Starkschall, G. (1984). A constrained least-squares optimization method for external beam radiation therapy treatment planning. *Med. Phys.*, **11**, 659–65.

Starkschall, G. and Horton, J.L. (ed.) (1991). *Quality assurance in radiotherapy physics.* Medical Physics Publishing, Madison, USA.

Tsien, K.C. (1955). The application of automatic computing machines to radiation treatment planning. *Br. J. Radiol.*, **28**, 432–39.

Williams, J.R., Bradnam, M.S., McCurrach, G.M., Deehan, C., and Johnston, S. (1991). A system for the quality audit of treatment dose delivery in radiotherapy. *Radioth. Oncol.*, **20**, 197–202.

Chapter 9

Treatment planning for external beam therapy: advanced techniques

A.T. Redpath and S.G. McNee

1. CT planning

1.1 Scanning techniques

1.1.1 CT scanning

It is now accepted that computerized tomography (CT) has a major role in treatment planning. Its diagnostic worth in the detection of malignant disease is significant, and the assessment of the extent of the disease may be vital in determining the choice of treatment. The specification of the anatomy of the patient in three dimensions, as a map of electron density values, allows accurate calculation of the dose distribution. It also permits accurate localization of the planning target volume and of critical normal structures.

CT scanning is the same as any simulation technique in that the patient must be placed in the treatment position, and this means that a flat insert for the curved CT couch-top is required. Although the diameter of the reconstruction circle (normally a maximum of 50 cm) is usually adequate to contain the patient tomogram, the physical size of the scanner aperture may provide problems for patient positioning, for example, in the treatment of breast where the arm is placed in the abducted position. The majority of modern scanners have a 70-cm diameter aperture. Any immobilization devices that will be used for treatment, such as beam direction shells, incline boards, body cradles, or foot-stocks must also be present during scanning. Care must be taken when using contrast agents to ensure that CT numbers are not altered to an extent that will influence the calculation of the dose distribution, and it is good practice to obtain scans with and without contrast to measure its effect. Modern scanners have short scan acquisition times of the order of 1–2 seconds per slice. However, treatment times cover several respiration cycles and, therefore, a long scan acquisition time is desirable in order to average patient movement, although this will result in a reduction in the quality of the image. This is rarely available, and a practical compromise is to obtain the scans under conditions of shallow breathing.

Lasers are normally used to assist in patient positioning. Two lateral and one sagittal laser are aligned so that they define the horizontal axis passing through the centre of the reconstruction circle. The sagittal laser is used to position the patient centrally on the CT couch, and all three laser lines are marked on the patient both with tattoo marks and by radio-opaque markers. Cardiac catheters or thin, high density wire (such as solder wire) can be used as radio-opaque markers and these can be visualized on the CT images. After the planning process, the position of the isocentre can be specified by an anterior/posterior and a lateral movement relative to these markers. A further marker placed on the anterior surface of the patient can be seen on a scout view and allows the longitudinal movement of the isocentre to be determined. The isocentre can be positioned during verification on the treatment simulator by making these movements after setting up to the tattoo marks.

A 'scout' or 'transmission' scan is taken prior to scanning, so that the superior and inferior limits for scanning can be determined. After the slice separation has been specified, the position of the scans to be taken are displayed on the scout view. A slice separation (and width) of 10 mm is normally adequate in the thorax and pelvis, but 5 mm is often used in the head and neck regions where greater accuracy is required. When beam shaping with customized blocks or multi-leaf collimation is to be used, a slice separation of 5 mm is recommended, especially in the region of the planning target volume. The accuracy to which the planning target volume can be specified at its superior and inferior limits is equal to half the slice separation and this should be remembered when deciding what separation to use. The number of CT scans taken will normally be in the range 20–50 and with 512 pixel resolution will contain up to 25 megabytes of data. They can be transferred to the planning computer by the use of magnetic media, but the preferred and more efficient method is over a local area network. It is vital to check the integrity of image data transfer to the treatment-planning system. As well as scaling factors, slice order and spacing, the transfer must correctly orientate the slices for all possible scan positions, e.g. supine, head first, prone, feet first.

Spiral scanning has become available more recently. This method of scanning records transmission data continuously as the patient moves through the scanner, and any required slice can then be reconstructed after interpolation of the necessary transmission data. This versatility has obvious advantages but results in a slight loss of resolution.

1.1.2 Simulator CT and the CT simulator

There are two main disadvantages in the use of CT scanners for treatment planning. First, the localization of the planning target volume is not carried out at the time of scanning, and second, as already stated, there may be a problem in placing the patient in the treatment position due to the limitation of the aperture size on the CT scanner. Both these problems can be overcome by using the treatment simulator to obtain CT data. A number of groups have developed simulator CT facilities (Kotre *et al.* 1984; Redpath and Wright 1985) and the technique has been described in Chapter 7, Section 7.2. However, there are disadvantages to this approach. Design and manufacturing constraints limit the 360° gantry rotation time, and hence the scan acquisition time, to a minimum of 1 minute. This is long enough to produce an average image over several respiration cycles, but imposes a limit on the number of scans that can be taken, not only due to the acquisition time but also the power constraints on the X-ray tube. It is unusual for more than three slices to be taken on any individual patient. The most common method employed to collect the transmission data is to digitize the video signal from the image intensifier. With low-resolution systems, the image quality is sufficient to delineate body outlines, the position of the lungs, and large bone masses with acceptable accuracy. The bulk inhomogeneity method for correcting dose calculations is used after assigning densities to these structures. Caution should always be taken in using these systems to provide diagnostic information. Commercially produced systems use high-resolution video digitizers and good quality images are available, comparable with those produced from CT scanners about a decade ago. Electron density information is also available and is sufficiently accurate to be used for treatment planning. A spatial resolution better than 2 mm and a density resolution better than 1% is claimed. More recently, some manufacturers have used solid-state detector arrays as used in diagnostic CT technology and claimed a further improvement in image quality.

Another approach that has been developed by some manufacturers (e.g. Picker, Medical High Technology International) is that of the CT Simulator. The equipment uses a CT scanner based in the radiotherapy department. A large diameter aperture (90 cm) is available making it possible to place the patient in the required treatment position for a higher proportion of cases. It uses the concept of virtual simulation, where CT images are used as a virtual patient and advanced computer graphics software is used instead of the treatment simulator. The computer software produces high-resolution digitally reconstructed radiographs, analogous to portal X-ray films on the simulator, with a beam's eye view of the target volume overlaid, allowing the shaping of beam portals. Software is also available for the three-dimensional manipulation of image data, and provides utilities for enhancing the visualization of the data. Externally mounted lasers are used to identify the location of markers placed on the external surface of the patient. Beam portals, geometrically determined for the treatment beam direction, can be marked on the patient's surface using a gantry mounted laser.

1.2 Outlining and target drawing

1.2.1 Outlining

After transferring the CT slices to the treatment planning system, the patient's external contour, the target(s) to be irradiated, and any internal organs of interest are outlined. Treatment-planning systems have facilities for the automatic outlining of the external body contour, which work by searching for boundaries in the matrix of CT numbers. In general they perform satisfactorily, but it is essential to examine outlines slice by slice to detect possible artefacts. These include external fiducial markers, the CT couch or positioning aids that may be contained within the outline. In the vicinity of the oral and nasal cavities, the generated contour may track along internal surfaces. Where there is a gap between the patient's skin surface and an immobilization device, such as a head shell, the operator may have to decide whether to outline the shell or the skin. This may depend on the ability of the dose calculation algorithm to calculate correctly for the effect of the air gap.

Ideally, treatment-planning systems allow bolus material to be added to the patient outline as part of the modelling process. In some systems, the use of bolus has to be anticipated and included as part of the external body outline. This may require an element of trial and error where the thickness of bolus is not known in advance, for example, in treatment with electrons. Automatic outlining tools work well for some internal organs, such as lung and bone, but have limited success for other organs. Outlining of brain tissue can be quickly achieved by selecting automatic outlining for bone and searching for the internal surface of the skull. In a similar manner, outlining the inner bone surface of the spinal column can

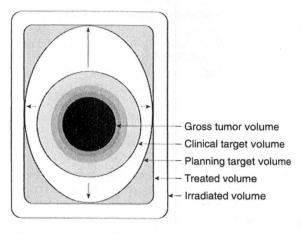

— Gross tumor volume
— Clinical target volume
— Planning target volume
— Treated volume
— Irradiated volume

Figure 9.1 ICRU (1993) definitions of target volumes.

speed up outlining of the spinal cord. Internal organs are outlined for two main reasons. First, they can be visualized in three-dimensional views, beam's eye views or reconstructed planes. Second, it enables the computation of the dose within the organ. Outlining is generally only performed for organs that are considered to be dose limiting. These are mainly spinal cord and eyes, but in three-dimensional planning may include lungs, liver, kidneys, rectum, bladder, brain, pituitary, and other organs.

Treatment-planning systems allow dose computation from CT density values (see Section 1.5.1). If this facility is not to be used, then tissue heterogeneities (such as lung, bone, and air cavities) have to be outlined and average values of density entered for each region. CT images can be severely distorted due to the presence of materials of high density, for example, dental fillings or replacement hip joints. Not only does this result in errors in dose calculation but positional geometry can also be distorted. Ideally, such slices should be excluded from the data set. Accumulation of radiological contrast agents (in oesophagus, stomach or bowel) is less likely to distort the image, but will affect dose calculation. In these circumstances, a facility to edit CT density values within defined areas can be beneficial.

1.2.2 Target drawing

Drawing of the target is of fundamental importance to the success of radiotherapy. Target definition using CT differs greatly from the traditional simulator-based technique. Where complex treatment techniques are to be used, additional factors have to be considered. A helpful description of the target is given in ICRU Report 50 (1993) and is represented in Figure 9.1. Malignant tumour that is visible to the eye, by palpation or by imaging techniques is known as the gross tumour volume

(GTV). The density of malignant tumour cells is greatest in the GTV. Surrounding the GTV is a zone in which the tumour cells infiltrate, and across which tumour cell density decreases. The clinical target volume (CTV) includes the GTV plus a margin to include this microscopic spread of tumour. Other sites of suspected subclinical spread of disease, such as regional lymph nodes, are also part of the CTV. The planning target volume (PTV) includes the CTV with a margin to allow for internal organ movement and treatment set-up errors. The latter may be due to machine tolerances or patient positioning reproducibility. The treated volume is that which receives a dose equal to or greater than the minimum prescribed therapeutic dose, and is greater than the PTV because of the geometric relationship of the beams to the PTV. The irradiated volume is that which receives a dose considered significant in relation to normal tissue tolerance.

Proposed changes to ICRU Report 50 (1993) include the separate identification of margins that are patient or machine related and the application of margins when outlining critical organs.

It is not essential to draw all these targets in all cases. Normally the clinician will draw the PTV, but in some centres the clinician draws the CTV and the treatment planner applies specified margins at various edges to define the PTV. The aim is to produce a plan in which all the PTV is enclosed by a particular isodose line, e.g. 95% of the dose at the centre of the PTV. In reality, the aim is that all the CTV is irradiated to the specified minimum dose, after allowing for organ movement and set-up errors. One of the major challenges to the clinician is to determine the correct margins for target drawing, and much investigative work is in progress. By its very nature, the extent of microscopic disease is impossible to define with certainty. In some sites, there may be a natural boundary defined by bony structures, e.g. in the skull. In other sites clinical assumptions may be made, for example, that the disease is confined within the wall of the bladder and that all the bladder must be irradiated. Generous margins may be allowed along the length of the oesophagus but tighter margins applied for lateral spread. In the absence of reliable diagnostic information, the necessity to irradiate the sites of possible nodal spread of disease, e.g. in the chest or pelvis, is a difficult clinical decision.

Other margins can be assessed more directly. The tolerances for linear accelerator performance are generally well established (see Chapter 5). Of particular importance are the movement of the isocentre with rotation of gantry, couch and diaphragm system, couch sag, and the calibration of the radiation beam size. Many studies have been performed using portal imaging (with X-ray film or with electronic imaging devices) to determine both systematic and random components of treatment set-up variation. Such studies rely on a comparison of the radiation field positions relative to bony structures. In general, field placement errors for pelvic irradiation are mostly up to 5 mm but may be as much as 10 mm. Using standard immobilization shells, the corresponding values for head and neck irradiation are 4 and 7 mm (Hanna *et al.* 1999). The main criticism of such studies is that they do not allow visualization of internal organ movement. Repeated CT scanning shows that the prostate may move by up to 20 mm in the anterior–posterior direction and by about 5 mm in the lateral and superior–inferior directions (Ten Haken *et al.* 1991; Van Herk *et al.* 1995) and depends upon bladder and rectal filling. Fluoroscopy on a simulator can be used to demonstrate movement of certain lung tumours during the breathing cycle, or of the larynx during swallowing. Two main challenges result from these points. First, the necessity to develop protocols to minimize movement and set-up errors, and second, the need to learn how to deal with the various uncertainties in drawing optimized CTVs and PTVs.

Target drawing for CT planning differs in many aspects from simulator-based planning. In many cases, the tumour can be visualized directly on the CT image, but this is not always possible with simulator planning, for example, in the bladder where only contrast agent is visible on the fluoroscopy display or a radiograph. The position of the tumour has to be deduced from diagnostic information. Determination of the extent of the bladder is even more difficult as beam sizes are probably based as much on clinical convention as on physical evidence. Comparative studies of CT and simulator planning have shown (Dobbs *et al.* 1983) that the latter often results in a geometric miss of part of the bladder. Target drawing is fundamental to the eventual success of CT treatment planning and therefore radiotherapy. For optimum CT planning, all CT slices should be transferred to the treatment-planning computer and targets drawn individually on all relevant slices using a mouse, light pen, or tracker-ball. A recent audit (McNee *et al.* 1998) showed that the implementation of CT planning in the UK was less than optimal. It was suggested that this was perhaps due to a lack of confidence in drawing optimal target outlines and to the extra time required for CT planning. Well-designed software tools that allow target outlines to be projected onto adjacent slices and then moved or modified, can greatly improve the speed and efficiency of this process. Sometimes it can be useful to be able to project outlines between transverse slices, and reconstructed sagittal or coronal sections.

Special attention must be given to the significance of the PTV drawn on the end slices. The most common practice is to scan with contiguous slices, e.g. 10-mm wide slices at 10-mm spacing. The target could be considered to end at the middle of the slice, or it may be more appropriate to consider the edge of the PTV to be at the edge of the CT slice. The choice depends on the margins that have been applied by the clinician. However, it should be remembered that there is an uncertainty of half the CT slice width at both the superior and inferior limits of the PTV. It is important that there is clear communication between the clinician and the planner on this aspect, as it affects the choice of beam length selected, and the adequacy of target coverage. Target drawing on the end slices is important in other ways. It is relatively simple to measure dimensions within CT slices to check the margins between PTV and CTV or GTV. It is more difficult to check the margins when projecting longitudinally, especially if the target shape is irregular (Stroom and Storchi 1997). Non-coplanar beams cut across the scan plane and the choice of beam length is very dependent on the target shape drawn on the end CT slices. Treatment of a pharyngeal tumour with latero-superior oblique beams is illustrated in Figure 9.2. At the superior, the PTV outline has been reduced in size when projected to the end slices. At the inferior, the PTV has been maintained in size. In covering to the corners of the PTV, substantially more normal tissue is irradiated to high dose at the inferior than at the superior, and this is perhaps unnecessary. It should be recognized that drawing targets on end slices is especially difficult, as these usually contain no visible disease.

Many treatment planning systems have tools for applying margins and initially most of these worked in two-dimensions. Some applied radial growth from a geometric centre and others imagined a ball of set diameter rolling around the perimeter of the target. Growth algorithms that work in three-dimensions have now been developed (Stroom *et al.* 1998). If the target shape is irregular, these methods give different final answers, particularly due to growth in the longitudinal axis and 3-D algorithms are to be preferred. Differences may be within the clinical uncertainties, but it is recommended that the clinician always views and verifies the final target shape.

Some tumours are poorly imaged with CT, even when using contrast-enhancing agents. MRI has shown superior imaging quality with respect to CT for some tumours in a variety of sites, especially brain and pelvis. However the following difficulties are associated with using MRI for radiotherapy dose calculations:

(1) no tissue density information is available;

(2) the images often display spatial distortion, particularly around the periphery and at interfaces;

(3) bone is not imaged, leading to difficulties in identifying landmarks and verifying the accuracy of set-up.

For planning purposes, it is recommended that the target is 'mapped' from an MRI image set to a CT image

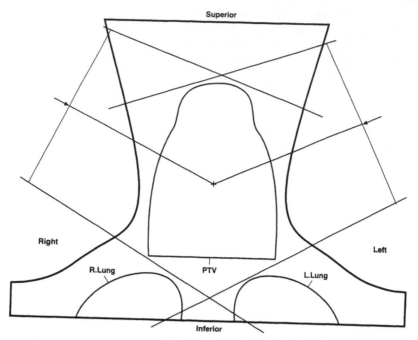

Figure 9.2 Latero-superior oblique beams treating pharyngeal tumour. Better conformation is achieved at the superior where the target shape is rounded, than at the inferior where the target shape is square.

set, and the latter used for dose calculation. This map, or transformation, can be based upon corresponding anatomical points or external fiducial markers, and has even been performed automatically. Alternatively, it is possible to fuse surfaces, such as the skull outline. Some systems require that for both CT and MRI the patient is in the same position and the slice positioning and spacing are matched. Other mapping tools permit three-dimensional scaling and rotation of images. One benefit of this is the possibility of using a diagnostic MRI study with a planning CT study, thereby removing the need to repeat MRI. This could be particularly useful for brain tumours, as internal organs stay in the same relative position when the head is moved, but problems could arise in the pelvis if the degree of bladder or rectal filling differed between scans. The success of the mapping process depends on the degree of image distortion and the development of advanced algorithms to correct for distortion. At present, image-mapping tools are more readily available on diagnostic workstations but it is highly desirable that they are developed for planning systems. In the future, there may be a need to match other image sets, such as SPECT or functional PET images.

1.3 Tools available for 3-D planning

Three-dimensional treatment planning must allow the calculation of the dose distribution in three-dimensions,

and allow the treatment beams to enter the patient from any direction. This implies that the calculation and set-up of non-coplanar treatment beams is possible, and therefore the planning software must deal with treatment couch and diaphragm rotation. Non-coplanar treatments are especially useful in treating lesions in the head and neck regions and may prove to be useful in the thorax with the development of conformal techniques. However, they pose added problems in the treatment-planning process, especially in the selection of beam direction as two rotational degrees of freedom are allowed. More sophisticated planning tools are essential both for the selection of beam direction and the assessment of the large amount of dose data that is calculated. Although the following tools were not specifically developed for non-coplanar planning, it is safe to say that full three-dimensional planning is not practical without their availability.

1.3.1 Beam's eye view (BEV)

Beam's eye view is probably the most useful tool that has been developed for three-dimensional planning. In this approach, the observer is placed at the radiation source, and the projection of the contour of any structure that has been outlined on a CT image set, is displayed on a plane normal to the central axis of the beam passing through the isocentre. The beam portal is also displayed. An

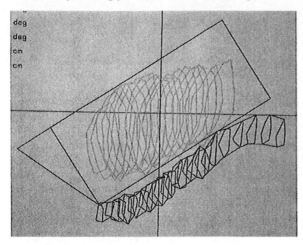

Figure 9.3 Beam's eye view for a target lying close to the spinal cord. See also colour plate section.

example for a target volume lying close to the spinal cord is shown in Figure 9.3. The BEV image is calculated as follows.

In a CT co-ordinate system with the origin at the isocentre, a point lying on an outline is specified by co-ordinates x, y on a CT slice at a distance z from the isocentre. The point can be transformed using three-dimensional co-ordinate geometry to a beam co-ordinate system by two rotations about the isocentre: first, for gantry angle and, second, for table angle. The co-ordinates of the point are then given by x_1, y_1, and the point lies on a plane normal to the central axis of the beam at a distance z_1 from the isocentre. The co-ordinates x_2, y_2 of the projection of this point onto the plane passing through the isocentre are given by:

$$x_2 = x_1 S/(S - z_1)$$
$$\text{and} \quad y_2 = y_1 S/(S - z_1)$$

where S is the isocentric distance of the treatment machine. This transformation allows the BEV of any structure to be calculated. Depth shading, as a function of z_1 is normally used to assist in displaying the image. Beam divergence means that any individual contour is displayed with perspective.

The calculation of BEV is sufficiently fast to allow dynamic display. This provides considerable assistance during the treatment-planning process for the selection of gantry angle, table angle and field size, specifically when trying to avoid vital structures. The definition of field size can include the position of asymmetric diaphragms, and the drawing of any beam blocks required by the use of interactive computer graphics. Wedge direction is also displayed, as shown in Figure 9.3. BEV is an essential tool in conformal therapy for determining the required

field shape. Algorithms are available that will automatically give a specified margin around whatever target volume has been specified, but it should be remembered that the size of the margin required may vary with direction. The field shape obtained can be used to manufacture customized blocks, or can be used to determine automatically the required position of the leaves of a multi-leaf collimator. Some computer-planning systems allow the beam's eye view to be displayed superimposed on a digitally reconstructed radiograph, as described in the next section.

1.3.2 Digitally reconstructed radiographs (DRR)

Treatment beam direction and size has conventionally been verified on the treatment simulator, and recorded by the use of radiographic film. More recently, digital radiography has begun to replace film and high resolution (1024×1024) images can be produced. It is also possible to compare or register these images with those taken at the time of treatment using electronic portal imaging (EPI) techniques. A third type of image, known as a digitally reconstructed radiograph (DRR) can also be produced at the time of treatment planning. It can be used both to assist with the planning process, and as a further method of verification either at simulation or at the time of treatment.

DRRs are calculated from CT data once the isocentre position and beam direction have been determined. The size of the image to be reconstructed is usually related to the size of the beam portal, and will include a predetermined margin around the portal. The time for calculation is directly related to the area of the image and to the resolution required, and is therefore minimized by keeping the reconstructed area as small as possible. The beam is modelled as a set of rays of equal angular increment in two orthogonal directions over the area of the radiograph. DRRs require the calculation of the effective path length d_{eff} in unit density material that each ray will traverse as it passes through the three-dimensional CT matrix and this requires ray tracing techniques (Siddon 1985). Alternatively, if a spherical beam model is used (Redpath 1995), where the CT number is interpolated at each voxel given by r, θ, ϕ, then a summation along r for each value of θ, ϕ will give the effective path length. This method has the advantage of allowing the DRR to be determined automatically at the time of dose calculation with virtually no increase in computational time. The relative transmitted intensity $I(\theta, \phi)$ along any ray can be determined simply from:

$$I(\theta, \phi) = \exp(-\mu d_{\text{eff}})$$

where μ is the linear attenuation coefficient appropriately chosen to provide optimum contrast within the image.

Image-processing techniques can be used to improve further the quality of the image. High resolution is essential for these images and a pixel size no greater than 1 mm should be used. DRRs can be displayed with the beam portal superimposed together with the BEV image if required. DRRs are an essential component of the concept of virtual simulation, and are used extensively in the CT simulator as described earlier.

1.3.3 Dose–volume histograms (DVH)

Three-dimensional treatment planning produces a large amount of dose information which can be difficult to interpret if displayed as a set of two-dimensional dose distributions. For that reason different methods of displaying the dose distribution have been developed. The dose distribution throughout individual organs, for example, the target volume or anatomical structures of interest, can be displayed as histograms. A conventional histogram shows the total number of voxels receiving a dose in a specified dose interval against a set of equally spaced dose intervals. If the total volume of the voxels is plotted instead of total number, the histogram is referred to as a differential dose–volume histogram. However, it has become more usual to plot the volume of the organ that receives a dose greater than a specified dose against that dose over the full dose range given by the treatment. These histograms are known as dose–volume histograms (or cumulative dose–volume histograms) and an example is shown in Figure 9.4. The volume may be specified as absolute volume or more commonly as a percentage of the total volume. In a similar manner dose may be specified as absolute dose or as a percentage of the prescribed dose.

DVHs have a number of uses. In the target volume they show if the dose uniformity is acceptable. In individual organs they show the percentage of the total volume of the organ that receives less than a stated percentage of the prescribed dose, and it has become common for such statements to appear in treatment protocols, especially in conformal therapy. They are very useful for comparing treatment plans and choosing the best from a selection of plans. The DVH for the total irradiated volume can show the presence of hot-spots in the dose distribution. However, it must be emphasized that DVHs give no positional information. DVHs have been used to calculate tumour control probability (TCP) and normal tissue complication probability (NTCP) (Lyman and Wolbarst 1987; Webb and Nahum 1993). A great deal of investigation is required to establish a correlation between these computed numbers and observed clinical outcomes.

It is important to remember that the full extent of any organ of interest must be both CT scanned and outlined if accurate DVHs are to be calculated. The three-dimensional anatomical representation of any organ will consist of a set of two-dimensional outlines that have been drawn on a sequence of CT slices. Various methods of determining the volumes from these data have been developed, for example, the use of a polyhedral approximation (Cook *et al.* 1980) or considering the volume to consist of a three-dimensional matrix of voxels (Drzymala *et al.* 1991). The latter is particularly relevant to the calculation of DVHs, where voxels can be specified by the pixel size on the CT slice and the slice separation. The volume is then considered as a set of contiguous slabs centred on the CT slices. Some planning systems will consider the first and last slab to have a thickness equal to half the scan spacing when calculating total volume but this is questionable. The voxel size used is important in calculating DVHs accurately and, in general, the smaller the structure then the smaller is the voxel size required. Ideally the voxel size should be adjusted to the size of the structure. Accurately determining the voxels that lie within the organ is important as it obviously has a direct effect on the calculation of the DVH. It has been shown that small changes in the DVH lead to significant differences in the calculation of TCP and NTCP (Drzymala *et al.* 1991). In some cases, dose–area histograms (DAHs) may be more relevant than DVHs, for example, the wall of the rectum or the surface of the bladder. DAHs are more difficult to calculate and for that reason are not so widely used.

Although the accurate calculation of DVHs is difficult and time consuming, it should be stated that in the comparison of different plans on the same patient the need for accuracy is reduced, as it is the change in the DVH that is used to assess the quality of the plans.

1.4 Dose display and reporting

It is highly desirable in radiotherapy to use a common system for reporting doses. This facilitates comparison of reported studies and enables consistent dose prescription between clinicians within and between centres. The

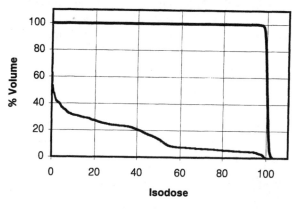

Figure 9.4 Example of a dose–volume histogram for a treatment of the bronchus. The upper curve is the PTV and the lower curve is the DVH for the lung.

system described in ICRU Report 50 (1993) is probably the system most widely used. It is necessary to report the prescribed target dose, dose uniformity, dose to critical organs, and the treatment technique. The point chosen for reporting target dose, the 'ICRU point', is that which can be calculated most accurately and most reproducibly. In most circumstances, it is the point of intersection of the beam central axes. For two opposing beams, it is the mid-separation point on the central axes or, alternatively, at the centre of the target, if this is offset from the mid-plane. Other treatment techniques are described in detail in the report (ICRU 1993). The distribution of dose can be described by dose–volume histograms or by reporting maximum, minimum, average, median, or modal values. These are usually based on a matrix of calculated dose points and values can vary significantly depending upon the matrix spacing and the planning system used. They are also affected if the target encroaches into the build-up zone, if edges of the target are not properly covered by the beam, and by the calculation techniques (e.g. single or multiple slice, two- or three-dimensional). Other details necessary to allow the treatment to be reproduced elsewhere should also be reported. These include the beam type and energy, beam sizes, beam configuration, fractionation schedule, patient preparation and positioning.

Optimization of the dose plan depends on a clear presentation of the distribution of dose, usually super-imposed upon the CT images, and this should be examined slice by slice. In this way, it is possible to see that the PTV is adequately treated, that the treated volume is minimized, that the variation in dose within the PTV is acceptable, that hot spots of dose are not excessive, and that critical organ doses are within stated limits. Other methods of displaying or assessing doses are also useful. Calculation of doses in orthogonal planes (sagittal and coronal sections) can give some indication of the need for wedging in the longitudinal direction. However, hot-spots often appear in the corners of the target and are not seen on these sections. For some treatment sites (such as the oesophagus), where the target and spinal cord are rotated in the A–P view, the dose can be usefully viewed on a reconstructed oblique plane. Isodose surfaces can be presented in three-dimensions, but the success of this depends on the computing power available and the ability to support detailed graphic displays. One method is to present an isodose line as a wire frame for each relevant slice, along with wire frame outlines of the target and structures, but such presenta-tions often lack clarity. A better approach is to use colour rendering of the surfaces of these structures. A percep-tion of depth can be added with shading, brighter for foreground surfaces and dimmer for background. An-other useful feature is to use colour-coding to highlight areas of regret, for example, parts of the target that receive doses lower or higher than desired. In this way,

attention is drawn to these areas and the suitability or otherwise of the plan can be assessed and possibly action taken to improve the plan. Another useful addition to computer simulation of the treatment is the room's eye view (REV), where the treatment machine, couch, treatment beams, and patient are displayed as seen by an observer who can be positioned at any point in the treatment room. It is useful in assessing the feasibility of a treatment set-up and in selecting beam directions to avoid critical structures.

In two-dimensional planning, a hard copy of the isodose display of the central plane with a note of the maximum dose to critical organs provides the clinician with an adequate record of dose. In three-dimensional planning, the dose display is ideally examined slice by slice at the computer by the clinician and the treatment planner together, as it is often difficult to present the full dosage information in hard copy form. Dose statistics are useful, such as the dose maximum, minimum, and mean or a dose–volume histogram for the target and structures of interest. Their major limitation is that they contain no positional information, e.g. the location of hot- or cold-spots, and such factors can affect the clinical accept-ability of a plan. For hard copy records, it is recommended that one to three representative transverse slices be printed, or alternatively the three cardinal sections (axial, sagittal, and coronal) through the target centre. In each case, the isodose distribution super-imposed on the CT image or a reconstructed CT image, will provide the clinician with extra information for assessing the dose distribution and for verifying the accuracy of beam position at simulation.

At present there is interest in assessing plans based on radiobiological factors rather than absorbed dose dis-tributions. Biological dose could be calculated using a suitable algorithm from the prescribed dose and fractionation schedule. A discussion of this issue is beyond the scope of this chapter and the subject is still under development. The choice of biological model (the linear quadratic model is probably the most widely used) and of tissue-specific parameters (such as alpha/beta ratios) are of prime importance. A potentially useful approach is to use a biological model to predict the tumour control probability (TCP) and normal tissue complication probability (NTCP) (Lyman and Wolbarst 1987; Webb and Nahum 1993). Whilst no model can, as yet, correctly predict absolute values for these para-meters, they may be useful tools for assessing the relative merits of alternative plans.

1.5 Dose-calculation algorithms

1.5.1 Conversion of CT numbers to electron density

After CT scanning, the images are transferred to the treatment-planning computer, but before their use the CT numbers must be converted into electron densities, and this requires a calibration curve for the scanner. A calibration curve is usually incorporated into the software supplied with commercial planning systems, but it is important that its accuracy is checked by scanning a phantom with inserts of known electron density. Although the random uncertainty in the CT numbers produced from a modern CT scanner is sufficiently small that it will not affect the dose calculation, a systematic error can produce a problem. A typical calibration curve is shown in Figure 9.5, which shows the relationship between CT number and electron density. A linear relationship holds up to relative electron densities slightly greater than 1.0, which covers air, lung, and soft tissue, all with similar atomic numbers. A different relationship is found at higher relative electron densities, and this represents structures that are bone-related with a higher atomic number. Again care must be taken, for any calibration curve will only apply for the X-ray generating voltage used and will vary from one scanner to another.

The main heterogeneities that affect the dose calculation occur in the lower part of the calibration curve shown in Figure 9.5 and it is important to ensure that this is correct. It is normal to set a CT number of −1000 for air (zero density) and a CT number of zero for water (unit density). Problems will occur from artefacts in the images such as beam-hardening effects or the presence of contrast material and these may produce reconstruction artefacts, such as streaking. Parker *et al.* (1979) stated that the systematic uncertainty in the CT value produced

Table 9.1 Algorithms for dose calculation in a heterogeneous medium

Type	Algorithm	Accounts for
1	One-dimensional (see manual methods)	Effective depth
2	Two-dimensional Tissue–air ratio power law	Distance between heterogeneity and point of calculation
3	Three-dimensional ETAR 3-D scatter correction Volume integration of DSARs	Position and shape of heterogeneity
4	Convolution Superposition Monte Carlo	As Type 3 but includes electron disequilibrium at interfaces

from their scanner altered calculated doses by less than 2% over a depth ranging from 8 to 12 cm and an energy range from ^{60}Co to 8 MV, and this is encouraging. Finally dual energy scanning can be used to obtain a direct estimate of electron density. Although more accurate, the improvement does not warrant the increased effort required.

1.5.2 Types of calculation algorithms

The dose-calculation algorithms that use electron density values derived from CT images are sufficiently complex to require computer processing. For routine treatment planning by computer it is not necessary to know how these algorithms work, however, the physicist responsible for the purchase of new planning software should understand the limitations and accuracy of the calculations used. The types of algorithms that are available are summarized in Table 9.1, and can be divided into four types that are essentially a compromise between speed and accuracy.

Moving down Table 9.1, the algorithms produce greater accuracy at the expense of greater computational time. Types 1–3 essentially calculate the dose distribution in a homogeneous water-equivalent medium, and correct this dose distribution for the presence of heterogeneities. Type 4 algorithms can calculate the dose distribution directly in the heterogeneous medium.

The first type of algorithm can be used manually, but only if heterogeneous regions are outlined on the CT images and average electron densities calculated for these regions. Occasionally these algorithms are used in computer calculations. They are one-dimensional and only correct for the effective depth of a point, considering only changes in the primary component of dose. These have been discussed in Chapter 8, Section 3.

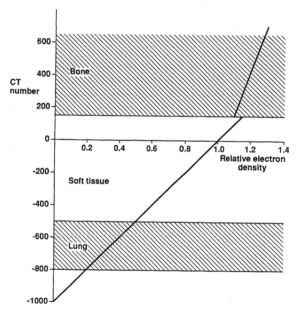

Figure 9.5 Typical calibration curve for a CT scanner relating CT number to electron density.

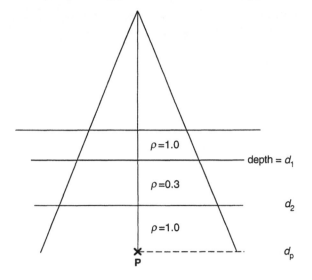

Figure 9.6 The power-law tissue–air ratio method for the inhomogeneity correction for a point in tissue of density 1.0 beneath a slab of material of density 0.3.

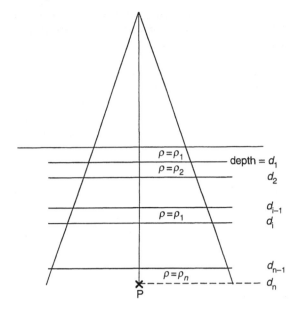

Figure 9.7 Inhomogeneity corrections for multiple slabs of different density materials.

1.5.3 Tissue–air ratio power-law algorithm

The second type of algorithm takes account of the position of the calculation point with respect to the heterogeneity, but considers the heterogeneity to be of uniform thickness over the beam width. This is known as the tissue–air ratio (TAR) power-law method (Sontag and Cunningham 1977), or the Batho method, and is the most frequently used method in computer planning systems. It is a two-dimensional method and only requires a knowledge of the tissue electron densities between the radiation source and the calculation point. The algorithm uses the ratio of two TARs raised to a power dependent on the electron densities of the tissues involved. Both the thickness and composition of the heterogeneity are accounted for, as well as the position of the calculation point with respect to the heterogeneity. In its most simple form, the method can be explained by Figure 9.6 where P is a calculation point lying in unit density material at depth d_p from the surface. P lies below a heterogeneity of density 0.3, which is assumed to be of uniform thickness $d_2 - d_1$ and of infinite lateral extent. The general form of the expression for the correction factor C_F to be applied to the depth dose at P is:

$$C_F = \left[\frac{\text{TAR}(d_p - d_2, r)}{\text{TAR}(d_p - d_1, r)} \right]^{0.7} \tag{1}$$

where r is the effective radius of the beam.

It should be noted that C_F is independent of the thickness of the material overlying the heterogeneity.

The equation only applies if the heterogeneity has the same atomic number as soft tissue.

The example given in Figure 9.6 represents a situation that frequently occurs in treatment planning, and the equation could be evaluated by hand for a limited number of points. However, when the method is used with CT data, a more generalized formulation of the method is needed. Figure 9.7 shows n layers of materials of different densities with a calculation point P situated within the nth layer of density ρ_n at a depth d_n from the surface. The ith layer has a density ρ_i and d_i is the depth of its rear surface. The general form for the correction factor is:

$$C_F = \prod_{i=1}^{n-1} \text{TAR}(d_n - d_i, r)^{\rho_{i+1} - \rho_i} \tag{2}$$

where Π denotes a multiplication of the terms in the resulting expression.

In general, the power-law TAR method predicts the dose to points close to heterogeneities with acceptable accuracy. However, it has shortcomings for heterogeneities of small lateral dimensions and when used with high-energy X-rays. Large errors can also result when the method is used for calculations within heterogeneities for large field sizes. The method should be used with caution if the distance of the calculation point from the heterogeneity is less than the build-up distance d_{max} for the energy of the radiation used. In this case, values of the TAR can be extrapolated into the build-up region from available values beyond the build-up region.

Alternatively, Thomas (1991) proposed that the distance from the point P to the boundary of the interface should be increased by d_{max}, therefore, in equation (2), $d_n - d_i$ would be replaced by $d_n - d_i + d_{max}$. This gives significantly better results and has become known as the modified Batho method.

1.5.4 Three-dimensional methods

The third type of algorithm takes into account the three-dimensional shape of the heterogeneity. The equivalent TAR method (ETAR) was developed by Sontag and Cunningham (1978), who extended the TAR method (Chapter 8, Section 3.2.4) so that the correction factor C_F for the dose in a heterogeneous medium is modified in the numerator not only for the effective depth but also for an effective field size. C_F is given by:

$$C_F = \frac{\mathrm{TAR}(d_{eff}, r_{eff})}{\mathrm{TAR}(d, r)}. \tag{3}$$

The parameters are the same as in the TAR method, except that r_{eff} is the radius of a circular field that, when incident on unit density material, produces the same scatter dose to a particular calculation point as is obtained in the heterogeneous situation. The method was developed from an idea by O'Conner (1957), who stated that a beam irradiating a medium of uniform but non-unit density, will produce the same dose to a point as a beam irradiating a unit density medium, with the depth and field size scaled in proportion to the density.

Redpath and Thwaites (1991) have developed a three-dimensional scatter correction algorithm based on the principles of the ETAR method. Fundamental to the method is a model that predicts the relative amount of scattered radiation that reaches a dose calculation point from any other point in the irradiated volume. The method uses the Klein–Nishina formulae to model Compton scatter, and both single and multiple scatter are considered. The relative amount of scatter reaching a calculation point is evaluated for the heterogeneous situation, and for a homogeneous unit density medium at normal incidence and the same SSD as the heterogeneous situation. The ratio of these estimates produces a correction factor giving a measure of the change in the scatter component of dose to the calculation point resulting from the heterogeneous nature of the medium. This correction factor can then be applied to the scatter component of dose calculated for the homogeneous unit density medium, using a table of differential scatter–air ratios (Cunningham 1972) and a sector integration technique (Clarkson 1941). The scatter component of dose is added to the primary component obtained from the zero-area TAR at the effective depth of the point.

Both this algorithm and ETAR use a similar procedure to reduce the calculation from three-dimensions to two-dimensions in order to speed up calculation times. This procedure coalesces the electron density information from the CT slices on either side of the calculation plane onto a single plane located at a distance z_{eff} from the calculation plane. A simplified explanation is that the scatter dose reaching the plane at z_{eff} is an average of the scatter dose to all planes throughout the treatment volume. This procedure is also applied if the calculation is taking place in two-dimensions, where only one CT slice is available for calculation and it has to be assumed that it is representative of the patient throughout the treatment volume. However, the speed of modern computer hardware may make it feasible to consider the change in scatter dose throughout the treatment volume without these approximations.

Sontag and Cunningham (1978) claim that an average accuracy of 2.5% can be achieved with ETAR over all megavoltage energies used in radiotherapy. Redpath and Thwaites (1991) showed that their algorithm performed significantly better than ETAR in extreme situations that were designed to provide a rigorous test of the algorithms. Although this type of algorithm is sufficiently accurate for dose calculation, it does not account for electron transport at the interface between media of different densities. However, Woo *et al.* (1990) have proposed an extension of these methods to situations in which conditions of electron equilibrium are not satisfied.

Cunningham (1972) developed the idea of scatter–air ratios (SARs), which are derived from TARs. The idea was developed further to show how SARs could be differentiated to produce differential SARs, and these represent the amount of scattered radiation reaching a point from a volume element (voxel) elsewhere in the irradiated volume. In three dimensions it is necessary to differentiate the SARs with respect to depth, radius, and angle. The scatter originating from any voxel is proportional to both the electron density of the voxel and to the primary fluence at the voxel, and is weighted accordingly. The effective path length to the scattering voxel has to be calculated in order to correct the incident primary fluence for the presence of heterogeneities. In a similar manner, the effective path length from the scattering voxel to the point of calculation is required in order to modify the scatter for the presence of heterogeneities. This calculation has to be summed over the whole of the treatment volume to estimate the total scatter dose to a point. Larson and Prasad (1978) have successfully implemented this algorithm, named the delta–volume method, although it has not been implemented clinically due to the large computation times required.

1.5.5 Convolution methods

The final two methods allow for electron disequilibrium. An approach developed recently uses convolution methods, where the energy deposited in a homogeneous medium is obtained by convolving the primary fluence at a point with a total energy deposition (or pencil beam) kernel (Ahnesjö *et al.* 1992), describing how the energy is distributed around the point. Pencil beam kernels have been produced by one of two methods:

(1) by deconvolving an experimentally measured beam profile in a homogeneous medium (measured for a large field size) with the primary distribution; or

(2) by using Monte Carlo simulations.

The approach is useful in computing the dose in irregular shaped fields in three dimensions. One of the methods described in Sections 1.5.3 and 1.5.4 is used to correct for the presence of heterogeneities. The use of convolution methods in a heterogeneous medium has been investigated by calculating kernels for the primary, singly scattered and multiply scattered components of the dose and convolving each separately with the primary fluence (Mackie *et al.* 1987). The effect of the heterogeneities is taken into account by scaling the magnitude of the kernels by the physical density at the interaction point. Density scaled kernels have also been used in superposition techniques, where the energy deposited throughout a medium resulting from the interaction at any point, is summed over all points to give the total dose distribution (Boyer and Mok 1986).

1.5.6 Monte Carlo techniques

Monte Carlo techniques predict the dose distribution from a beam of radiation passing through a patient by simulating the behaviour of a large number of photons that make up the beam. Random numbers are used to determine, for example, the interaction processes that occur, the distance that a photon will travel along a particular path, and the way in which the photon is finally absorbed. The absorbed dose resulting from photon interactions is due to the secondary electrons produced, and the calculation must also follow the fate of these electrons. This is a complicated procedure due to the many electron interactions that take place, and much simplification is needed. The main problem is that a very large number of random samples is required to achieve an acceptable accuracy for the resultant dose distribution. Photon histories must be followed until the statistical uncertainty in the resultant dose distribution is acceptable, and this is likely to require several million histories.

The above is possible with current Monte Carlo computer codes such as the EGS4 code (Nelson *et al.* 1985), and will give accurate answers to dose calculations in a heterogeneous medium. With current computer hardware the computation times are too long for routine treatment planning. The method is used for benchmark-ing in testing the performance of other dose-calculation algorithms, and for calculating energy deposition kernels for superposition and convolution techniques. Several groups are currently involved in using multi-processor parallel computing in an attempt to reduce computational times to a level that could make routine planning a possibility.

2. Conformal therapy

2.1 Definition and rationale

It is known that a significant proportion of treatments fail to control the primary disease. It is logical to conclude that if the target dose could be increased, then cure rates could be improved. The tolerance of normal tissues limits the dose that can safely be delivered, and is dependent upon the volume of tissue that is irradiated. Thus, by minimizing the treated volume, the dose delivered to the PTV could be increased, offering the possibility of improved cure rates with no increase in complication rates (Leibel *et al.* 1991; Armstrong *et al.* 1995). For these reasons, there is much interest in implementation of what has become known as conformal radiotherapy, where beam portals are individually shaped to the PTV. There is probably no simple, uniformly accepted definition of conformal radiotherapy; in fact radiotherapy has always been conformal in making use of whatever technology was available.

The first essential element of conformal radiotherapy is the outlining of the patient, the target, and any organs of interest as three-dimensional structures in the correct geometrical relationship to each other. In practice, this is usually achieved using a CT study. The second element is the positioning of the radiation beams in three-dimensional space to match optimally the beams to the target shape, to minimize the treated volume, and to keep doses to critical organs within acceptable limits. This involves the use of blocked beams and non-coplanar beams, where necessary. The third element is to prescribe a higher target dose whenever possible. There is evidence that escalation of dose can be implemented without excessive morbidity, but clinical trials are required to demonstrate what clinical improvement can be achieved (Read 1998). Successful implementation of conformal radiotherapy relies on the determination of optimal treatment margins, and as yet these are not well established. The extent of microscopic infiltration is more a matter of clinical judgement than of scientific measurement. Data are available on internal organ movement, but cannot be measured for every individual patient. Set-up errors can be more readily measured and minimized by proper quality assurance of treatment machines and the use of patient immobilization. Even if

(a)

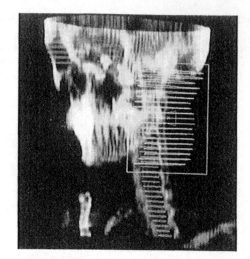

(b)

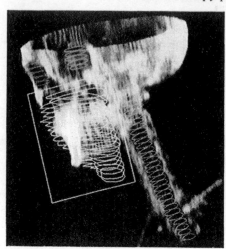

Figure 9.8 Beam's eye view of non-coplanar beams used to treat a tumour of the left parotid. PTV, spinal cord and eyes are outlined (a) anterior oblique beam, (b) posterior-superior oblique beam. See also colour plate section.

each of these parameters is known with reasonable precision, it is still not clear how they should be combined when drawing the PTV (e.g. in quadrature or linearly). If margins are set too small, then the outcome might be tumour underdosage and a failure to control the disease. The investigation of treatment margins is of key importance to the success of conformal radiotherapy and will be an important area of research for some time to come (Mageras *et al.* 1999).

2.2 Selection of beam directions

After the structures have been outlined, the next step is to select the beam directions. Until now, the constraints of treatment planning computers have meant that most conformal radiotherapy is delivered with coplanar beams. The choice of beam directions is often defined by departmental conventions, e.g. the use of a four-field box technique for pelvic tumours, or by the need to avoid critical organs. Three-dimensional planning provides the possibility of using non-coplanar beams. However, it is unlikely that it will ever be possible to test the benefits of non-coplanar beams by clinical trial, or to prove which beam directions are optimal. Instead, it will be for the treatment planner to demonstrate that there is some perceived improvement by the use of non-coplanar beams. For example, the treated volume may be minimized or the DVH for the target or for critical organs may be improved.

For some tumours of the head and neck, it may not be possible to design a satisfactory plan with coplanar beams. Figure 9.8 shows the treatment of a tumour of the left parotid using two beams. The anterior oblique field is coplanar to the plane of the CT slices. A coplanar

posterior oblique field would exit through the right eye, and could not treat all the PTV without also irradiating the spinal cord. By rotating the couch through 25° and the diaphragm by 20°, the beam neatly conforms to the PTV, misses the spinal cord and exits below the eyes. There would be no significant improvement in conformation with the use of blocking. This treatment could not be prescribed by conventional simulator methods and this highlights the importance of target drawing in three-dimensional conformal planning.

2.3 Asymmetric collimators

Certain aspects of the use of asymmetric collimators have been covered in Chapter 8. Asymmetric setting may be used to minimize treatment margins where three or more non-orthogonal treatment beams are used. The example shown in Figure 9.9 is a bronchial tumour of irregular cross-sectional shape. Where symmetrical beams are used, an excessive amount of tissue is irradiated at the medial/anterior edge of the target. Using asymmetric collimator settings on the left anterior beam achieves better conformation to the target shape. An alternative solution, which requires the use of two isocentre positions, would be slower and less reliable to set up. Drawbacks associated with the use of asymmetric collimators are the extra care required to ensure correct transfer of data to the treatment machine, and the need to establish and verify a method of dose calculation.

2.4 Customized blocking

Optimal shaping of beams is achieved by manufacturing customized blocks made of low melting-point alloy. A mould is prepared by milling the desired shape out of a

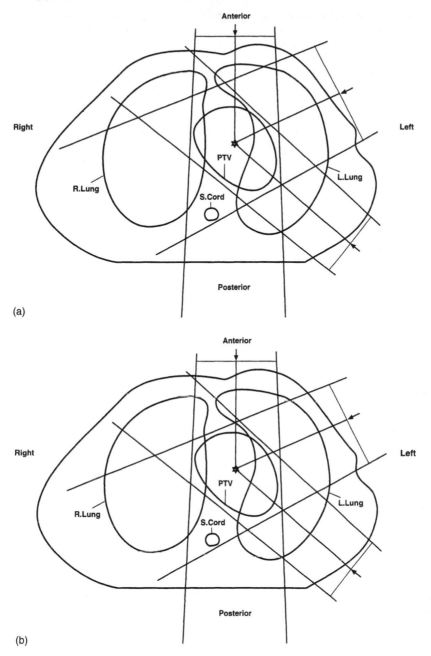

Figure 9.9 Irradiation of a bronchial tumour: (a) all beams are symmetric; (b) collimators are set asymmetrically for the left anterior oblique beam, thereby achieving improved conformation to the PTV.

Styrofoam sheet of suitable thickness. Molten alloy is poured into the mould, and the Styrofoam sheet is mounted on a slide that can be located in the shadow tray on the head of the treatment machine. The shape of the block can be defined on a simulator radiograph or by using a beam's eye view facility on the treatment-planning computer. The cutting of the Styrofoam can be accomplished by exporting data from the planning computer to an automated block milling machine. Alternatively, a 'hot-wire cutter', a device with a pointer linked by a wire to a focal point can be used. Placing the radiograph, or a plot of the BEV, at the correct distance from the focus reproduces the geometric setting of the beam. The Styrofoam is placed at the distance corresponding to the shadow tray on the treatment machine. Thus the edge of the block is matched to the divergence of the radiation beam, thereby minimizing penumbral edges. The block may simply shield at one or more edges of the beam, or may define the entire field shape as a portal within the block. The thickness of the block depends on the degree of dose reduction required, but is often restricted by the clearance available on the shadow tray and the physical weight of the block.

The ability to create any shape with customized blocking is ideal for use with conformal radiotherapy. The extent to which the treated volume can be minimized depends on the treatment site, the beam configuration and the shape of the PTV in the BEV. Reduction in treatment volume can be considerable. For example, using a three-field box technique to treat a tumour of the prostate, where the CTV includes the prostate gland and seminal vesicles, the volume of tissue irradiated to 95% of the dose to the ICRU point can be reduced by up to 40%. It is for clinical judgement to determine what amount of dose escalation might be possible as a result of this amount of reduction in treated volume, but it would be highly dependent upon the type of tissue irradiated.

2.5 Multi-leaf collimators (MLC)

Manufacture of alloy blocks is labour intensive, and they are cumbersome to use because of their weight. Multileaf collimation (MLC) is a facility that allows beams to be shaped without the need to manufacture blocks. The standard diaphragms are used to define a rectangular beam and the MLC used to shape the treatment portal within this. The MLC consists of opposing pairs of tungsten leaves, usually about 60 mm thick, which can be driven independently across one axis of the beam. In one design of accelerator, MLCs replace one pair of diaphragms. A number of design features of the MLC have a significant bearing on its clinical use. They are described below.

The width of the leaf is usually 10 mm at the isocentre plane, although micro MLCs are now available, for which the leaf width is 3–5 mm. The maximum length of field for which the MLC can be used will obviously depend on the number of pairs of leaves and the leaf width, but is generally in the range of 20–40 cm. The length of each leaf and the maximum extent of its travel across the beam limit the size and shape of field that can be defined. Due to physical constraints of weight and space, the thickness of the leaves is less than that of the diaphragms. Typically, the primary transmission through the leaves will be about 2%. Another problem is with leakage of radiation between adjacent pairs of leaves. This is minimized by various design features, such as

interlocking of leaves, but can still result in doses of up to 5% to small areas. Problems of leakage between opposing leaves when fully closed should be avoided by closing down the diaphragms. The closing faces of the leaves are usually curved to achieve an element of focusing and therefore a constant penumbra width at all positions of the leaves. This results in a penumbra width across the face of the leaf that is slightly larger (approximately 1 mm) than for the diaphragms. It might be thought important for dose computation to know whether it is the MLC or the diaphragm that forms the effective beam edge. In reality, the accuracy of dose computation in this area is reduced due to the presence of steep dose gradients, set-up errors and patient movement and a 1 mm discrepancy may be of no importance.

Detailed measurements of the dose distributions across the boundary formed by the MLC are of help in determining the optimal positioning of the leaves relative to the edge of the PTV. The isodose lines display a ripple pattern, following the stepped shape formed by the MLC as shown in Figure 9.10. In general, the 50% isodose coincides with the projection of the centre of the leaf edge.

The dose profile across the boundary of an irregular MLC shape shows characteristic stepping (Figure 9.10), which is only improved by reducing the leaf width. Setting leaf positions relative to the PTV is best done in beam's eye view in which a contour line with defined margins (of about 6 mm laterally and 10 mm craniocaudal) is set around the perimeter of the PTV. This would coincide with the edge of customized shielding blocks, if used. Most treatment planning systems allow automatic fitting of the MLC leaves to this contour line. Often, the centre of each leaf is set to coincide with the contour line. The corner of the some of the leaves may intersect the PTV and individual repositioning of these leaves is required.

Best conformation is achieved when the angle formed between the outline of the PTV and the direction of movement of the MLC is minimal (Zhu *et al.* 1998). The closeness of fit of the MLC to the PTV will, therefore, be dependent upon the selection of collimator angle. Some planning computers have software features that 'optimize' the fit by selecting the most appropriate collimator angle. This may have the effect of using much larger diaphragm settings than normal, and result in noncoplanar treatments as the major axes of the diaphragms for the different beams are no longer coplanar. The extra complexity introduced, both in terms of dose calculation and verification of set-up, should be considered before use.

In practice, the setting of MLC positions is made more complex by the use of wedges and by the close proximity of critical organs. If wedges are required in order to achieve a satisfactory dose distribution, the freedom to

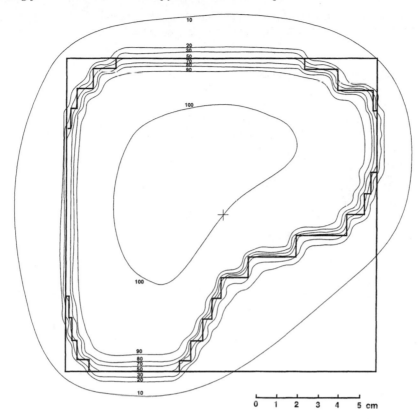

Figure 9.10 Isodose distribution, in a plane perpendicular to the beam axis, using a multi-leaf collimator (leaf width = 10 mm).

rotate collimators may not be available as the MLC orientation rotates with the collimator. This can prove to be a significant restriction to the satisfactory use of the MLC. For some linear accelerators, the MLC moves parallel to the wedge direction whilst for others it is orthogonal. More usefully, for some linear accelerators the wedge can be inserted in any of the four principal directions.

These factors are illustrated by the example in Figure 9.11, of a tumour in the post cricoid region that is curved along the edge of the cervical vertebrae with spinal cord in close proximity. The wedge axis is perpendicular to the direction of leaf movement. The beam shown is with a gantry rotation of 70° from the vertical. In Figure 9.11 four treatment options are shown. These are with the collimator leaves moving in the cranio-caudal direction and at 90° to that, and with and without collimator rotation to the angle of the PTV. Figures 9.11a and b have no collimator rotation. With the leaves in the cranio-caudal direction, Figure 9.11a, conformation to the PTV is poor and there is inadequate shielding of the cord. Figure 9.11b shows the leaves in

the vertical orientation with the wedge direction cranio-caudal. A large beam size is set and a large proportion is 'blocked' using the MLC. This is not ideal, because of leakage and transmitted radiation. Conformation to the PTV is acceptable but where the spinal cord is at an angle of about 45° to the horizontal, shielding by the MLC is inadequate. Conformation to the PTV is poor and the shielding of spinal cord is unacceptable with the collimator rotated 20° from the horizontal and with the leaf movement in the cranio-caudal direction (Figure 9.11c). Figure 9.11d provides the best solution both in term of conformation to the PTV and shielding of the cord. In this case the wedge axis is in the cranio-caudal direction.

Similar problems arise when planning is not with CT and MLC positions are defined on simulator radiographs. Where areas to be shielded are rectangular, one edge may fall along the centre of a leaf. It may be necessary to choose between over-shielding or under-shielding by half a leaf width. A possible solution might be to offset the field centre and to use asymmetric collimator settings with the MLC.

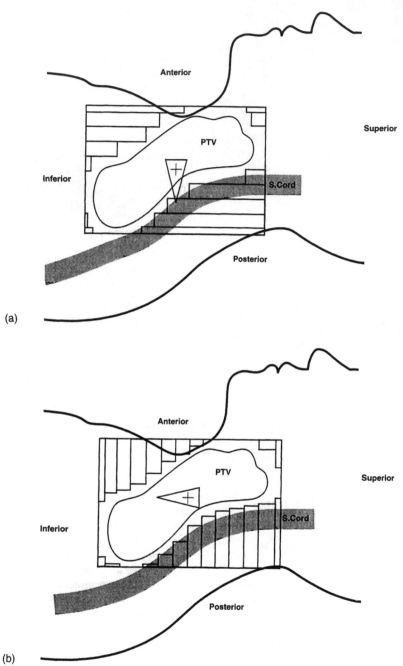

Figure 9.11 Treatment of a tumour of the post cricoid region using MLC when the wedge axis is perpendicular to the direction of leaf movement: (a) poor conformation to PTV and inadequate shielding of spinal cord; (b) good conformation but suboptimal spinal cord shielding; (c) inadequate conformation and spinal cord shielding; (d) satisfactory set-up.

For ease of use, it is essential that the MLC positions are set automatically from the linear accelerator's computerized record and verify system. Keyboard entry of all of the MLC positions for each beam would be tedious, slow, and prone to error. Digitizing tablets on some systems allow some degree of automation of data entry (e.g. if the shape is defined on a simulator radiograph or a beam's eye view). Ideally, the data

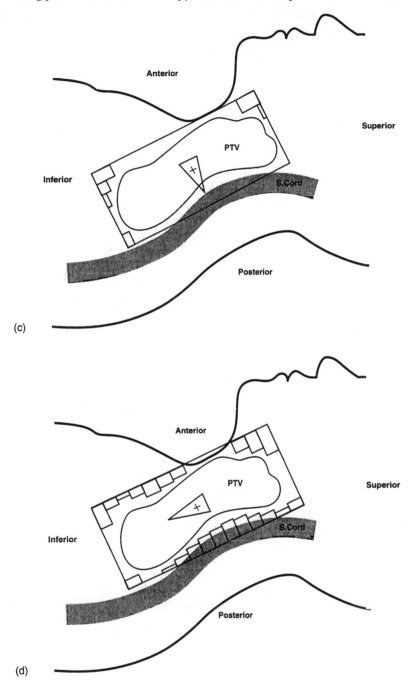

(c)

(d)

Figure 9.11 (*continued*)

should be transferred over a network link between the treatment planning computer and the linear accelerator record and verify system. Alternatively, data transfer can be made using floppy disks.

2.6 Treatment set-up and verification

Treatment margins are minimized when using conformal therapy, and it is clear that procedures taken to minimize set-up errors and verify treatment set-up must be more rigorous. Patient positioning errors can be minimized in many circumstances by the use of immobilization devices, such as stereotactic frames, moulded thermoplastic shells, and vacuum bags, and in all cases, care has to be exercised when positioning the patient (Mubata *et al.* 1998). Video-imaging devices (such as Osiris) are available that help to ensure that the external body position is accurately reproduced between simulation and treatment. This might also reduce internal organ movement.

It is essential to verify treatment set-up. This is generally performed using a radiotherapy simulator, and subsequently on the treatment machine using portal radiographs or electronic portal-imaging devices (EPIDs). These techniques are useful for minimizing systematic set-up errors in beam positioning. Images taken during treatment are usually compared with simulator images, and beam registration is performed relative to bony structures. The quality of digitally reconstructed radiographs (DRR) superimposed on a beam's eye view from treatment-planning systems is now of much improved quality. Perhaps this, rather than the simulator radiograph, should be used as the reference image. For some beam directions (such as a direct superior field to the head), it is not possible to acquire an image on the simulator or treatment machine. This means that a greater dependence is placed upon the geometrical accuracy of the treatment-planning system, as well as the treatment-machine movements. It is vitally important to establish that the isocentre is correctly located within the patient. As much information as possible from the planning CT study, regarding the position of the beams, the target and critical structures, must be made available for comparison with simulator or treatment machine images. It can be useful to transfer machine images back into the planning computer where tools may be available for comparison with BEV images. Alternatively, this can be done at an imaging workstation.

The interactive use of EPIDs has been successfully employed to minimize set-up errors on a treatment by treatment basis. This process can be automated, with computerized matching of the images and a specification of the translational or rotational movements required to relocate the isocentre correctly (Van de Steene *et al.* 1998). The accuracy of treatment set-up can be quantified, and intervention criteria established should the required accuracy not be achieved. The limitation of these verification procedures is that they are measured by the position of bony structures, and the target and other internal organs are usually not imaged. As stated in Section 1.2.2, the use of the fluoroscopy unit on a simulator can give valuable dynamic information on the extent of movement of lung tumours during the breathing cycle, or of oropharyngeal structures during swallowing. Radiographs may give misleading information by 'freezing' the position of the structures at one extreme of movement. Information on the movement of internal organs is available from repeat CT studies but these cannot be performed regularly on every patient.

3. Dynamic therapy

3.1 Arc therapy

The origins of arc or rotation therapy date back to the 1940s before megavoltage energies were available. At orthovoltage energies it was difficult to obtain a high target to non-target dose ratio for deep-seated lesions without using a large number of static beams. The logical development was to use one beam aimed at the target with the radiation source rotating around the patient about an axis passing through the centre of the target. This was equivalent to using the maximum number of beams for the treatment. Arc therapy was used widely both at orthovoltage and ^{60}Co, but almost disappeared with the availability of megavoltage energies where an acceptable target to non-target dose ratio could be achieved with a relatively small number of static beams. However, arc therapy has recently undergone something of a revival in that it has been used in dynamic conformal therapy (Wang and Redpath 1994), where the beam portal is dynamically shaped to the target using asymmetric or multi-leaf collimation during the arc. Electron arc therapy has been used to treat superficial target areas in curved surfaces, such as the chest wall (Chapter 10, Section 7).

A variety of methods for calculating the dose distributions resulting from arc therapy have been developed, but it is now accepted that computer calculation is required. A treatment arc can be simulated adequately by a number of equally spaced static beams. The smaller the angle between the beams, the more accurate is the calculation, but a beam separation of $5°–10°$ is sufficiently small to give an accurate simulation of the dose distribution. Care must be taken in the calculation to ensure that the changes in depth dose and beam weighting, resulting from the variable SSD for each of the simulating beams, are taken into account. The first and last of the beams simulating the arc should be given half-weight.

Even at megavoltage energies, the dose distributions resulting from arc therapy have some merits compared to those from static beam therapy. For example, high-dose regions are more regular, approximating to cylindrical or ellipsoidal in shape, and the fall-off in dose outside the high-dose region is more rapid. Incident doses are lower, and the relatively high-dose volumes under the beam portals are averaged out over the whole of the irradiated volume. However, as stated, at megavoltage energies an acceptable target to non-target dose ratio can be obtained with three or four fields even in the pelvis, making the treatment planning, treatment set-up, and verification considerably simpler than for arc therapy. For these reasons static field therapy is preferred.

3.2 Dynamic wedge

A dynamic wedge differs from a physical wedge in that no external beam modifier is used to create the wedged dose distribution. Instead, the process of dynamic intensity modulation is used, where the wedge effect is produced by the motion of one of the asymmetric diaphragms from the open to the closed position while the beam is on (Leavitt *et al.* 1990; Elder *et al.* 1995). The total dose to any point is determined by the integration of the dose deposited during the motion of the diaphragm, and as different parts of the beam are irradiated for different times, a wedge effect is produced. The relations between collimator position and beam machine units delivered is defined by a segmented treatment table (STT), and this is accurately followed under computer control to create a wedged field of desired wedge angle. All dynamic wedge treatments give some fraction of the total dose before the diaphragm starts to move, the smaller the wedge angle required the larger is this fraction. The fraction also varies with field size and beam energy. During the dynamic part of the treatment, the number of machine units delivered varies with diaphragm position, and depends on the wedge angle and beam energy. This is achieved by varying the dose rate or the diaphragm drive speed under computer control.

The STT for a 20-cm wide symmetric wedged field is shown graphically in Figure 9.12. The example produces a 60°-wedged beam, where the total number of machine units given is 100. The STT specifies machine units and diaphragm position at 21 discrete points (the example is taken from a 6 MV Varian 600C linear accelerator), and the computer control system ensures that there is a linear progression from one STT value to the next. Dose rate and diaphragm speed between each segment is constant and the slope of the segment defines their values. Either one of these is maintained at its maximum value thus ensuring that the treatment is executed in the shortest possible time. It should be noted that the moving diaphragm stops 5 mm away from the stationary diaphragm.

It is only necessary to store the STT for the maximum field size and wedge angle for each photon beam energy. The STT for any required wedge angle θ can be calculated from the STT table for the maximum angle θ_{max} from the following equation:

$$STT(\theta) = (1 - \alpha) + \alpha STT(\theta_{max}) \quad (4)$$

where $\alpha = \tan(\theta)/\tan(\theta_{max})$.

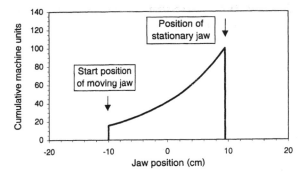

Figure 9.12 Graphical representation of a segmental treatment table for a dynamic wedge.

This equation is applied to each point defining the STT. The STT table for the required field width (symmetric or asymmetric) is obtained simply by truncation of that derived for the maximum field width. The values in the STT are then normalized, so that the final value in the table is the total number of machine units required for the beam. The control computer then calculates the dose rate and diaphragm speed required for each segment of the dynamic wedge treatment.

By appropriate design of the STT it is obviously possibly to choose the shape of the wedge isodoses produced. In general, the STT is designed to give the chosen wedge angle over as large a fraction of the beam width as possible, and this is particularly noticeable at large field sizes. Beam profiles orthogonal to the wedge direction are not subjected to the beam hardening effect resulting from the use of manual wedges, and this means that profiles for unwedged fields can be used for off–axis dose calculations. Using the same argument, it would be expected that central axis depth doses for dynamic wedges would be very similar to those for unwedged fields. In practice there is a small increase in depth dose with increasing wedge angle of approximately 2–3% of the local dose at a large depth in a large field size. If a dynamic wedged beam is considered to be the summation of a number of asymmetric beams, then the consideration in the change in scatter dose can explain this increase.

Wedge factors for dynamic wedges decrease both with increasing wedge angle and field width (Beavis *et al.* 1996) as shown by the example in Figure 9.13. Wedge factors are defined in the same way as for manual wedges. The decrease with increasing wedge angle is relatively small at small field widths, but at large fields widths can reach approximately a factor of two. The decrease in wedge factor with increasing field size is much larger for dynamic wedges than for manual wedges, and again can be as much as a factor of two for large wedge angles. However, the variation with field size is generally very smooth and continuous although

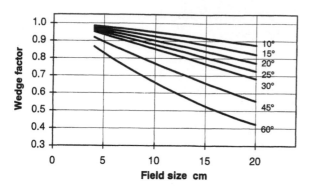

Figure 9.13 Wedge factors for a dynamic wedge.

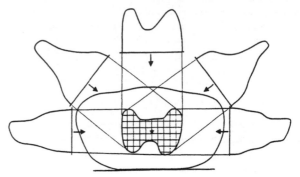

Figure 9.14 An example of a treatment situation where intensity modulation is beneficial.

this may not be the case for some earlier designs. It is relatively simple to calculate wedge factors for a dynamic wedge if they are defined at the reference point where scatter dose is a small proportion of the total dose. They can be calculated from the STT for the beam as follows:

$$\text{wedge factor} = (MU_B + P \times MU_A)/(MU_B + MU_A) \quad (5)$$

where MU_B is the number of monitor units given before the diaphragm crosses the reference point, MU_A is the number of monitor units given after the diaphragm crosses the reference point, and P is the fractional primary transmission through the diaphragms.

The majority of modern linear accelerators are equipped with a dynamic wedge facility.

3.3 Beam-intensity modulation

A new approach to radiotherapy has been developed recently, which although not widely used clinically at present, may revolutionize treatment in the near future. It is based on the principle of allowing the beam intensity to vary over the beam portal (Webb 1992; Stein *et al.* 1994). This is not new in that it is seen in the use of compensators to correct for patient shape and heterogeneities. What is different is that the dose distribution can be shaped so that high-dose volumes are produced conforming to planning target volumes that are concave in shape. This can be important in sparing critical organs that lie close to the target volume.

Conventional treatment planning is considered as a 'forward problem', where the dose distribution resulting from a particular beam configuration is calculated and assessed. The beam parameters are varied, often by a trial and error process, until an acceptable dose distribution is obtained. Mathematical optimization techniques can be used to assist the process. However, it can be argued that treatment planning is an 'inverse problem', where the required dose distribution is specified by the clinician. The planning process then consists of determining the

beam configuration, and the shape and intensity distribution for each individual beam. The methods used to determine the beam intensity profiles are well established. Each beam is considered to consist of a two-dimensional array of pencil beams, where each pencil beam can have an intensity independent of the others. A simple solution is to set the intensity to the thickness of the target volume along a ray specifying the direction of the pencil beam. An example of the problem to be solved is shown in Figure 9.14 for a two-dimensional situation, with the beam intensity profiles shown in one dimension.

The problem of determining the intensity profiles necessary to produce the required dose distribution is analogous to the reconstruction of CT images from their projections. In practice it is the inverse problem, where the projections correspond to the intensity modulated beam profiles, and the electron density distribution to the dose distribution. The two main algorithms used for CT reconstruction, namely filtered backprojection and iterative reconstruction, have been studied by Bortfeld *et al.* (1990). The main problem in these approaches is the physical restriction that the intensity of the pencil beams are not allowed to be negative. For practical reasons it is desirable to keep the number of beams as small as possible, and it has been found that of the order of five to nine beams are required to give satisfactory results depending on the complexity of the problem. An odd number of beams are used because opposing fields do not improve the dose distribution. Other methods that have been used are that of simulated annealing by Webb (1989), and a convolution technique using inverse back projection by Brahme (1988).

A number of different methods have been proposed for the delivery of the required beam intensity profiles in a treatment situation. The simplest of these is to manufacture individual compensators for every beam, but the practical consequences of this approach makes it unsuitable for routine treatment. An alternative approach is to use a dedicated scanned beam linear accelerator, where the electron, and consequently the photon beam, is steered under computer control. Intensity modulation can be achieved by varying the scanning speed over the beam portal. Linear accelerators using scanned electron-beam techniques are not common, which reflects the limited development of this approach. A more widely accepted solution is to use dynamic multi-leaf collimation. In this, each pair of leaves can be considered independently, as the one-dimensional intensity modulation they produce is directly transferable to two dimensions. It is evident that both leaves must be able to move independently across the field. If motion is restricted to one leaf, then the intensity distribution will increase across the beam towards the static jaw as in the dynamic wedge. If the leaves close or open from a point then the intensity profiles will have a maximum at that point. Both leaves must be able to traverse across the field with independent motion so that a variable width slit can be moved across the field. Convery and Rosenbloom (1992) have developed an algorithm that optimizes the motion of the leaves such that the desired profile is produced with the minimum irradiation time. Their technique provides a practical solution to the delivery of intensity modulated beams for conformal therapy.

An alternative approach has been proposed by Boyer *et al.* (1994) who used a beam segmentation technique described as a discrete step beam modulation procedure. An aperture is set at one edge of the field width required for each pair of leaves, and a small dose is given. The beam is switched off, and the leaves are then driven to form a second aperture and irradiated again to a small dose. The process is continued for 10–30 steps, and these dose segments are accumulated as the variable aperture progresses across the field. This will produce the required dose profile, but such 'step and shoot' techniques are not efficient in terms of beam irradiation time.

3.4 Automated treatment

Beam intensity modulation controlled by a segmented treatment table (STT) was introduced in the concept of the dynamic wedge. The STT defines the relationship at discrete points between machine units delivered and the position of an asymmetric diaphragm. Linear interpolation is used to execute the movement from one point in the STT to the next. A logical extension of this concept is to include more of the machine parameters that can be varied in the STT, for example, the position of all diaphragms, gantry, and collimator angles, as well as the number of machine units delivered. This will allow the automatic execution of a multiple beam coplanar treatment by setting up a single STT. Movement from one static beam to another is achieved by altering the gantry angle without incrementing the machine units delivered; arc therapy is achieved by incrementing the

machine units. Dynamic wedge beams can be incorporated as part of the STT. Automatic treatments of this type are possible at present. Non-coplanar treatments are possible by including couch rotation in the STT, and conformal therapy by including the setting up of a multi-leaf collimator. Beam intensity modulation using dynamic multi-leaf with arc therapy is the ultimate goal for this technique.

4. Stereotactic radiotherapy

Stereotactic radiotherapy has become an increasingly popular technique for the treatment of small lesions, most commonly located in the brain. The technique is based on the precise localization of a target within an independent three-dimensional co-ordinate system defined by a stereotactic frame fixed uniquely to the patient's head.

The technique was originally devised for functional neurosurgery but was adapted by Leksell (1951) into a precision radiotherapy technique for the treatment of small inoperable brain lesions. An invasive frame was attached to the skull and the lesion irradiated using a specially devised treatment unit known as the Gamma Knife (Leksell 1971). A modern gamma knife unit contains 201 small ^{60}Co sources distributed evenly over a hemispherical treatment head. The beam from each source is finely collimated and the beams converge at an isocentre. The stereotactic frame attached to the patient's head, is itself attached to a helmet which provides secondary collimation for every source, and any source can be blocked according to the requirements of the treatment plan.

Treatment to a dose in the region of 20 Gy is normally administered in one fraction and takes approximately 10 minutes. Such a dose, if delivered in a conventional fractionated schedule, would be well within the tolerance limit of normal tissue due to tissue repair processes. When this dose is delivered in a single fraction, tissues in the high-dose region become necrosed. Because of this, the technique relies on very high accuracy of beam positioning to minimize the irradiation of normal tissues. The technique has a role in the treatment of arteriovenous malformations (AVMs), which are benign lesions usually treated with surgery or embolization. Where these techniques are not feasible, stereotactic radiotherapy may be appropriate. Because of this surgical-like operation, Leksell defined the term 'radiosurgery' to mean the stereotactic localization and treatment of small lesions in a single fraction.

The gamma knife has the advantage of a very steep fall off in dose outside the treatment volume and a high degree of accuracy in positioning. The disadvantages are its high cost and that it is limited to treating a maximum lesion diameter of around 20 mm in a single fraction. As a result, stereotactic techniques for linear accelerators have been developed (Heifetz *et al.* 1984) based on the use of small, well-collimated beams of circular cross-section. To achieve this, tertiary collimators are attached to the head of the linear accelerator, providing beams of up to 40-mm diameter with a narrow penumbra. Additional quality assurance procedures on linear accelerators are required to ensure the necessary degree of precision for this application. A stereotactic frame is used to attach the patient's head either to the couch or to a floor stand separate from the couch. One advantage of linear accelerator-based stereotaxy is the possibility of fractionation using non-invasive relocatable frames, such as that developed by Gill and Thomas (Gill *et al.* 1991). Attachment of the Gill–Thomas frame to the patient utilizes an impression of the upper dentition and a mould of the occiput. Relocatability has been measured to be within 1 mm by matching to bony anatomy using orthogonal radiographs (Graham *et al.* 1991).

Treatment is delivered using three to six non-coplanar arcs. Thomson *et al.* (1990) developed a planning technique based on angiography films and an approximation to the size and shape of the skull. He suggested that the term 'stereotactic multiple arc radiotherapy' (SMART) should be used as an alternative to radiosurgery. Modern three-dimensional planning systems utilizing advanced graphics help in the selection of treatment arcs that do not pass through critical structures. These planning systems reconstruct the head and internal anatomy from CT data. Angiography is used to delineate the target in the treatment of AVMs, although this process has problems (Bova and Freedman 1991). In the treatment of small malignancies, it is normal to outline the CTV using CT scans. Although MRI can aid localization, the effects of any image distortion must be determined. The optimal method of delineating the target and sensitive structures is to use image fusion (Van Herk and Kooy 1994), either within the planning system or imported from an imaging workstation.

Planning systems usually require the measurement of central axis depth doses or TMRs, off–axis ratios and outputs for every available collimator. Measurement of these data is particularly difficult, firstly because of the lack of electronic equilibrium in small field sizes, and secondly because the size of the detector may be comparable with the size of the field. Diamond detectors have been shown to be suitable because of their small spatial resolution and near tissue-equivalence (Rustgi 1995), but problems in the manufacturing process has made these difficult to acquire and prohibitively expensive. Alternatively, it has been recommended that a variety of small detectors such as ionization chambers, diodes or film should be used, and the relative merits of each assessed for any particular measurement situation

(Rice *et al.* 1987). Beam data have also been calculated using Monte Carlo simulations.

The use of static conformal fields, in conjunction with a stereotactic frame has also been investigated. Fields can be conformed by the use of individualized conformal blocks or a micro MLC. In terms of the volume of normal brain irradiated and conformity to the target, static conformal blocks perform better for irregular target shapes when compared with multiple non-coplanar arcs. More complex methods of treatment delivery also exist. Dynamic stereotactic radiotherapy involves the simultaneous movement of both the gantry and the couch (Podgorsak *et al.* 1988). Dynamic field shaping involves the movement of the leaves of an MLC within the stereotactic collimator during gantry rotation. The Peacock system (Carol *et al.* 1992) utilizes dynamic field shaping with intensity modulation for the administration of a stereotactic treatment. Stereotaxy has also been applied to non-cranial lesions (such as solitary liver metastases) using a stereotactic body cradle.

Acknowledgement

The authors would like to thank Ms. C. McKerracher for her contribution to the section on stereotactic radiotherapy.

5. References

Ahnesjö, A., Saxner, M., and Trepp, A. (1992). A pencil beam model for photon dose calculation. *Med. Phys.*, **19**, 263–73.

Armstrong, J.G., Zelefsky, M.J., Leibel, S.A., Burman, C.M., Han, C, Harrison, L.B. *et al.* (1995) Strategy for dose escalation using 3-dimensional conformal radiation therapy for lung cancer. *Annals Oncol.*, **6**, 693–7.

Beavis, A.W., Weston, S.J., and Whitton, V.J. (1996). Implementation of the Varian EDW into a commercial RTP system. *Phys. Med. Biol.*, **41**, 1691–1704.

Bortfeld, Th., Bürkelbach J., Boesecke, R., and Schlegel W. (1990). Methods of image reconstruction from projections applied to conformation radiotherapy. *Phys. Med. Biol.*, **35**, 1423–34.

Bova, F.J. and Freedman, W.A. (1991). Stereotactic angiography: an inadequate database for radiosurgery? *Int. J. Rad. Oncol. Biol. Phys.*, **20**, 891–5.

Boyer, A.L. and Mok, E.C. (1986). Calculations of photon dose distributions in an inhomogeneous medium using convolutions. *Med. Phys.*, **13**, 503–9.

Boyer, A.L., Bortfeld, T.R., Kahler, D.L., and Waldron, T.J. (1994). MLC modulation of X-ray beams in discrete steps. In *Proceedings 11th international conference on the use of computers in radiation therapy* (ed. A.R. Hounsell, J.M. Wilkinson, and P.C. Williams), pp. 178–9. Christie Hospital NHS Trust, Manchester.

Brahme, A. (1988). Optimization of stationary and moving beam radiation therapy techniques. *Radiother. Oncol.*, **12**, 129–40.

Carol, M.P., Tergovnik, H., Smith, D., and Cahill, D. (1992). 3-D planning and delivery system for optimized conformal therapy. *Int. J. Rad. Oncol. Biol. Phys.*, **24**, Supplement 1, 158.

Clarkson, J.R. (1941). A note on depth dose in fields of irregular shape. *Br. J. Radiol.*, **14**, 265–8.

Convery, D.J. and Rosenbloom, M.E. (1992). The generation of intensity-modulated fields for conformal radiotherapy by dynamic collimation. *Phys. Med. Biol.*, **37**, 1359–74.

Cook, L.T., Cook, P.N., Lee, K.R., Batnitzky, S., Wong, B.Y.S., Fritz, S.L. *et al.* (1980) An algorithm for volume estimation based on polyhedral approximation *IEEE Trans. on Biomed, Eng.* **27**, 9, 493.

Cunningham, J.R. (1972). Scatter-air ratios. *Phys. Med. Biol.*, **17**, 42–51.

Dobbs, H.J., Parker, R.P., Hodson, N.J., Hobday, P., and Husband, J.E. (1983). The use of CT in radiotherapy treatment planning. *Radiother. Oncol.*, **1**, 133–41.

Drzymala, R.E., Mohan, R., Brewster, M.S., Chu, J., Giotein, M., Harms, W. *et al.* (1991). Dose–volume histograms. *Int. J. Rad. Oncol. Biol. Phys.*, **21**, 71–8.

Elder, P.J., Coveney, F.M., and Walsh, A.D. (1995). An investigation into the comparison between different dosimetric methods of measuring profiles and depth doses for dynamic wedges on a Varian 600C linear accelerator. *Phys. Med. Biol.*, **40**, 683–9.

Gill, S.S., Thomas, D.G.T., Warrington, A.P., and Brada, M. (1991). Relocatable frame for stereotactic external beam therapy. *Int. J. Rad. Oncol. Biol. Phys.*, **20**, 599–603.

Graham, J.D., Warrington, A.P., Gill, S.S., and Brada, M. (1991). A non-invasive, relocatable stereotactic frame for fractionated radiotherapy and multiple imaging. *Radiother. Oncol.*, **21**, 60–2.

Hanna, C.L., Slade, S., Mason, M.D., and Burnet, N.G. (1999). Accuracy of patient positioning during radiotherapy for bladder and brain tumours. *Clin. Oncol.*, **11**, 93–8.

Heifetz, M.D., Wexler, M., and Thompson, R. (1984). Single-beam radiotherapy knife. *J. Neurosurg.*, **60**, 814–8.

International Commission on Radiation Units and Measurements (1993). *Prescribing, recording and reporting photon beam therapy. Report 50.* ICRU, Bethesda.

Kotre, C.J., Harrison, R.M., and Ross, W.M. (1984). A simulator-based CT system for radiotherapy treatment planning. *Br. J. Radiol.*, **57**, 631–5.

Larson, K.B. and Prasad, S.C. (1978). Absorbed dose computation for inhomogeneous media in radiation treatment planning using differential scatter-air ratios In *Proceeding 2nd annual symposium on computer applications in medical care*, p. 93. IEEE, Piscataway, NJ.

Leavitt, D.D., Martin, M., Moeler, J.H., and Lee, W.L. (1990). Dynamic wedge field techniques through computer-controlled collimator motion and dose delivery. *Med. Phys.*, **17**, 87–91.

Leibel, S.A., Ling, C.C., Kutcher, G.J., Mohan, R., Cordon-Cordo, C., and Fuks, Z. (1991). The biological basis for conformal three-dimensional radiation therapy. *Int. J. Rad. Oncol. Biol. Phys.*, **21**, 805–11.

Leksell, L. (1951). The stereotaxis method and radiosurgery of the brain. *Acta. Chir. Scand.* **102**, 316–9.

Leksell, L. (1971). *Stereotaxis and radiosurgery: an operative system.* Charles C Thomas, Springfield.

Lyman, J.T. and Wolbarst, A.B. (1987). Optimization of radiation therapy, III: a method of assessing complication probabilities from dose-volume histograms. *Int. J. Rad. Oncol. Biol. Phys.*, **13**, 103–9.

Mackie, T.R., Ahnesjö, A., Dickof, P., and Snider, A. (1987). Development of a convolution/superimposition method for

photon beams. In *Proceeding 9th international conference on the use of computers in radiation therapy* (ed. I.A.D. Bruinvis, P.H. van der Giessen, H.J. van Kleffens, and F.W. Wittkämper), pp. 107–10. Elsevier Science, Amsterdam.

Mageras, G.S., Fuks, Z., Liebel, S.A., Ling, C.C., Zelefsky, M.J., Kooy, H.M *et al.* (1999). Computerized design of target margins for treatment uncertainties in conformal radiotherapy. *Int. J. Rad. Oncol. Biol. Phys.*, **43**, 437–45.

McNee, S.G., Rampling, R., Dale, A.J., and Gregor, A. (1998). An audit of 3D treatment planning facilities and practice in the UK. *Clin. Oncol.*, **10**, 18–23.

Mubata, C.D., Bidmead, A.M., Ellingham, L.M., Thompson, V., and Dearnaley, D.P. (1998). Portal imaging protocol for radical dose-escalated radiotherapy treatment of prostate cancer. *Int. J. Rad. Oncol. Biol. Phys.*, **40**, 221–31.

Nelson, W.R., Hirayama, H., and Rogers, D.W.O. (1985). *The EGS4 code system. Slac Report 265.* National Technical Information Service, Springfield, VA.

O'Connor, J.E. (1957). The variation of scattered X-rays with density in an irradiated body. *Phys. Med. Biol.*, **2**, 352–69.

Parker, R.P., Hobday, P.A., and Cassell, K.J. (1979). The direct use of CT numbers in radiotherapy dosage calculations for inhomogeneous media. *Phys. Med. Biol.*, **24**, 802–9.

Podgorsak, E.B., Olivier, A., Pla, M., Lefebvre, P.-Y., and Hazel, J. (1988). Dynamic stereotactic surgery. *Int. J. Rad. Oncol. Biol. Phys.*, **14**, 115–26.

Read, G. (1988). Conformal radiotherapy: a clinical review. *Clin. Oncol.*, **10**, 288–96.

Redpath, A.T. (1995). A beam model for three-dimensional radiotherapy planning. *Br. J. Radiol.*, **68**, 1356–63.

Redpath, A.T. and Thwaites, D.I. (1991). A 3-dimensional scatter correction algorithm for photon beams. *Phys. Med. Biol.*, **36**, 779–98.

Redpath, A.T. and Wright, D.H. (1985). The use of an image processing system in radiotherapy simulation. *Br. J. Radiol.*, **58**, 1081–9.

Rice, R.K., Hansen, J.L., Svensson, G.K., and Siddon, R.L. (1987). Measurements of dose distributions in small beams of 6 MV X-rays. *Phys. Med. Biol.*, **32**, 1087–99.

Rustgi, S.N. (1995). Evaluation of the dosimetric characteristics of a diamond detector for photon beam measurements. *Med. Phys.*, **22**, 567–70.

Siddon, R.L. (1985). Fast calculation of the exact radiological path for a three-dimensional CT array. *Med. Phys.*, **12**, 252–5.

Sontag, M.R. and Cunningham, J.R. (1977). Corrections to absorbed dose calculations for tissue inhomogeneities. *Med. Phys.*, **4**, 431–6.

Sontag, M.R. and Cunningham, J.R., (1978). The equivalent tissue-air ratio method for making absorbed dose calculations in a heterogeneous medium, *Radiology.* **129**, 787–94.

Stein, J., Bortfeld, T., Dörschel, B., and Schlegel, W. (1994). X-ray intensity modulation by dynamic multi-leaf collimation. In *Proceedings 11th international conference on the use of computers in radiation therapy* (ed. A.R. Hounsell, J.M. Wilkinson, and P.C. Williams), pp. 174-5. Christie Hospital NHS Trust, Manchester.

Stroom, J.C. and Storchi, P.R.M. (1997). Automatic calculation of three-dimensional margins around treatment volumes in radiotherapy planning. *Phys. Med. Biol.*, **42**, 745–55.

Stroom, J.C., Korevaar, G.A., Koper, P.C.M., Visser, A.G., and Heijmen, B.J.M. (1998). Multiple two-dimensional versus three-dimensional PTV definition in treatment planning for conformal radiotherapy. *Radiother. Oncol.*, **47**, 297–302.

Ten Haken, R.K., Forman, J.D., Heimburger, D.K., Gerhardsson, A., McShan, D.L., Perez-Tomayo, C. *et al.* (1991). Treatment planning issues related to prostate movement in response to differential filling of the rectum and bladder. *Int. J. Rad. Oncol. Biol. Phys.*, **20**, 1317–24.

Thomas, S.J. (1991). A modified power-law formula for inhomogeneity corrections in beams of high-energy X-rays. *Med. Phys.*, **18**, 719–23.

Thomson, E.S., Gill, S.S., and Doughty, D. (1990). Stereotactic multiple arc radiotherapy. *Br. J. Radiol.*, **63**, 745–51.

Van de Steene, J., Van den Heuvel, F., Bel, A., Verallen, D., De Mey, J., Noppen, M. *et al.* (1998). Electronic protal imaging with on-line correction of set-up error in thoracic irradiation: clinical evaluation. *Int. J. Rad. Oncol. Biol. Phys.*, **40**, 967–76.

Van Herk, M. and Kooy, H.M. (1994). Automatic three-dimensional correlation of CT–CT, CT–MRI, and CT–SPECT using chamfer matching. *Med. Phys.*, **21**, 1163–78.

Van Herk, M., Bruce, A., Kroes, A.P.G., Shuman, T., Touw, A., and Lebesque, J.V. (1995). Quantification of organ motion during conformal radiotherapy of the prostate. *Int. J. Rad. Oncol. Biol. Phys.*, **33**, 1311–20.

Wang, Q. and Redpath, A.T. (1994). Computer Controlled Dynamic Conformal Therapy. In *Proceeding 11th international conference on the use of computers in radiation therapy* (ed. A.R. Hounsell, J.M. Wilkinson, P.C. Williams), pp. 212–5, Christie Hospital NHS Trust, Manchester.

Webb, S. (1989). Optimization of conformal radiotherapy dose distributions by simulated annealing. *Phys. Med. Biol.*, **34**, 1349–70.

Webb, S. (1992). Optimization by simulated annealing of three-dimensional, conformal treatment planning for radiation fields defined by a multileaf collimator: II. Inclusion of two-dimensional modulation of the X-ray intensity. *Phys. Med. Biol.*, **37**, 1689–1704.

Webb, S. and Nahum, A.E. (1993). A model for calculating tumour control probabilities in radiotherapy including the effects of inhomogeneous distributions of dose and clonogenic cell density. *Phys. Med. Biol.*, **38**, 653–66.

Woo, M.K., Cunningham, J.R., and Jezioranski, J.J. (1990). Extending the concept of primary and scatter separation to the condition of electronic disequilibrium. *Med. Phys.*, **17**, 588–95.

Zhu, X-R., Klein, E.E., and Low, D.A. (1998). Geometric and dosimetric analysis of multileaf collimation conformity. *Radiother. Oncol.*, **47**, 63–8.

Chapter 10

Electron beam treatment-planning techniques

D.I. Thwaites

1. Introduction

The attractive feature of electron beams for a variety of clinical applications is the shape of the depth–dose curve, characterized by a relatively steep fall-off and a finite range. This enables reasonably uniform doses to be delivered to a well-defined region extending from the surface, whilst at the same time sparing underlying tissue. Above about 20 MeV the fall-off of the curve becomes progressively less steep with energy, and the separation of the high-dose and spared regions becomes increasingly blurred. Energies higher than this can be used for deeper-seated tumours in a manner similar to megavoltage photons. However, the majority of linear accelerators that provide clinical electron beams provide energies within the range 4–20 MeV and this chapter is mainly concerned with their use. Discussion is limited to the parameters affecting either the dose distribution or the link between monitor units (mu) and dose. Calculation methods are considered, where appropriate, but no detailed discussion is given of more complex algorithms. Simple manual methods are outlined as these illustrate the physical principles involved in planning electron treatments and can be used to give simple checks of more sophisticated algorithms.

Electron beams of 4–20 MeV deliver high doses (greater than about 90% depth dose) to depths from 1 to 6 cm. Common applications include skin and lip cancers, chest wall, and peripheral lymphatic areas in breast cancer, additional boost doses to limited volumes, such as scar areas and nodes, certain head and neck cancers, and other sites lying at these depths below the surface. The most widely used beams are generally those of medium energy. Most electron treatments are given as normally incident single fields at fixed SSD. At lower energies full dose distributions are often not calculated. However, they may be required more frequently at medium and higher energies and in situations involving inhomogeneities, surface obliquity, or where beam edges are positioned close to critical structures or to other

irradiated areas. Generally, the major problem in planning such treatments is to account for electron scatter.

It may be emphasized that many of the parameters of interest for electron beams depend much more strongly on the design of the accelerator head than is the case for megavoltage photons. These variations can occur between machines of the same manufacturer and between individual collimators on the same machine. Thus, planning calculations must be based on extensive measurements in all beams on each machine. For many non-routine treatments, special measurements may be required in order to verify calculations (Chapter 4, Section 5).

2. Beam characteristics

The beam characteristics necessary to select beam energy and size are briefly outlined here. Further details are given in Chapters 2–4, ICRU (1984), and AAPM (1991).

2.1 Depth dose

Figure 10.1 shows central axis depth–dose curves for electron beams from 5 to 20 MeV, measured for a moderately large field size. The therapeutic range is generally taken to be the depth of the 90 or 85% dose, depending on local practice, and can be roughly estimated in centimetres of water or soft tissue as one-third of the beam energy in MeV. The mean energy at depth in water or soft tissue falls by approximately 2 MeV cm^{-1}, giving a practical range in centimetres of approximately half the beam energy in MeV. The 50% depth is approximately midway between these two. Beyond the practical range, a small dose is contributed by the bremsstrahlung component, arising mainly from interactions in the machine head. This is typically between 1 and 5%, becoming larger as beam energy increases. The penetration, represented by practical

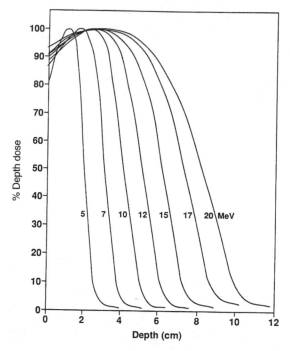

Figure 10.1 Central axis depth–dose curves for various electron beam energies.

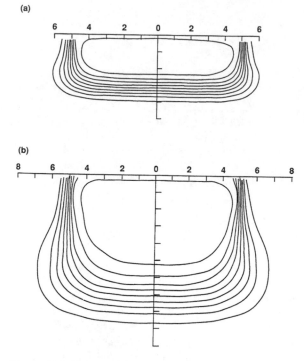

Figure 10.2 Typical electron isodose distributions in water for (a) a 7.5 MeV and (b) a 17 MeV beam.

range, increases with energy, whilst the falling parts of the curves become less steep at higher energies.

Surface dose, conventionally stated at 0.5 mm depth, is usually in the range of 75–80% for lower energy beams, and up to around 95% for higher energy beams. Thus, skin sparing is small. The build-up of dose from the surface to dose maximum is caused by the increasing obliquity of the electron paths due to scatter. This increases the electron fluence with depth and also the mean path length traversed per unit depth into the material and, therefore, it increases the energy deposited per unit depth. The fall-off of dose beyond the depth of dose maximum is due to the removal of electrons from the beam following full absorption, remembering that the significant scatter effects cause the electrons to follow tortuous paths, with a low probability of travelling through without scatter. The position of dose maximum varies with energy, but not necessarily in a straightforward monotonic way, and with field size and can depend strongly on machine design.

Differences in depth doses can be evident between machines using scattering foils to produce the clinical field and those using scanning beam techniques, the latter generally having 'cleaner' beams with steeper fall-off and, therefore, a rather greater therapeutic range for a given energy.

2.2 Isodoses

Figure 10.2 shows isodoses (90–10%) for a 10 × 10 cm² field for two electron beams, of 7.5 and 17 MeV, illustrating the characteristic flat closely-spaced isodose lines in the central region of the field. Close to the surface, the 50% isodose line approximately follows the geometric beam edge. Lower value isodose lines bulge significantly outward due to scattered electrons. Therefore, significant doses can be delivered to significant distances outside the beam edge. Correspondingly, the higher value isodose lines are pulled in at depth. This has the consequence that the high-dose volume is reduced in width as depth increases and can be considerably narrower at the depth of therapeutic range than at the surface. For the isodoses shown this is approximately 2E mm for the 90% isodose on each side of the field, where E is in MeV, and this is a reasonable general guide to the estimation of the high-dose region (90%) pull-in. However, the exact value will vary with beam energy, machine design and field size. In addition it will be greater on the diagonal of a square or rectangular field.

2.3 Field-size variations

At moderate and large field sizes, central axis depth doses do not vary very much, with the possible exception of the region from the surface to the position of dose maximum. However, the depth–dose curves become less steep as the field dimensions are reduced below the value necessary to give side-scatter equilibrium at the central axis. More electrons are scattered away from the central axis, reducing the fluence and therefore the energy deposition, than are scattered in. The dose maximum and other relatively high depth–dose values are pulled closer to the surface and the surface dose increases. However, the practical range is hardly changed, as this represents those electrons that travel through virtually unscattered. This is illustrated in Figure 10.3a for a 10 MeV beam (see also Chapter 4, Figure 4.7 for a 20–MeV beam). In addition, as field size decreases the isodose distribution narrows, until the two penumbral regions merge and the high-dose volume is then increasingly constricted in width at depth as fields get even smaller. This is in accord with the reduced penetration (Figure 10.3b). This loss of side-scatter equilibrium occurs for field dimensions that are less than some critical value, which depends on beam energy but is also affected by machine design. Frequently this dimension is approximately the same as the practical range of the electron beam.

These effects must be clearly appreciated when prescribing and planning small-field electron treatments. This includes small applicators, small shaped fields and larger fields, where one dimension, or part of the irradiated area, is less than this critical value. A suitably wide range of planning data must be available to enable correct calculations. Alternatively, specific measurements must be made in order to plan the individual treatment. For rectangular fields of sides $a \times b$, the depth dose (%DD) at a given depth can often be estimated from related square field information, using:

$$\%DD(a, b) = [\%DD(a, a) \cdot \%DD(b, b)]^{1/2},$$

provided the variation in collimator scatter is small.

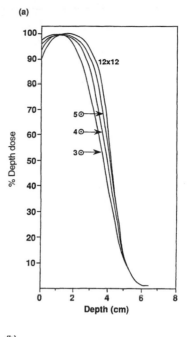

(a)

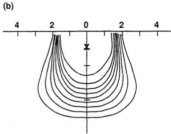

(b)

Figure 10.3 Effect of small beam area on 10 MeV electron dose distributions: (a) variation of the central axis depth–dose curves with beam size; (b) isodose distribution for a 3.5 cm circular applicator.

3. Choice of energy and beam size

Beam energy is generally chosen so that the 90% (or 85%) isodose line encompasses the target volume at depth. For chest-wall irradiation, a lower value, e.g. 70–80%, may be chosen to lie at the lung surface in order to reduce penetration into lung and hence overall lung dose, noting that the penetration into lung will be approximately inversely proportional to electron density. If any critical structure, e.g. spinal cord, lies beneath the target volume, then careful consideration of the relative doses is required, both at the inner limit of the target and at this structure, to make an appropriate clinical choice of the optimum beam energy.

If superficial target volumes are involved, but a low-energy beam gives a surface dose that is too low, then a higher energy may be selected and used in conjunction with an appropriate energy degrader (decelerator) in contact with, or close to, the patient surface. By suitable choice of the combination of energy and degrader thickness, the 90% dose can be adjusted to the required depth and an acceptable surface dose can be obtained. The steepness of the dose fall-off will be reduced compared to using the lower energy beam, but this is generally not significant. Degraders used include wax or commercial flexible tissue-substitute materials moulded to the patient surface. Alternatively, rigid sheets of plastic (e.g. PMMA) may be used provided that air gaps are minimized. Appropriate equivalent thicknesses should be used, taking into account the differences in electron density from water as verified by measurement.

Field size should be chosen to ensure that the required planning-target volume is enclosed by an acceptable high-dose region. It is usual to aim for coverage by the

90% isodose, but in some cases the considerations outlined above dictate a lower value. Because of the constriction of the higher isodoses at depth, this generally entails using a larger surface field size than may have been selected for the same site using a photon beam. Frequently, a reasonable balance between coverage at depth and increased coverage at the surface is to add a 1-cm margin on all sides, but this must be based on an examination of the isodose curves for the machine and energy used, and must also take into account the clinical requirements. Particular care is required to ensure adequate coverage for any fields involving small dimensions. Attention must also be given to the dose outside the geometric beam edge, particularly where the beam is to be placed close to a critical structure. In this situation, some compromise on field size and positioning may be necessary.

4. Field shaping

Electron fields can be shaped simply using cut-outs of lead or low melting-point alloy attached to the end of the applicator (cone) or on the patient surface. As a guide, the required thickness of lead in mm is about half the surface energy of the beam in MeV. For low melting-point alloy, shield thicknesses should be increased from the lead value by a factor of 1.2. Generally these give adequate shielding with less than 5% transmission at low energies to about 10% at 20 MeV. The highest doses under the shielding are on the skin and experimental verification should, therefore, be carried out at the surface of a phantom using a thin-walled parallel-plate chamber. If the shielding used is too thin, the skin dose can be increased as compared to the open-field values. If a collection of standard cut-outs is prepared, it is advisable to make these in one thickness to match the highest energy available in order to prevent inadvertent use of a cut-out that is too thin. Alternatively two easily identifiable thicknesses may be used, one for lower energy beams only and one for any beam up to the maximum energy.

The sharpest field definition can be maintained by using shields in close proximity to the patient surface. However, some compromise may be necessary, depending on the treatment site, the shield weight and patient tolerance, the applicator design, and the standard air gap. Normal electron field edge effects occur at a shield edge and, therefore, field restriction and scatter under the shield should be considered, particularly if close to a critical structure and also where the shielded area may be subject to scattered electrons from more than one direction.

Small-field problems require consideration in the event that any dimension of a shaped field is small (see Section 2.3). Dose distributions and dose/mu may be significantly changed. Planning must be based on direct measurement if there are inadequate data available to predict effects. Film dosimetry is a convenient technique for this, but it requires very careful use and interpretation (ICRU 1984; see also Chapter 4, Section 5.2). It is advisable to obtain distributions for the standard open applicator and the shaped field on the same film, so that calibration problems and variations between films or due to processing can be minimized. In this way the two are developed in identical conditions and the open-field image serves as a calibration. In this situation care must be taken that scatter or leakage from one field does not affect the film at the position of the second field.

5. Output factors

In many cases, the only remaining planning procedures for electron treatments are the selection of the output factor and the calculation of the treatment machine setting for the prescribed dose. For standard open applicators this is straightforward. A set of applicator (cone) outputs or factors relative to a standard applicator size (usually 10×10 cm^2) must be measured for planning (see Chapter 4, Section 5.2). If the machine uses a fixed side-scattering cone mount or a fixed X-ray collimator setting, with a range of add-on field-defining applicators, the factors usually vary relatively smoothly with field size at a given energy. For machines that have differing pre-set X-ray collimator positions for each combination of applicator and energy, as set up at installation to optimize field profiles, the variation of dose/mu with field size may be less predictable and calculations must be based on more detailed measurements. For variable trimmer systems, the output varies relatively smoothly with field size so that a limited set of measurements may allow interpolation to intermediate settings.

The dose/mu at dose maximum on the central axis varies with collimator/head scatter and scatter from the applicator, as well as phantom scatter. If further field shaping is used, there may be additional scatter from the edge of the shield. The relative contributions of these components may vary with:

(1) beam energy;

(2) the depth of dose maximum (itself energy and field size dependent);

(3) the individual standard applicator involved;

(4) the X-ray collimator position;

(5) the overall size and shape of any modified field, including the distance of the shaping material from the central axis.

This represents a complex combination. Depth–dose data and output factors must be measured for a range of cut-outs on each applicator. Output factors for cut-outs must relate to the particular dose maximum of the field produced, noting that measurements at different depths (e.g. at different dose maximum positions for open field and for cut-out) require different stopping power ratios, etc., to convert to dose. The factors may be expressed relative to the output of the particular open applicator at its dose maximum, or to the standard applicator, depending on local practice. Measurements should be carried out under the conditions to be used clinically. Thus, if the applicator design and the position of field shaping material require changes in the nominal treatment distance, this is included in the factor. Because of the various components contributing to output when cut-outs are used, the relative output factors may not be smooth or monotonic in behaviour and prediction for unmeasured fields must be carried out with care and verified by measurement.

For shaped fields where the dimensions are greater than that required to provide side-scatter equilibrium, the output factors may be little changed from that of the open applicator, for example, when shaping corners or areas on beam edges that are small compared to the total beam area. For other shaped fields, one of a number of approaches can be used to estimate output factors (see Chapter 4, Section 5.2). In many cases equivalent area approaches have been shown to be accurate to within 2 or 3%. For rectangular fields similar accuracy can be achieved by using:

$$OF(a, b) = [OF(a, a) \cdot OF(b, b)]^{1/2}$$

where the output factors (OF) are relative to those for the open applicator and all the field sizes are produced on the same standard applicator. Output factors have also been determined by Clarkson scatter integration and by pencil beam approaches (Bruinvis and Mathol 1988). The limitations of any of these methods, and any corrections required for their application, must be determined experimentally before they are used in treatment planning.

Prescription depends on clinical requirements. Generally, it is to the position of dose maximum but other levels may be used. In some circumstances, low-energy scatter components may give a dose maximum quite close to the surface and this may influence the position of dose prescription. Note that electron prescription recording and reporting was specifically dealt with in ICRU Report 29 (1978). Whilst the recommendations for photon beams were updated in ICRU report 50 (1993), there have been no specific parallel recommendations for electron beams, although this is to be addressed in a supplement to ICRU Report 50.

It should be noted that experience derived from photon-beam therapy is often not directly applicable to electron beams. Thus, the particular requirements for the individual patient must be carefully discussed between clinician and planning staff, and planning should be based on a detailed consideration of the dosimetric information that is applicable for the specific treatment conditions. This is true even for the simpler situations that have been considered so far.

6. Non-standard treatment distances

For some treatments, non-standard (generally increased) distances are required because of surface irregularities in the area to be treated. In these cases the incident dose for a given machine setting is reduced by the increased distance. Because of electron scatter this reduction is more rapid than the inverse square law (ISL) predicts. Correction may be based on the use of an effective source position (see Chapter 4, Section 5.2 and AAPM 1991). However, this position varies with energy and field size and the ISL may only be applicable over a limited range of extended treatment distances. Alternatively, the ISL correction may be based on a nominal or virtual SSD, combined with air-gap correction factors based on measurements (see Chapter 4, Section 5.2 and AAPM 1991). For some lower energy beams, a power law distance correction with an exponent equal to 2.4 or 2.5 has been found to represent the data. Planning calculations require clear information on the approach to be used and on its limitations.

Non-standard treatment distances also alter the dose distribution. Generally, for changes in SSD of less than 10 cm, the depth–dose curve is not altered significantly in the region of the steeply falling part of the curve and the standard depth doses can be used, although the depth of therapeutic range should be checked. However, the air gap may alter the surface dose and the detail of dose build-up from surface to dose maximum. An example is given in Chapter 4 (Figure 4.10). In addition, the distribution across the beam can be altered significantly. In particular, increasing gaps produce wider penumbra due to electron scatter in air, such that increasing SSD does not generally produce wider high-dose regions. Instead these may remain approximately constant or may even be reduced in width. Beam flatness across the remaining flattened area may also be altered by increased SSD, particularly in those designs in which electron scatter off the collimator system is used to improve flatness. Sharp penumbra can be regained by using field shaping at the patient surface, but the maximum field size for acceptably uniform dose is still determined by the scatter behaviour. Therefore, unlike photon beams, extending SSD does not usually allow larger areas to be treated uniformly. Large areas need to be treated with combined fields (Section 10), with electron arc therapy (Section 11), or by using specialized techniques such as total skin electron irradiation (Section 12).

Typical machine and applicator designs have the applicator base either in contact with the patient surface or with a small standard air gap of up to 5 cm. Increased air gaps should be avoided where possible and even where unavoidable should not normally be more than 10 cm (see above). Where gaps are due to surface irregularities, the field direction should be chosen so as to equalize gaps at extreme points in the field, provided that this does not conflict with other clinical considerations. The effects on the beam-edge distribution and high-dose volume should always be considered.

7.   Oblique incidence

Stand-off due to surface irregularity is almost inevitably accompanied by oblique incidence. This also alters the distribution due to changes in the effective penetration of the electrons and due to scatter effects. For angles of less than about 30°, isodose lines tend to follow the surface contour. However, the penumbra region is widened at edges away from the collimator. At larger angles the depth dose increasingly changes, pulling the curve towards the surface in the region of the therapeutic range and giving increased relative doses near the surface and near R_p due to scatter (see Figure 10.4). Therefore, whilst dose is generally reduced due to the increased distances involved, hot-spots can be produced near the surface and penetration worsens due to the angled

surface. Khan *et al.* (1985) discuss the use of obliquity correction factors to provide a framework for dealing with these effects. Pencil-beam models provide the best accessible method for dealing with the scatter hot-spots.

A common example of this is in the treatment of the chest wall. Where other clinical requirements or adjacent treated areas allow, it is advisable to choose the beam angle so that the obliquity is equalized at opposite ends of the treated area. This ensures that the maximum obliquity at any part of the field is minimized. The reduced depth doses at the more oblique edges of the field should then be considered when choosing the appropriate energy to give sufficient depth of coverage at these positions. Typically this results in the surface dose at the extremes of the field being too low and the penetration in the centre of the field being too high, with a gradual variation between these situations across the field. Variable thickness bolus can be designed to improve this, preferably using the treatment-planning system. A thin layer can increase the surface dose at the edges, whilst a thicker central bolus gradually tapering out to the edges can modulate the penetration to match the required isodose to the inner aspect of the target volume. If the obliquity is sufficiently pronounced there may be small scatter hot-spots under the surface towards the edges of the target volume (Figure 10.5).

Sharp irregularities in surface shape can produce significant local hot- or cold-spots from scatter imbalance at the tissue/air boundaries. To minimize these problems, such edges can be made less steep using bolus. For

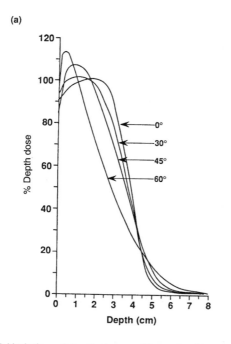

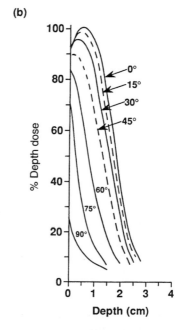

Figure 10.4 Variation of depth doses with angle of incidence: (a) measured along the central axis for 10 MeV electrons; (b) measured perpendicular to the surface for a nominal 4.5 MeV surface energy beam used for total skin treatment.

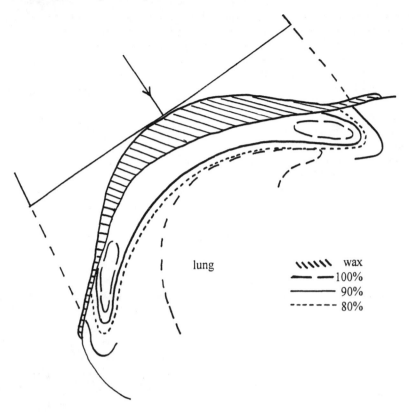

Figure 10.5 Example of variable thickness bolus used to improve a single-field electron dose distribution for chest-wall treatment. The 90% isodose from a 12-MeV beam is matched to the required target volume.

similar reasons, the edges of energy degraders, which would otherwise be parallel to the beam, should also be sloped or tapered if they are positioned to lie within the beam. This is one particular example of interface scatter effects, as discussed in the next section.

8. Inhomogeneities

Inhomogeneities in composition and in shape modify dose distributions in two ways, both of which need to be considered in treatment planning. The first is the effect on absorption and the consequent shift in isodose lines, and is most pronounced through and beyond large inhomogeneities. The second is due to scatter differences between different materials and is most pronounced for small inhomogeneities or near the edges of larger heterogeneities. The resultant distribution depends on the size, shape, and composition (atomic number and electron density) of the inhomogeneity, as well as on the energy and field size of the beam. In current practice they are best considered by using pencil-beam algorithms and,

increasingly, by using Monte Carlo techniques. Simpler methods are outlined here that can be used to estimate the magnitude of effects and to provide an approximate check of more sophisticated calculations.

8.1 Absorption (bulk) effects

A number of empirical approaches have been used to predict the shift in isodoses due to the presence of non-water equivalent media. For example, the coefficient of equivalent thickness (CET) method calculates equivalent water thicknesses, in terms of electron absorption from the surface to the point of interest, taking account of the different materials along the path. The effective depth, d_{eff}, is given by:

$$D_{eff} = d - t(1 - CET)$$

where d is the physical depth of the point, t is the thickness of inhomogeneity traversed, and CET is the ratio of water thickness to that of the heterogeneity, which will produce the same dose transmission. Strictly this is for a non-diverging beam. CET varies with energy and depth, but frequently single representative values can be used to give estimates of changes to within about 10%, at least away from beam edges or structure edges. These ratios are often taken to be the ratios of electron densities in the different media. For compact bone, a CET of 1.65 can be used, whilst for spongy bone the value is close to unity. For lung, CET values close to the relative density of lung can be used to give a reasonable approximation to the isodose line shift. The equivalent distance of the point is used to select a depth–dose value that can then be corrected for ISL, where necessary. Scatter effects can modify these corrections, due to differences in both forward scatter and back scatter at the interface lying across the beam. For example, at a chest wall/lung interface, dose in the chest wall close to the lung, and in the initial lung layers, may be reduced from that measured in a homogeneous water medium due to the reduction in lung scatter. As the depth into the lung increases, the increased penetration outweighs this and the dose at depth becomes increasingly greater than at the same depth in soft tissue or water.

8.2 Scatter (edge) effects

A scatter perturbation is produced when the junction of two materials of different composition is struck tangentially, or at a large oblique angle, by an electron beam. More electrons are scattered away from the higher density material towards the lower density material giving rise to hot-spot scatter lobes into or under the lower density medium. There are correspondingly low-dose areas in or under the higher density region, reflecting a relative loss of electrons. These can give large local changes in dose and should be taken into account in planning. These perturbations have been widely studied theoretically and experimentally and have been shown to be maximum at an angle α (Figure 10.6), which is approximately 60° at 5 MeV, 30° at 10 MeV, and 15° at 20 MeV, where the energies are mean values at the depth of the interface. The effects decrease with lateral distance from the interface to become negligible at a second angle β, beyond which edge effects are not significant and the distribution is only influenced by differences in absorption. β is approximately 2.2–2.5 times α in the energy range 10–30 MeV. Maximum changes in dose, whether reductions or increases as compared to the dose at the equivalent point in a homogeneous water phantom, may be estimated along either line at angle α. They are found to increase with increasing energy at the depth of the interface, e.g. varying from approximately 4% at 5 MeV, to 8% at 10 MeV, and 14% at 20 MeV for a bone/water interface. For air/water interfaces, the figures are approximately 1.8 times these values.

These effects may need to be considered at, for example:

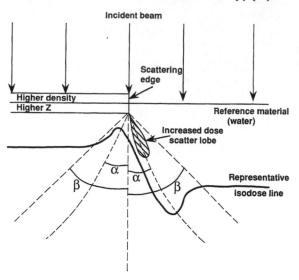

Figure 10.6 The general form of scatter perturbation effect on dose distributions beneath an interface, following Klevenhagen (1985).

(1) interfaces between different media due to internal structure, e.g. lung, bone, air cavities;

(2) the edges of pronounced surface irregularities, e.g. nose, ear canal, bolus or degrader edges;

(3) the edges of lead used for shielding or shaping.

Where small inhomogeneities or irregularities are present, the effects may be reinforced by the overlapping of more than one scatter perturbation from more than one interface. In general, air cavities give rise to greater effects than bone cavities. The ear canal is an illustrative case; here incident electrons can be scattered off the tissue/air interface a number of times, effectively channelling down the canal. This can be prevented by using a wax plug or a water-soaked plug of cotton-wool or cotton swab, or similar.

For many simpler treatment situations, where scatter effects are involved, these approximate manual methods provide an acceptable estimate of the dose distribution with an accuracy approaching 10%. However, scatter is such a significant process for electrons that for complex situations the errors may be much greater. Currently, pencil-beam models provide the standard technique for calculating edge effects to an acceptable accuracy, although Monte Carlo approaches are becoming increasingly used (Section 14). Figure 10.7 illustrates the general form and magnitude of the scatter perturbation effects in a few clinical situations.

8.3 Bolus

Bolus, or energy degraders, may be introduced deliberately at the patient surface and this may represent an

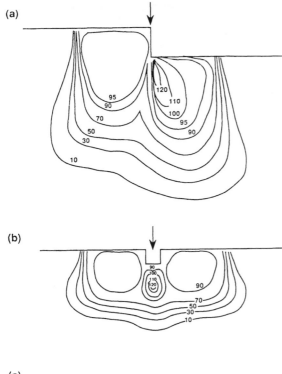

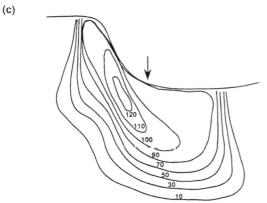

Figure 10.7 Illustrative examples of scatter perturbation effects on dose distribution (similar effects occur at internal interfaces): (a) a 20-MeV beam incident on a sharp irregularity on the surface, such as bolus or surface projection; (b) a 10-MeV beam incident on a narrow air cavity (surface depression); (c) a 17-MeV beam incident on a neck/chin contour.

inhomogeneity, even though materials are generally selected to be close to tissue in their absorption and scattering properties (see Sections 3 and 7). Any differences in density, etc., should be taken into account in the thickness calculations. Variable bolus thicknesses can be calculated manually in simple situations, but this is also relatively straightforward using treatment-planning systems. These calculations should initially be checked against measurement to give confidence in the predictions.

The three reasons for using such materials are summarized below.

1. To improve surface dose, as discussed in Section 3. If plastics that have different absorption properties to water are used, the thickness must be scaled by the relative electron density to produce the required surface dose and penetration in the patient.

2. To improve dose distributions when problems arise due to surface shape by smoothing sharp surface irregularities to minimize scatter perturbations, in-filling less pronounced surface irregularities to produce regular isodose curves over the target volume, providing side-scatter to a treated area where necessary, or improving the variation of penetration caused by oblique incidence.

3. To shape the isodoses by positioning shaped wax or other materials over part of the field to modulate the penetration to conform more closely to the required target volume. Any sharp edges produced that are parallel to the beam should be smoothed by tapering where possible to reduce scatter perturbations.

9. Internal shielding

Internal shielding is occasionally required to spare structures lying below the target volume, for example, in treatments involving lip, cheek, ear, or eyelids. Given space restrictions, the minimum thickness to provide the required shielding should be used for the field size and depth involved. Any shielding material will produce backscatter, which will increase the dose at the tissue/shield interface. This excess dose increases as the atomic number of the scattering material increases and as the mean energy at the position of the shield (E_s) decreases. For lead, Klevenhagen *et al.* (1982) give the empirical relationship:

$$EBF = 1 + 0.735 \exp(-0.052E_s)$$

where the electron backscatter factor (EBF) gives the relative increase in dose at the surface of the back-scattering shield compared to the dose at that point in the absence of the shield. Dose enhancement can be up to 65% for E_s of 3 or 4 MeV. Lambert and Klevenhagen (1982) have reported the transmission of backscattered electrons through suitable thicknesses of lower atomic number material, which can be added between the shield and the overlying tissue to attenuate the backscatter sufficiently to produce an acceptable dose distribution through the irradiated tissue. Wax, or a similar material, is generally suitable, but when space is restricted, aluminium may be preferred, which will itself contribute up to about 10% backscatter. When tissue-similar material is used, Lambert and Klevenhagen (1982) also provide an exponential expression to estimate the transmission of the backscattered electrons at t mm upstream from the shield:

$$\mathrm{EBS}(t) = Ae^{-kt}$$

where A is unity for energies of 1–9 MeV and $k = 0.61 \, E_s^{-0.62}$. This allows thicknesses of wax, etc., to be calculated to satisfy the distribution requirements. Frequently in such calculations the mean energy at the shield is found to be around 3–4 MeV and a shield of 2 mm of lead is sufficient with around 5 mm of wax applied in the upstream direction.

In some situations, space restrictions dictate a compromise on added thickness and, therefore, on distribution, which must be calculated at the planning stage and verified for acceptability. In extreme cases, such as internal shields under the eyelids, no extra material can be accommodated. In this case, planning calculations must estimate the dose variations through the overlying volume, combining the incident and the backscatter components. It may be necessary to use external shields for part of the treatment time to ensure the area does not receive an unacceptably high dose when the dose enhancement due to backscatter is taken into account.

10. Adjacent fields

The problem of matching fields for photon therapy is generally well understood (e.g. see Chapter 8, Section 2.1.4). It is markedly more difficult for electrons because of the shape of the isodose distribution. Simple matching of 50% on the surface results in hot-spots at depth, whilst matching at depth results in cold-spots on the surface. The choice of gap between the two beams is, therefore, determined by taking into account the distribution across the target volume and the clinical acceptability of any such hot- or cold-spots. Even small variations in the relative position of the beams can significantly change the size of these regions and consideration should be given to the effect of any variations in surface topography at different points along the join. If the fields are angled towards each other, e.g. around a chest wall, the problems become more acute. Adjacent electron fields should be avoided whenever possible. However, there are situations when they may be necessary such as:

(1) to provide varying penetration by using different energy electron beams for adjoining areas;

(2) to treat a larger area than standard applicators allow;

(3) to treat irregular topography, e.g. chest wall, head, etc.;

(4) when an adjacent area is having other treatment (electron or photon) or has already had previous treatment.

In these situations, the join should be positioned away from critical areas. Staggered joins (i.e. shifting joins at different treatment fractions) may be considered, if this is practical. The matching can be improved by using a moderately extended SSD or a small angulation of the fields away from each other on the match-line, to utilize the broadened penumbra regions produced. This necessitates on-surface shaping of the other field edges to restore sharp penumbra and may well lead to loss of beam flatness. Alternatively, small plastic blocks, or wedges, can be used along one or both field edges to be joined, again in order to broaden the penumbra. The particular methods are dependent on the applicators and the overlap or gap will still need careful investigation.

McKenzie (1998) has proposed a simple but effective method using 'spoiler' slabs of plastic (e.g. PMMA) across the whole of the beams to be matched, intended to spoil or broaden the penumbra. Matching fields with wider penumbra is then not so critical, the light field edges (50%) can be abutted (i.e. no overlap or gap is required) and, typically, the hot-spots are reduced to acceptable levels. Small added strips of absorber can be laid along the match line to reduce these even further, if necessary, e.g. on curved surfaces where hinge angles are large. There is no dependence of the spoiler design on the particular applicator, SSD or angle, and treatment-planning programmes can be used without modification or additional measurement to calculate the spoiler effect. A higher beam energy must be selected, such that the combination of energy and spoiler bring the therapeutic isodose back to the required depth. The spoiler thickness should be selected to be the minimum that produces an adequately wide penumbra, e.g. a 10-mm spoiler for a 9–10 MeV chest wall irradiation. As the spoiler broadens all field edges, it may be necessary to add shielding around the other sides of the treated area to restore sharper edges and shield adjacent tissues. It should be noted that predicted doses should be tested experimentally for curved surface matching, as scatter could significantly affect the final distributions.

11. Electron arc therapy

Large field treatment areas have been shown to present problems of obliquity and matching. One solution for relatively superficial target areas along curved surfaces, such as the chest wall, is to use an arc technique. The implementation of these methods requires significant effort and cannot be covered in detail here. Reviews of electron arc therapy methods and requirements can be found in AAPM (1981), Leavitt *et al.* (1985), and Leavitt (1996). Factors requiring attention are given below.

1. The choice of beam energy: arcing modifies the effective depth–dose curve, giving an increase in apparent penetration and in the contribution of bremsstrahlung at depth and giving a reduction in surface dose.

2. The isocentre position: this should be approximately equidistant from surface points around the treated area to minimize the changes in FSD. It should be positioned at a depth greater than the electron range (R_p) and preferably around $2R_p$ to prevent the superposition of dose at the same point.

3. The beam width: the arc technique is aimed at taking the complete beam profile over any point. Beam widths of around 5 cm projected to isocentre are recommended. This ensures acceptable dosimetry requirements, the beam being roughly parallel to the surface at all points and, therefore, producing minimal obliquity problems, and also without causing too much bremsstrahlung accumulation at the isocentre. A special arc therapy secondary collimator is required, mounted in the accelerator accessory holder to ensure adequate clearance at all points around the arc.

4. Beam shaping: if the skin curvature varies away from the central plane, the secondary collimator can be shaped to produce a varying-width beam to compensate. In this case, a narrower or wider beam passes over the various points producing varying distributions. Trapezoidal shapes are often necessary. More recent facilities allow shaping with multi-leaf collimators.

5. Treated-field shaping: as the beam should be arced completely over the treatment area, the edges of the area should be delineated using tertiary shielding on the patient's surface to produce sharp definition. The poorer distribution at the other edges can be sharpened in this way aided by additional shaping of the secondary collimator.

6. The dose per arc and the dose distribution: this may be obtained by direct measurement or from an integration of stationary beam data. Planning is currently best carried out using a pencil-beam algorithm

12.   Total skin electron irradiation

Special techniques have been developed for total skin electron irradiation (TSEI) for mycosis fungoides and other skin conditions. Here the aim is to achieve uniformity of dose around the patient and also from head to toe, with uniformity of penetration to a depth selected on the basis of the stage of the disease, and also ensuring that the bremsstrahlung X-ray contamination, which contributes a whole-body dose, is acceptably low.

Some patient-related or clinical problems include:

(1) variations in surface shape, body cross-section, etc.;

(2) the inevitability of self-shielding of some areas by others;

(3) whether the patient can take up the positions required for the relatively long treatment times;

(4) the problem of whether or not to omit non-involved areas;

(5) the positioning of any necessary shielding in contact with, or close to, the patient surface, e.g. for finger nails, toe nails, eyes, etc., or previously irradiated areas;

(6) the potential requirement for variable depth penetration, e.g. if there are thick plaque lesions in addition to the generalized areas with only thin superficial involvement: in some circumstances, patients may be referred who have already had a number of areas treated either with small field electron beams or kV X-rays.

The physics problems in attempting to meet the clinical requirements include the following.

1. The choice of general technique to provide full coverage, involving multiple beams, around the patient and some means of covering the full length of the patient in a uniform manner. Longer SSDs than normal will result in significantly poorer beam edges and beam flatnesses due to scatter, and also in loss of energy as the beam passes through significant distances of air (approximately 0.25 MeV per metre)

2. The choice of beam energy to provide both the required surface dose and depth of penetration, taking into consideration that the combination of beams from different directions around the patient involves oblique incidence at a range of angles up to the extreme of tangential incidence. This modifies the effective depth doses in different ways at different positions around the patient, which will depend on the technique chosen. The more beam directions used, the better will be the uniformity of penetration. To produce a high surface-dose requires a beam degrader/scatterer close to the patient surface. Typical incident beam energies at the patient surface will be around 4–6 MeV and will produce effective therapeutic ranges (85–90%) between about 3 and 5 mm.

3. The addition of fields around the patient also produces a dose variation around the circumference of the patient, which may vary with body cross-

section. Again the more beam directions used, the more uniform will be the surface dose distribution around any given body section.

4. X-ray contamination contributions from each beam direction around the patient will be additive at the centre of the body

5. Doses may need to be monitored at the treatment position, either in terms of the beam, using an ion chamber, or in terms of patient dose, using TLD. This is required for safety reasons if high-dose rate modalities are used for long FSD techniques, but separate safety interlocks for the selection of this modality are also needed.

6. Boost doses may be required later in areas that receive lower dose from the TSEI, such as self-shielded areas (e.g. perineum), areas that are not presented to the beams (e.g. soles of feet, if the patient is standing), areas where all beams are tangential (e.g. the top of the head), etc.

Many techniques have been proposed as solutions to the problems. Some of these are based on large-field and long-SSD, utilizing two beams angled at ±10–20° to the horizontal, so that the combined distribution is uniform over the height of a standing patient. Others use medium SSDs and either add adjacent fields or employ translation of the patient or arcing of the beam. Beam directions around the patient have varied from 2 (which does not provide adequate distributions) to 8, with the ultimate being the rotational technique (Podgorsak *et al.* 1983). All such techniques are specialized time-consuming treatments, requiring extensive development and careful dosimetry, planning, and execution. A review of some of the techniques and of some of the physics approaches can be found in AAPM (1987).

13. Other techniques

Electrons can be combined with megavoltage photons to give modified dose distributions, for example to decrease skin dose while maintaining a high dose to a relatively well-specified depth, or to provide a boost to a relatively superficial volume, combined with a lower dose to a greater volume. Combining parallel opposed electron beams has been shown to give useful distributions compared to photon beams in some instances (ICRU 1984), but this has used beams of higher energies than those commonly available. This is not advisable when using lower energy beams for sites with a small separation because the steep dose gradients can lead to very significant under- and over-dosing, due to inhomogeneities or irregular body surfaces.

Developing techniques involving both lower and higher energy electron beams, either alone or mixing

energies, or in combination with photon beams, can be found in an increasing body of literature (e.g. Karlsson and Zackrisson 1997; Korevaar *et al.* 1998). Here the aim is to improve dose distributions over the target volume for specific clinical situations, e.g. depth doses, penumbral widths, or surface doses for simpler cases, or, more generally, intensity modulation both in terms of beam profile and of penetration. Multi-leaf collimation of electron beams is also being explored, in both static and dynamic mode (e.g. Klein 1998; Korevaar *et al.* 1998).

14. Electron-beam algorithms

A range of algorithms have been used for predicting the dose distributions from electron beams, all of which suffer from inaccuracy to a greater or lesser extent, due to the strong influence of scatter and the difficulties in modelling it. In particular, there are significant problems resulting from inhomogeneities and from both scattered electrons and secondary photons produced in the treatment head. Comprehensive reviews of the state of this developing subject can be found in Nahum (1985) and Jette (1996).

Early calculation algorithms were based on *isodose shift methods*, such as the CET approach as outlined in Section 8. These did not consider scatter perturbations and, therefore, did not cope well with surface variations or inhomogeneities and, in general, were not particularly accurate. More recent work, providing relatively successful calculation models have been based on *pencil-beam models*, incorporating age-diffusion theory or multiple-scattering (Fermi–Eyges) theory. Building on the approximate Gaussian spread of a narrow electron beam, the dose is calculated at a point by summation of contributions to that point from a matrix of spreading elemental pencil beams making up the applied beam at the surface. Variations over the incident beam, changes due to surface shape and irregular fields, and effects due to inhomogeneities can be taken into account for each pencil individually, in order to calculate dose distributions. The *Fermi–Eyges approach* incorporates multiple-scattering theory explicitly and accounts for both lateral and angular dispersion of the pencil beam. It has been widely applied as the basis of practical dose-calculation models, starting with the work of Hogstrom *et al.* (1981) and of Brahme *et al.* (1981), and subsequent developments.

The Fermi–Eyges theory is a small-angle scatter approximation and so does not deal with backscattered electrons at all. It breaks down completely towards the end of the range and it does not account for bremsstrahlung. The *Hogstrom algorithm* (Hogstrom *et al.* 1981) circumvented some of the limitations of the basic theory by normalizing to measured data in the homogeneous situation. It simplified the behaviour in the treatment head by replacing the real situation by an appropriate weighting of zero angular dispersion pencil beams at the final collimator level and then propagating these through any remaining air gap to the surface and then into the patient. Therefore, it could produce reasonable accuracy in modelling the actual beam and for depths beyond that at which Fermi–Eyges might be expected to break down. Hogstrom provided a practical approach, formulated to deal directly with CT information, which was implemented in a number of treatment-planning systems in one form or another. Lax and co-workers (Lax *et al.* 1983; Lax and Brahme 1985) have improved on the small-angle scatter approximation, by modelling radial dose profiles to include large-angle scatter, using three Gaussian functions with parameters obtained from Monte Carlo calculations or from experimental data, producing the *generalized Gaussian model.*

The Fermi–Eyges theory is applicable to layered geometries. Therefore, a significant limitation, common to any implementation of these approaches, is that inhomogeneities are dealt with only along the central ray of each pencil, i.e. they are assumed to be larger in extent than the spread of each individual pencil beam. Thus, effects due to narrow inhomogeneities are not predicted accurately, in particular at depths where the pencil beam has spread significantly. *Redefinition algorithms* (Storchi and Huizenga 1985; Shiu and Hogstrom 1991) improve performance for inhomogeneities of limited extent and at depth. They redefine the pencil beams at appropriate depths close to both the medium and calculation points of interest, propagating from one layer to the next using CT data to ensure that multiple scatter is more correctly accounted for than simply using a single pencil beam that begins at the surface. The Shui and Hogstrom (1991) approach also accounts for the associated energy changes.

An alternative algorithm is the *phase space evolution* (PSE) method (Huizenga and Storchi 1989; Janssen *et al.* 1994), a numerical calculation method that incorporates large-angle scattering, energy straggling and secondary electron and bremsstrahlung production. It begins with a pre-calculated initial phase space state, describing the positions, energies, and directions of all the incident electrons and evolves from this initial state by repeated redistributions of these parameters, based only on the physical interaction processes, from one phase space element to the next, until no energetic electrons remain. The calculation time is reported as significantly less than Monte Carlo methods.

Currently implemented algorithms on treatment-planning systems have been investigated by a number of workers (e.g. Lax 1986, 1987; Cygler *et al.* 1987; Mah *et al.* 1989; Shiu and Hogstrom 1991; Kawrakow *et al.* 1996). They have generally been shown to be accurate to about ±5% and/or ±5 mm over a range of applications, with later algorithms improving the performance compared to earlier ones. In the simpler situations, accuracies of ±2% or ±2 mm can be achieved, in accordance with the requirements for photon algorithms (ICRU 1987). However, discrepancies of the order of 10% (and potentially up to several tens of per cent in extreme cases) are often observed for narrow inhomogeneities, particularly those with long edges parallel to the beam and at large depths, e.g. discrepancies of up to around 14% have been observed for 15 MeV electrons in a spinal phantom (Dominiak *et al.* 1991). Lax (1987) notes that the original Hogstrom algorithm tends to overestimate local doses, whilst the generalized Gaussian algorithm tends to underestimate. The redefinition algorithms improve accuracy for narrow and deep inhomogeneities over the earlier Fermi–Eyges models, approximately reducing discrepancies by a factor of two in the situations where the earlier algorithms performed worst. Janssen *et al.* (1994) report comparisons of the PSE method to Monte Carlo calculations in situations incorporating 3-D inhomogeneities, showing generally good agreement.

As there are a number of different approaches and implementations on current treatment-planning systems, the user must ensure that the details and limitations of the particular approach are well understood. The system should be extensively tested against measurement. Test methods and criteria for commissioning electron-beam algorithms and for quality assurance are provided in Shiu *et al.* (1992), van Dyk *et al.* (1993), IPEMB (1994), and AAPM (1998).

Monte Carlo (MC) methods are widely used already to provide input to some of the algorithms, to provide benchmark values to test other algorithms against, and to model specific situations, e.g. treatment heads (Udale-Smith 1992; Rogers *et al.* 1995). The main drawback is perceived to be the long calculation times necessary to achieve data with reasonable uncertainties. Various methods have been implemented to reduce calculation times, e.g. the macro-MC method (Neuenschwander and Born 1992; Neuenschwander *et al.* 1995) or the voxel based MC algorithm (Kawrakow *et al.* 1996), some involving approximations. However, the continuing improvements in hardware speed and capacity, and the development of techniques to improve the statistics without increasing the times involved or to reduce the times without significant loss of accuracy, have meant that times for treatment-planning calculations have rapidly approached practical values, in particular for electron beams where frequently only single beams are involved and the volumes are limited. Thus, whilst the pencil-beam approach is currently the method of choice for practical electron treatment-planning calculations, Monte Carlo electron treatment planning is now feasible and will soon be commonplace on treatment-planning systems.

15. References

American Association of Physicists in Medicine (1981). *Proceedings of the symposium on electron dosimetry and arc therapy* (ed. Paliwal, B). AIP, New York

American Association of Physicists in Medicine (1987). *Total skin electron therapy: technique and dosimetry.* Report of AAPM Task Group 30. AAPM Report, no. 23. AIP, New York.

American Association of Physicists in Medicine (1991). Clinical electron beam dosimetry. Report of AAPM Task Group 25. *Med. Phys.*, **18**, 73–109.

American Association of Physicists in Medicine (1998). Quality assurance for clinical radiotherapy treatment planning. Report of AAPM Task Group 53. *Med. Phys.*, **25**, 1723–829.

Brahme, A., Lax, I., and Andreo, P. (1981). Electron beam dose planning using discrete Gaussian beams: mathematical background. *Acta Radiol. Oncol.* **20**, 147–58.

Bruinvis, I.A.D. and Mathol, W.A.F. (1988). Calculation of electron beam depth–dose curves and output factors for arbitrary field shapes. *Radiother. Oncol.*, **11**, 395–404.

Cygler, J., Battista, J.J., Scrimger, J.W., Mah, E., and Antalok, J. (1987) Electron dose distributions in experimental phantoms: a comparison with 2D pencil beam calculations. *Phys. Med. Biol.*, **32**, 1073–86.

Dominiak, G.S., Starkschall, G., Shiu, A.S., and Hogstrom, K.R. (1991). Dose in spinal cord following electron irradiation. *Med. Phys.*, **18**, 848 (Abstract).

Hogstrom, K.R., Mills, M.D. and Almond, P.R. (1981). Electron beam dose calculations. *Phys. Med. Biol.*, **26**, 445–59.

Huizenga, H. and Storchi, P.R.M. (1989) Numerical calculation of energy deposition by broad high-energy electron beams. *Phys. Med. Biol.*, **34**, 1371–96.

Institution of Physics and Engineering in Medicine and Biology (1994). *A guide to commissioning and quality control of treatment planning systems.* IPEMB Report 68. IPEMB, York.

International Commission on Radiation Units and Measurements (1978). *Dose specification for reporting external beam therapy with photons and electrons.* Report 29. ICRU, Washington, DC.

International Commission on Radiation Units and Measurements (1984). *Radiation dosimetry: electron beams with energies between 1 and 50 MeV. Report 35.* ICRU, Washington, DC.

International Commission on Radiation Units and Measurements (1987). *The use of computers in external beam radiotherapy procedures with high-energy photons and electrons.* Report 42. ICRU, Washington, DC.

International Commission on Radiation Units and Measurements (1993). *Prescribing, recording and reporting photon beam therapy.* Report 50. ICRU, Washington, DC.

Janssen, J.J., Riedeman, D.E., Morawska-Kaczynska, M., Storchi, P.R., and Huizenga, H. (1994). Numerical calculation of energy deposition by high-energy electron beams: III. Three-dimensional heterogeneous media. *Phys. Med. Biol.*, **39**, 1–16.

Jette, D, (1996). Electron beam dose calculations. In *Radiation therapy physics* (ed. AR Smith). Springer-Verlag, Berlin. 95–121

Karlsson, M. and Zackrisson, B. (1997). Exploration of new treatment modalities offered by high energy (up to 50 MeV) electrons and photons. *Radiother. Oncol.*, **43**, 303–9.

Kawrakow, I., Fippel, M., and Friedrich, K. (1996). 3D dose calculation using a voxel based Monte Carlo algorithm (VMC). *Med. Phys.*, **23**, 445–57.

Khan, F., Deibel, F., and Soleimani-Meigooni, A. (1985). Obliquity correction for electron beams. *Med. Phys.*, **12**, 749–53.

Klein, E.E. (1998). Modulated electron beams using multi-segmented multileaf collimation. *Radiother. Oncol.*, **48**, 307–11.

Klevenhagen, S.C. (1985). *Physics of electron beam therapy.* Medical Physics handbook 13. Adam Hilger, Bristol.

Klevenhagen, S.C., Lambert, G.D., and Arbabi, A. (1982). Backscattering in electron beam therapy for energies between 3 and 35 MeV. *Phys. Med. Biol.*, **27**, 363–73.

Korevaar, E.W., van Vliet, R.J., Woudstra, E., Heijmen, B., and Huizenga, H. (1998). Sharpening the penumbra of high energy electron beams with low weight narrow photon beams. *Radiother. Oncol.*, **48**, 213–20.

Lambert, G.D. and Klevenhagenn, S.C. (1982). Penetration of backscattered electrons in polystyrene for energies between 1 and 25 MeV. *Phys. Med. Biol.*, **27**, 721–5.

Lax, I. (1986). Inhomogeneity corrections in electron-beam dose planning: limitations with the semi-infinite slab approximation. *Phys. Med. Biol.*, **31**, 879–92.

Lax, I. (1987). Accuracy in clinical electron beam dose planning using pencil beam algorithms. *Radiother. Oncol.*, **10**, 307–19.

Lax, I. and Brahme, A. (1985). Electron beam dose planning using Gaussian beams: energy and spatial scaling with inhomogeneities. *Acta Radiol. Oncol.*, **24**, 75–85.

Lax, I., Brahme, A., and Andreo, P. (1983). Electron beam dose planning using Gaussian beams: improved radial dose profiles. *Acta Radiol.* Supplement **364**, 49–59.

Leavitt, D.D. (1996). Physics of electron arc therapy. In *Radiation therapy physics* (ed AR Smith). Springer-Verlag, Berlin. 139–154

Leavitt, D.D., Peacock, L.M., Gibbs, F.A., and Stewart, J.R. (1985). Electron arc therapy: physical measurement and treatment planning techniques. *Int. J. Radiat. Oncol. Biol. Phys.*, **11**, 987–99.

Mah, E., Antolak, J., Scrimger, J.W., and Battista, J.J. (1989). Experimental evaluation of a 2D and 3D electron pencil beam algorithm. *Phys. Med. Biol.*, **34**, 1179–94.

McKenzie, A.L. (1998). A simple method for matching electron beams in radiotherapy. *Phys. Med. Biol.*, **43**, 3465–78.

Nahum, A.E. (ed.) (1985). *The computation of dose distribution in electron beam radiotherapy.* Umea University, Sweden.

Neuenschwander, H. and Born, E.J. (1992). A macro Monte Carlo method for electron beam dose calculations. *Phys. Med. Biol.*, **37**, 107–25.

Neuenschwander, H., Mackie, T.R., and Reckwerdt, P.J. (1995). MMC-a high-performance Monte Carlo code for electron beam treatment planning. *Phys. Med. Biol.*, **40**, 543–74.

Podgorsak, E., Pla, C., Pla, M., Lefebvre, P.Y., and Heese, R. (1983). Physical aspects of rotational total skin electron irradiation. *Med. Phys.*, **10**, 159–68.

Rogers, D.W.O., Faddegon, B.S., Ding, G.X., Ma, C-M., We, J., and Mackie, T.R. (1995). BEAM: a Monte Carlo code to simulate radiotherapy treatment units. *Med. Phys.*, **22**, 503–24.

Shiu, A.S. and Hogstrom, K.R. (1991). Pencil-beam redefinition algorithm for electron dose distributions. *Med. Phys.*, **18**, 7–18.

Shiu, A.S., Tung, S., Hogstrom, K.R. Wong, J.W., Gerber, R.L., Harms, W.B., *et al.* (1992). Verification data for electron beam dose algorithms. *Med. Phys.*, **19**, 623–36.

Storchi, P.R.M. and Huizenga, H. (1985). On a numerical approach of the pencil beam model. *Phys. Med. Biol.*, **30**, 467–73.

Udale-Smith, M. (1992). Monte Carlo calculations of electron beam parameters for three Philips linear accelerators. *Phys. Med. Biol.*, **37**, 85–105.

Van Dyk, J., Barnett, R.B., Cygler, J.E., and Shragge, P.C. (1993). Commissioning and quality assurance of treatment planning computers. *Int. J. Radiat.* Oncol. Biol. Phys., **26**, 261–73.

Chapter 11

Treatment verification and *in vivo* dosimetry

W.P.M. Mayles, S. Heisig, and H.M.O. Mayles

1. Introduction

In this chapter, the problem of ensuring that radiotherapy treatments are carried out as they were intended is considered. The principal focus is on external beam therapy but some reference is also made to brachytherapy.

The treatment plan for a patient will be the result of careful work and interaction between the planning technicians and the radiation oncologist (radiotherapist). The prescribed dose may be the mid-target dose, as recommended by the ICRU, or frequently some other means of specification may have been used. A dose distribution may have been calculated. However, at every step in the process and in the treatment delivery, uncertainties will be introduced. These may include the following:

(1) uncertainties in the position and extent of the target volume;

(2) inaccuracies in the computer dose-calculation algorithm;

(3) inaccuracies in the treatment-machine calibration;

(4) inaccuracies in the mechanical alignment of the treatment machine;

(5) inaccuracies in the patient set-up;

(6) patient movement (which may be unavoidable, as in respiration);

(7) variability of the patient's internal anatomy;

(8) errors in the treatment machine settings.

A comprehensive treatment-verification programme should include verification of dose, verification of field position, and verification that the correct treatment machine parameters are set.

2. Dose verification

Verification of dose is perhaps the most obvious way to check the accuracy of patient treatment. It is widely accepted that treatment doses need to be accurate to within 5% or even 3%. *In vivo* dosimetry has been in use since the days when skin erythema was the only form of dosimetry available. In the present day, skin erythema is a much underrated dosimetry technique and an unexpected skin reaction should always be carefully investigated. It can provide an indication of gross calibration errors and can alert staff to the need to improve skin sparing, for example, by cutting out the beam entry ports in treatment shells. It can also give a clear indication of the accuracy and reproducibility with which a treatment field has been set up.

The WHO (1988) publication on *Quality Assurance in Radiotherapy*, recommends that *in vivo* dosimetry should be carried out on all patients. However, it is necessary to balance the costs of carrying out such procedures against the quality-assurance benefits.

The principal techniques used for *in vivo* measurements are thermoluminescence dosimetry (TLD) and semiconductor dosimetry. Before discussing these systems in detail, a description is given of how dosimetric accuracy can be assessed.

2.1 Accuracy and precision

Considerable care needs to be taken to make a dose measurement accurately, and it is often not possible to achieve this in the pressured environment of the treatment room. For this reason, the physicist must be fully conscious of the accuracy achievable and resist the temptation to replace accurate calculations of dose with inaccurate measurements. Equally, consideration of the expected accuracy is important to prevent *in vivo* measurements being dismissed as inaccurate, when they in fact reflect an error in the dosimetry.

Accuracy and *precision* are two concepts that are very important to the proper conduct of *in vivo* dosimetry. *Precision* encompasses the statistical reproducibility of measurements and the resolution of the measuring instrument. Reproducibility can be measured by carrying out repeated measurements from which the *standard deviation*, SD, can be calculated. This is defined as:

$$SD = \left[\frac{1}{n-1} \sum_{i=1}^{n} (R_i - \text{mean})^2 \right]^{\frac{1}{2}}$$

where *n* is the number of readings carried out and R_i are the individual readings. For a normally distributed variable, 68% of the readings will fall within one standard deviation of the mean and 95% within 2 standard deviations. A set of *m* measurements of the dose at a point may be made, and the mean of the set will be a more precise measure of the 'true' mean than an individual reading. If *m* sets of measurements were made, their means would be distributed about the 'true' mean with a standard deviation of $SD/\sqrt{m}$, which is the *standard error* of the mean. However, the precision of the measurement cannot be increased beyond the resolution of the measuring instrument. For example, the precision of an instrument reading of 33 mGy is limited to 3%. This can be a problem in low dose rate TBI dosimetry. It is also important to be sure that the conditions for repeat measurements are subject only to random variations. This will not be the case if, for example, the machine output drifts.

The *accuracy* of a measurement describes the difference between the measured result and the true answer. A combination of factors may contribute to the inaccuracy of a measurement, such as the perturbation of the radiation field caused by the dosimeter or the fact that the dosimeter cannot be placed at the point at which we wish to measure the dose. For such reasons, the result, however precise, may not be accurate. To estimate the accuracy of a measurement we must combine the effect of all sources of error, whether systematic or random. If two or more independent random variables need to be added or subtracted to obtain the result we have:

$$\text{standard error of result} = \left[\sum SE_i^2 \right]^{1/2} \quad (1)$$

where the SE_i are the standard errors of each variable. If the standard error of a ratio of two variables is required, it may be obtained as a per cent of the result by substituting per cent standard errors for their absolute values in equation (1). Estimation of the size of the systematic errors requires a good understanding of the physical principles of the measurement and sensible estimates of the magnitude of the uncertainties. In combining systematic errors, it is safer to assume that they are directly additive and so estimate the maximum uncertainty.

2.2 Thermoluminescence dosimetry

2.2.1 Basic principles

TLD relies on the fact that in certain materials electrons, when provided with sufficient energy, may be trapped in metastable states. By heating the material, these metastable electrons may be given sufficient energy to escape from their unstable state and, in reverting to a stable state, they emit an optical photon. The optical photons are detected by a photomultiplier and the light output can be measured. Dosimeters can be re-used once they have been subjected to a process of annealing to eliminate any residual thermoluminescent signal (see Section 2.2.9). For annealing and calibration, dosimeters are grouped together in 'batches'.

2.2.2 Choice of TLD material

TLD materials come in many physical and chemical forms. The most commonly used material in radiotherapy is lithium fluoride doped with traces of magnesium and titanium (LiF:Mg,Ti). The production process was originally patented by Harshaw (now Harshaw/Bicron) who manufacture the material as extruded ribbons, which are then cut into chips about 3 mm square and 0.9 mm thick (actually 0.125 in square by 0.035 in thick). This material is available as TLD 100 containing lithium with natural abundance (i.e. 92.5% lithium-7), TLD 600, which contains 95.6% lithium-6, and TLD 700, which is almost pure lithium-7. ^6LiF is sensitive to thermal neutrons and ^7LiF is not, so a combination of the two can be used for differential detection of neutrons. For routine photon dosimetry, TLD 100 is satisfactory. Other manufacturers supply similar products. The Bicron/NE version is fabricated by pressing ^7LiF into pellets and then sintering them, which produces a circular dosimeter that is 4.5 mm in diameter and 0.8 mm thick. Many other thermoluminescent materials have been used, but for most medical uses the only others of interest are calcium fluoride, calcium sulphate, and lithium borate. $CaSO_4$ and CaF_2 are more sensitive than LiF:Mg,Ti and can be used for measuring very low doses. $LiBO_4$ has an effective atomic number that is very close to that of tissue, so that its sensitivity increases by only 3% at low-photon energies, compared to about 30% for LiF:Mg,Ti. Its drawback is that it is deliquescent (absorbs moisture) and very sensitive to ultraviolet radiation, and is consequently difficult to use. A newer material, lithium fluoride doped with about 2% of phosphorus and traces of magnesium and copper (LiF:Mg,Cu,P), may supplant these other materials (Horowitz 1993). It is up to 30 times more sensitive than LiF:Mg,Ti and, for reasons that cannot be explained by cavity theory, is almost as energy independent as $LiBO_4$. LiF:Mg,Cu,P is very sensitive to incorrect thermal treatment (Furetta *et al.* 1994), so for

Table 11.1 Properties of TL dosimeters commonly used in medicine

	Lithium Fluoride	Lithium Fluoride	Lithium Borate	Calcium Sulphate	Calcium Fluoride
Most common doping material	Mg, Ti	Mg, Cu, P	Mn	Dy	Dy
Effective atomic number (tissue 7.4)	8.14	8.14	7.4	15.6	16.6
Density	2.64	2.64	2.3	2.61	3.18
Stopping power (ratio to water)					
at 100 keV	0.808	0.808	0.846	–	0.781
at 10 MeV	0.809	0.809	0.849	–	0.831
Mass energy absorption coefficient ratio					
at 100 keV	0.875	0.875	0.865	–	0.875
at 10 MeV	0.859	0.859	0.883	–	1.100
Temperature (°C) of dosimetry peak	190, 210	230	200	220	200, 240
Other peaks (°C)	70, 130, 170, 235, 260	140, 190, 270	50, 90	65, 105, 250	120, 140
Wavelength (nm)	400	400	600	478, 571	460, 483, 576
Fading in 1 month (approx.)	<1%	Negligible	5%	1%	13%
Annealing cycle	1 h at 400°C 16 h at 80°C	10 min at 240°C	30 min at 300°C	1 h at 500°C	1 h at 600°C
Sensitivity relative to LiF: Mg, Ti	1	~20	0.15	20	30
Linear up to	1 Gy	10 Gy	1 Gy	30 Gy	10 Gy
Minimum measurable dose	100 μGy	1 μGy	1000 μGy	1 μGy	10 μGy
Maximum dose	1 kGy	1 kGy	10 kGy	1 kGy	10 kGy

routine radiotherapy use, LiF:Mg,Ti still has advantages. Table 11.1 gives a summary of the properties of these materials. The discussion that follows is based on the properties of LiF:Mg,Ti, but the principles apply to any thermoluminescent dosimeter.

Traditionally, LiF was used in powder form but subsequently, other more practical physical forms have been developed. Discs of LiF mixed with Teflon are widely used in radiation protection dosimetry, but the variability of sensitivity within a batch, and the upper limit of 300°C on the temperature at which the discs can be annealed, limit their use in radiotherapy. The two most useful forms are the chips already described and microrods. The latter are made of extruded material that is formed into rods 1 mm in diameter and 6 mm long. Chips are possibly easier to handle, but for some applications microrods are particularly convenient, as they can be accurately inserted into small cylindrical holes. (In what follows, the word 'chip' will be used for any compressed form of dosimeter.)

2.2.3 Read-out

The two requirements to read out the dose given to a TLD sample are: a reliable form of heating and a method of measuring the light output. In one form of reader (e.g. the Rialto reader manufactured by Bicron/NE) the dosimeter is placed on a planchette and then pushed into the reader. A heater is then brought into contact with the underside of the planchette. Another form of reader (e.g. the 5500 reader manufactured by Harshaw/Bicron)

uses hot gas to heat the dosimeter. Both types of reader are available with automatic sample changers. The advantages of the heated-tray method are as follows:

(1) any form of dosimeter, including powder, can be read;

(2) the heating cycle can be accurately controlled.

The advantages of the hot-gas method are as follows:

(1) transfer of heat to the dosimeter is fast;

(2) temperature control is not dependent on good thermal contact with the tray;

(3) automatic readers have no dependence on the reflectivity of the tray and the mechanical arrangements are simpler.

The significance of these factors will become apparent during the discussion of the procedures that follows.

The light output of the dosimeter is measured with a photomultiplier. As the temperature of the dosimeter is increased, the light output will vary (see Figure 11.3). The area under the curve, i.e. the total light output, is proportional to dose. The reading may be modified in two ways.

1. The voltage applied to the photomultiplier can be altered. An increased voltage produces a larger signal and better resolution, but this may saturate the system.

2. A multiplication factor can be applied to the result in order to convert the reading to dose.

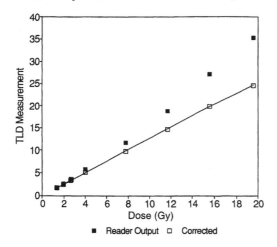

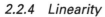

Figure 11.1 Variation of TLD output with dose: ■, raw TLD readings; □, readings corrected according to equation (2).

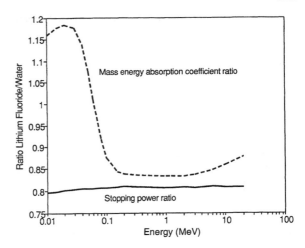

Figure 11.2 Variation with energy of mass energy absorption coefficient and stopping power ratios of LiF to water. Data from Hubbell (1982) and ICRU (1984), respectively.

2.2.4 Linearity

The light output of LiF:Mg,Ti is linearly related to dose up to about 1Gy, but after that it becomes supralinear. The necessary correction can be established by plotting the TL reading against dose as in Figure 11.1. A useful empirical formula to correct for the supralinearity is:

$$C_{supralin} = (1 + 0.0278D - 0.000265D^2)^{-1} \quad (2)$$

where D Gy is the dose given and $C_{supralin}$ is the factor by which the reading must be multiplied to correct for supralinearity. (It should be noted that D is the dose and not the TLD reading, but $C_{supralin}$ can be calculated iteratively if D is unknown.) This formula has been found to work satisfactorily up to 20 Gy. However, the properties of TLD materials are affected by their thermal treatment and, therefore, its applicability should be checked by measurement. The supralinearity correction should not alter as the chips age but it is wise to confirm this from time to time. The response of LiF:Mg,Cu,P is linear up to about 10 Gy, after which its response becomes sublinear.

2.2.5 Energy and quality dependence

Horowitz (1981) gives a useful review of the extensive, and often contradictory, literature on the energy dependence of LiF. The theoretical foundation is the Burlin formula for the ratio of the photon dose, D_{det}, recorded by a radiation detector to the dose D_{med} to the medium in which it is placed:

$$D_{det} = D_{med}[d\{\text{mass stopping power ratio}\} + (1 - d) \\ \{\text{mass energy absorption coefficient ratio}\}] \quad (3)$$

where d is a factor to allow for attenuation of secondary electrons in the detector. For a small detector (compared

to the secondary electron range) $d = 1$ and for a large detector $d = 0$ (see Ma and Nahum (1991) for further details). For an electron beam, only the first term in equation (3) applies, and d may be regarded as a perturbation correction (Nahum 1996). Figure 11.2 shows that for energies between 200 keV and 3 MeV both the stopping power ratio and mass energy absorption coefficient ration for LiF are almost unchanged. Mobit *et al.* have shown that, as expected from equation (3) and Figure 11.2, the differences in sensitivity of LiF at different megavoltage energies are small, both for photons (Mobit *et al.* 1996a) and for electrons (Mobit *et al.* 1996b), and in many situations LiF measurements may be easier to convert to dose than ion chamber measurements. The following conclusions may be drawn.

1. The simplest approach is to calibrate the chips against an ionization chamber using the beam quality that is to be used for the measurements. For photon beams, such calibrations should be carried out at the standard calibration depth for that energy rather than at d_{max}.

2. If a cobalt-60 beam is used for calibrations, the measured doses will need to be multiplied by a factor ranging from 1.01 for 6 MV X-rays to 1.025 for 25 MV X-rays (Mobit *et al.* 1996a) and from 1.04 for 2 MeV electrons to 1.03 for 20 MeV electrons (Mobit *et al.* 1996b). The necessary correction increases towards the end of the electron range (Robar *et al.* 1996).

3. If thicker TLD materials are used, or if dosimeters are stacked up, the correction factors will increase.

4. For X-ray energies below 300 kV, it is essential to calibrate the TLDs in the relevant beam. The calibration

factor will be expected to follow the variation in mass energy absorption coefficient ratio. LiF:Mg,Cu,P is a better dosimeter for use at these energies.

5. A particular problem arises for isotope sources such as iridium-192 (mean energy 346 keV) and iodine-125 (energy 27 keV) for which it is difficult to match the radiation exactly and for which point dose measurements with ion chambers are difficult. Close to iridium wires, the cobalt-60 calibration is appropriate, but the relative sensitivity increases for distances greater than 30 mm from the wire (Meigooni *et al.* 1988). For iodine-125 there is general agreement that a correction factor of 0.70 is appropriate (Huang *et al.* 1990).

6. The widely varying results obtained by different workers illustrates the need for careful consideration when the energy spectrum of the radiation is changing. However, such problems exist even when ionization chambers are used for dosimetry.

2.2.6 Angular dependence

The angular dependence of TLD is only a problem in so far as the orientation of the chips can affect the size of the cavity. This is more important for electrons and in brachytherapy, where the dose gradient may be high. However, it is always sensible to irradiate normal to the flat face of chips or to the long axis of microrods.

2.2.7 Fading

Fading is the term applied to the decrease in the thermoluminescent signal between irradiation and read-out. This is caused by electrons in the lower energy traps moving into the stable state. Fading is increased by exposure to UV light, especially for lithium borate. Because it is essentially a thermodynamic effect, it is the lower temperature traps that are most affected. The read-out cycle should include a pre-read-out anneal at about 80°C in order to eliminate the signal from the low-temperature peaks. If large numbers of chips are to be read out at one time, the duration of the read cycle can be reduced by annealing all the chips together at 80°C in a separate oven. To allow the lowest temperature peaks to decay, some people recommend waiting 30 minutes after irradiation before reading the dosimeters, but this should be unnecessary with a suitable read cycle.

2.2.8 Background signals

Some dose will be recorded even if the dosimeters have not been irradiated. Under normal circumstances, background signals will be no more 0.2 mGy. The background signal comes from several sources.

1. The dark current of the photomultiplier: this current increases with exposure to light and it is, therefore, important to leave the instrument for several hours to settle down whenever the photomultiplier is exposed to ambient light. Ideally, the power to the photo-multiplier should be permanently on. This also improves the stability of calibration. (The Harshaw 5500 reader uses Peltier cooling to eliminate the warm-up effect.)

2. Residual signals from previous irradiation: these can be removed by annealing (see next section). If dosimeters are to be used at the limit of their sensitivity, it is advisable to restrict the maximum dose to which they are exposed.

3. Background luminescence: unirradiated dosimeters produce a small luminescent signal. This may be due to chemical interactions in the surface of the dosimeters (chemiluminescence) or, particularly with powder, to movement in the crystal lattice (tribothermoluminescence). Background luminescence can be reduced by reading out the dosimeters in an atmosphere of oxygen free nitrogen. Although this is not really a problem for doses greater than 10 mGy, nitrogen also helps to reduce tarnishing of the trays and it is therefore advisable to use it as a matter of course.

The background signal should be checked first with the planchette on its own and then with an unirradiated chip. For most measurements in radiotherapy, background should not be a significant problem, but it is important to check that the residual TLD signal has been successfully eliminated by the chosen annealing cycle.

2.2.9 Annealing

The residual signal after the dosimeter has been read out is removed by heating the dosimeter to a temperature above the read-out temperature. A facility to do this is built into some readers. However, this increases the read-out time and is not fully effective, particularly if the dosimeters have been submitted to large doses, so it is better to use a separate annealing oven. Advice on suitable annealing cycles varies, but 400°C for 1.5 h followed by 16 h at 80°C has proved satisfactory with LiF:Mg,Ti. For LiF:Mg,Cu,P, it is important that the annealing temperature does not go above 240°C, as its sensitivity and energy independence will be reduced.

The annealing process not only removes residual signal, but also sets the sensitivity of the dosimeter. Therefore, batches of dosimeters should be subjected to an identical annealing cycle. This is achieved by putting all the dosimeters together into an oven in a tray made of stainless steel, glass, or anodized aluminium. (Ordinary aluminium may contaminate the dosimeters and should not be used). Metal trays have the advantage of conducting heat and, therefore, contributing to the uniformity of the heat treatment. Trays made in-house should have the holes counterbored so that the surface is smooth and flat, and all traces of oil must be removed.

The rate of cooling from 400 to 80°C determines the sensitivity of the dosimeters–the faster the cooling, the greater the sensitivity. It is advisable for quality assurance purposes to control the annealing process to maintain constant sensitivity from one annealing to the next. High sensitivity is not usually important for radiotherapy and, therefore, it is sensible to choose a slower cooling rate that can be controlled, if such a facility is provided on the oven.

2.2.10 Glow curves

The glow curve (Figure 11.3) is a plot of the output of the photomultiplier against time. It is usual also to superimpose a plot of the heater temperature (which, however, may differ from the temperature of the dosimeter). Most modern readers have a built-in computer interface that permits storage and display of the glow curves. This is a useful facility, as it allows retrospective analysis of the glow curve in the event of unexpected readings.

The heating cycle is in three phases: a low temperature pre-read-out anneal to eliminate the low-temperature peaks; the measurement phase, when the light output from the main peak is integrated; and a high-temperature post-read-out anneal. The latter is optional but it enables

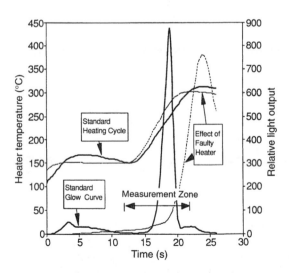

Figure 11.3 Standard glow curve and heating curve for lithium fluoride read in a Rialto reader. The left-hand axis shows the heater temperature and the right-hand axis the counts from the current-to-frequency converter. The counts are only integrated during the period marked 'Measurement Zone'. The effect of a faulty heater is also shown. The overshoot on the heater curve is related to the thermal inertia of the system.

a check to be made that read-out is complete. The duration and temperature of each of these phases can usually be adjusted by the user, but in most cases the cycle recommended by the reader manufacturer can be used. Regular monitoring of the glow curve is an important tool in the quality assurance of the TLD process. The heater curve should not vary, but small variations may be seen in the shape of the glow curve. The integration period of the instrument should be set to include the whole of the main peak. One of the most common faults is poor thermal contact with the heater (especially in the type of reader that uses electrical heating rather than hot nitrogen) and this can be detected by a shift and broadening of the peak, as shown in Figure 11.3.

Glow curve deconvolution can be carried out on glow curves stored in the computer to separate out the individual peaks mathematically (Pla and Podgorsak, 1983). This can enable a reduction in the read-out time, as the need for separation of the low-temperature peaks by the pre-heating period is reduced. It is also possible to use the ratio of the different peaks that fade at different rates to establish the time elapsed since irradiation and to eliminate errors due to fading (Section 2.2.7). These facilities are not essential for radiotherapy purposes.

2.2.11 Calibration

The calibration technique used depends on the form of dosimeter and the accuracy required. A detailed description will be given of the procedures appropriate to chips and microrods. The dosimeters are divided into calibration batches: these should be as large as possible because several of the dosimeters have to be used for calibration purposes. The maximum number is limited by the stability of the reader calibration and the need to ensure that the whole batch is subjected to an identical annealing cycle. An appropriate number is 120, for most purposes. Each new batch must be irradiated and annealed once or twice before reliable results are obtained, although for this purpose it is not essential that all the chips get the same dose. (It is believed that the effect of these preliminary irradiations is to fill up some traps permanently).

After the initial pre-irradiation at least three irradiations must be performed, taking care to give the same dose to each dosimeter. This is conveniently done in a cobalt-60 beam, laying out the chips side by side in a contiguous array. The array should be laid out on a clean sheet of paper on some appropriate built-up material and then covered with another sheet of paper and more build-up material. The deviation of the readings of each chip from the mean of the batch is then calculated, together with the variation of the readings of the individual chips. Subsequent action depends on the calibration method chosen.

1. Method A. All those chips whose calibration falls outside an acceptable calibration range are discarded and subsequent calibrations are carried out assuming that all chips are equally sensitive. This method achieves the least precision.

2. Method B. Chips are sorted into order of increasing sensitivity and are then put into pairs taking a chip from the most sensitive end and one from the least sensitive end. Provided that chips are then kept in their pairs, the average sensitivity of each pair will be approximately the same.

3. Method C. Sorted chips are placed into rows of 10 chips in which they are all numbered 1–10. Rows are labelled A, B, C, etc. Chips 5 and 6 of each row are then used as calibration chips for the row. Chips are normally irradiated in pairs in order to increase precision.

4. Method D. The identity of each individual chip is retained and a chip calibration factor, C_{chip}, calculated for it by the method described below. A number of chips are chosen at random to obtain the batch calibration factor, N_{batch}. (It should be noted that, while it is not essential, it is wise to sort the chips as in Method C, because this reduces the error introduced if neighbouring chips are inadvertently exchanged).

The precision achievable by Method A is limited by the batch variability. Method B is a simple way of improving precision. Method C is appropriate if chips are to be used for many different beam energies or for infrequent use, as each row may be calibrated as required. Method D is the most satisfactory method because it allows easier measurement and control of the variability of the data; this method will, therefore, be described in detail.

The n chips are annealed, irradiated to an equal dose and read out m times. Let R_{ij} denote the jth reading of the ith chip. The first step is to calculate the chip calibration factor, C_{ij}, for each individual chip, to convert its reading to the mean of the batch:

$$C_{ij} = \frac{\sum_{i=1}^{n} R_{ij}}{nR_{ij}}.$$

The average calibration factor for each chip, C_i, is then:

$$C_i = \frac{\sum_{j=1}^{m} C_{ij}}{m}.$$

The per cent standard deviation of C_{ij} can also be calculated:

$$SD = \frac{100}{C_i}\left[\frac{1}{m-1}\sum_{j=1}^{m}(C_i - C_{ij})^2\right]^{1/2}.$$

There is no reason to suppose that the standard deviation for any one chip is any different from that of any other, so it is appropriate to calculate a pooled estimate:

$$SD = 100\left\{\frac{\left[\sum_{j=1}^{m}\sum_{i=1}^{n}(C_i - C_{ij})^2\right]^{1/2}}{n(m-1)}\right\}$$

when estimating the precision of an individual measurement made subsequently (the mean value of C_i is 1.0 by definition). It should be noted that the per cent standard deviation of the whole batch SD_{batch} is in general greater and is given by:

$$SD_{batch} = \left[\frac{1}{n}\sum_{i=1}^{n}(C_i - 1)^2\right]^{1/2}.$$

SD_{batch} is a measure of the precision to be obtained by Method A. However, if chips have been selected from a larger batch by the manufacturer, the batch may not follow a normal distribution and statistical calculations may then be misleading. If $SD_i > 3SD$ it is an indication that there is something wrong with the individual chip. If the chips are read out after the first one or two irradiations and these calculations are performed, it will be noted that the variability of C_{ij} will be greater, but it will eventually settle down. SD should be around 2.5% of the mean, but it is claimed that some dosimeters and readers can achieve a standard deviation as low as 1%.

Each time the chips are annealed, a number p of dosimeters are selected at random and given a known dose of radiation, in order to measure the conversion factor to Gy to water, $N_{w,batch}$. This calibration should be carried out using the radiation quality to be used for the subsequent measurements. However, a cobalt-60 beam is often used because of its stability, in which case an energy correction should be applied for other beam qualities (see Section 2.2.5). A jig should be made so that the dosimeters can be irradiated simultaneously with an ionization chamber placed at the same depth. The depth should be beyond the depth of dose maximum to avoid problems of ion chamber calibration at d_{max} (see Section 2.3.8). The ion chamber and dosimeters should be placed in a circle about the centre of the radiation beam. For maximum accuracy, a Perspex tube with a hole to contain the TLDs can be made to fit into the Perspex phantom used to intercompare ionization chambers at a depth of 50 mm. This allows a direct substitution to be made between the TLD and the ion chamber. At kilovoltage energies, the dosimeters should be on a line perpendicular to the central axis of the tube to avoid the heel effect. If R_i are the readings of the chips and D_i is the dose given to each, then:

$$N_{w,batch} = \frac{1}{p} \sum_{i=1}^{p} \frac{D_i}{R_i C_i}$$

p should be at least 6, as this allows a reasonably accurate independent estimate of the standard deviation (SD) that will alert the user to problems with the system. The other $n-p$ dosimeters may be used to carry out dose measurements. The dose is given by:

$$D = (R - \text{background})N_{w,batch} \cdot C_i \cdot C_{supralin} \cdot C_{energy}$$

where $C_{supralin}$ and C_{energy} are supralinearity and energy corrections as discussed in Sections 2.2.4 and 2.2.5, respectively.

The standard error to be expected for an individual measurement can be calculated as follows. Suppose that q chips are used for the measurement. Then the per cent standard error (SE) of the final result is:

$$SE = \left(\frac{SD^2}{p} + \frac{SD^2}{q} + \frac{SD^2}{m}\right)^{1/2}. \quad (4)$$

Equation (4) is important because it demonstrates the equal importance of m, p, and q in determining the precision of the final result. Equation (4) allows an estimate also of the precision for Methods B and C, if we equate the process of sorting to that of establishing an individual C_i. For Method A, the per cent standard error of a measurement is given by:

$$SE = \left[\left(\frac{SD_{batch}}{p}\right)^2 + \left(\frac{SD_{batch}}{q}\right)^2\right]^{1/2}. \quad (5)$$

Comparison of the results of equations (4) and (5) provides an objective criterion for choosing the calibration method to be adopted.

The use of powder is described in detail by McKinlay (1981). Equal quantities of the powder are dispensed into sachets before irradiation using a special dispenser. After irradiation, all the powder from each sachet is transferred to the planchette and read-out. For the greatest accuracy, portions of powder sufficient for several read-outs are put in the sachet and then dispensed directly onto the planchette after irradiation, but this is too time consuming for routine work. Several samples from each batch are given a known dose and a calibration factor can then be derived as for Method A.

2.2.12 Packaging and handling

Some ways of packaging TLD materials are shown in Figure 11.4. The walls of the packaging material should be as tissue-equivalent as possible, so that they do not affect the energy response. UV radiation can have an effect in increasing both the background and fading. Neither effect is likely to be a problem with lithium

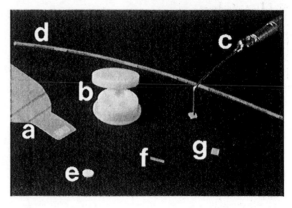

Figure 11.4 Different forms of TLD materials and appropriate packaging for *in vivo* measurements: (a) plastic sachet into which two chips are sealed – suitable for eye-dose measurement; (b) rigid containers used for TBI measurements; (c) vacuum 'tweezers' used to handle chips; (d) LiF microrods in polythene tubes suitable for intracavitary measurements; (e), (g) two forms of LiF chips; (f) LiF microrod.

fluoride for therapeutic doses, but it is advisable to avoid exposure to UV light and to store the dosimeters in the dark. However, in most cases it is critical to be able to place the dosimeters at exactly the spot at which the measurement is required. For this reason, the packaging for *in vivo* measurements should be transparent. Loose powder should be stored in a dark glass bottle, which should be shaken before the powder is dispensed.

It is essential that TLD materials do not become contaminated, especially with grease. They must, therefore, not be touched by hand. The only really satisfactory method of handling rigid materials is to use vacuum tweezers (see Figure 11.4c). If chips become contaminated, they should be washed in pure methanol and rinsed in deionized water. However, it is not recommended that this should be a frequent procedure. Severely contaminated dosimeters should be discarded. Planchettes should be cleaned in a similar way.

Planchette reflectivity may change the measured light output by several per cent and cleaning should not, therefore, take place between read-out of the batch calibration chips and the measurement chips. Variation in reflectivity between planchettes is a problem for automatic readers. A non-reflecting planchette would solve this problem, but a suitable material has so far proved elusive. Higher precision can be achieved in manual mode with only one planchette, or by associating specific chips with specific planchettes (Wood and Mayles 1995).

2.2.13 Quality control

A check-list of quality assurance procedures is given in Table 11.2. Good records are essential and these should

Table 11.2 Regular checks on TLD systems

Check	Frequency	Notes
Standard deviation	Each Anneal	Based on Calibration chips
Glow curves	Monthly	Against reference curve
Planchette cleanliness	Daily	
Internal light source	Daily	Stability within 2%
Background without chip	Daily	Before use
Background with unirradiated chip	Monthly	
Oven temperature	On acceptance	And if a problem is suspected
Batch calibration stability	Each anneal	Stability within 2%
External light source	3 monthly	Not possible for all readers

be set up so that changes in reader sensitivity and reproducibility can be detected quickly.

If TLD records are kept in a computer, it should be easy to monitor the standard deviations of chips used for batch calibrations. The ratio of the readings of chips irradiated in pairs can also be monitored. If SD is the expected standard deviation of dosimeter readings (see Section 2.2.11) the standard deviation of the ratio of the two chips will be approximately $SD\sqrt{2}$. It will probably be a little greater than this in practice because some chip pairs may not have been given identical doses.

With accurate temperature control of the oven, the batch calibration factor $N_{w,batch}$ should remain constant within 1 or 2%. Although stability of $N_{w,batch}$ is not essential for dosimetry purposes, it is a very sensitive measure of the reproducibility of the annealing cycle. Provided that $N_{w,batch}$ remains constant and the TLD background signal is low, there is no need for further checks on the oven. However, when installing a new oven, it is wise to carry out an independent check of the temperature.

Most readers have an internal light source and the readings obtained with this should be monitored. An external light source is also useful as it provides an independent check of the reader sensitivity. In dual-channel readers it is necessary to check that the two channels have the same sensitivity by reading out a number of chips that have been given a known dose in both channels. All such checks carried out on the instrument should be recorded, together with records of any repairs carried out and of any changes made to the settings of the reader.

2.3 Semiconductor dosimetry

Semiconductor diodes are useful in radiation dosimetry because of their high-radiation sensitivity relative to the ionization volume. Therefore, the measuring volume can be very small, leading to good spatial resolution, particularly when compared with a conventional air-filled ion chamber. Semiconductor diodes offer many advantages for clinical dosimetry: high sensitivity, real-time read-out, simple instrumentation, robustness, and air

pressure independence. However, a rigorous dosimetry system cannot be developed unless many parameters associated with the diode output are taken into consideration. Many data on the properties of diodes are available (see, for example: Rikner and Grusell 1987, Dixon and Ekstrand 1982). Some of these properties are considered below.

2.3.1 Theory of operation

Most semiconductor diodes are made from silicon that is either n type (silicon doped with group V material, e.g. phosphorus) or p type (silicon doped with group III material e.g. boron). To form a detector, a p–n junction must be created.

During irradiation, electron-hole pairs are created. Not only are they formed in the depletion region (which has a built-in voltage across it) but also carriers are created outside it in the body of the detector, which may diffuse into the depletion region. The charge carriers are swept across the depletion region and collected rapidly under the action of the field that exists across it. In this way a current is generated, flowing in the reverse direction to normal diode current flow. The rise time can be fast enough (approximately 1000 times faster than in an ion chamber) to see individual pulses of a linear accelerator, but it is dependent on the way the detector is operated.

Diodes for dosimetry are operated without an external reverse bias voltage to minimize leakage. Without external bias, the output signal of the diode can be measured in short-circuit mode (current) or open-circuit mode (voltage); a simple electrometer can be used in each case. The short-circuit mode is the mode of choice since it has the advantage of producing a linear relationship between the charge generated in the diode and the dose. In the short-circuit mode, the electrometer must have a low dynamic input impedance, as is provided by an operational amplifier with a feedback loop and a low offset voltage (Figure 11.5). As the diode signal is quite high, the electrometer used needs only to have moderate gain. Several multi-channel electrometers are available commercially.

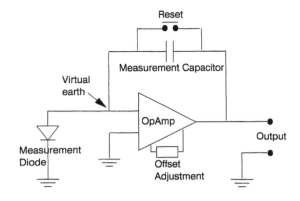

Figure 11.5 Simple short-circuit mode electrometer suitable for dose measurement with diodes.

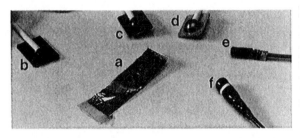

Figure 11.6 A selection of diodes for patient measurements: (a) an unencapsulated diode; (b) an encapsulated diode but without build-up; (c) diode for cobalt-60 (can also be used in electron beams); (d) diode for 4–6 MV (similar diodes are available for 8–10 MV); (e), (f) cylindrical diode encapsulations suitable for both surface and depth measurements.

2.3.2 Diode encapsulation

Diodes are fragile and need to be encapsulated, as shown in Figure 11.6. For most patient measurements, peak doses are required and the diode encapsulation can be designed to incorporate the necessary build-up material. If unit density material were used it would be inconveniently bulky. To reduce the bulk, stainless steel can be used as part of the build-up. The construction of such a diode suitable for patient measurements is shown in Figure 11.7.

2.3.3 Temperature effects

The internal resistance of a diode decreases as the diode temperature increases. The sensitivity usually increases with temperature but has also been found to decrease. This is due to changes in parameters such as carrier mobility and the number of traps in the detector crystal. The variation of sensitivity with temperature depends on the accumulated dose received by the diode. Typically, the sensitivity will increase with temperature by less than

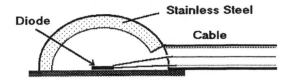

Figure 11.7 The construction of a Scanditronix EDP-10 diode for surface measurements in photon beams.

0.1% per °C when the diode has not been irradiated, but after a dose of 6 kGy with 20 MeV electrons (more with photons) this may increase to 0.4% per °C. (It should be noted that some manufacturers usually supply pre-irradiated diodes, as this reduces the initial rate of change of the calibration factor). When a diode is placed on a patient its temperature will rise by about 10°C from room temperature in 2–3 minutes and then reach a steady state. If the sensitivity variation is found to be significant, the diodes should be left to reach body temperature for at least 3 minutes before the measurement is begun and a correction made for the difference in temperature between calibration and measurement. Diodes can be calibrated at body temperature using a water phantom containing warm water.

2.3.4 Background signal

Even in the unbiased mode of operation, a diode will generate a 'dark' current due to thermally generated charge carriers. This is only a problem when low doses and dose rates are being measured and if the input offset voltage of the electrometer is not zero. The background signal is strongly temperature dependent and some diodes generate increasingly high currents as the temperature rises, even at reasonably low accumulated doses. The background signal can change by 4 mGy min^{-1} between room temperature and body temperature. The effect appears to be greater for n-type diodes than for p-type diodes. Although the current can be zeroed out before measurements are taken, several minutes are necessary to obtain a satisfactory background measurement and any subsequent change in temperature will upset the balance of the circuit and cause a change in diode response.

2.3.5 Radiation damage

Radiation damage occurs when silicon atoms are displaced from their lattice sites. This introduces recombination centres, which capture charge carriers leading to a reduction in sensitivity and an increased dose rate dependence. p-type diodes are less affected by radiation damage than are n-type diodes, which show a pronounced drop in sensitivity with accumulated radiation dose (Figure 11.8). The amount of damage for a given dose is dependent on radiation quality, for example, 20 MeV electrons are 20 times more damaging

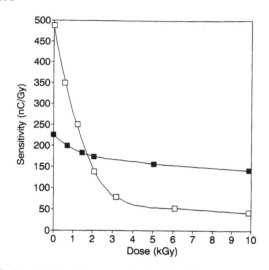

Figure 11.8 Variation in diode sensitivity with accumulated radiation dose for p-type diodes (■) and n-type diodes (□). Plotted from data supplied by Scanditronix.

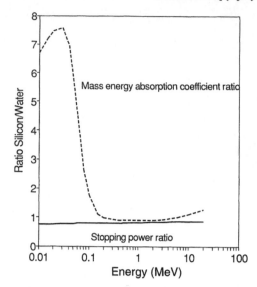

Figure 11.9 Variation with energy of mass energy absorption coefficient and stopping power ratios of silicon to water. The difference in scale compared with Figure 11.2 should be noted.

than 8 MV photons. When subjected to radiation damage, n-type diode response becomes non-linear with dose rate. Therefore, the more expensive p-type diodes are recommended for general use, as they show a linear response with dose rate, even after very high dose irradiation, and have a smaller sensitivity drop with accumulated dose. n-type diodes can be used in cobalt-60 beams. They can be pre-irradiated to overcome the initial sensitivity drop, if they are not being used in situations where the dose rate will vary significantly.

2.3.6 Energy dependence

As can be seen from Figure 11.9, silicon is far from being tissue-equivalent, especially for low-energy radiation. For this reason, energy-compensated diodes (as described by Rikner and Grusell (1985)) must be used for water-phantom dosimetry in photon beams. The stainless steel used to provide the build-up material for surface dose measurements also has the effect of shielding the diode from low-energy scattered radiation. Care must be taken when making measurements at depth or in TBI fields, where low-energy scattered radiation contributes a substantial fraction of the dose.

2.3.7 Angular dependence

For domed diodes (as in Figure 11.6c and d, directional dependence does not become a significant factor until the radiation is angled greater than 30° from a line perpendicular to the diode base-plate. The actual dependence is related to the shape and construction of the diode. In most applications, the diodes will be placed on a surface perpendicular to the radiation beam axis and so correction factors can be neglected. However, the

diodes do exhibit an asymmetry of calibration that can be as much as 15% when irradiated from the flat side compared to irradiation from the domed side. Cylindrical diodes (as in Figure 11.6e and f) have a cylindrically symmetrical response, but the response reduces by about 15% towards the tip.

2.3.8 Calibration

Calibration of diodes is in two parts: calibration against an ion chamber in a standard set-up to establish the diode calibration factor for absorbed dose to water $N_{w,diode}$ and the establishment of a series of correction factors to account for calibration differences when measurements are performed under various experimental conditions. The values of $N_{w,diode}$ for individual diodes may vary widely, but the correction factors will usually be close to 1.0 and will be similar for diodes of the same type. For diodes that are to be used for surface dose measurements, the ion chamber should be placed at the depth of peak build-up and the diodes on the surface of the phantom. If the ion chamber is calibrated to read accurately at 5-cm deep, with its effective point of measurement taken as its geometric centre (as is the case for National Physical Laboratory calibrations), a correction must be applied (about 1%) when the chamber is placed at d_{max}. Care must be taken that the diodes do not affect the dose to the ion chamber. A circular arrangement should be used to exploit the circular symmetry of most radiation beams. (The circular symmetry can be checked by repeating the calibration at different orientations of the phantom). If D is the absorbed dose to water received by the ion

Table 11.3 Correction factors needed to enable diodes to be used for *in vivo* dose measurements

Factor	Symbol	Frequency of checks	Notes
Standards corrections			
Diode sensivity	N_i	Weekly	Daily for maximum accuracy
Dark current	I_o	Daily	May be temperature dependent
Dark current at body temperature	I_{temp}	3 monthly	Only important for low dose rates
Temperature	C_{temp}	6 monthly	May need to be more frequent
Angle of incidence	C_{angle}	Annually	Unlikely to change. Depends on encapsulation
Dose rate	C_{pulse}	Annually	Only a problem in pulsed beams
Energy	C_{energy}	Annually	
Factors specific to entry and exit dose measurements			
Field size	C_{field}	Annually	Should be close to 1.0 if the diode build-up is sufficient
Wedge	C_{wedge}	Annually	Affected by change in dose per pulse and in the energy spectrum
SSD	C_{SSD}	Annually	In addition to inverse square correction
Exit dose	C_{exit}	Annually	Specific to exit doses
Patient thickness	$C_{thickness}$	Annually	Usually 1.0 for entrance doses

chamber, R_i is the reading of ith diode and d_{max} the depth of dose maximum, the calibration factor $N_{w,i}$ of an individual diode is given by:

$$N_{w,i} = \frac{D}{R_i} \frac{(\text{SSD} + d_{max})^2}{\text{SSD}^2}.$$

Diodes that are to be used inside a phantom can be placed at the same distance from the source as the ion chamber, and the SSD correction is not then necessary. In this case, it is appropriate to carry out the calibration at a depth of 50 mm. Table 11.3 lists factors for which corrections may need to be established. Experience has shown that type tests are not sufficient, as large differences can be seen between diodes of the same type. Therefore, each radiotherapy centre should establish the responses of their diodes under the various conditions encountered and monitor them as the cumulative dose to the diodes increases. C_{energy} corrects from the standard set-up at the standard energy to the standard set-up at the measurement energy. C_{pulse} is difficult to measure directly but is effectively included in other corrections such as C_{wedge}.

In measuring entrance and exit doses, the positions of the diode and the ion chamber are the same as in the calibration set-up but with different field size, etc. The correction factors are each measured relative to the standard set-up. When an entrance dose measurement is made, the dose D for a diode reading R is calculated according to the formula:

$$D = (R - I_{temp})N_{w,i}C_{wedge}C_{SSD}C_{field}C_{temp}C_{thickness}. \quad (6)$$

Although each correction factor needs to be measured for every diode, it is usually possible to use a single factor for all diodes. For entrance doses, $C_{thickness}$ can usually be ignored. C_{exit} is the ratio, corrected for the difference in SSD, of the dose to an ion chamber at the peak depth on the exit side of the phantom to the reading of the diode placed on the exit surface at the standard field size. It is a combination of the effects of the different backscatter conditions and the angular dependence for radiation incident on the flat face of the diode. The appropriate factor will depend on whether the exit surface is in air or on a couch-top. C_{wedge}, C_{SSD}, C_{field}, and $C_{thickness}$ will have to be measured again for the exit surface. Typical values for these factors and further details will be found in Leunens *et al.* (1990), Heukelom *et al.* (1991), and Van Dam and Marinello (1994), although their definitions differ in respect to inclusion of SSD corrections.

2.3.9 Quality control

Table 11.3 shows the frequency at which corrections need to be checked. For critical applications, such as TBI dosimetry, the sensitivity should be checked daily. Frequency of checks may be adjusted according to the frequency of use of the diodes and the variability encountered.

2.4 Other dosimetry systems

One alternative system uses the electron spin resonance (ESR) due to free radicals induced in alanine (Regulla and Deffner 1982). Alanine is almost perfectly tissue-equivalent and has a density of 1.1. In addition to its tissue-equivalence, the ESR signal is stable for years without fading and read-out of the ESR signal does not destroy the information. The problems with what seems to be an ideal system for *in vivo* dosimetry are that the ESR spectrometer needed is expensive and the minimum useful dose is about 1 Gy, but the National Physical Laboratory will provide and read out dosimeters.

Much work has been done in recent years to find alternative methods of dosimetry. The radiation damage to MOSFETs alters their threshold voltage, which is approximately linearly proportional to the dose delivered (Soubra *et al*. 1994). Since the damage is permanent, the detectors can provide a permanent record of the dose delivered. In order to improve the linearity of the response it is necessary to provide a small bias voltage while the detectors are irradiated, but unlike diodes they do not have to be connected to the read-out system during irradiation. Precision in the region of 3% can be achieved for cumulative doses up to about 10 Gy. The minimum dose increment that can be conveniently measured is around 500 mGy.

Diamonds have also been used for dosimetry, either as a TLD material or as an ionization detector (Heydarian *et al*. 1996). Carbon is a good dosimeter material as its response is moderately energy independent.

It is possible to use photographic film for *in vivo* dosimetry. If the dose information on a film is to be useful, it requires careful control of the processor. Most radiotherapy departments have now dispensed with their manual developing systems and frequently use small automatic processors. Control of these is usually less satisfactory, partly because the low volume of films processed results in less frequent replacement of the chemicals. For this reason, film may be unsuitable for routine dosimetry. Film is calibrated by exposing different areas of the film to different doses. (An optical sensitometer, which exposes a small area of the film to an optical step wedge, can be used to monitor film sensitivity thereafter). The optical density of the film is proportional to the logarithm of the radiation dose above a threshold level. However, it is just as easy to plot optical density against dose and fit a smooth curve rather than rely on the logarithmic nature of the relationship. Therapy verification film is ideal for dosimetry purposes because a dose of around 1 Gy can be given. A full discussion of photographic dosimetry is given by Becker (1973).

In addition to photographic film, a new material called GafChromic film (Chiu-Tsao *et al*. 1994) has become available. This film is only slightly sensitive to optical radiation but changes colour and optical density when irradiated with X-rays. Ideally, the resulting optical density of the film should be measured at a wavelength of around 630 nm. If red light is used, the dose response

is more nearly linear and the film is more sensitive. The film is relatively expensive but because it does not require blackout conditions, it can be useful for measurements in phantoms to verify dose distributions in unusual situations. However, Zhu *et al*. (1997) report problems with recent batches.

Much recent interest has been shown in using ferrous sulphate (Chan and Ayyangar 1995) or, more recently, BANG gels (Maryanski *et al*. 1996) for volume dosimetry. These gels can be formed into appropriately shaped phantoms. They are then irradiated and a three-dimensional dose distribution may then be obtained by magnetic resonance imaging. The magnetic resonance signal is approximately proportional to dose. Accuracy claimed with ferrous sulphate gels (Chan and Ayyangar 1995) is only around 5%, but BANG gels can give better accuracy (Maryanski *et al*. 1996). This provides the only method of obtaining a fully three-dimensional dose distribution in a phantom.

2.5   Clinical situations

2.5.1   Practical considerations for in vivo measurements

Accurate *in vivo* dosimetry is a particularly demanding area of radiotherapy physics that is all too often treated as a trivial routine task. The following are the factors to be considered before any *in vivo* measurement.

1. What is the aim of the measurement? Is it the skin dose, the peak dose, or the dose at a point deep in tissue that is required? If it is the 'skin' dose, at what depth should this be measured?

2. Can the expected dose be estimated?

3. Is the measurement point in an area of high-dose gradient?

4. What is the most appropriate dosimeter and how should it be packaged?

5. How accurate does the measurement need to be and what precautions are needed to achieve this level of accuracy?

6. Should a separate measurement be made for each treatment field?

Figure 11.10 shows a possible format for reporting the measurements. Typical results are given in the first column. The following should be considered in preparing the report.

1. Application of the appropriate correction factors.

2. Comparison of the result with the expected result. Non-medical staff should be aware of what constitutes an acceptable reading, so that ways of solving a problem can be considered at the earliest opportunity.

IN VIVO DOSIMETRY

Patient Name: Hospital Number:

Consultant:

Date of measurement	1st June 1997		
Site	Left eye		
Dosimeter identification	A1 Batch G		
Build-up used	1cm wax		
Field(s) treated	All		
Changes to original field?			
Dose delivered to prescription point:	1.8 Gy		
Expected dose at measurement site:	0.1 Gy		
Reader output	0.31		
Measured dose	0.25 Gy		
Standard error	± 0.01 Gy		
Dose as percentage of dose to prescription point	13.9%		
Comment	Field to close to eye?		
Checked by	A. Physicist		
Is dose acceptable?	No		
Proposed action	Move field 3 mm posteriorly		
Radiotherapist signature	A. Radiotherapist		

Figure 11.10 A possible format for recording and reporting routine *in vivo* dose measurements.

3. Consideration of the precision achieved. Differences between duplicate readings may indicate that the dosimeters were in an area of high-dose gradient. If two readings differ, there is a temptation to reject the one that is least satisfactory without any strong scientific justification. This temptation should be resisted.

4. Follow-up of differences between the observed and expected results and of imprecise readings. For example, the measurement may not have been carried out as planned. The likelihood of an incorrect reading must be balanced against the risk of giving a further excess dose and consideration given to repeating the measurement rather than changing the set-up on the basis of an inaccurate result.

5. Checking the results by a second person.

Table 11.4 lists some of the advantages and disadvantages that may influence the choice between the different methods of dosimetry.

2.5.2 Routine quality assurance by in vivo dosimetry

Entrance or exit-dose measurements may be made on a regular basis as the ultimate test of the treatment-

Table 11.4 Advantages and disadvantages of some dosimetry systems for radiotherapy dosimetry

Dosimeter	Advantages	Disadvantages	Uses	Comments
TLD	Small – easily inserted into cavities Detector-elements are cheap Reasonably tissue-equivalent Can record many simultaneous results Versatile packaging No wires	No permanent record Easy to lose a reading Accurate results require care Read-out and calibration time consuming Statistical precision poor	General *in vivo* dosimetry Eye doses TBI dosimetry Solid-phantom measurements Protection measurements	
Diodes	Small size High sensitivity Instant read-out No bias voltage Simple instrumentation	Requires connection cables Background signal for low dose rates Long-term calibration drift Variability of calibration with temperature Unreliable	Water tank dosimetry TBI dosimetry Electron measurements Eye doses General *in vivo* dosimetry	MOSFETs similar, but are less precise. Connecting wires are not needed. They can be used for *in vivo* dosimetry when high doses are expected.
Film	High spatial resolution Very thin – so does not perturb beam	Processing hard to control Must be kept dark Difficult to use with patients Sensitivity varies across film Variation between films and batches	Electron phantom dosimetry Phantom measurements	GafChromic film similar, but requires high doses. It does not require to be handled in the dark and is more tissue equivalent. It is expensive.
MR gels	3-D dose distributions Good spatial resolution	Difficult to handle Requires MR scanner	Phantom measurements – particularly for conformal therapy	
Ion chamber	Accurate and precise Necessary corrections well understood Reliable Instant read-out	Connection cables needed Requires high voltage Requires temperature and pressure corrections Large measurement volume Fragile	Output calibrations Water-phantom measurements Absolute-dose measurements	
Alanine	Very tissue-equivalent Signal not erased with read-out	Very large capital cost Not commercially available in hospitals High doses needed	Absolute-dose measurements Solid-phantom measurements Treatment-dose measurements	

planning and delivery process. Entrance-dose measurements can provide a check of the following:

(1) machine calibration;

(2) wedge filters and other beam modifiers;

(3) patient position in relation to the accelerator.

Exit-dose measurements check the above factors, as well as beam alignment, and the radiological thickness of the patient (i.e. the thickness corrected for differences in attenuation at the energy of interest). A useful review of the application of *in vivo* dosimetry is given in Essers and Mijnheer (1999).

Diodes are most commonly used and a description of the calibration procedures is given in Section 2.3.8. Most of the corrections described would also be needed if measurements were made with TLD dosimeters, although the correction factors are likely to be smaller. For comparison with the measurements, it is necessary to calculate the expected entrance and exit doses for each beam. The entrance dose is simply the peak dose for the field size corrected for any accessories used. Exit-dose calculations must account for the lack of backscatter beyond the exit surface of the patient; this is not a correction to the dose reading, but rather a correction to the planning-computer calculation. When measuring entrance doses, the build-up material on the dosimeter will perturb the beam significantly (the dose at 100 mm deep may be reduced by up to 5%) and will increase the skin dose. Therefore, it is advisable to limit entrance-dose measurements to a small proportion of the total number of fractions. Exit doses do not present this problem, but are harder to interpret because so many different factors contribute to them. When entrance and exit doses are being measured simultaneously, the diode on the exit surface should be placed away from the centre of the beam, so that it is not affected by the diode on the entrance surface.

2.5.3   Total body irradiation

Doses for TBI are difficult to calculate accurately from first principles because of the very large fields employed, the increased effect of scattered radiation, and the need to correct for tissue inhomogeneities. For this reason it is essential to make confirmatory measurements, even if calculation is to be the method of determining the treatment time. It is usual for the treatment technique to be designed to bring the dose maximum to the surface (e.g. by the use of a Perspex screen). The dose measured on the surface is a measure of the maximum dose delivered to the patient. If the mid-point dose is required, a conversion factor dependent on the radiological thickness of the patient must be applied. This may be measured by making both entrance- and exit-dose measurements. If the dose prescription is based on lung tolerance, the maximum dose to lung is the appropriate measurement to make. TLD is the most straightforward dosimetry method because the calibration does not depend on beam direction and energy, but diode measurements offer the advantage of giving immediate results. The correction factors described in Section 2.3.8 must be measured under TBI conditions. For low dose rate, single-fraction TBI, the diode dark current, and particularly its variation with diode temperature, has proved a significant problem. A useful account of TBI dosimetry is given by Sánchez-Doblado *et al.* (1995).

2.5.4   Skin-dose measurement

The surface dose is affected by the field size and the presence of beam-modifying devices and is consequently difficult to calculate accurately. It is important to decide at what depth the dose is to be measured and, if necessary, to apply an appropriate thickness of build-up material. TLD chips are well suited to skin-dose measurements because they are the appropriate thickness to represent the sensitive layers of the skin. Examples of situations where skin doses are of interest are measurements to determine the adequacy of build-up material (e.g. over scar tissue or superficial tumours) and monitoring the loss of skin sparing due to beam direction shells or shadow trays.

2.5.5   Eye doses

One of the most common measurements is that of the lens dose in situations where the treatment field comes close to the eye (e.g. Chapter 8, Section 6.7). Here it must be borne in mind that the sensitive tissue is the lens and not the eyelid, where doses are most easily measured. A phantom study carried out by Harnett *et al.* (1987) suggests that for lateral irradiation, a dosimeter placed on the outer canthus may give a more accurate estimate of lens dose than one placed on the eyelid, but even that may seriously underestimate the lens dose. If anterior beams are used, the surface dose just outside the beam edge may actually overestimate the lens dose because of electron contamination of the radiation reaching the dosimeter (an effect that can easily be demonstrated if a film is exposed at the edge of a megavoltage beam with build-up material covering only half of the film). The inaccuracy in the measurement of the lens dose will be less significant if the determination of the dose limit was based on measurements performed in a similar way. Diodes can be used, as well as TLD, and have the advantage of enabling the contribution of individual fields to be determined, but care needs to be taken in interpreting the results because of the directional response.

2.5.6 Field matching

Diodes are well suited to determination of the position of the beam edge and ensuring satisfactory matching on the surface. It is not necessary to place a diode at the 50% point exactly, because fall-off in dose with distance from the beam centre in the penumbra region is approximately linear (about 10% reduction per millimetre for an accelerator). When matching two beams, the dosimeter should be left in place while both beams are treated because a small inaccuracy in placement of the dosimeter may give a false result. Surface-dose matching is not necessarily an appropriate index of the success of matching at depth (see Chapter 8, Section 2.1.4).

2.5.7 Dynamic therapy

The advent of computer-controlled linear accelerators raises the possibility of more complicated treatment arrangements aimed at better conformation of the treatment volume to the target volume. The confidence to place the necessary reliance on the control software will be based on verification by *in vivo* measurements. When the collimator jaws are moved dynamically, the dose delivered is proportional to the collimator opening. Therefore, verification of dose is particularly important. (This contrasts with traditional arc therapy for which the dose rate at the isocentre is insensitive to the beam direction, so that deviations in the speed of gantry rotation have only a second-order effect on the dose distribution). A similar problem is presented by scanning-beam accelerators. Multiple diodes are useful for verification of such treatments because they permit the monitoring of both instantaneous dose rate and total dose. Phantom measurements will also be necessary (see Section 2.6.3).

2.5.8 Rectal-dose measurements

One of the dangers in treating the cervix with brachytherapy is that of giving a high dose to the rectum. To guard against this, it is advisable to use a rectal probe at the time of insertion of the applicators. Diodes mounted at the end of a rigid rod are ideal for this purpose. The rod is graduated, so that the depth of insertion can be monitored, while measurements are made at several points in the rectum to ensure that the maximum dose rate is determined. With remote after-loading techniques, low-activity source trains can be used to make the measurement. It is important to carry out rectal measurements while it is still possible to adjust the packing of the sources, if the results of monitoring require it. Because radiation damage to the detector is unlikely to be a problem and the maximum available sensitivity is required, n-type silicon can be used. In many centres, it is felt that a more satisfactory determination of rectal dose can be made by taking

radiographs with contrast medium in the rectum. However, if this method is used, it will be more inconvenient to adjust the packing of the sources to reduce the rectal dose.

2.5.9 Iridium implant dosimetry

The accuracy that can be achieved with flexible iridium implants depends on the stability of the implant during the course of the treatment and on the accuracy of dose calculation. In addition, the dose to the skin surface overlying the implant is of interest. For this purpose, TLD microrods contained in a nylon tube can be used (see Figure 11.4d). The microrods can also be inserted into the nylon tubes used for implantation as described by Dawes *et al.* (1988).

2.6 Phantom measurements

2.6.1 Phantom materials

Details of suitable phantom materials can be found in ICRU (1989). Water is an appropriate material: it has the advantage of conducting electricity – as required for electron measurements (Galbraith *et al.* 1984) – and is universally available. However, for radiation from isotope sources used in brachytherapy, it may not match particular tissues as well as expected and it is difficult to simulate irregular contours. Epoxy-resin-based tissue substitutes can be made following the detailed instructions given by White *et al.* (1977), but in practice it may be simpler to purchase the phantom.

Elliptical, oval, or cylindrical phantoms of the appropriate radii are useful for simulating body and limb cross-sections. However, homogeneous phantoms with regular shapes are not a good representation of real patients and can give a misleading impression of the accuracy of computer calculations. Humanoid phantoms, made of tissue-equivalent material and containing material to represent inhomogeneities (Figure 11.11), are available but are expensive. For the most accurate measurements, it is necessary to be able to insert an ionization chamber into the phantom.

2.6.2 Confirmation of in vivo measurements

In some clinical situations, *in vivo* measurements can give unexpected results, even when the uncertainties in the measurements have been accounted for. For example, an unexpected high eye-dose may be recorded, despite apparently correct field-edge placement and lead-shielding positioning. Phantom measurements will give information on whether the dose is as a result of some form of electron contamination or due to internal or external scattered radiation. Daily set-up inaccuracies can also be excluded as a source of error. Phantom

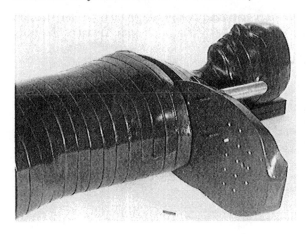

Figure 11.11 'Rando' anthropomorphic phantom. The phantom is divided into sections that allow the insertion of TLD dosimeters in plugs.

measurements are necessary to establish the relationship between surface-dose measurements and doses at depth.

2.6.3 Checks on dose calculations

Phantom measurements should be made to ensure that new treatment techniques are satisfactory in terms of dosimetry before they are used for patient treatments. Computer calculations often give inaccurate results when calculating the dose to a critical structure outside the plane of the treatment plan and may not represent the effect of patient contour and tissue inhomogeneities accurately.

Treatment-planning algorithms should be verified by designing appropriate phantoms to test potential weaknesses. For example, electron-calculation algorithms have difficulty simulating isodoses immediately below sharply changing contours, as might be found when additional build-up material is used to boost a skin dose. Step phantoms can be used to measure the potential calculation error in these situations.

In vivo measurements can be made but, because they introduce additional uncertainties, surface doses are not a useful test of dose-calculation algorithms. If a convenient body cavity is available, TLD dosimeters can often be inserted in an appropriate package (e.g. microrods inside a naso-gastric tube). Dynamic treatments should be verified before using them on a patient. This can be done by calculating a similar plan for a phantom. Film is a convenient way of measuring the dose distributions produced, especially as its continuous nature means that localized hot-spots will be easily identified. Manufacturers are developing new approaches to these problems and recent developments include multiplexed diode arrays and thin flexible sheets of TLDs spaced on 5 mm centres, which are read out in a special reader.

3. Verification of positional accuracy

There is increasing awareness that positional accuracy is at least as important as dosimetric accuracy in radical radiotherapy. This is especially important when field sizes are being minimized in order to allow an increase in the dose. The traditional method of assessing positional accuracy has been to take a port film, but the use of digital imaging methods is increasing.

3.1 The nature of set-up errors

ICRU (1993) identifies three components of the target volume in radiotherapy:

(1) the overt tumour – the gross tumour volume (GTV);
(2) an allowance for microscopic spread of the tumour (the biological margin) leading to the clinical target volume (CTV);
(3) an allowance for set-up variability and inaccuracy (the technical margin) leading to the planning target volume (PTV).

The margin between the CTV and the PTV should include an allowance for movement of the target within the patient, which is more difficult to quantify. This is expressly recognized in the new concept of the internal target volume (ITV) being developed by ICRU. The CTV–ITV margin should not simply be added to the ITV–PTV margin because both internal movement and set-up errors are random variations and should, therefore, be combined in quadrature. In order to deliver an adequate dose to the PTV, an additional margin is required between the field edge and the PTV to allow for the fall-off in dose in the beam penumbra. In modern radiotherapy the aim is to reduce the technical margin to the minimum width since, for a typical 60 mm diameter target volume, an increase of 5 mm (8%) in the margin will increase the volume of tissue irradiated by 27%. It is nevertheless essential that the CTV is adequately treated and a reduction in the PTV must be accompanied by improved geometric accuracy of treatment delivery. Similar consideration in analysing set-up errors should also be given to the necessity of margins around organs at risk.

The aim of the treatment set-up process is to place the centre of a radiation field of the correct shape in the intended position. The treated field may be in error, relative to the PTV, in one or more of the following ways:

(1) the shape of the field may be incorrect;
(2) the field centre may be transposed in either (or both) of the two directions orthogonal to the beam axis;
(3) the field may be rotated about the axis of the beam;

(4) the direction of the field may be rotated about the axis of rotation of the gantry, a so called 'out-of-plane rotation'.

These errors are called 'field placement errors', although in practice it is usually the PTV, or the patient, that is incorrectly positioned rather than the beam.

If the patient is treated on a number of occasions, the magnitude of these errors will vary randomly according to the precision of set-up and it is these random errors that are allowed for in the margin between the PTV and the CTV. In addition, there may be a systematic difference between the intended and actual set-up. Verification seeks to correct any systematic error and to determine the size of the technical margin required to allow for the random errors. Two secondary possibilities arise. First, if it were possible to obtain an instant indication of the field placement error, it would be possible to adjust the set-up to correct the error. Second, because a portal image is essentially an attenuation map of the patient, there is the potential for dose verification through transmission dosimetry.

3.2 Limitations to verification

The major difficulty in verification is that megavoltage beam images have inherently poor contrast. A 10-mm thick bone that produces a contrast of 18% at 50 kV will produce a contrast of only about 2% at 6 MV. Since it is often impossible to identify the tumour on a diagnostic film, it is almost always impossible to identify it on a megavoltage film. Radio-opaque markers have been inserted into tumours in order to overcome this difficulty (Vigneault *et al.* 1997), but it is usual to base decisions on bony landmarks and air cavities that may be separated from the PTV by several centimetres. One way of overcoming these limitations is to attach a diagnostic tube to the head of the therapy machine so that, by rotating the gantry through a fixed angle, an exact replication of the therapy situation can be achieved (Biggs *et al.* 1985), but this is rather cumbersome. The use of a low-energy target in the accelerator head has also been proposed (Tsechanski *et al.* 1997).

A second limiting factor is that a film of a therapy portal is a two-dimensional image, whereas the treatment volume is three-dimensional. This is not quite as serious a limitation as it might at first appear because errors in the distance of tissue from the source will only have a secondary effect on the dose. (For example, a 10 mm error parallel to the beam axis will only affect the dose by a few per cent, whereas a similar error perpendicular to the beam at the beam edge may reduce the dose by 90%).

3.3 Therapy verification films

A number of specially designed verification films are available for taking portal images at high energies.

Although the best images are obtained with specially formulated films, such as Kodak XOmat TL, it is possible to obtain satisfactory images with less expensive film suitable for industrial radiography (Roberts 1996). These films require about 20 mGy for a satisfactory image, can be used both to verify the set-up before the patient is treated and as a confirmatory check, and are suitable for dual exposure techniques (see Section 3.5). Very slow films that can be left in the beam throughout the treatment are also available. These are particularly useful for reproducibility studies.

In order to reduce the dose needed to form an image, a cassette with lead screens can be used. The screen generates secondary electrons to produce build-up and high-density materials are used so that these secondary electrons are generated in close proximity to the film. Some improvement in the image is achieved with a copper screen on the patient side, and such a cassette is available commercially (Kodak L). When the film is placed very close to the patient, the lead screen also has the advantage of stopping secondary electrons and some low-energy scattered radiation produced in the patient. A new cassette film combination, Kodak EC-L, uses a fluorescent screen and provides significantly increased contrast.

3.4 Digital imaging devices

A useful review of electronic portal imaging devices (EPIDs) is given by Boyer *et al.* (1992). There are obvious advantages associated with digital imaging devices rigidly attached to the treatment machine and all linear accelerator manufacturers now market some such device. Most of the devices are based on a video camera (Munro *et al.* 1990) which, with the aid of a 45° mirror, views a phosphor-coated metal plate. Such devices have inherently good resolution and have the advantage that, with frame averaging, the time necessary to obtain an image can be chosen depending on whether the primary requirement is a rapid image or a noise-free image. However, they are bulky and may impede the use of the machine. Another commercial device uses a matrix ionization chamber filled with an organic liquid (Van Herk and Meertens 1988). By switching the high voltage from one cell to another it is possible to read out each of the 256 × 256 cells of the detector. This device inherently uses signal averaging over about 1 second because of charge storage in the liquid.

3.5 Improving image quality

The position of the image detector relative to the patient can affect image quality. Traditional radiological practice is to place the film as close to the patient as possible to improve the sharpness of the image. In making a megavoltage image this is not usually the best solution.

Bissonnette *et al.* (1994) have shown that for TV camera-based systems optimization of modulation transfer function is achieved with a magnification of around 1.6, while for optimization of the signal to noise ratio a magnification of at least 2 is better. For film, both considerations are optimized with minimum magnification (i.e. with the film as close to the patient as possible). An additional consideration is the effect of scatter, which can be reduced by increasing the distance between the patient and the image detector. A separation of 0.4 m is sufficient for this (Swindell *et al.* 1991). This is an important consideration for transit dosimetry.

3.6 Quality control

Quality control of EPIDs is very important. The 'Las Vegas' phantom (Herman *et al.* 1994), which is simply an aluminium plate with circular cut-outs of varying thickness and diameter, is a widely used method of assessing achievable contrast, but analysis of the results is somewhat subjective. An objective test phantom, the images from which can be automatically analysed by a computer, has been developed by Rajapakshe *et al.* (1996). This includes grids to demonstrate spatial resolution as well. This is important, as a common fault with TV-based devices is that the camera lens focus is inaccurately set.

In addition to the image quality, it is also necessary to verify the geometric accuracy of the system. A simple phantom consisting of a grid of wires mounted so that it can be rotated about the axis of rotation of the treatment machine has been developed by Kirby (1995). This phantom can also be used to verify the relationship between the centre of the image and the centre of the radiation field for those EPIDs that are rigidly mounted to the gantry (so that this relationship should be constant).

3.7 Measurement of field-placement errors

3.7.1 Establishment of the reference image

Field-placement errors must be measured relative to some agreed 'correct' field position. This is usually done from simulator check films taken as the final verification of the treatment plan. However, there are a number of pitfalls that must be borne in mind if these are to be a reliable basis for the analysis of set-up errors. In the first place, many target volumes will have been defined on the basis of CT data. The sagittal position of the centre of the target volume may be identified from a 'scanogram' (also called a 'topogram' or 'scout view' – the image generated by moving the patient through the stationary fan-beam). A scanogram differs from a simulator film in being formed by a beam that is divergent only in the transverse plane, whereas the simulator beam diverges in both directions. For this reason, structural relationships

will only be the same at the beam centre. Second, simulators are subject to inaccuracies in the same way as the treatment machines. This is a particular problem in the case of older simulators, where the tolerances specified were often significantly less severe than those specified for treatment machines. Third, it is often difficult to establish the correctness of an oblique view taken on a simulator on the basis of direct comparison with CT, and these views are commonly taken on trust. Finally, the assumption is made that the patient was in the same position on the simulator as on the CT scanner. As they become more familiar with the hospital environment, patients often become more relaxed and this may affect the relationship of the tumour to the bony landmarks that are used to check the beam alignment on the simulator. Although not all these problems can be overcome, the fundamental rule should be to try to relate back to the criteria used by the radiotherapist when defining the target volume.

The analysis of the portal images will be based on the identification of bony landmarks, so it is necessary to establish the relationship of these to the target volume. Comparisons with CT-based field definitions should ideally be made on the basis of digitally reconstructed radiographs (DRR) (Sherouse *et al.* 1990; Wong *et al.* 1990), although these, like the CT data themselves, suffer from inherently poor resolution in the sagittal direction. For this reason, it is often more important to have a smaller CT slice spacing at the edge of the target volume than at the centre – the reverse of traditional practice. For satisfactory DRRs, a maximum slice spacing of 5 mm is required. Some centres are using CT simulation, where the patient is marked up for treatment on the CT scanner couch and the simulator verification films are replaced altogether with DRRs (see Chapter 7, Section 6). However, the simulator still has the advantage of being able to show movement of the internal anatomy. The ultimate form of verification is to take a CT image in the treatment position on the therapy machine (Lewis *et al.* 1992), but this technology is still under development and the limitations of machine time will probably restrict its use to particularly critical applications and to specific studies of accuracy.

3.7.2 Creating the image

In order to make it easier to relate the portal image to the patient's anatomy, it is common practice to use a double-exposure technique. An initial exposure is made with the treatment field size and any additional shielding. The field is then opened up to produce a 50-mm border and a second exposure made with no additional shielding. In carrying out such procedures, it is important to avoid giving excess dose to particularly sensitive structures, such as the eyes, which should remain shielded. The double-exposure technique may be appropriate to establish a reference portal image, but it is clearly impractical for multiple images throughout the course of treatment.

An independent verification of the position of the field centre can be achieved by temporarily mounting a plate containing a metal cross on, or below, the shadow tray of the accelerator while the image is being taken. The detector must be held normal to the radiation beam to prevent image distortion. Operation is simpler if the detector is rigidly fixed in relation to the beam.

3.7.3 Imaging processing

Portal images have inherently poor contrast and basic processing is helpful to improve the contrast. The simplest way to do this is to adjust the windowing, so that the full dynamic range of the display is used. This is most conveniently done using histogram equalization. Various forms of processing have been developed to improve the visibility of image features (Leszczynski *et al.* 1990). It may also be necessary to correct distortion in images captured electronically.

3.7.4 Measurement techniques

Portal films can be compared with a reference image by visual inspection, but to use all the information available in the image is very time consuming. The advent of electronic portal imaging devices has lead to rapid development of techniques for computer assisted analysis of portal images. However, these techniques are not limited to portal images obtained with electronic devices, since good quality digital images can also be obtained by scanning film – indeed some studies have suggested that film images are superior to EPID images. Analysis packages are supplied with imaging devices, but device independent packages are also available (Wong *et al.* 1995; Shalev *et al.* 1996).

The first step in the analysis of a portal image is to establish the position of the field borders, and this should be done before applying image enhancement techniques. Numerous methods for extracting the edges have been described. At the simplest level, this involves finding the isodose line at 50% of the average dose in the field (Evans *et al.* 1992) or the steepest dose gradient. For noisy images and for non-uniform dose distributions, more sophisticated methods are needed (Gilhuijs *et al.* 1995; Wang and Fallone 1995). Having identified the position of the field edge the orientation can be matched to that of the reference image and the magnification corrected if necessary, assuming that the field shape is approximately correct.

There are several techniques for manual matching of the portal image to the reference image. The simplest is to identify points (at least three) on each image and then to calculate the rotation and translation necessary to align them. Alternatively, outlines of the anatomy can be drawn on the two images. The outlines can then be compared either automatically by chamfer matching (which seeks to minimize the discrepancy between the lines) or manually by moving the template drawn on the reference image so that it aligns with the portal image. A more direct approach is to match the two images visually. This can be done by alternating the two images on the screen, while moving the position of one of them until the apparent movement between the two images disappears (Evans *et al.* 1992), or by using a look-through technique, as in the PIPS system (Shalev *et al.* 1996).

Ideally, image matching would be carried out automatically by the computer, but it has proved difficult to achieve this reliably, particularly with small fields. Chamfer matching has been used successfully to match the reference template to edges extracted automatically from the portal image (Fritsch *et al.* 1995; Gilhuijs *et al.* 1995). Some success has also been achieved with cross-correlation of greyscale images (Dong and Boyer 1995), but this approach will be sensitive to the presence of artefacts, such as bowel gas, in the image.

3.7.5 Correction of field placement errors

Correction of field placement errors must be carried out with care. For inter-treatment corrections, it is the systematic component of the error that is to be corrected. If the random set-up errors are greater than the systematic error, a correction based on a single portal image may actually result in a less accurate treatment. Shalev has suggested reducing the correction made by a 'factor of maximum likelihood' defined as:

$$\sigma_s^2 / (\sigma_s^2 + \sigma_r^2)$$

where σ_s and σ_r are the standard deviation of the systematic errors and the random errors, respectively. The threshold, α, for making corrections should be proportional to:

$$\sigma_r / \sqrt{n}$$

where n is the number of measurements made (Bel *et al.* 1996). Pouliot and Lirette (1996) combining these approaches found that the optimum policy was to use a threshold of:

$$2 \, \sigma_r / \sqrt{n}$$

and to carry out repeat measurements on the two subsequent fractions following correction. There is conflicting evidence as to whether the mean set-up position remains stable throughout the course of treatment. If it does not, it is clearly necessary to repeat measurements at intervals during the treatment.

Some studies have been carried out looking at the possibility of measuring and correcting the set-up error at the start of each treatment (Gildersleve *et al.* 1994). This significantly improves the accuracy of treatment delivery and eliminates the need to distinguish random and systematic errors, but has a significant time penalty at present.

3.8 Portal image dosimetry

The radiation dose measured at the detector is related to the attenuation through the patient and to the input dose. If the dose distribution expected at the detector is calculated, this can be compared with the measured dose distribution (Wong *et al.* 1990). A more ambitious approach is to backproject the portal image into the patient and to recalculate the dose distribution (Hansen *et al.* 1996).

If the detector is sufficiently far from the patient to reduce scatter to a minimum, the image should give an accurate estimate of the radiological thickness of the patient. In the case of parallel opposed beams, these data can be used to design compensators (Evans *et al.* 1995).

4. Treatment machine verification

There is abundant evidence that mistakes in treatment set-up occasionally occur even with highly trained staff. Computer verification of treatment parameters allows such errors to be corrected before the machine is turned on. In this section, the factors necessary to derive the maximum benefit from such systems are considered.

Further information can be found in Podmaniczky *et al.* (1985).

4.1 Verification of machine operation

Traditionally, the principal monitoring circuits have been directed towards ensuring that the machine is working correctly. Examples include mechanical position interlocks, electronic beam flatness monitors, and two-channel dosimetry systems, where the magnitude of the difference between the channels is monitored. Malfunctions of such monitoring systems are not uncommon, and in a busy department there will be pressure to override them. On some machines an override key is provided for this purpose, while on others the same effect can be achieved more subtly by adjusting the gain of the detector circuits. Such action should only be taken as a last resort and then only after a thorough investigation of the causes of the fault. Even if the fault is relatively minor, correction should be a matter of priority as it is dangerous for use of the override facility to become routine. Several machine malfunctions that have led to incorrect patient doses have occurred when fault warnings have been overridden.

4.2 Verification of treatment parameters

A computerized verification system aims to compare the dose and the set-up parameters with the prescription.

Table 11.5 Verification parameters and recommended tolerance tables for routine use

Patient identification
Mode of treatment (photons or electrons) and treatment technique (static or arc therapy)
Treatment plan, treatment field, and fraction numbers
Beam energy and dose rate
Monitor units – open field and wedged field
Daily target and reference point doses (optional)
Cumulative dose (optional)
Wedge number and blocking tray number (optional)
Gantry stop angle and increment angle (for arc therapy)

	Units	Tolerance table number:			
		1	2	3	4
Gantry angle	Degrees	1.0	1.0	1.0	20.0
Collimator	Degrees	1.0	1.0	10.0	20.0
Field X and Y	mm	1	2	5	10
OFFSET X and Y	mm	1	1	1	
Couch height	mm	10	20	20	(*)
Couch lateral and longitudinal	mm	10	200	200	(*)
Couch rotation	Degrees	1.0	1.0	10.0	(*)
Floor rotation	Degrees	1.0	(*)	(*)	(*)

1. Smallest tolerances: for accurate treatments with the patient immobilized on the couch.
2. Small tolerances except on couch lateral and longitudinal movement: for isocentric treatments where patients are not immobilized on the couch.
3. Wide tolerances on all parameters: for palliative parallel opposed treatments.
4. Maximum flexibility: for static electron treatments.
*No verification of these parameters.

Patient identification data, machine parameters, and dose prescription are entered into the computer beforehand. At the time of treatment, the patient is first identified and the machine set-up parameters are recalled from the data base. After the field has been set up, the computer gives a warning (and usually inhibits treatment) if there is a difference between the parameters set and those in the database. Table 11.5 lists the machine parameters that a typical system will verify. (Some of these may not apply to particular machines).

To allow for patient variations from day to day, verification systems must be able to accept minor deviations from the data base value. This is achieved by defining tolerances for each parameter depending on the type of treatment. A complete set of tolerances is called a 'tolerance table'. For each treatment, an appropriate tolerance table is specified. Recommended values are given in Table 11.5. To avoid confusion, it is wise to limit the number of tolerance tables, but some additional tables may be required for specialized treatments.

Some systems use a default tolerance table, unless one is specifically selected. The default table should be the most restrictive, to ensure that wide tolerances are not selected unintentionally.

4.3   Computer assisted set-up

Verification systems have been slow to become accepted for several reasons:

(1) entry of data is time consuming;

(2) system malfunctions were common;

(3) mistrust of computers.

Key factors in their increasing acceptance are a greater awareness of safety, an increase in sophistication of techniques, and the availability of computer assisted set-up. Assisted set-up allows the computer to set the machine parameters once the patient is positioned on the couch. This facility is most useful for setting the collimator jaw positions, gantry angle, and collimator rotation. On some machines, the couch can also be set automatically, but this is only useful when the patient is at the same point on the couch each day. Local procedures for using assisted set-up should include the following:

1.   The isocentre position must be at the desired point in the patient (or the patient in the correct position on the couch, if couch movements are to be computer controlled) before activating the 'auto set-up' facility.

2.   After using assisted set-up, the field position must be checked on the patient (e.g. field light position and SSD indicated by the optical indicator) before leaving the room.

3.   The first treatment should be set-up manually.

4.   The operator must be alert throughout to the possibility of collision.

The assisted set-up facility can also be used from the treatment console to move the machine between fields. This will substantially reduce the time for which the patient has to lie on the couch and so reduce patient movement errors. When using this facility, the following additional guide-lines should be adhered to.

1.   The patient must be warned that the gantry and collimators will move during the treatment and reassured that there is no danger.

2.   The position of the patient must be monitored throughout using closed-circuit TV and laser axis lights.

3.   If computer control of couch movements is to be included, a dummy run should be carried out before leaving the treatment room because of the increased risk of collision.

4.   Parameters that are allowed to be changed under computer control must be monitored by two independent circuits. Sometimes the resolution of the secondary monitor is not as high as that of the primary monitor, so that the degree of security is not as high as it seems.

5.   The gantry should not be moved from outside the room if lead trays or electron applicators are attached to the head.

4.4   Recording patient data

In addition to storing the preset values for the parameters that are being verified, the computer can also keep a record of the actual machine settings used and any overrides or machine failures that occurred. As with any data base, it is essential, indeed, in the UK, a legal requirement of the Data Protection Act, that the data base is correct. It may be necessary to make entries manually when patients are treated on more than one treatment machine. A printed record should also be kept, ideally on a patient record card and on a daily record sheet of all treatments carried out.

A worthwhile option is the recording of cumulative target dose as treatment progresses by summing the contribution from all the fields. This gives the machine the ability to identify when the prescribed target dose has been reached. However, maintaining the accuracy of this record can require considerable effort if machine break-downs lead to inaccurate data. The associated option to calculate cumulative doses at other sites, such as the spinal cord, is less useful.

4.5   Networks

Some form of data transfer from the simulator or the treatment-planning computer is desirable if the maximum benefit is to be obtained from computerization, although there is a danger that staff will become less vigilant (see Section 4.6.1). If several treatment machines are to be networked together, sufficient data must be stored locally in each accelerator to enable it to operate in stand-alone mode for at least a day in the event of failure of the network.

Data protocols independent of treatment machine manufacturers are essential, because a high proportion of departments have machines from more than one manufacturer. Standardization has finally been achieved with the publication of the DICOM 3 standard, which now has a radiotherapy-specific section (DICOM 1997). This defines the order in which patient-specific information is required to be transmitted and also specifies the network protocol for transmission of the data. A rather simpler protocol to implement is the AAPM format (Baxter *et al.* 1982), which provides patient data in ASCII format with a series of standard field names, which are included in the file, such as 'Patient name:='.

Properly designed networks can bring many advantages, including immediate access to the current state of a patient's treatment by a doctor in the clinic. Additional features include booking patients efficiently on machines, allocating clinic times to patients, and producing statistical data. In order to avoid the need for duplicate entries, the radiotherapy network should ideally be linked to the main hospital patient administration system.

4.6 Practical considerations

4.6.1 Data checking

Any mistakes made at the data entry stage are likely to be carried through the whole treatment and, therefore, have graver consequences than random mistakes made during the course of a treatment. For this reason, data must be entered by qualified staff and then checked by a second authorized person. Incidents of data corruption must be thoroughly investigated and the causes eradicated, although corrupt data will usually prevent treatment rather than cause it to be delivered incorrectly. Data transferred automatically from the planning computer may not have the correct machine angle settings, for example, a couch angle may be simulated on a two-dimensional coronal plan as a gantry angle. Carefully thought out procedures must be written to ensure that data that has been transferred automatically is appropriate. Digital data-checking protocols can help with this, but should not be relied on exclusively. When data have been transferred from the planning computer, the most secure system is for the operator to retype the data into the verification system, which can then verify the entries (but this concept must be supported by the manufacturers). Particular care must be taken to ensure that items,

such as wedge orientation, are correct as they may not be correctly set on the simulator. A system that simply involves visual comparison of two sets of numbers is prone to error (as anyone who has proof read text will testify). Ways of ensuring active comparison of the data should be encouraged.

4.6.2 Improving patient throughput

Verification systems can reduce patient throughput significantly. However, some measures can be taken to prevent this:

1. A second terminal can be supplied, so that the data base can be updated while the machine is being used to treat patients.

2. Single-character data entry can be used for standard text items like consultants' names.

3. It should be possible to copy beam data to a second beam and then edit any different parameters.

4. For the initial data input, rapid transfer of the treatment machine set-up parameters into the data base, by copying the parameters that have been manually set, should be provided.

5. Maximum use should be made of assisted set-up.

4.6.3 System administration

Most systems require a system manager whose role can include data back-up, the assignment of passwords, and customization of the user interface. It is essential that this person be familiar with computers. The system manager should become thoroughly familiar with the system, since apparent drawbacks of the system frequently prove to be due to lack of knowledge by the users.

Proper staff training is essential to the successful implementation of computer verification. Formal arrangements must be made to ensure that operators new to the machine are properly trained, rather than just picking it up as they go along. This also applies to physics staff.

To ensure that patient data are properly safeguarded, the verification system should be password protected. Different passwords can be allocated to allow different levels of access. If required, password access can also be used to prevent junior staff from entering or changing patient data. For security to be effective it is important that users log out when the machine is unattended.

4.6.4 Verification films

The taking of therapy verification films (see Section 3.5) can be particularly difficult with computerized accelerators if a well thought out facility is not provided. The requirement is to make a short exposure with the treatment field size, to open each jaw by a fixed amount (about 50 mm), and then to make a second exposure;

both exposures should be taken without a wedge. The number of monitor units required may be different for different situations and must, therefore, be easily adjustable. Ideally, the dose given should be deducted from the monitor units for that field. However, the contribution to the total dose will usually be relatively small and the increased complication may not be justified.

4.6.5 System override

There will be times when the field settings need to be modified at treatment time. In this case, an override facility allows treatment to proceed even though the parameters are not those in the data base. A record should be kept of the reason for the override. If the change is to be permanent, the data base must be updated as soon as possible.

5. Summary and conclusions

In vivo dosimetry is an important part of the quality-control process in radiotherapy, but verification of dose should also extend to establishing that the beam is irradiating the desired target volume. Thermoluminescence dosimetry is the most accurate form of *in vivo* dosimetry, but diodes are more precise and, provided that they are appropriately calibrated, are a convenient alternative. Without improved verification methods, attempts to reduce the margin between the biological target and the treated volume may result in reduced local control because of inaccurate delivery.

6. References

Baxter, B.S., Hitchner, L.E., and Maguire, Jr, G.Q. (1982). *A standard format for digital image exchange*. AAPM Report 10. American Institute of Physics, New York.

Becker, K. (1973). *Solid state dosimetry*. CRC Press, Cleveland, OH.

Bel, A., Vos, P.H., Rodrigus, P.T.R., Creutzberg, C.L., Visser, A.G., Stroom, J.C. *et al.* (1996). High-precision prostate cancer irradiation by clinical application of an offline patient setup verification procedure, using portal imaging. *Int. J. Radiat. Oncol. Biol. Phys.*, **35**, 321–32.

Biggs, P.J., Goitein, M., and Russell, M.D. (1985). A diagnostic X-ray field verification device for a 10 MV linear accelerator. *Int. J. Radiat. Oncol. Biol. Phys.*, **11**, 635–43.

Bissonnette, J.P., Jaffray, D.A., Fenster, A., and Munro, P. (1994). Optimal radiographic magnification for portal imaging. *Med. Phys.*, **21**, 1435–45.

Boyer, A.L., Antonuk, L., Fenster, A., Van Herk, M., Meertens, H., Munro, P. *et al.* (1992). A review of electronic portal imaging devices (EPIDs). *Med. Phys.*, **19**, 1–16.

Chan, M.F., and Ayyangar, K.M. (1995). Confirmation of target localization and dosimetry for 3D conformal radiotherapy

treatment planning by MR imaging of a ferrous sulfate gel head phantom. *Med. Phys.*, **22**, 1171–5.

Chiu-Tsao, S.T., de-la-Zerda, A., Lin, J., and Kim, J.H. (1994). High-sensitivity GafChromic film dosimetry. *Med. Phys.*, **21**, 651–7.

Dawes, P.J., Aird, E.G., and Crawshaw, I.P. (1988). Direct measurement of dose at depth in breast cancer using lithium fluoride. *Clin. Radiol.*, **39**, 301–4.

DICOM. Part 3, Supplement 11. (1997). National Electrical Manufacturers Association, Washington DC.

Dixon, R.L., and Ekstrand, K.E. (1982). Silicon diode dosimetry. *Int. J. Appl. Radiat. Isot.*, **33**, 1171–6.

Dong, L., and Boyer, A.L. (1995). An image correlation procedure for digitally reconstructed radiographs and electronic portal images. *Int. J. Radiat. Oncol. Biol. Phys.*, **33**, 1053–60.

Essers, M., and Mijnheer, B.J. (1999). *In vivo* dosimetry during external photon beam radiotherapy. *Int. J. Radiol. Biol. Phys.*, **43**, 245–59.

Evans, P.M., Gildersleve, J.Q., Morton, E.J., Swindell, W., Coles, R., Ferraro, M. *et al.* (1992). Image comparison techniques for use with megavoltage imaging systems. *Br. J. Radiol.*, **65**, 701–9.

Evans, P.M., Hansen, V.N., Mayles, W.P., Swindell, W., Torr, M., and Yarnold, J.R. (1995). Design of compensators for breast radiotherapy using electronic portal imaging. *Radiother. Oncol.*, **37**, 43–54.

Fritsch, D.S., Chaney, E.L., Boxwala, A., McAuliffe, M.J., Raghavan, S., Thall, A. *et al.* (1995). Core-based portal image registration for automatic radiotherapy treatment verification. *Int. J. Radiat. Oncol. Biol. Phys.*, **33**, 1287–300.

Furetta, C., Leroy, C., and Lamarche, F. (1994). A precise investigation on the TL behavior of Lif:Mg,Cu,P (GR-200A). *Med. Phys.*, **21**, 1605–9.

Galbraith, D.M., Rawlinson, J.A., and Munro, P. (1984). Dose errors due to charge storage in electron irradiated plastic phantoms. *Med. Phys.*, **11**, 197–203.

Gildersleve, J.Q., Dearnaley, D.P., Evans, P.M., Law, M., Rawlings, C., and Swindell, W. (1994). A randomized trial of patient repositioning during radiotherapy using a megavoltage imaging system. *Radiother. Oncol.*, **31**, 161–8.

Gilhuijs, K.G., Touw, A., van Herk, M., and Vijlbrief, R.E. (1995). Optimization of automatic portal image analysis. *Med. Phys.*, **22**, 1089–99.

Hansen, V.N., Evans, P.M., and Swindell, W. (1996). The application of transit dosimetry to precision radiotherapy. *Med. Phys.*, **23**, 713–21.

Harnett, A.N., Hirst, A., and Plowman, P.N. (1987). The eye in acute leukaemia. 1. Dosimetric analysis in cranial radiation prophylaxis. *Radiother. Oncol.*, **10**, 195–202.

Herman, M.G., Abrams, R.A., and Mayer, R.R. (1994). Clinical use of on-line portal imaging for daily patient treatment verification. *Int. J. Radiat. Oncol. Biol. Phys.*, **28**, 1017–23.

Heukelom, S., Lanson, J.H., and Mijnheer, B.J. (1991). Comparison of entrance and exit dose measurements using ionization chambers and silicon diodes. *Phys. Med. Biol.*, **36**, 47–60.

Heydarian, M., Hoban, P.W., and Beddoe, A.H. (1996). A comparison of dosimetry techniques in stereotactic radiosurgery. *Phys. Med. Biol.*, **41**, 93–110.

Horowitz, Y.S. (1981). The theoretical and microdosimetric basis of thermoluminescence and applications to dosimetry. *Phys. Med. Biol.*, **26**, 765–824.

Horowitz, Y.S. (1993). LiF:Mg,Ti versus LiF:Mg,Cu,P: The competition heats up. *Radiation Protection Dosimetry*, **47**, 135–41.

Huang, D.Y., Schell, M.C., Weaver, K.A., and Ling, C.C. (1990). Dose distribution of ^{125}I sources in different tissues. *Med. Phys.*, **17**, 826–32.

Hubbell, J.H. (1982). Photon mass attenuation and energy-absorption coefficients from 1 keV to 20 MeV. *Int. J. Appl. Radiat. Isot.*, **33**, 1171–6.

International Commission on Radiation Units and Measurements (1984). *Stopping powers for electrons and positrons*. ICRU Report 37. ICRU, Bethesda, MD.

International Commission on Radiation Units and Measurements (1989). *Tissue substitutes in radiation dosimetry and measurement*. ICRU Report 44. ICRU, Bethesda, MD.

International Commission on Radiation Units and Measurements (1993). *Prescribing, recording and reporting photon beam therapy*. ICRU Report 50. ICRU, Bethesda, MD.

Kirby, M.C. (1995). A multipurpose phantom for use with electronic portal imaging devices. *Phys. Med. Biol.* **40**, 323–34.

Leszczynski, K.W., Shalev, S., and Cosby, N.S. (1990). An adaptive technique for digital noise suppression in on-line portal imaging. *Phys. Med. Biol.*, **35**, 429–39.

Leunens, G., Van Dam, J., Dutreix, A., and Van der Schueren, E. (1990). Quality assurance in radiotherapy by *in vivo* dosimetry. 2. Determination of the target absorbed dose. *Radiother. Oncol.*, **19**, 73–87.

Lewis, D.G., Swindell, W., Morton, E.J., Evans, P.M., and Xiao, Z.R. (1992). A megavoltage CT scanner for radiotherapy verification. *Phys. Med. Biol.*, **37**, 1985–99.

Ma, C., and Nahum, A.E. (1991). Bragg-Gray theory and ion chamber dosimetry for photon beams. *Phys. Med. Biol.*, **36**, 413–28.

Maryanski, M.J., Ibbott, G.S., Eastman, P., Schulz, R.J., and Gore, J.C. (1996). Radiation therapy dosimetry using magnetic resonance imaging of polymer gels. *Med. Phys.*, **23**, 699–705.

McKinlay, A.F. (1981). *Thermoluminescence dosimetry*. Adam Hilger, Bristol.

Meigooni, A.S., Meli, J.A., and Nath, R. (1988). Influence of the variation of energy spectra with depth in the dosimetry of ^{192}Ir using LiF-TLD. *Phys. Med. Biol.*, **33**, 1159–70.

Mobit, P.N., Mayles, P., and Nahum, A.E. (1996a). The quality dependence of LiF-TLD in megavoltage photon beams: Monte Carlo simulation and experiments. *Phys. Med. Biol.*, **41**, 387–98.

Mobit, P.N., Nahum, A.E., and Mayles, P. (1996b). The energy correction factor of LiF thermoluminescent dosimeters in megavoltage electron beams: Monte Carlo simulations and experiments. *Phys. Med. Biol.*, **41**, 979–94.

Munro, P., Rawlinson, J.A., and Fenster, A. (1990). Therapy imaging: a signal-to-noise analysis of a fluoroscopic imaging system for radiotherapy localization. *Med. Phys.*, **17**, 763–72.

Nahum, A.E. (1996). Perturbation effects in dosimetry: Part I. Kilovoltage X-rays and electrons. *Phys. Med. Biol.*, **41**, 1531–80.

Pla, C., and Podgorsak, E.B. (1983). A computerized TLD system. *Med. Phys.*, **10**, 462–6.

Podmaniczky, K.C., Mohan, R., Kutcher, G.J., Kestler, C., and Vikram, B. (1985). Clinical experience with a computerized record and verify system. *Int. J. Radiat. Oncol. Biol. Phys.*, **11**, 1529–37.

Pouliot, J., and Lirette, A. (1996). Verification and correction of setup deviations in tangential breast irradiation using EPID: gain versus workload. *Med. Phys.*, **23**, 1393–8.

Rajapakshe, R., Luchka, K.B., and Shalev, S. (1996). A quality control test for electronic portal imaging devices. *Med. Phys.*, **23**, 1237–44.

Regulla, D.F., and Deffner, U. (1982). Dosimetry by ESR Spectroscopy of alanine. *Int. J. Appl. Radiat. Isot.*, **33**, 1101–14.

Rikner, G., and Grusell, E. (1985). Selective shielding of a p-Si detector for quality independence. *Acta Radiol. Oncol.*, **24**, 65–9.

Rikner, G., and Grusell, E. (1987). Patient dose measurements in photon fields by means of silicon semiconductor detectors. *Med. Phys.*, **14**, 870–3.

Robar, V., Zankowski, C., Pla, M.O., and Podgorsak, E.B. (1996). Thermoluminescent dosimetry in electron beams: energy dependence. *Med. Phys.*, **23**, 667–73.

Roberts, R. (1996). Portal imaging with film-cassette combinations: what film should we use? *Br. J. Radiol.*, **69**, 70–1.

Sánchez-Doblado, F., Quast, U., Arráns, R., Errazquin, L., Sánchez-Nieto, B., and Terro[']n, J.A. (1995). *Total body irradiation prior to bone marrow transplantation*. European group for Blood and Marrow Transplantation, Seville.

Shalev, S., Gluhchev, G., Chen, D., and Luchka, K. (1996). In *Quantitative imaging in oncology*, Ch. 5, p. 123. Proceeding, 19th L.H. Gray Conference. British Institute of Radiology, London.

Sherouse, G.W., Novins, K., and Chaney, E.L. (1990). Computation of digitally reconstructed radiographs for use in radiotherapy treatment design. *Int. J. Radiat. Oncol. Biol. Phys.*, **18**, 651–8.

Soubra, M., Cygler, J., and Mackay, G. (1994). Evaluation of a dual bias dual metal-oxide semiconductor field effect transistor detector as radiation dosimeter. *Med. Phys.*, **21**, 567–72.

Swindell, W., Morton, E.J., Evans, P.M., and Lewis, D.G. (1991). The design of megavoltage projection imaging systems: some theoretical aspects. *Med. Phys.*, **18**, 855–66.

Tsechanski, A., Bielajew, A.F., Faermann, S., and Krutman, Y. (1997). A target port for high quality portal imaging in linear accelerators. *Med. Biol. Eng. Comput.*, **35**, Supplement, Part 2, 1064.

Van Dam, J., and Marinello, G. (1994). *Methods for in vivo dosimetry in external radiotherapy*. Physics for Clinical Radiotherapy, Booklet no. 1, ESTRO/Garrant, Leuven.

van Herk, M., and Meertens, H. (1988). A matrix ionization chamber imaging device for on-line patient set-up verification during radiotherapy. *Radiother. Oncol.*, **11**, 369–78.

Vigneault, E., Pouliot, J., Laverdière, J., Roy, J., and Dorion, M. (1997). Electronic portal imaging device detection of radio-opaque markers for the evaluation of prostate position during megavoltage irradiation: a clinical study. *Int. J. Radiat. Oncol. Biol. Phys.*, **37**, 205–12.

Wang, H., and Fallone, B.G. (1995). A mathematical model of radiation field edge localization. *Med. Phys.*, **22**, 1107–15.

White, D.R., Martin, R.J., and Darlison, R. (1977). Epoxy resin-based tissue substitutes. *Br. J. Radiol.*, **50**, 814–21.

Wong, J.W., Slessinger, E.D., Hermes, R.E., Offutt, C.J., Roy, T., and Vannier, M.W. (1990). Portal dose images. I: Quantitative treatment plan verification. *Int. J. Radiat. Oncol. Biol. Phys.*, **18**, 1455–63.

Wong, J., Yan, D., Michalski, J., Graham, M., Halverson, K., Harms, W. *et al.* (1995). The cumulative verification image analysis tool for offline evaluation of portal images. *Int. J. Radiat. Oncol. Biol. Phys.*, **33**, 1301–10.

Wood, J., and Mayles, W.P.M. (1995). Factors affecting the precision of TLD dose measurements using an automatic TLD reader. *Phys. Med. Biol.*, **40**, 309–13.

World Health Organization (1988). *Quality assurance in radiotherapy*. WHO, Geneva.

Zhu, Y., Kirov, A.S., Mishra, V., Meigooni, A.S., and Williamson, J.F. (1997). Quantitative evaluation of radiochromic film response for two-dimensional dosimetry phantom. *Med. Phys.*, **24**, 223–31.

7. Additional reading

McKinlay, A.F. (1981). *Thermoluminescence dosimetry*. Adam Hilger, Bristol.

Oberhofer, M. and Scharmann, A. (ed.) (1979). *Applied thermoluminescence dosimetry*. Adam Hilger, Bristol.

International Commission on Radiation Units and Measurements (1987). *Use of computers in external beam radiotherapy procedures with high-energy photons and electrons.* ICRU Report 42.

International Commission on Radiation Units and Measurements (1989). *Tissue substitutes in radiation dosimetry and measurement.* ICRU Report 44.

Proceedings of the 8th international conference on solid state dosimetry. (1986). Oxford.

Radiation protection dosimetry **17** (1986). Nuclear Technology Publishing.

White, D.R. and Constantinou C. (1982). Anthropomorphic phantom materials. In *Progress in medical radiation physics 1.* (ed. C.G. Orton), pp. 133–89. Plenum Press, New York.

Chapter 12
Brachytherapy

E.G. Aird, J.R. Williams, and A. Rembowska

1. Introduction

Brachytherapy makes use of radioactive sources placed directly into, or immediately adjacent to, the volume of tissue to be treated. The main advantage of this type of therapy is that the very short source–tumour distance allows a high dose of radiation to be given to the tumour, while the surrounding normal tissues receive a low dose. There are three distinct types of brachytherapy: interstitial, intracavitary, and surface applicator.

In interstitial therapy, the sources are introduced surgically and are, therefore, in a form that is of small diameter to allow penetration into tissue. The most common sites treated are the tongue, the breast, the vulva, and the anus. Other less accessible sites, such as the prostate, can be treated by using special, localized techniques generally with iodine-125 seeds.

The use of radioactive sources in the uterus, around the cervix, and in the vagina for the treatment of gynaecological malignancies is the most common intracavitary brachytherapy technique. The sources can be in the form of tubes placed within rubber applicators, or they may be placed in shaped spacers made from rubber or other material in order to fit within the cavity to be treated and to reduce the dose rate to the tissues closest to the source. Several standard applicator systems have been developed for gynaecological treatments. Alternatively, and now more commonly, special applicators may be used that permit the loading of sources after the applicators have been placed within the patient. Afterloading systems are discussed in Section 5. Other sites into which sources may be introduced include the bronchus and the oesophagus.

Surface applicators, or moulds, were formerly an important area of sealed-source therapy. The rapid fall-off in dose into tissue made these especially suitable for those superficial tumours lying above particularly sensitive normal tissues. Their usefulness has diminished with the increasing availability of electron therapy units. One particular example of surface applicators has been in the treatment of ocular tumours, in which beta-emitting radionuclides may be used as well as photon emitters.

In all types of brachytherapy there are different methods by which the sources can be handled. Originally, all sources were manipulated by the surgeon or radiotherapist in theatre, which meant that all theatre staff could be exposed to high radiation doses. Most radiotherapy centres now have some form of afterloading, particularly for the higher activity sources used in gynaecological treatments. Manual afterloading for gynaecological treatments entails the placing of an applicator in the patient in theatre, while for iridium wire treatments, flexible tubes are implanted. The sources are loaded into the applicator after check radiographs have been taken and the patient has returned to the ward. For manual afterloading, the ward staff and others who may be in close contact with the patient are liable to receive unwanted doses of radiation. To eliminate this, and to make it possible to treat with even higher activity sources, remote afterloading systems are used in which the applicator is connected to a machine by catheters through which the sources can be moved, using either cable drivers or compressed air. Machines of this type are now available that allow the complete range of brachytherapy, from low dose-rate implants or insertions to high dose-rate treatment of the bronchus and other sites to be performed, without any significant dose to staff (Section 5).

Typically, conventional brachytherapy is given at the following dose rates over periods of 2–10 days: interstitial therapy at 7–20 Gy per day (30–90 cGy h^{-1}) to the prescribed point or isodose, or intracavitary treatment at 13–17 Gy per day (50–70 cGy h^{-1}). For this low dose-rate (LDR) therapy, treatment may be given on the wards if lead screens are used and working practices are carefully controlled. However, when higher dose rates are used with remote afterloading, the patient must remain within a separate protected cubicle. The dose rate to the target volume may then be 30–40 Gy per day (1.2–1.8 Gy h^{-1}), which is referred to as medium dose rate (MDR), or the high dose rate (HDR) of 1–5 Gy min^{-1} (60–300 Gy h^{-1}).

LDR treatments have been given since radium was isolated by the Curies in the early years of the twentieth century. Systems of source distribution and dosimetry are well established and there are extensive clinical data to assess the outcome of therapy. Dosimetry systems will be discussed in Section 6. HDR treatments have been developed in recent years because of the availability of miniature high-activity sources and the development of afterloading systems, and the shorter treatment time is of considerable benefit to the patient. It is recognized that the biological effects of treatment, i.e. tumour control and the incidence of morbidity, are significantly affected by dose rate. Radiobiological models have been employed to establish the optimum dose–time relationship for these higher dose rates based on LDR experience. These will be discussed in Section 8. Clinical experience gained with HDR treatments is needed to establish the validity of the models used.

In some sites it is common to combine brachytherapy with external beam radiotherapy, for example, in gynaecological treatment or conservative treatment of breast cancer. However, the combination of LDR brachytherapy with HDR fractionated external beam therapy is a complex radiobiological problem that is probably best tackled by analysing clinical results. The issue is simplified if both types of therapy are given at a high dose rate.

Most brachytherapy applications involve treatment over a period of several days given in one or possibly two fractions. With HDR therapy the treatment time is reduced to minutes and several fractions may be given. There are a few types of treatment for which shorter-lived radionuclides may be used for permanent implants, and these are generally in sites for which repeated surgery for the removal of sources is undesirable. The sources usually have a relatively short half-life. Permanent implants produce particular radiation protection problems.

2. Sealed radioactive sources

A sealed source is one in which the radioactive material is encapsulated, so that the material cannot be lost under any foreseeable degree of physical or chemical stress. Generally, the material is encapsulated within a metal casing. The metal wall serves the combined function of preventing the escape of radioactivity (particularly in the case of radium, which has a gaseous daughter product, radon) and of absorbing the unwanted beta particles. It must provide the highest possible integrity together with the minimum attenuation of the required irradiation. The International Organization for Standardization (ISO) has

produced a system of classification of sealed sources based on safety requirements for typical use (ISO 1990a). All sources used in brachytherapy should be issued with a certificate from the manufacturer to show that they conform to this standard. All sources used in brachytherapy are sealed sources (in that the radioactivity is totally sealed by metal welds), except for iridium-192 in the form of wire or hairpins. This is classified as a closed source, since its radioactive core is exposed when the wire, or hairpin, is cut. ISO has also issued a report that specifies 'leak test methods' for sealed sources (ISO 1990b). Most of these are performed by the manufacturers (and reported on the certificate), but some, such as wipe tests and leakage tests, are recommended to be carried out a the local level.

In the early days, radium-226 was the only source used extensively. This was because it was the only naturally occurring radionuclide with a reasonably high specific activity, i.e. the activity per unit mass of the material. Radium was an extremely practical source, and it should be noted that much of the clinical experience gained with radium is still of interest today. However, it has several disadvantages, mainly concerned with radiation hazards. Not only does it decay by alpha emission but, more importantly, its daughter product, radon-222, is a gas that is also an alpha emitter with a short half-life and it decays to other short-lived alpha emitters. The advent of nuclear reactors and cyclotrons in the 1940s enabled the production of artificial radionuclides, many of which have equal or better characteristics for brachytherapy. Thus, the use of radium diminished considerably in the 1960s and 1970s. Today it is no longer used and it will not be considered further in this chapter.

Sources in common current use, and their physical characteristics, are shown in Tables 12.1 and 12.2. These will now be considered in more detail.

2.1 Caesium-137

Caesium-137 is the most commonly used source for brachytherapy at the present time. It decays with a half-life of 30.0 years and emits both beta particles and 662 keV gamma rays. Normally, the beta particles are absorbed in a thin layer of metal encapsulation; this is usually stainless steel or an iridium-platinum alloy with a thickness of approximately 0.5 mm. Caesium-137 may be supplied in the form of tubes to be used in gynaecological applicators, needles for implants, and cylindrical or spherical beads to be used in afterloading systems.

One of the advantages of caesium is its long half-life, which means that sources can be kept for many years. In practice, manufacturers recommend a maximum working life for sources; in the case of caesium, this recommendation is usually about 10 years, due partly to decay but

Table 12.1 Radionuclides used in brachytherapy

Radionuclide	Photon energy (MeV)		Half-life	Attenuation in lead (approx.) (mm)		AKR constant[a] (μGy m^2 GBq^{-1} h^{-1})
	Mean	Maximum		HVL	TVL	
^{60}Co	1.25	1.33	5.27 years	12	45	309
^{137}Cs	0.662	0.662	30.0 years	6.5	22	78
^{192}Ir	0.37	0.61	74 days	4.5	15	113
^{125}I	0.028	0.035	60 days	0.03	0.1	33 (35.8[b])
^{103}Pd	0.021	0.023	17.0 days	0.03	0.1	35.0[b]
^{198}Au	0.42	0.68	2.7 days	3	11	55.5
^{226}Ra	ca. 1	2.4	1600 years	16	45	195

HVL, half-value layer; TVL, tenth-value layer.
[a]Data from Trott (1987).
[b]Data from Nath *et al.* (1995).

Table 12.2 Some common sealed sources for brachytherapy with typical source strengths

Radionuclide	Type/use	Size (mm)	Nominal activity (MBq)	Reference AKR (μGy h^{-1})
^{60}Co	Pellet/HDR remote afterloading	2.5 (diameter)	Up to 18.5×10^3	Up to 5.7×10^3
^{137}Cs	Needle/implant	15–45 (active length)	3.7 or 7.4 per mm	3.5–22
^{137}Cs	Tube/gynaecological insertion	13.5 (active length)	460–2300	36–180
^{137}Cs	Miniature cylinder/ manual afterloading	3.3 (active length)	550–1300	42–100
^{137}Cs	Pellet/LDR or MDR remote afterloading	2.5 (diameter)	370–1480	28–115
^{192}Ir	Wire	0.3 (diameter) 500 (length)	1.1–11 per mm	0.13–1.3 per mm
	Hairpin	0.6 (diameter) 60 (length)		
^{192}Ir	Miniature cylinder/ HDR remote afterloading	3 (active length)	Up to 370×10^3	Up to 42×10^3
^{125}I	Seed/permanent implant	3–4.5	4–180	0.15–6
^{125}I	Seed/permanent implant	active/total length	180–1500	6–50
^{198}Au	Seed/permanent implant	2.5 (length)	Up to 1460	Up to 80

also taking into account possible wear of the source encapsulation.

2.2 Iridium-192

Iridium-192 undergoes beta decay with a half-life of 74 days and its principal gamma ray has an energy of 370 keV. It is generally supplied in the form of wire, which combines flexibility with strength. The wire has a core of an iridium-platinum alloy and an outer sheath of platinum 0.1 mm thick, which is required to absorb the beta principles.

Strictly, iridium-192 in this form is not a sealed source because the outer sheath is slightly active and the process of cutting the wire potentially leads to a loss of the radioactive material, which constitutes a potential contamination hazard. This hazard is not usually realized in practice and so these sources are classified as closed sources.

Iridium wire normally has an outer diameter of 0.3 mm. Thicker source material (0.6 mm diameter) is supplied in the form of pins, which may be single or double; the latter are commonly described as hair-pins. The advantage of wire is that it can be cut to any length to fit the tumour volume. For treatment, the wire is loaded into a plastic tube.

The process of cutting the wire and loading it into the tube requires some skill, and the operator may receive a high radiation dose to the fingers. An alternative form of iridium is as seeds that are preloaded into nylon ribbons.

These generally contain 12 seeds spaced at 1-cm intervals, the seeds themselves being approximately 3 mm long. The seeds are encapsulated in stainless steel and, therefore, constitute a genuine sealed source.

HDR sources are available as very small cylinders (0.6 mm diameter and 3.5 mm long with a 3 mm active length) for use in remote afterloading systems.

Typical applications of iridium are for breast implants (wire), tongue implants (hairpins), and various HDR intracavitary and interstitial treatments.

2.3 Cobalt-60

Cobalt-60 is a less common source. It undergoes beta decay with an associated emission of 1.33 and 1.17 MeV gamma rays, and its half-life is 5.27 years. Cobalt-60 has been used in the form of wire, but this has been discontinued because of the tendency of the wire to break. It has been used for ophthalmic applicators and, in some countries, in needles and tubes. It is also used in HDR afterloading systems for gynaecological treatments in the form of beads.

2.4 Gold-198

Gold-198 has a short half-life of 2.7 days and, therefore, is suitable for permanent implants. It has a number of gamma ray energies, but the dominant energy is 412 keV. Gold is normally supplied in the form of cylindrical grains or seeds with an outer diameter of 0.8 mm and length equal to 2.5 mm. The outer part of the gold grain is a 0.15 mm encapsulation of platinum. Gold grains have been used for small-area moulds but, more commonly, for permanent implants. These are for sites, such as the prostate, which would otherwise require surgical procedures for both the insertion and removal of sources. In addition, they may be used in sites, such as the tongue, for which a needle implant could be particularly uncomfortable.

2.5 Iodine-125

Iodine-125 decays via electron capture to the first excited state of tellurium-125, with a half-life of 59.4 days. This undergoes 93% internal conversion and 7% gamma emission of a 35.5 keV photon. The electron capture and internal conversion processes give rise to characteristic X-rays: 27.4 and 31.4 keV.

Two types of individual seeds are available in the UK. Type 6711 consists of a welded titanium capsule containing I-125 adsorbed onto a silver rod, with an active length of 3.0 mm and an overall length of 4.5 mm. The silver rod acts as an X-ray marker. The high-activity type 6702 seed has no such marker, and the I-125 is adsorbed on anion resin spheres. The dose distribution around both types of individual seed is not isotropic (Nath *et al.* 1995).

A more recent development is the provision of I-125 seeds in a carrier (Rapid Strand™ by Nycomed Amersham). The standard configuration consists of 10 type 6711 seeds, with a centre-to-centre distance of 10 mm contained in a braided stiffened suture. This can be cut to length and accommodated in a standard 18-gauge implant needle. These sources not only decrease needle loading and preparation time, when 100 seeds may need to be loaded, they also minimize seed migration within the implanted volume.

The low-energy photons from I-125 ensure that surface dose rate from a patient is generally insufficient to cause any restrictions on their movement, and it is, therefore, safe for use in permanent implants without increasing hospital stay.

The AAPM Radiation Therapy Committee Task Group No. 43 (Nath *et al.* 1995) recommended an air kerma rate constant $(\Gamma_\delta)_k$ of 0.0358 μGy m^2 MBq^{-1}h^{-1}. This is 8.5% greater than the value recommended by Trott 1987 (Table 12.1).

2.6 Palladium-103

Palladium-103 also decays via electron capture, mostly to the first and second excited states of rhodium-103, with a half-life of 17.0 days. Rh-103 undergoes internal conversion leading to the production of characteristic X-rays (20.1 and 23.0 keV). There is also some gamma emission. The average photon energy is about 21 keV.

Palladium-103 sources are similar in size and encapsulation to I-125 sources. The active material is coated onto two graphite pellets 0.9 mm long and 0.6 mm in diameter. Between the active pellets is a 1-mm long lead marker for radiographic visibility. The encapsulation is 0.05 mm titanium tube that is laser welded on the ends.

These sources can be used in permanent implants to treat faster growing tumours of the prostate.

2.7 Beta-ray sources

The use of these sources is relatively infrequent and they will be discussed in this one brief section. They have been used principally for the treatment of lesions in the eye for which their short treatment range is particularly advantageous.

Strontium-90 is a radionuclide that has a long half-life (28.7 years), but only a low-energy beta particle (546 keV); however, its daughter product, yttrium-90, emits a high-energy beta particle (2.27 MeV). The short half-life of yttrium-90 (64 hours) is of no concern because its activity is maintained by the decay of strontium-90. Ophthalmic applicators with strontium-90 are used to treat malignant melanoma and corneal vascularization. It should be noted that the dose rate from these sources is difficult to measure and reference should be made to Sayeg and Gregory (1991).

3. Sealed-source dosimetry

This section is concerned with the specification of source strength and the calculation of dose to a point in the medium in which the source is located. The measurement of source strength is considered in Section 4.2.

3.1 Source strength

Historically, source strength was specified in terms of the mass of radium. This was effectively also a specification of activity, since the curie (Ci) was defined in terms of the activity of 1 g of radium. Most dosimetry systems considered standard source distributions. Treatment was prescribed as the product of mass of radium and the time of treatment in units of milligram hours (mg h); the only modifying factor required was the thickness of filter surrounding the sources. Other isotopes were accommodated by specifying their strengths in terms of their radium equivalent, i.e. the mass of radium which gave the same exposure rate. This system of source specification has now been superseded.

Source strength can be specified in terms of either the source activity or its radiation output at a specified distance. Activity of the intact source in its housing cannot be measured directly. For dosimetry purposes, activity has to be converted to a dose rate at a point in a medium, which requires factors that may not be known with sufficient accuracy. Dose rate is the quantity of interest clinically; when two different isotopes are compared, activity does not provide a means of direct comparison. For these reasons, source strength is now specified in terms of radiation output. It should always be accompanied by the date (and time) of specification.

The standard definition of source strength is the reference air kerma rate, which is the air kerma rate (AKR) at a distance of 1 m from the source in free space. There are inconsistencies in the literature with regard to the units for this quantity. The AAPM recommends the use of air kerma strength defined as the product of air kerma rate and the square of the reference distance in units of μGy m^2 h^{-1} denoted by the symbol U (AAPM 1987). For this specification, the reference distance is 1 m and it is, therefore, numerically equal to reference AKR. However, the units of the latter quantity should omit distance, and are simply μGy h^{-1}. This convention is followed in this text. It should be noted, however, that the omission of m^2 from the unit may cause some confusion when using equations to calculate AKR at some other distance, since the reference distance (1 m) may not be explicitly included in the equation. Reference AKR has the advantage of being directly measurable, apart from a small correction due to attenuation and scatter in air. However, it should be noted that this measurement is not trivial, particularly in the hospital environment. The measurement at 1 m must be under scatter-free conditions, which requires substantial laboratory space. In addition, the reference AKR associated with LDR brachytherapy sources is typically in the range 10–100 μGy h^{-1}. This may be compared with typical dose rates in external beam therapy of the order of 100 Gy h^{-1}. This indicates that dosimeters used for external beams are inadequate for these sources; in particular, the volume of the ion chamber is too small to provide sufficient sensitivity (see Section 4.2.2).

Specification of reference AKR is for a standard geometry. For line sources, such as needles, and for seeds, the AKR on a line bisecting the axis of the source and perpendicular to it is required. For wires the strength is normally specified per millimetre of wire length.

The source strength indicates the output (AKR) in free space at a distance of 1 m. For dosimetry, the quantity of interest is the absorbed dose rate at distances of approximately 1 cm in a tissue-equivalent medium. The following section will consider this conversion for line sources.

3.2 Air kerma rate calculations

In order to understand the way that the dose at any point in a medium varies with distance d from a sealed source, it is necessary to revert to consideration of the activity A of the source and the use of the AKR constant Γ. The equation relating the two is:

$$\text{AKR} = \frac{A_E \Gamma}{d^2}. \tag{1}$$

It should be noted that in this equation the symbol A_E is used to indicate that this is the apparent or equivalent activity. It is the activity of a bare source with no self-absorption of the gamma radiation, which would give the same AKR. Values of Γ are given in Table 12.1. Many computer algorithms for brachytherapy treatment planning still require these factors (A_E and Γ) as the starting point for dose calculations. Different values of Γ from those listed in Table 12.1 may be found in the literature. This is not a problem as long as the factors that are used in the programme to convert from activity to AKR and dose rate are consistent with those used to derive activity from the stated AKR. Certain texts refer to the exposure rate constant in units of R h^{-1} mCi^{-1} cm^2. To convert to air kerma rate constant in μGy m^2 Gbq^{-1} h^{-1}, the values should be multiplied by 23.6.

3.2.1 Unfiltered line source

In order to consider how dose rate is determined from a line source, it is easier to begin with an unfiltered source. If each segment of source has a length dx, then AKR at point P at a distance d from the centre of the source segment (Figure 12.1) is given by:

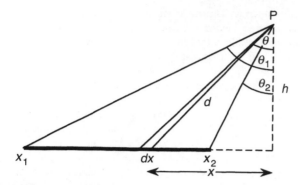

Figure 12.1 Calculation of dose at point P for an unfiltered line source.

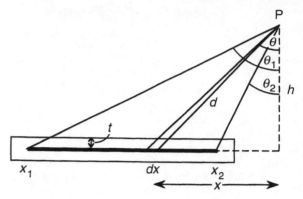

Figure 12.2 Calculation of dose at point P for a filtered line source.

$$d(\text{AKR}) = \frac{A}{L} dx \frac{\Gamma}{d^2} \quad (2)$$

where L is the length of the source and A is its activity. By integrating over the length of the source, the total AKR at P is given by:

$$\text{AKR} = \int_{x_2}^{x_1} \frac{A\Gamma}{Ld^2} dx. \quad (3)$$

By changing to polar co-ordinates using $d = h \sec \theta$ and $x = h \tan \theta$, it can be shown that:

$$\text{AKR} = \frac{A\Gamma}{L} \int_{\theta_2}^{\theta_1} \frac{d\theta}{h} \quad (4)$$

$$= \frac{A\Gamma}{Lh} (\theta_1 - \theta_2). \quad (5)$$

3.2.2 Filtered line source

In the derivation of the above equations, it was assumed that there is no attenuation in the source casing. Figure 12.2 shows that the degree of attenuation in the casing is a function of angle and is given by $\exp(-\mu t \sec \theta)$, where t is the wall thickness and μ is the linear attenuation coefficient. Equation (4) now becomes:

$$\text{AKR} = \frac{A\Gamma}{Lh} \int_{\theta_2}^{\theta_1} \exp(-\mu t \sec \theta) d\theta \quad (6)$$

which can be rewritten as:

$$\text{AKR} = \frac{A\Gamma}{Lh} \left[\int_0^{\theta_1} \exp(-\mu t \sec \theta) d\theta \right.$$
$$\left. - \int_0^{\theta_2} \exp(-\mu t \sec \theta) d\theta \right]. \quad (7)$$

Integrals of the type appearing in equation (7) are known as Sievert integrals after the author who first tabulated their values. A more recent tabulation has been given by Shalek and Stovall (1969). It should be noted that for $\theta < 0.35$ rad (20°) the approximation:

$$\int_0^{\theta} \exp(-\mu t \sec \theta) d\theta = \theta \exp(-\mu t) \quad (8)$$

can be used for the source wall thicknesses normally encountered in brachytherapy. With computer systems, a summation instead of an integration can be performed quickly by dividing the source into a large number of segments. Beyond the end of the source, the Sievert integral method breaks down, but this is usually for a region that has less clinical significance.

In general, the filtration correction, which includes self-absorption, is given the symbol, $f_1(d,\theta)$, so that equation (6) becomes:

$$\text{AKR} = \frac{A\Gamma}{Lh} \int_{\theta_2}^{\theta_1} f_1(d,\theta) d\theta. \quad (9)$$

3.3 Absorption and scattering in a medium

The equations given above apply strictly to a source *in vacuo*. In a medium, the photons will be scattered and absorbed by varying amounts depending on their energy and the path length in the medium. For many years these factors were ignored because, fortuitously, the amount of absorption is closely balanced by the scattered radiation over the few centimetres for which calculations are needed.

The ratio of AKR from a point source in a medium to that *in vacuo* can be described by the function:

$$f_2(d) = B \exp(-\mu_m d) \quad (10)$$

Table 12.3 Coefficients to be used in the quadratic function $f_2(r) = 1 + ar + br^2$ for describing the net effect of attenuation and scattering in water at a radial distance r cm, from a point source (from Sakelliou *et al.* 1992)

Radionuclide	a	b
Cobalt-60	−0.1335 E-01	−0.3451 E-03
Caesium-137	−0.5767 E-02	−0.8628 E-03
Gold-198	0.6678 E-02	−0.1527 E-02
Iridium-192	0.1250 E-01	−0.1834 E-02

in which d is the distance from the source, B is a build-up factor to take account of scattering in the medium, and μ_m is the linear attenuation coefficient of the medium.

The attenuation coefficient for each photon energy can be obtained from standard compilations of attenuation data and interpolated for the particular radionuclide. However, the scatter correction is more complex. It has been derived by several authors either by measurement or through Monte Carlo calculation. It has been shown (Berger 1968) that the build-up factor can be fitted to equations of the form:

$$B = 1 + a(\mu_m d)^K \qquad (11)$$

in which a and K are constants for a given radionuclide. An evaluation of these constants has been made by Kornelsen and Young (1981). More recently, Sakelliou *et al.* (1992) have determined the composite factor $f_2(d)$ for a number of commonly used radionuclides, and some of their data fitted to second-order polynomials are shown in Table 12.3. These data were calculated for water with the source at the centre of a 20-cm sphere. Care should be taken in using the data at distances that are close to the edge of the medium. For iodine-125 sources (type 6702 and 6711), the calculated values of the build up factors were fitted to third-order polynomials. The coefficients can be found in Sakelliou *et al.* (1992).

An alternative approach, used in several brachytherapy-planning systems, is to describe $f_2(d)$ in terms of a third-order polynomial in d fitted to experimental and theoretical data derived by Meisberger (1968) for distances less than 10 cm.

In comparing data from different authors, it should be noted that some normalize to unity at a distance of 1 cm from the source rather than reporting the absolute values as calculated from the coefficients in Table 12.3. There may also be small differences depending on whether the ratio is expressed relative to an evaluation of AKR *in vacuo* or in air.

Although there may be some uncertainty in the values of $f_2(d)$ to be used, its consequences are small relative to the major attenuating mechanism of distance. For example, the AKR at 4 cm from a point source falls to 6.25% of its value at 1 cm due to the inverse square law. The correction for

attenuation and scatter at this distance is not less than 0.94 for the radionuclides listed in Table 12.3. However, for iodine-125 corrections of 0.56 and 0.50 are required relative to that at 1 cm for type 6702 and 6711 sources, respectively.

The foregoing discussion is concerned with a point source. For extended sources, the function has to be integrated over the whole source. For a line source, the function can be written as $f_2(d,\theta)$ to indicate that its value varies over the source length. The product $f_1(d,\theta) f_2(d,\theta)$ must then be integrated to give the AKR at point P in Figure 12.2, when the point is in a medium. This calculation method is readily incorporated into computer systems, which carry out the calculations by summation over a large number of source segments.

3.4 Absorbed dose calculation

A third factor f_3 is required to convert AKR to absorbed dose rate in water. This is given by:

$$f_3 = \frac{(\mu_{en}/\rho)_{water}}{(\mu_{en}/\rho)_{air}}(1 - g) \qquad (12)$$

in which $(\mu_{en}/\rho)_{water}$ and $(\mu_{en}/\rho)_{air}$, are the mass energy absorption coefficients for water and air, respectively, and g is the fraction of the energy transferred, which leads to bremsstrahlung production. The last factor is generally ignored since, for the radionuclides used in brachytherapy, g is very small (0.3% or less). For all the radionuclides in Table 12.1, f_3 is equal to 1.11, except for iodine-125 for which it is 1.02.

In summary, for a point source the absorbed dose rate $D(d)$ at a distance d can be calculated from the activity by:

$$D(d) = \frac{A\Gamma}{d^2} f_1 f_2(d) f_3. \qquad (13)$$

For the point source within a spherical casing, the attenuation factor f_1 is independent of position and is equal to $\exp(-\mu t)$. It is not necessary to use this factor when source strength is specified in terms of the reference AKR (AKR$_0$) and the equation may be rewritten as:

$$D(d) = \frac{AKR_0}{d^2} f_2(d) f_3. \qquad (14)$$

For a line source, equation (7) has to be combined with the correction for absorption and scatter and kerma has to be converted to absorbed dose to give the absorbed dose rate $D(d,\theta)$ at a distance d and angle θ as:

$$D(d, \theta) = \frac{A\Gamma}{Lh} f_3 \left[\int_0^{\theta_1} f_1(d, \theta) f_2(d, \theta) d\theta \right.$$
$$\left. - \int_0^{\theta_2} f_1(d, \theta) f_2(d, \theta) d\theta \right]. \qquad (15)$$

To convert this equation for the reference AKR source specification, use can be made of the approximation in equation (8). At the reference distance of 1 m, equation (7) can be used to give:

$$AKR_0 = \frac{2A\Gamma}{L} \exp(-\mu t) \tan^{-1}\left(\frac{L}{2}\right) \quad (16)$$

in which the active length L of the source is in metres. For source lengths that are less than 15 cm, the last term is approximately equal to $L/2$, which leads to the equation for a line source:

$$D(d,\theta) = \frac{AKR_0}{Lh} f_3 \exp(\mu t)\left[\int_0^{\theta_1} f_1(d,\theta)f_2(d,\theta)d\theta\right.$$
$$\left. - \int_0^{\theta_2} f_1(d,\theta)f_2(d,\theta)d\theta\right]. \quad (17)$$

Example

The following example for a caesium needle with 0.5 mm Pt filtration, an active length of 45 mm, and reference AKR of 10 μGy h^{-1}, illustrates the use of this equation. With reference to Figure 12.2, the point at which the dose is to be calculated is at a distance of $h = 2$ cm from the source axis and is 1 cm from the end of the activity. Values of the Sievert integrals were taken from Shalek and Stovall (1969).

$$\theta_1 = \tan^{-1}(5.5/2) = 70°$$
$$\theta_2 = \tan^{-1}(1/2) = 27°$$
$$\mu t = 0.0625$$
$$f_3 = 1.11$$
$$\int_0^{\theta_1} f_1(d,\theta), d\theta = 1.1186$$
$$\int_0^{\theta_2} f_1(d,\theta), d\theta = 0.4416.$$

Therefore:

$$D(d,\theta) = \frac{10}{0.02 \times 0.045} \times 1.11 \times 1.065$$
$$\times (1.1186 - 0.4416) \times 10^{-3}$$
$$= 8.89 \text{ mGy h}^{-1}.$$

Absorption and scattering in the medium has been ignored in this calculation.

4. Radiation protection and quality assurance

One of the overriding principles of radiation protection is that the use of ionizing radiations should be optimized in terms of the unwanted dose to any person who may be irradiated. This has been summarized as a requirement to keep doses as low as reasonably achievable, the ALARA principle, and has been incorporated into radiation protection legislation of most countries. In this section, radiation protection will be considered, with the emphasis on practical methods of reducing the dose to patients, staff, and others to a minimum. Detailed regulations are not considered, as these may vary from country to country.

The ALARA principle is the overwhelming argument that can be used in favour of adopting afterloading systems because they result in a considerable reduction in dose to staff without, in principle, a detrimental effect on the quality of treatment. Such systems are now commonly in use in Europe and North America. It should be noted that the ICRP qualifies its statement on optimization by stating that 'economic and social factors' should be taken into account. In economically weaker countries, the cost of purchase and maintenance of afterloading equipment, particularly remote systems, may be prohibitive, and if manual systems were not used, patients would not receive the benefits of this form of treatment.

ALARA is concerned with unwanted dose, but an equally important factor in radiotherapy is the optimization of the wanted dose to the patient being treated. The potential benefit will not be realized if treatment is given incorrectly. Therefore, this section is also concerned with quality control.

The requirements for safety and quality assurance are different for manual and remote systems of brachytherapy delivery. Some detail for both is given. More extensive information for HDR can be found in Kubo *et al.* (1998).

4.1 Storage of sources

The employer should appoint a custodian of radioactive sources to be responsible for the security and storage of all radioactive substances and for all necessary records. Radioactive sources issued from a store should be in the care of responsible individuals at all times until their return. The local rules should state the responsibilities of individuals, including patients, for the care of radioactive sources.

Sources should be stored in the preparation area in a safe shielded with a thickness of 5–10 cm of lead or its equivalent, depending upon the amount and type of radioactivity stored. The safe should be compartmentalized to permit easy access and control over individual sources. A detailed inventory of sources is necessary. Each source should be identified individually with the following details: isotope, type of source, strength, calibration date, date of purchase, and serial number. The inventory should include a record of its acceptance and leakage tests.

4.1.1 Record keeping

It is essential that the location of every source is known at all times. One system of achieving this is to have a log-book in which an entry is made on each occasion that a source is moved, for example, from the safe to the theatre or from the theatre to the ward. Each week the contents of the safe should be checked against this record. This does not necessarily involve the checking of every drawer or compartment within the safe. A reliable system of checking that reduces the dose to staff to a minimum makes use of drawers that are designed to operate an indicator (a 'flag') when opened. The weekly check is then a matter of inspecting which drawers or compartments have been opened and checking the contents of these against the records. Inspection of sources in the safe should be achievable without the need to look directly at the sources; a mirror or a lead-glass screen makes this possible. A full audit of the sources against the inventory should be made annually.

4.1.2 Disposal of solid sources

A source that is no longer in use can be sent either to a person authorized to dispose of that type of source or to a manufacturer of that type of source, provided that records are kept showing the radionuclide and its activity, the date of disposal, and the name and address of the person who receives the source.

4.2 Checking sources on receipt

Sources will be delivered from the manufacturers with a certificate of source strength for a particular day (and time in the case of very short-lived radionuclides). After a check-measurement of source strength has been made, it is important to reconcile this measurement with that on the certificate and to establish the date (and time) as a baseline from which to calculate the source strength for use at future dates. For long-lived radionuclides, such as caesium-137, it is usual to alter standard treatment tables every 6 months (or monthly for cobalt-60), which corresponds to a decay of about 1%. For sort-lived radionuclides, it is important to calculate the source strength for the time of use. In the case of iridium-192, a correction must also be made for the decay over the period of treatment, if this is several days.

When sources are received they will be supplied with a calibration certificate from the manufacturer. In general, the strength stated on this certificate is used for dose calculations because almost invariably the manufacturer can provide a more accurate calibration service than that in a hospital. However, in view of the critical dependence of dose on source strength, it is prudent to check that an error has not been made. This check may be performed only once during the lifetime of the source, which may be as much as 10 years in the case of caesium-137, during which time many hundreds of patients may be treated with any one source. Therefore, it is essential that the check is carried out correctly, and that an accurate record is retained that clearly indicates the technique used and the various calculation steps. Where applicable, the distribution of activity should also be checked.

Source strength is specified in terms of AKR at a distance of 1 m. For the reasons indicated in Section 3, this is a non-trivial measurement requiring large-volume ionization chambers and a scatter-free geometry. For routine hospital use, simpler techniques are required than those carried out in the calibration laboratory. Usually a re-entrant ionization chamber is used, or it may be necessary to measure AKR, usually at a distance which is less than 1 m.

4.2.1 Re-entrant ionization chambers

Re-entrant ionization chambers are used in isotope calibrators for the measurement of activity. This is not a direct measurement, as they require calibration with standard sources whose calibration is traceable to a standards laboratory. The calibration is strongly dependent on energy and on the particular isotope being used; therefore, a range of calibrated sources is required together with conversion tables for those radionuclides for which calibrated sources are not available, in particular for short-lived radionuclides. Energy dependence is only one factor that may lead to measurement error. Other factors are source geometry, source position, source holder, effect of scatter from the external shielding, and source activity. It is the last of these factors that is most critical in the context of HDR brachytherapy sources. With the conventional isotope calibrator there is significant loss of signal with very high activity sources, owing to recombination effects within the ionization chamber. It then becomes necessary to adopt an alternative means to measure source strength by using a thimble ionization chamber to determine the AKR at a known distance (see Section 4.2.2).

The most satisfactory way in which a re-entrant ionization chamber can be used is to have a calibrated source of the same approximate activity and the same geometry. A jig is required to ensure that the source is held in the centre of the chamber. A calibration factor can then be derived for the re-entrant chamber for this particular source geometry. Without a calibrated source or a method of transferring the calibration of one source geometry to the geometry of the sources being used, the re-entrant ionization chamber can only be used for relative measurements. This is useful when batches of sources are purchased. Checks of response in the chamber will indicate whether the relative strength of each source corresponds to the calibration certificate. Such measurements should be compared with existing sources of the same geometry or sources that are being replaced. These measurements should be reconciled and any discrepancies investigated. A record of this calibration should be maintained in the sealed-source inventory.

Iridium wire is commonly supplied in the form of 50 cm coils or 25 cm loops of varying strengths. It is important that the strength of the wire is measured on receipt. This is a relative measurement that can be compared with previous supplies. Similarly, the source strength of iridium hairpins and single pins should be measured and compared with previous records and the manufacturer's certificate. It should be noted that calibrated iridium-192 wire can be obtained and this provides a calibration with an overall uncertainty of ±3.5% (Löffler 1989). Such a standard presents problems because of its relatively short half-life, requiring it to be replaced several times each year. However, it can be used for a single calibration to be compared with a measurement using a longer-lived source, such as a caesium-137 needle. The measurement with the caesium needle, corrected for decay, can then be used for iridium-192 calibrations with the underlying assumption that the energy–response characteristics of the chamber do not change with time. This can be checked by repeat iridium-192 calibrations at longer time intervals (1 or 2 years).

Gold grains arrive in a standard magazine in which they must be measured and kept until used. Similarly, iodine-125 seeds that have not been packed in ribbons are very difficult to handle and it is impossible to identify individual sources and strengths; therefore, the complete batch is kept together and the total strength measured.

4.2.2 High dose-rate systems

The calibration of high-activity sources, in particular the intense iridium-192 sources used in the remote afterloading systems that require to be replaced and, therefore, to be recalibrated every 3 months, presents a special problem. For these HDR sources (reference AKR greater than about 5 mGy h^{-1}), the use of a special re-entrant ionization chamber is required. This type of chamber is an extremely useful instrument for routine checks of sources, provided it is checked periodically (at least annually) against a method of calibrating HDR sources such as that described below.

The AKR can be measured either in air at distances between 100 and 500 mm or in a water phantom between 50 and 150 mm. The measured value can then be converted to reference AKR at 1 m by the application of the inverse square law. The measurements in water need to be made at the small distance for which scatter and attenuation corrections are small and subject to less uncertainty. However, at these distances the chamber dimensions become significant and appropriate corrections need to be made. Further details of these measurements in water are given in Jones and Bidmead (1989). At the longer distances used for the in-air measurements, the chamber dimensions are less significant but the ion current may approach the limit of measurement for the system. Therefore, great care is needed to ensure low noise levels and stable conditions. For the measurements it is essential to use a rigid jig with a precisely controlled geometry to hold the chamber and the applicators from the afterloading equipment.

The method recommended in the UK (BIR 1993) can be summarized. An ionization chamber with a graphite wall and build-up cap to serve as an electron filter should be used. The build-up cap for 2 MV X-rays is suitable for this purpose. It should be calibrated in terms of air kerma against an NPL secondary standard. Until an iridium-192 calibration is available, it is recommended that the calibration factor for heavily filtered 280 kV X-rays is applied.

The ion chamber should be held in a Perspex jig centrally between two plastic source catheters. The jig should be of a light-weight design. This arrangement should be positioned in the centre of the room to reduce scatter, 1 m above the floor, and 1.5 m away from the walls. Typically, exposure times of 300 s should be used if the source-to-chamber distance is 100 mm.

Using the formalism in BIR (1993), AKR$_0$ is then found from:

$$\dot{K}_{\mathrm{r}} = RF_{\mathrm{c}}F_{\mathrm{tp}}F_{\mathrm{s}}F_{\mathrm{g}}F_{\mathrm{e}}F_{\mathrm{is}}F_{\mathrm{m}}/t \qquad (18)$$

where:

R is the instrument reading;

F_{c} is the air kerma calibration factor;

F_{tp} is the temperature/pressure correction factor ($= T/P \times 1013/293.2$), where T is the temperature in °kelvin and P the pressure in millibar;

F_{s} is the correction for scatter produced in the jig and its support (this should be less than 0.3% and can be tested by adding similar quantities of material in the vicinity of the catheters),

F_{g} is the dose gradient correction factor for the ion chamber ($= 1.004$ for a 0.6 cm^3 Farmer chamber at 100 mm);

F_{e} is the electron filter correction ($= 1.017$ for a 2 MV build-up cap);

F_{is} is the inverse square scaling from 1 m ($= 10^{-2}$ for measurements at 100 mm);

F_m is the gray to microgray conversion factor (10^6);

t is the time in seconds for each reading.

4.2.3 Linear activity

The simplest method of testing the distribution of activity in a source is by means of autoradiography. The source is placed in contact with a film to produce an image of the activity distribution. Hairpins should be autoradiographed in their delivery foil. The film speed should be sufficiently slow that insignificant exposure takes place during the placement of the sources. With LDR sources, e.g. caesium needles and tubes, and iridium wire or hairpins, the slow-speed verification film Kodak X-Omat V with exposure times of between 5 and 15 minutes is suitable. Following film processing, it is possible to see whether there are any cold or hot areas. For the low-activity caesium beads used in the Selectron, this method can be used to check the position and loading within the treatment catheter. The applicator is placed over the film and sources are exposed for a short time, usually for about 2 minutes for reference AKR per bead of 100 μGy h^{-1}. More accurate measurements of linear activity can be made with special techniques, such as those developed for use with iridium wire. The wire can be passed behind a lead aperture of 5-mm diameter through which the radiation can pass to a sensitive detector such as a Geiger–Muller counter, so that any variation in activity can be located.

4.2.4 Preparation of sources and quality control

The strength of every source should be checked prior to its being administered to the patient. Long-lived sources, such as caesium needles, will have been measured and checked against the manufacturer's certificate on delivery to the hospital. Each source is then checked against the inventory at the time that it is removed from store. Sources should be identified during their preparation by some means of colour coding, such as the silk thread used to keep them in place.

For iridium wire or hairpins, a measurement will have been made on the complete coil and each hairpin on delivery. In theory, provided that the autoradiograph of the wire is satisfactory, a length of wire cut from this coil should have the desired activity as a proportion of the total. However, it is advisable to make a check-measurement of source strength and an autoradiograph of each cut length to be used in the patient.

If a centre is using iridium wire frequently, it may be desirable, and cost-effective, to store cut lengths of wire within the nylon sheath for re-use. A careful inventory is then required to keep account of this stock of iridium wires. One limitation of the re-use of loaded wire is the radiation damage to the nylon tubing, which becomes brittle and has to be replaced. The shelf-life of these loaded wires has been found to be about 40–60 days (Mayles *et al.* 1985).

4.3 Protection in theatre and wards

It is a requirement of United Kingdom legislation that areas in which dose rates exceed certain levels should be classified as controlled areas. Entry to controlled areas must be under a written system of work. Legislation in other countries may be different, but these regulations can be used to illustrate good practice.

4.3.1 Controlled areas and room design

A temporary controlled area must be established in any theatre or recovery room in which radioactive sources are handled or in which there is a patient carrying radioactive sources. The area can be returned to a non-controlled status after all the radioactive sources have been removed. The designation as a controlled area must be indicated by a notice on all doorways giving access to the theatre or recovery room.

Wherever possible, treatment should be carried out in specially designed rooms containing only one or two beds, and these ward areas should be controlled areas whilst occupied by patients treated with radioactive sources. Lead screening should be used around the bed if there are other patients in the room. People in the adjoining rooms should be adequately protected; ideally, the dose rate should not exceed 2.5 μGy h^{-1} at any time.

The maximum dose rate at a distance of 1 m from each patient undergoing treatment should be calculated in order to determine times for safe working procedures and systems of work. These calculations are simplified with the new source strength specification, since the relevant dose rate is simply the sum of all the reference AKRs of the sources used. This assumes no attenuation within the patient. These times are particularly important for nurses, who may need to perform nursing operations on patients, and to porters who move patients around the hospital.

Beds in which there are patients undergoing treatment with radioactive sources should carry a notice that includes a radiation warning sign. Nursing staff should be given details of the number and nature of sources, the total source strength, and the time and date of application and intended removal. The patient should be confined to bed-rest. It is important that nursing staff are properly trained in the precautions necessary with sealed sources. Regular refresher courses should be held, particularly in those units where there may be a high staff turnover.

When LDR/MDR afterloading systems are used, the typical total reference AKR is 1–3 mGy h^{-1}. This requires a special protected room. For caesium-137 sources with this output, wall thicknesses of up to 40 cm of concrete or 4 cm lead would be required. There should be a simple maze entrance, so that the door is not directly irradiated. An interlock to withdraw sources to the safe, if the door is opened when the sources are in the patient, should be provided. In addition, there should be an independent gamma-alarm system to indicate when sources are out of the safe.

HDR systems using cobalt-60, with total reference AKR up to 130 mGy h^{-1}, require even more wall protection, but the other requirements are very similar. These units have frequently been used in existing teletherapy rooms, since a minimum thickness of 1 m concrete is generally required in the walls.

The maximum source strength for iridium-192 HDR treatment is typically 40 mGy h^{-1}, but the penetrating power of the gamma rays is less than that of cobalt-60 and a wall thickness of 45 cm of concrete or 5 cm of lead is sufficient. All the thickness given above are approximate and based on a minimum distance of 3.5 m between the sources and the area outside the room.

When designing protection for treatment rooms, attention should always be paid to the construction of floors and ceilings, which may need additional protection.

4.3.2 Systems of work for entry to controlled areas

Systems of work are needed to establish working procedures, which ensure that the radiation dose to staff is minimized. Some general points are summarized below.

Theatres

Theatre staff should not send for sources until they are required. Sources must be removed from the transit trolley or lift and put behind a protective barrier as soon as they arrive in the theatre area. Sources must be checked against the information sheet and a receipt document signed. Special tools or surgical instruments that keep some distance between the hands and the sources should always be used when sources are being prepared or administered to patients. All instruments should be monitored and cleaned after use.

Wards

Where remote afterloading is not used, the ward sister must limit, as far as is reasonably practicable, the times spent by staff and visitors in the controlled area around the patient. A typical limitation on nursing procedures in close proximity (about 0.5 m) to a patient treated with radioactive sources for cancer of the cervix would be to keep the time below 10 minutes per 9-hour day. Visitors should normally be asked to stay at least 2 m away from the active sources and to restrict each visit to not more than 30 minutes per day.

The number and position of removable sources in or on the patient should be checked against the record sheet on arrival in the ward, followed by regular checks using a procedure that minimizes dose to staff. A shielded container should be placed near the patient's bed. If a source becomes accidentally displaced, it should be transferred to the container using forceps and a note made of the time that this occurred. Dressings and excreta from patients receiving treatment should not be disposed of until monitoring has shown that they do not contain live sources. This is particularly important for seed implants, which are more readily lost from the treatment site. All containers, such as rubbish bins, soiled dressings bins, and laundry baskets coming from a ward where such sources are employed, should be tested for radioactivity with a monitoring instrument.

The time of removal of the sources must be noted and the number of sources removed must be checked. If any source is missing, the contingency plans outlined below must be followed immediately. Sources should be removed carefully to avoid patient trauma (sometimes this needs to be carried out under anaesthetic). When taking out iridium wire, special care must be taken not to cut through it. The cut should be made between the nylon ball and the lead washer. Following removal of the sources into a lead container, the patient must be checked with a portable radiation detector to ensure that no sources (in particular pieces of iridium wire) are left *in situ*. The operation of the radiation monitor should be checked before this measurement is made.

Patients with sources in or upon their bodies should not leave the ward or treatment room without the approval of the appropriate doctor and radiation protection supervisor (RPS). Patients with temporary implants must not leave hospital. For patients leaving hospital with a permanent implant, similar rules apply as with unsealed sources. They may be found in the appropriate guidance documents such as NRPB (1988).

In the United Kingdom, patients may leave hospital subject to consideration of the method of travel. For gold grains, the limits on the maximum AKR are 22 μGy h^{-1} (400 MBq) if the patient needs to travel by public transport, and 110 μGy h^{-1} (2000 MBq) if private transport is used. The latter figure is a special exemption to enable patients treated with gold grains to be sent home within a reasonable time period. Permanent iodine-125 implants will always be below the exemption level, although contact with a partner or children should be restricted for a specified period of time. Any other restrictions are detailed in NRPB (1988).

4.3.4 Contingencies arising from the use of sealed sources

All staff should be aware of the seriousness of incidents in which a source or sources may be lost, and the instructions for dealing with them should be clearly laid down. If a source is lost, all movement of items from the vicinity of the patient must be prevented by the member of staff in charge. The RPS and Physics Department must be informed without delay. The radiation protection adviser (RPA) and Head of Department will need to be informed also. Physics or RPA staff must conduct a thorough search using a suitable radiation monitor.

Any perceptible bending, breakage, or damage to a sealed source must be reported to the responsible physicist. The source must be checked for leakage of activity and then stored separately in a shielded container until it can be removed for repair or disposal.

There should be a readily available and up-to-date list of all places in the establishment where radiation sources are located or could be located. Arrangements should be made with the fire officer for the local fire brigade to visit the establishment to obtain information about the layout of the premises, warning notices, and the location of sources.

4.4 Transport of radioactive sources

Transport of radioactive materials is governed by national and international regulations and is normally divided into two categories: transport within the institution, in this case the hospital, and transport outside the institution by means of road, rail, or air.

For internal transport, radioactive sources should be moved only by staff who have received adequate training. Procedures should be written so that it is clear who is responsible for the sources at any time.

Records should be kept of the issue, distribution, and return of all sources – not just from the safe store but at each stage, e.g. arrival in theatre and arrival on the ward. While being transported, a container of sources must not be left unattended in areas accessible to the public or staff not concerned with its use. Containers should be labelled correctly giving details of the sources within. Care should be taken to remove labels form empty containers.

Generally, the only occasion when it would be necessary to transport radioactive sources outside the hospital is when they need to be returned to the supplier. However, it may be necessary to transport sources to another hospital. In either case, reference must be made to the relevant national regulations, particularly the following:

(1) identify the radionuclide and its source strength;

(2) establish the type of packing required (and ensure that it has been type-tested);

(3) after packing the sources correctly, measure the dose rate on the surface and at 1 m from it, and calculate the transport index which is the dose rate in mSv h^{-1} at a distance of 1 m multiplied by 100 (the IAEA has set a limit on the transport index of 10 and a maximum surface dose rate of 2 mSv h^{-1});

(4) label the package with the correct transport label, showing radionuclide, activity, and transport index;

(5) fill in all transport documents;

(6) ensure that drivers have been trained and have placards that specify the hazard clearly displayed within their vehicle.

4.5 Precautions after death of a patient containing sealed sources

Information about any radioactive substances remaining in a patient's body should always be available. Whether the patient dies in the hospital or at home, appropriate instructions should be given to those responsible for the handling and disposal of the body.

Temporary implants should be removed from corpses as soon as possible after death and before the body is released for post-mortem examination or disposal. If a permanent implant is involved, no special precautions are necessary provided that the total reference AKR of the sources does not exceed certain specified values. For gold-198 grains these are 0.55 μGy h^{-1} (10 MBq) for post-mortem or embalming, 22 μGy h^{-1} (400 MBq) for burial, and 5.5 μGy h^{-1} (100 MBq) for cremation. For iodine-125 seeds the values are 1.3 μGy h^{-1} (40 MBq), 1300 μGy h^{-1} (400 MBq), and 1300 μGy h^{-1} (4000 MBq), respectively for the three situations. If the reference AKR is greater than these values, then the RPA should be consulted.

5. Afterloading systems

Afterloading systems are designed to reduce the radiation dose to staff. Afterloading refers to any method whereby empty source containers can be placed in the tissues or in a body cavity and the sources loaded later in a simpler and quicker procedure. This has the advantage that time and care can be taken over the implant or insertion without the theatre staff receiving any radiation exposure. Radiographic checks on source positions can be made using dummy sources, or simply using the applicator itself, to provide the contrast on the radiograph. The sources are then positioned in the applicator when these checks have been made and the patient has returned to the ward or, in the case of HDR sources, to the treatment room. Sources can be loaded either manually or remotely.

There is increasing pressure for the use of afterloading systems because of the recognition that brachytherapy is the main source of radiation to which staff working in hospital radiotherapy departments are exposed. In future, manual systems may not be accepted as good practice, and even manual afterloading systems for LDR gynaecological treatments may be discouraged.

5.1 Manual afterloading

Examples of manual systems are the use of pre-implanted catheters for iridium wire treatments and certain applicator systems for gynaecological insertions. The main disadvantage of manual afterloading is that, although the theatre staff and surgeon receive no radiation, the ward staff are still exposed to radiation during nursing procedures. The maximum total source strength that can be handled safely in this way is of the order of reference AKR 800 μGy h^{-1}. HDR and MDR can only be used with remote afterloading.

5.2 Remote afterloading

For remote afterloading, the sources are contained in a lead safe by the patient's bed on the ward, from which they can be loaded automatically into the applicator from outside the room. Source transfer systems are either pneumatic or via drive cables through delivery tubes connected to the machine and the catheter or applicator in the patient. The sources can be removed from the patient whenever a nursing procedure is necessary.

The choice of afterloading equipment is strongly influenced by clinical applications and preferences. For gynaecological treatments, the main choice is between LDR (or MDR) and HDR. This has important radiobiological implications (see Section 8), so that the decision is likely to be made mainly on clinical grounds. The advent of HDR iridium-192 systems has facilitated the treatment of new sites, such as the bronchus and oesophagus. However, such systems may not be able to manage a large gynaecological workload. In addition, many therapists prefer LDR therapy with conventional doses and fractionation for gynaecological treatments. Therefore, the ideal may be to have an LDR (or MDR) system for this work and an HDR system for other applications. However, this may be economically prohibitive and some treatments at LDR may continue to need manual afterloading systems.

5.2.1 Low/medium dose-rate systems for gynaecological tumours

LDR and MDR systems deliver dose rates to point A for gynaecological treatments typically in the range 0.5–1.5 Gy h^{-1}. Three systems are considered here.

1. The Selectron, manufactured by Nucletron, in which the active caesium-137 sources are contained within steel spheres, which are 2.5 mm in diameter. These, together with inactive spheres, form a linear array of 48 sources of any combination. Once a safe connection has been made between the applicator and the lead safe using a special tube, the sources are loaded by compressed air. Special applicators are available to match conventional dosimetry systems,

and up to three applicators are generally used for a treatment.

2. The Curietron uses individually designed source trains consisting of caesium-137 sources and spacers loaded into long stainless steel springs and closed at one end, which can be driven automatically from the safe on the end of a cable inside a catheter into the applicator.

3. The Buchler system makes use of a single iridium-192 source for the uterine tube, which oscillates to produce the same radiation distribution as a train of sources. It is used in conjunction with two fixed ovoids if the standard three-source arrangement of sources is required for gynaecological treatment.

A fourth system, which is known as pulsed dose rate (PDR), should be mentioned here. This can simulate the physical dose rate of LDR and MDR by using a relatively high strength source of iridium-192 (reference AKR approximately 4 mGy h^{-1}), but loading it for only a few minutes every hour. The complete treatment can then extend over several hours or days instead of minutes, thus producing an average dose rate similar to that of an LDR system (typically 0.5 Gy h^{-1}). However, the radiobiology of late effects is more complicated and still being clinical tested.

5.2.2 High dose-rate systems

The dose rate for HDR systems is generally up to 5 Gy min^{-1} (instantaneous dose rate). In these systems, activities are increased so that treatment times are in minutes rather than hours. In order that the sources retain the same physical dimensions as for LDR and MDR, the use of caesium is excluded because of its relatively low specific activity. The radionuclides used are cobalt-60 and iridium-192.

There are three commonly used systems: source trains of cobalt-60 loaded on drive cables (as in the Cathetron, which is no longer manufactured), beads of cobalt-60 loaded using compressed air (as in the Selectron-HDR, Nucletron), and a miniature iridium-192 source that is moved automatically to produce any distribution required in a single line or multiple lines (as in the MicroSelectron-HDR or GammaMed, Isotopen-Technik Dr Sauerwein GmbH).

All these remote afterloading systems have the major advantage of versatility of source position and time, as well as the radiation safety aspect of their use.

5.2.3 Low dose-rate interstitial systems

Typically, these treat at a dose rate of 0.3–0.9 Gy h^{-1}. They use sources that can be loaded into fine catheters or needles that are already in place in the patient. At present, the sources available are iridium wire or seeds and caesium seeds. A variety of suitable lengths of wire or source trains of seeds must be available to the clinician. A typical remote afterloading system has 15 channels with 15 drive motors for up to 15 individual sources simultaneously loaded. Alternatively, the pulsed (PDR) Selectron described above can be used.

6. Dosimetry systems

In external beam therapy, absorbed dose to a point, such as the treatment isocentre, can be used to represent the dose to the tumour because it is relatively easy to deliver a uniform dose over the target volume. Dose to a point does not have the same meaning in brachytherapy. The problem is much more complex because the dose varies considerably in the region of the sources. Second, it is not always possible to deliver the treatment exactly as planned because of the difficulty in positioning sources in tissues in a precise manner. A third difficulty, historically, was an inability to make comprehensive fast calculations of the dose distribution around the source array.

For these reasons a number of dosimetry systems have been developed that provide rules to answer such questions as the following.

How close should the sources be to each other?

What activity should be chosen?

How should the activity be distributed?

How is the dose specified?

In this chapter, two interstitial dosimetry systems will be described. The Paterson–Parker or Manchester dosage system, which has been in use since the mid-1930s, was developed for radium sources but can be applied to caesium needles and tubes. The Paris system has been in use since the 1960s and was primarily developed for iridium wire. These systems are intended for standard-source arrangements based on the volume to be treated. Precalculated tables are available to derive the total time required to deliver a treatment dose defined in a way that is specific to the dosimetry system. Many systems have been developed for gynaecological brachytherapy; the Manchester system is described in Section 6.7.

6.1 Dose prescription and reporting

When radium was first used, clinicians prescribed a quantity of radium to be put in place for a specified time depending on the site of the tumour, whether it was interstitial or intracavitary treatment, and the treatment volume. This is the origin of the source-related prescription given in the units milligram hours (mg h).

As dosimetry systems developed in parallel with the developments in dose quantities and units, prescription methods evolved in terms of exposure or dose within the standard dosimetry system. For example, in the Manchester system for gynaecological treatment, the specification changed from milligram hours to the exposure to point A. In the Paterson–Parker system for interstitial planar implants, the average dose to the treatment plane at a distance of 0.5 cm from the source is used as a basis for prescription. In other systems the minimum peripheral dose for a given target volume was specified, and the more recent Paris system utilizes 85% of the mean value of defined dose minima in a central plane. Thus, when doses to tumours and dose rates used for brachytherapy are discussed, a particular system should always be quoted, otherwise the meaning of dose is very imprecise. A particular example concerns the HDR iridium sources, where dose rates and doses are frequently quoted without any explanation of their precise meaning. The instantaneous dose rate from such a source may be, for example, of the order of 5 Gy min^{-1} at 1 cm. However, if the source is moved throughout treatment, the average dose rate will be different and will depend on the movement parameters.

With the availability of brachytherapy computer-planning systems, which can rapidly calculate and display isodose curve patterns for any source arrangement, it may seem appropriate to use these to choose an isodose rate curve in the same way that an isodose curve is chosen from an external beam plan. However, there is a vast difference between these two types of plan. In external beam therapy, fairly uniform doses are achieved throughout the target volume with a relatively rapid fall off at the periphery. It is usual to prescribe to an isodose such that the maximum dose within the target volume is no more than 5–10% greater. For brachytherapy, the dose within the target volume is very inhomogeneous; the dose to tissue in contact with the sources can be very high. At the periphery an isodose rate curve can be chosen for prescription, but the dose rate may change by a factor of 2 or more over distances of a few millimetres. Therefore, although computer systems are attractive tools with which to produce isodose rate curves in three dimensions around a source array, dosimetry systems continue to have an important role, in particular as the starting point in the planning/prescribing process. This is true even if the final precise calculation is made by computer. One of the benefits of computers is that they permit a degree of optimization of source arrangement, or dwell times, to be made quickly, which was not possible with traditional systems.

Standard dosimetry systems are likely to continue to be used for gynaecological treatments since the source arrangements and strengths for these treatments are based on many years of clinical experience, and changes in method, particularly dose rate, can compromise results significantly. The currently recommended method for reporting gynaecological brachytherapy treatment in full is given in ICRU Report 38 (ICRU 1985). This is discussed in Section 6.7.3.

The full reporting of interstitial brachytherapy is the subject of ICRU Report 58 (ICRU 1997), which includes the following:

(1) the mean central dose (the arithmetic mean of the local minimum doses between sources in the central plane(s));

(2) the total reference air kerma, i.e. the product of source strength and treatment time;

(3) the regions of low and high dose within the target volume, where high dose is greater than 150% of the mean central dose and low dose is less than 90% of the prescribed dose;

(4) clinical target volume (CTV) and treated volume concepts (similar to external beam therapy, see Chapter 7, Section 2) are also included.

The Paris method of determining the 85% isodose rate curve relative to the minimum central dose gives consistency to implant-therapy prescribing and reporting, but any of the systems of dosimetry, where there is a large clinical base of evidence that the prescription produces the right result, is preferable to the arbitrary choice of isodose rate curve from the computer print-out.

6.2 Interstitial therapy: Manchester system

The Manchester system is summarized in Meredith (1967). This gives a useful guide to the rationale of brachytherapy-dosimetry systems, even though much of the discussion deals with the calculation for moulds, which are not very relevant now and will not be considered in this chapter. However, the physical principles of the system, particularly regarding the development of the distribution rules to ensure a uniform dose over the treatment plane, are most clearly set out in the chapter on moulds in this reference. It is important to understand this concept of homogeneity of dose in brachytherapy. The basis of the Manchester system is that the dose throughout the treatment plane should be constant to within ±10%, except for localized high spots.

6.2.1 Single-plane implants

For single-plane implants, the treatment plane is defined as being 5 mm on either side of the source array. It should be noted that the basis of this was that:

> Experience has shown that the arbitrary choice of 0.5 cm as the treating distance leads to results which are clinically satisfactory, and at the same time allows a sufficient number of needles to be used in order to produce an arrangement of sources conforming with the distribution rules (Meredith 1967).

The rules for implant are a considerable simplification of the corresponding mould rules. This was necessary as the

Table 12.4 Relative proportion of total source strength to be placed in the periphery and the area of a planar implant (Manchester system)

Area (cm^2)	Periphery	Area
<25	2/3	1/3
25–100	1/2	1/2
>100	1/3	2/3

range of needles available is limited and the source arrangements stipulated for moulds are generally impracticable for implants. However, it was emphasized that, wherever possible, the mould rules should be applied, since they give better distributions.

For implants, the needles should be positioned in a parallel array. In order to prevent a fall in dose at the ends of the needles, additional sources should, if possible, be placed across the ends of the implant. These are referred to as crossing needles. The rules for the distribution of activity depend on the area of the implant. They are shown in Table 12.4, which gives the relative source strengths in the periphery of the implant and within the central area. The dose calculation is also based on the area and will be described later.

Many users of the Manchester system miss some of the more subtle points, partly because the range of use of needle implants is now restricted compared with the time when the rules were first derived.

It is interesting to note some of these points in Meredith (1967), particularly when it comes to making a comparison with the Paris system.

1. The area of the surface of the slab of tissue to be implanted, and not the area outlined by the needles, is considered as the area of the implant. These are not the same when the needles lie in a curved plane.

2. There is an emphasis on considering the peripheral activity and central area activity separately, which derives from the Manchester system's rules for moulds.

3. Within the parallel array, the needles should normally be about 1 cm from each other and never more than 1.5 cm; in practice, separations between 0.8 and 1.2 cm are used.

4. The depth or thickness of the treated volume is always 1 cm for a planar volume regardless of area.

5. The width of the treated volume is the width of the implanted volume plus about 1 cm.

6. The length of the treated volume depends on whether crossing needles have been used.

This last point can cause problems for the inexperienced user, since the effects of crossing needles are not spelt out precisely. This is partly because there has to be some flexibility in the system, since it is often impossible to perform real implants exactly to the rules. Even in the examples given in Meredith (1967), there are slight variations as to where the crossing needle should be. The problem arises because the active length of the needle is significantly shorter than the overall length. Strictly, the crossing needles should cross the active ends of the area array. However, in practice (and in the illustrations in the book) they are often positioned across the physical ends of the needles.

If no crossing needles are used, the area to be used in the calculation is found from the area of the active part of the needle arrangement minus 20%, i.e. 10% for each uncrossed end. This means that the length of the treatment volume is also reduced by about this amount. If one end is crossed, the treatment volume is shortened by 10% at the uncrossed end of the implant but extends to the crossing needle at the other end, provided that the crossing needle is not further out than the physical end of the needle array. If the crossing needle is displaced form the end of the implant by a distance x, then the treated length extends to about $x/2$ from that end.

An alternative method of extending the treated length is to use differentially loaded needles. The original radium needles were given the names 'Indian club', when one end cell had an activity three times that of the others, and 'dumb-bell', when each of the end cells had a linear activity twice that of the other cells of the needle. In both cases, the area of the implant is taken to be the same as that for standardly loaded sources of the same length and no correction is made for the uncrossed end if the higher-activity cells are at the end of the needles.

Calculation of implant times to achieve the required dose utilizes tables, generally referred to as Paterson–Parker tables. These were originally determined by performing a large number of calculations based on integrating the dose received from each source across the area of the treated plane. The dosage tables derived in this way gave the number of milligram hours of radium required within the implanted plane to produce a 'dose' of 1000 R in the plane of calculation for different implant areas.

The tables are used at the pre-implant stage to determine the total activity required to deliver the prescribed dose in a given time for the specified area. Following implant and the measurement of the actual area of the implant, the tables give the total treatment time.

Since publication of the original Paterson–Parker tables, a number of changes in dosimetry, available sources, and physical constants have necessitated a review of these data. The data in Table 12.5 were taken

Table 12.5 Modified Paterson–Parker dose tables for the Manchester system to give air kerma at 1 m (reference AKR × treatment time) per unit absorbed dose (Gy) as defined for the Manchester system. For single and double plane implants, the treatment distance is 5 mm and the data are taken from Massey *et al.* (1985). The data for volume implants was derived from Meredith (1967). The data can be derived directly from the original Paterson–Parker tables in Meredith (1967) by applying a factor 108 to convert from the original exposure unit 'R' to absorbed dose in Gy and a factor 7.2 to convert from source strength in mg radium to reference AKR in $\mu Gy\ h^{-1}$

Single/double plane		Volume implants	
Area (cm^2)	$\mu Gy\ Gy^{-1}$	Volume (cm^3)	$\mu Gy\ Gy^{-1}$
6	138	10	123
8	160	15	161
10	183	20	195
12	203	25	227
14	224	30	256
16	245	40	310
18	266	50	360
20	286	60	407
22	305	70	450
24	324	80	492
26	343	90	533
28	362	100	571
30	381	110	609
32	399	120	645

from Massey *et al.* (1985) for a treatment distance of 5 mm. Data for other distances are given in the reference. Table 12.5 shows the product of reference AKR ($\mu Gy\ h^{-1}$) and implant time (hours) to deliver an absorbed dose of 1 Gy in the treatment plane. The data can be used for the sources commonly used for implants such as Cs-137 or Ir-192. However, in the latter case, some caution should be applied, since it is generally unlikely that the correct distribution of sources will have been used as required by the Manchester system. In particular, it is unlikely that a lower linear activity will be used over the central area of the implant.

The tables give a useful guide to overall activity/source strength required for a given target volume. Detailed calculations of the completed implant can be performed by computer, following reconstruction from radiographs.

An example of a single-plane implant has been adapted from Meredith (1967). It is required to treat a lesion (2 × 3 cm) of the external surface of the cheek by means of a single-plane implant at about 0.5 cm from the skin surface. The size of implant is to be 4 × 5 cm (to allow a 1 cm margin around the tumour, this is called the target volume). The planning steps are shown in

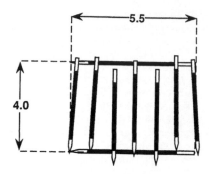

Figure 12.3 Implanted needles for the single-plane implant given as an example in Table 12.6.

Table 12.6, with the calculation of total time based on the implanted source distribution shown in Figure 12.3. In this example, the source strengths are specified in terms

of reference AKR, and it should be noted that the identification of sources follows the original Manchester convention for radium sources.

6.2.2 Double-plane implants

Single-plane treatments are used for lesions that are no more than 10 mm thick. For thicker volumes, a second plane of sources must be used. Dosage for two-plane implants is based on the average dose between the two planes. For a separation of 10 mm, the average is considered to be equal to the mid-plane dose for which the Paterson–Parker tables for single-plane implants can be used directly. For separations greater than 10 mm, the total source strength (or time) must be increased by the factor shown in Table 12.7, column 2. For separations greater than 15 mm, the dose on the mid-plane is significantly less than the average to the slab of tissue between the sources; the resultant dose reduction is

Table 12.6 An example of a single-plane implant (Manchester system)

Planning

Area of implant	4×5 cm = 20 cm^2
Prescription	60 Gy in 7 days (168 h)
Integrated source strength	286×60 = 17160 μGy (*Table 12.5*)
Total source strength	17160/168 = 102 μGy h^{-1}

Available sources

ID	Source strength (μGy h^{-1})	Active length (mm)	Total length (mm)
A1	3.5	15	25
A2	7	30	42
A3	10.5	45	58
B1	7	15	25
B2	4	30	42
B3	21	45	58

Date of source calibration	January 1995
Implant geometry	2/3 periphery, 1/3 area (*Table 12.4*)
	On each long side, $1 \times$ B3 (crossing needle)
	On each short side $1 \times$ B2
	Central area, $5 \times$ A2
	Needle separation = 5/6
	= 0.8 cm

Source strength

Periphery	$(2 \times 21) + (2 \times 14)$ = 70 μGy h^{-1}
Area	(5×7) = 35 μGy h^{-1}
Total	105 μGy h^{-1}

Calculation

True area of implant	4×5.5 cm = 22 cm^2 (*Figure 12.3*)
Integrated source strength	305×60 = 18300 μGy
Date of implant	July 1998
Decay correction	exp $(0.693/30.0 \times 3.5)$ = 1.08
Total time	$(18300/105) \times 1.08$ = 188 h

Table 12.7 Multiplicative factor to be applied to the activity or time for a two-plane implant with a separation greater than 10 mm (Manchester system) and the reduction in dose in the mid-plane for separations greater than 2 cm (Meredith 1967)

Plane Separation (cm)	Separation factor	Area (cm²)	Dose reduction in the mid-plane (%)
1.5	1.25		
2	1.4	0–25	20
		25–50	10
2.5	1.5	0–25	30
		25–80	20

shown in Table 12.7, column 4. Plane separations greater than 25 mm, corresponding to a total thickness of 35 mm, should not be used.

As an example of a two-plane implant, the calculations necessary prior to the treatment of an anal tumour are given in Table 12.8. In this case it is difficult to insert crossing needles, so that a correction has to be made for the uncrossed ends, assuming that differentially loaded needles are not available. The average area of the implanted sources should be used for the final calculation of the total treatment time based on the actual implanted source distribution.

6.2.3 Volume implants

A different rationale is used for volume implants, but the principle of applying distribution rules is very similar. The rules are more complex and depend on whether the shape of the volume can be described as a cylinder, sphere, or cuboid. Since volume implants are now rarely used, a full description of the rules is not given here and reference should be made to Meredith (1967). Table 12.5 includes data for dose calculations for volume implants. These were derived from Meredith (1967) using a net conversion factor of 0.778 to convert the original source and dose specifications to units of $\mu Gy\ Gy^{-1}$ (Gibb and Massey 1980; Massey *et al.* 1985). The method applies to volumes whose dimensions are equal in all directions. If this is not the case, an elongation factor that depends on the ratio of the longest to the shortest dimension should be used; these factors have the effect of increasing the overall treatment time.

The most common source for which the Manchester system for volume implants is still used is gold-198 in the form of seeds or grains, which are introduced into the tissues using a specially designed 'gun'. Grains give much greater flexibility than needles on the implant geometry. Gold-198 seeds also have the potential advantage of a short half-life, so that the implant can be left in place permanently.

In this case, the effective treatment time is derived by integrating the decay curve to infinite time. For the half-life of ^{198}Au (64.7 h), it can be shown that the effective treatment time is 93.4 h, which can be used in conjunction with the source strength at the time of implant.

Implants using gold seeds are difficult to carry out in accordance with the distribution rules and to the exact volume specified at the planning stage. It is particularly difficult to achieve an even distribution of seeds through the target volume. Once the seeds are in place the dose

Table 12.8 An example of a two-plane implant (Manchester system)

Planning	
Area of implant	4 × 4.5 cm = 18 cm²
Plane separation	2 cm
Prescription	60 Gy in 6 days (144 h)
Effective area	18 × 0.8 = 14.4 cm² (uncrossed ends)
Integrated source strength	228 × 60 = 13680 μGy (*Table 12.5*)
Separation correction	1.4 (*Table 12.7*)
Total source strength	(13680/144) × 1.4 = 133 μGy h^{-1}
Available sources	See *Table 12.6*
Implant geometry	On each short side, 1 × B3
	Central area, 3 × A3
	Needle separation = 4.5/4
	= 1.1 cm
Source strength (each plane)	
Periphery	2 × 21 = 42 μGy h^{-1}
Area	3 × 10.5 = 31.5 μGy h^{-1}
Total (both planes)	2 × (42 + 31.5) = 147 μGy h^{-1}

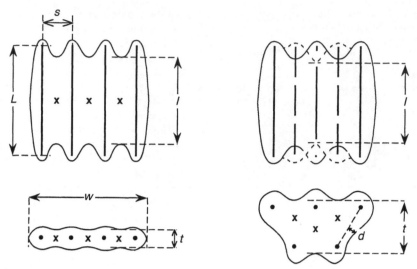

Figure 12.4 Definition of implant dimensions for the Paris system. A single-plane implant is shown on the left and a two-plane implant with a triangular arrangement of wires is shown on the right. The reference isodose is shown and the crosses represent the positions of the basal dose rate calculation.

delivered cannot be adjusted, which is the major disadvantage of a permanent implant.

6.3   Interstitial therapy: Paris system

Radioactive needles present a significant hazard to the surgeon or radiotherapist because they must be manipulated directly and both the fingers and the eyes can receive fairly high radiation doses. To reduce this hazard, manual afterloading systems have been developed using iridium-192 wires, which can be loaded either at the end of the operation or when the patient has returned to the ward. The fine diameter of iridium wire, while still maintaining a relatively high specific activity, makes this a very versatile technique. As well as wires inserted into implanted plastic tubing, hairpins and single pins can be used. Slotted steel guides are inserted into the patient; the radioactive hairpins or single pins can then be inserted and sutured into position, and the guides withdrawn.

The Paris system was developed primarily for iridium wire and is quite different from, and more flexible than, the Manchester system. Its rules for implant and dose specification are outlined below, but a more complete description is given in Pierquin *et al.* (1978).

6.3.1   Implant rules

Wires should be implanted according to the following rules.

1. Each wire should be continuous with a uniform activity and the lengths and activity of each wire should be the same.

2. The wires should be implanted so that, as far as possible, they are straight and parallel to each other.

3. The separation between the wires should be equal and depends on the volume to be treated. For small volumes, the spacing should not be less than 5 mm, and for large volumes it should not exceed 20 mm.

4. The wires should extend beyond the limits of the tumour volume at each end by about 20% for short wires and by about 30% for long wires. This contrasts with the Manchester system in which crossing needles are used. One end is partially crossed when hairpins are used, in which case the additional length is only required at the open end of the hairpin.

5. When more than one plane is used for volume implants, the wires are arranged so that the cross-sectional source distribution is either a series of equilateral triangles (Figure 12.4) or a series of squares.

6.3.2   Dose specification

The Paris system dose specification uses a basal dose rate, which is the average of the dose rates calculated at each minimum dose point in the central transverse plan of the implant. This is at the mid-point between wires in a single plane, or at the centre of the triangles or squares formed by wires in a multiple-plane implant. These points are shown for the single and triangular plane arrangements in Figure 12.4. The dose rate used for prescription is the reference dose rate, which is equal to

85% of the basal dose rate. Therefore, the treatment volume is delineated by the reference isodose curve, which corresponds to the reference dose rate.

6.3.3 Treatment volume

The dimensions of the treatment volumes for single-plane and two-plane implants are shown in Figure 12.4.

1. The length (*l*) of the treatment volume is defined parallel to the wires. It corresponds to the minimum distance across the reference isodose rate curve within the area bounded by the wires. For the ideal implant it occurs between the two outer wires. For a single plane it is measured in the plane of the wires, and for a two-plane implant it is measured half-way between the planes.

2. The width (*w*) of the treatment volume is only defined for a single-plane implant. It is the reference isodose width in the central transverse plane.

3. The lateral margin (*d*) is the alternative parameter used for multiple-plane implants to describe the distance that the reference isodose extends beyond the physical boundary of the implant in the central transverse plane. It is the minimum distance between the reference isodose and a line drawn joining two of the outermost wires, as shown for the triangular arrangement in Figure 12.4.

4. The thickness (*t*) is also defined in the central transverse plane of the implant. It is the distance between the two parallel lines that are tangents to the reference isodose curve and are parallel to the source positions in each plane. The tangents are chosen to minimize this distance (Figure 12.4).

The values of these parameters depend on the length (*L*) of the wires and their separation *s* and can vary with the number of sources. However, some empirical relationships have been established and are shown in Table 12.9. It should be noted that for multiplane implants, *s* is the separation between the wires and not the separation between the planes.

Table 12.9 Size of the reference isodose in the central plane of the implant for wires of length *L* and separation *s* (Paris system)

	Single plane	Double plane
Length, *l*	0.6*L*–0.75*L*	
Thickness, *t*	0.5*s*–0.6*s*	1.2*s* (triangles)
		1.5*s* (squares)
Width, *w*	(*n* − 1)*s* + 0.74*s* cm	–
Lateral margin, *d*	–	0.15*s* (triangles)
		0.28*s* (squares)

6.3.4 Dose calculation

The basal dose rate for standard implant geometries can be calculated from standard charts. These give the dose rate at varying distances for a range of wire lengths. Two types of chart are available.

1. The original method developed by the Paris group used 'escargot curves'. These were subsequently modified by Dutreix *et al.* (1982) to allow for the new source specification.

2. The Oxford system uses cross-plot charts (similar to the original radium charts) developed by Hall *et al.* (1966), which were subsequently converted to read absorbed dose (Walsh *et al.* 1983). These charts are based on the milligram radium equivalent specification of source strength.

The graphical methods are simple to use, but it may be preferable to use a direct calculation based on the formula for a line source. From the equations given in Section 3, it can be shown that the dose rate at a perpendicular distance *d* mm from the mid-point of an unfiltered line source is given by:

$$D(d) = 2\frac{\text{AKR}_0}{d}\tan^{-1}\left(\frac{L}{2d}\right)f_3 \qquad (19)$$

in which *L* is the source length. It can be shown that the units of $D(d)$ are Gy h^{-1}, provided that the reference AKR, AKR$_0$, has the units μGy h^{-1} mm^{-1}, i.e. source strength specification per millimetre wire length, and the wire length and the distance are also specified in millimetres. f_3 is the factor to convert air kerma to absorbed dose to water and is equal to 1.11 for iridium-192.

This equation is sufficiently accurate when planning implants provided that $L/2d$ is less than 5, for which errors of 5% or less are introduced due to the effects of oblique filtration. Corrections for this have been derived by Casebow (1985) for wires of thicknesses 0.3 and 0.6 mm.

An example of an iridium-wire plan for a single-plane treatment is given in Table 12.10. This is for the same area specified for the Manchester system example (Table 12.6), i.e. 4 × 5 cm. In this case, the length of the volume has been specified to be 4 cm with the outermost sources specified as being 5 cm apart. This orientation has been chosen to be comparable with the needle arrangement from Table 12.6. The arrangement of wires is shown in Figure 12.5 with the position of the basal dose rate calculation points. A range of source strengths is available from manufacturers and the closest to that calculated would be ordered taking into account any decay correction.

For the planning of iridium wire implants, it is also possible to use tables published by Casebow (1984,

Table 12.10 An example of the planning for a single-plane iridium wire implant to treat an area of 4 × 5 cm with five wires

Prescription	20 Gy in 48 h
Wire length, L	40/0.7 = 57 mm
Separation, s	50/4 = 12.5 mm
Implant thickness	12.5 × 0.55 = 7 mm
f_3	1.11
Calculation of wire reference AKR	
Position A (and D)	
Dose rate from wires 1 and 2	d = 6.25 mm
	AKR_0 (2/6.25)$\tan^{-1}$(28.5/6.25) × 1.11 = 0.481 AKR_0
Dose rate from wire 3	d = 18.75 mm
	AKR_0(2/18.75)$\tan^{-1}$(28.5/18.75) × 1.11 = 0.117 AKR_0
Dose rate from wire 4	d = 31.25 mm
	AKR_0(2/31.25)$\tan^{-1}$(28.5/31.25) × 1.11 = 0.053 AKR_0
Dose rate from wire 5	d = 43.75 mm
	AKR_0(2/43.75)$\tan^{-1}$(28.5/43.75) × 1.11 = 0.029 AKR_0
Total dose rate (A and D)	AKR_0(0.481 × 2 + 0.117 + 0.053 + 0.029) = 1.161 AKR_0
Dose rate at positions B and C	AKR_0(0.481 × 2 + 0.117 × 2 + 0.053) = 1.249 × AKR_0
Average basal dose rate	1.205 AKR_0
Reference dose rate	1.205 × 0.85 × AKR_0 = 1.024 AKR_0
Required source strength	(20/48)/1.024 = 0.407 μGy h^{-1}mm^{-1}

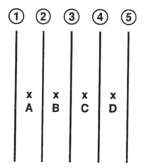

Figure 12.5 A single-plane implant for the example calculation in Table 12.10 showing the positions of the basal dose rate calculation.

1985). These give the source strength required for a range of implant sizes. In these publications, source strength is specified in reference exposure at 1 m in units of mR h^{-1}. These figures need to be multiplied by 8.76 to convert to the μGy h^{-1} specification.

6.4 Line sources

Although this subject has been dealt with theoretically in Section 3.2, it merits a further section since there is a resurgence of interest in the use of one or two line sources for treatments such as carcinoma of the oesophagus or bronchus. Both the Manchester and the Paris systems give guidance on the dosimetry of line sources and tables to calculate dose rates at various distances.

The isodose curves round a line source are virtually independent of the type of source except towards its ends, where the fall in dose depends on the geometry of the inactive end. For the purposes of prescription, however, the region beyond the active end is not generally of great significance. The following points should be noted.

1. The dose rate at the treatment distance is reasonably constant over about 75% of the active length of the source (it should be noted how this fits with the definition of the treated length in both the Manchester and Paris systems).

2. Opposite the end of the active length at the treatment distance, the dose rate falls to approximately 50% of the peak value.

3. For source lengths greater than 3 cm, the dose rate at 0.5 cm distance increases by only 1–2% for each centimetre increase in source length.

6.5 Comparison of the Manchester and Paris systems

In many radiotherapy departments, both iridium wire and caesium needles are used for different clinical applications. Therefore, it is not uncommon for both the Paris and Manchester systems to be used in one centre. Although computer programs are employed widely for brachytherapy, they are not necessarily very useful for the first stages of brachytherapy-treatment planning and it is essential for the physicist to know

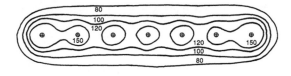

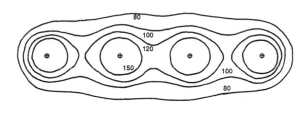

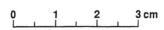

Figure 12.6 Central plane isodose distributions for two single-plane implants. The upper figure is for a Manchester implant for the example in Table 12.6. The lower distribution is for the Paris system to give a thickness of 10 mm. The 100% isodose represents the treatment dose rate.

and appreciate the rules of both the Manchester and Paris systems.

The Manchester system is for rigid needles forming rectangular, nowadays quite small, area implants. Because of the way in which this system evolved, the rules stress the formation of a rectangular box (the peripheral activity) and then the filling of the area with line sources of different linear activity, in order to achieve dose uniformity throughout the target volume and to counter the fall-off in dose at the margins of the volume.

This latter point particularly contrasts with the Paris system, where the array of wires inevitably shows a lower dose rate at its margins. This can best be illustrated by the isodose curves produced by single-plane implants shown in Figure 12.6. For the Manchester system implant, the isodose curves are for the examples shown in Table 12.6. For the iridium wire implant, four wires have been chosen rather than the five that were used in Table 12.10. These have a separation of 17 mm, which gives a treatment volume thickness of 10 mm, which is the same as the nominal thickness in the Manchester system. It can be seen that this inevitably produces a less uniform dose distribution throughout the target volume.

Volume implants are very different, with the emphasis in the Paris system being on a pattern of wires within the volume to maintain uniformity of dose, whereas the Manchester system again concentrates on the peripheral

activity with circular/cylindrical patterns of activity to obtain a uniform dose across the centre. The great advantage of iridium wire is that any length can be used, compared with the discrete lengths of caesium needles. In addition, a range of activities is available. Wire can be loaded into stainless steel needles for use in anal or vulval treatments. Several centres have also adopted a rigid-jig technique for use in treatments of breast tumours, rather than have the uncertainty of a flexible outer tube. Such rigid techniques become desirable when remote afterloading systems are used to ensure safe loading and unloading of the sources.

6.6 Seed implants

Differences in approach to brachytherapy between the UK and the USA have existed for at least 30 years. They are most strongly demonstrated in the use of seeds for interstitial brachytherapy. In the UK (and elsewhere in Europe), the use of needles and iridium wire and hairpins and their associated dosimetry systems have been maintained. Seeds have been used much less frequently, e.g. gold-198 grains. In the USA, seeds are much more commonly used, particularly iridium-192 but also iodine-125, and more recently palladium-103. An outline is given here of the dosimetry protocol developed by Task Group No. 43 of the AAPM for seed dosimetry (Nath *et al.* 1995) and some details of particular dosimetry systems.

6.6.1 AAPM seed dosimetry protocol

The dose rate from cylindrically symmetric sources is given by:

$$\frac{d(D)}{dt}(r, \theta) = S_k \Lambda \left[\frac{G(r, \theta)}{G(r_0, \theta_0)} \right] g(r) F(r, \theta) \quad (20)$$

where:

$\frac{dD}{dt}(r, \theta)$ is the absorbed dose rate at a distance r and angle θ to the source axis.

S_k is the air kerma strength (either in μGy m^2 h^{-1} or cGy cm^2 h^{-1}).

Λ is the dose rate constant, which is the dose rate to water at a distance of 1 cm on the transverse axis of a unit air kerma strength source in a water phantom.

$G(r, \theta)$ is a geometric factor based on the variation of relative dose due to the spatial distribution of activity within the source itself, it does not include the effect of encapsulation. When the distribution of radioactivity can be approximated by a point source $G(r, \theta)$ reduces to r^{-2}, when the distribution of radioactivity is a line source of constant linear activity $G(r, \theta)$ becomes $(\theta_2 - \theta_1)/Lr\sin\theta$, which is equivalent to the geometric factor in equation (5); r_0, θ_0 are the co-ordinates of the reference point; $r_0 = 1$ cm and $\theta_0 = \pi/2$.

$g(r)$ is the radial dose function accounting for the effects of absorption and scatter in the medium; $g(r)$ is normalized to unity at 1 cm from the centre of the source, unlike f_2 in equation (10).

$F(r, \theta)$ is an anisotropy function due to self-filtration in the source and oblique filtration through the encapsulating material. It is equivalent to $\int_{\theta_1}^{\theta_2} f_1(d, \theta)d\theta$ in equation (9).

For detailed information on this formalism and for data for specific sources, reference should be made to Nath *et al.* (1995).

This approach to the calculation of dose rate from a sealed source differs from the BIR method. AAPM use Λ and its relationship to air kerma strength (see Section 3.1). The BIR protocol places the emphasis on AKR at 1 m. The difference is particularly significant for seeds emitting low-energy photons, for which the dose rates at 1 cm in water have been measured. As such, the AAPM formulation is more accurate.

It is also recommended that liquid water should be used as a reference medium for describing dose-rate distributions around the source, and that the treatment-planning software should include data-entry options allowing single-source treatment-planning data to be entered in tabular form, to include calculated data for the above functions as included in the report.

AAPM have issued guidance on the practical implementation of the recommendations of Task Group No. 43 (AAPM 1997).

6.6.2 Seed-dosimetry systems

The calculation methods described above enable the dose distribution from an implant to be calculated retrospectively and, in the planning process, to determine the optimum distribution of sources and source strengths to treat a particular target volume. Dosimetry systems for brachytherapy provide general guidance on the distribution of sources to produce an optimized dose distribution based on target size. The Manchester system for the planning of volume implants using gold grains was described in Section 6.2.3. A system that is well established in the USA for seed implants requires the sources, of equal strength, to be spaced uniformly throughout the target volume. The dose prescription is based on an isodose surface that represents the minimum peripheral dose to the target volume. In practice, the isodose surface that just surrounds the implant (usually in the central plane perpendicular to the sources) is selected as the reference isodose for dose specification. The risk for such a system is that the selection of the prescription isodose is highly subjective because of the high dose gradients at the periphery of the implant. This may lead to uncertainty and error, particularly for inexperienced clinicians.

Because the sources are evenly distributed, the implant will be similar to a Paris distribution. However, many more sources will be used and this ensures that the dose distribution does not suffer large hot or cold regions. The dose uniformity is quoted as $\pm 5\%$, except for hot-spots close to sources.

The uncertainty of choice of isodose is minimized by designing the target volume before implanting with suitable margins around the tumour and implanting the peripheral sources on the outer surface of this target volume. The reference isodose curve is then selected, so that it just encloses the implant. This principle, which tends to increase the target volume by adding a greater margin around the tumour, ensures that overdose does not happen.

6.6.3 Iridium seeds

As an alternative to wire, iridium may be supplied in the form of seeds – usually spaced at 1-cm intervals in nylon tubes. The standard system for dosimetry was developed at Memorial Sloan Kettering, New York, and is based on the calculation of the minimum peripheral dose (Anderson *et al.* 1981). This is not discussed further here.

An alternative method of dealing with iridium seed implants could be to follow the Paris system. However, it has been shown that this is not valid unless the spacing between seeds is such that the ratio of the separation of the seed centres to the gap between the seeds is less than or equal to 1.5 (Marinello *et al.* 1985).

6.6.4 Iodine-125

Iodine-125 seeds have generally been used for permanent implants of the prostate and bronchus, although other sites have been investigated. The seeds have also been used for individually designed eye plaques to treat ocular melanomas. The rationale for developing a brachytherapy technique for iodine-125, which has a very low energy emission, has been primarily concerned with radiation safety. Prior to implantation, protection can be achieved using thin lead or tin foils. Tin is used because of the energy of its K absorption edge. In addition, relatively low activities of iodine-125 are needed for permanent implants due to the long effective treatment time (2080 h). Following the implant, the patient does not represent a radiation hazard. However, if the patient dies within about a year, there is a potential problem regarding the handling and disposal of the body.

There are several problems associated with the dosimetry of I-125 seeds. The low photon energy means that significant absorption occurs in the titanium encapsulating the seeds. In addition, use of the resin-bead type seeds introduces a degree of uncertainty in source positioning. Early estimations of dose were often normalized to the value of dose rate per unit activity at

1 cm on the transverse axis. The activity referenced here was that of an unencapsulated point source that would result in a transverse-axis exposure rate measured for the seed at a distance large enough for the inverse square law to be valid (Nath *et al.* 1995).

In addition, the absorption of primary photons by the medium is not matched by the build-up of scattered photons in a 10 cm range from the source. This is in contrast to the situation with higher energy photon sources, where there is much closer matching (see Table 12.3). There have also been inaccuracies in some of the early measurements of dose rate near I-125 sources in various phantom materials. Due to the predominance of the photoelectric effect at the I-125 photon energies, there are quite significant differences in penetration with even small variations in the atomic number of the medium.

For a more detailed review of developments in dosimetry for I-125 seeds, reference may be made to the recommendations of AAPM Task Group No. 43 (Nath *et al.* 1995).

One dosimetry system that was commonly used for permanent implants with iodine-125 seeds is the 'dimension averaging' system. In this system the total activity A mCi to be implanted is given by:

$$A = Kd_a \qquad (21)$$

in which K is a constant and d_a cm is the average dimension of the implant, i.e. the average of the sizes of the implant measured along three orthogonal axes, so as to encompass all the implanted sources. Originally, K was based on clinical experience and a value of 5 mCi cm^{-1} was recommended. This leads to a minimum peripheral dose (MPD) of approximately 150 Gy for small volumes, but lower doses for larger volumes. Therefore, as the system was developed, the constant became a function of d_a such that:

$$K = 5 \qquad\qquad d_a \leq 2.4$$
$$K = 3.87(d_a + 1)^{1.293} \qquad 2.4 < d_a \leq 3.24$$
$$K = 2.76(d_a + 1)^{1.581} \qquad d_a > 3.23.$$

Tables giving minimum peripheral and maximum central dose rates for cubic lattices are available (Krishnaswamy 1979). These are based on 1 mCi sources spaced at 1-cm intervals. In general, the source spacing should be between 1.0 and 1.5 cm. A nomogram for the calculation of the number of seeds and their spacing has been published (Anderson 1976). Rao *et al.* (1981) provide a useful summary of this system including tables of doses achieved from different sizes of implant.

It should be noted that this remains a somewhat empirical system, which does not satisfactorily produce a prescribed dose to the volume to be treated. One problem is the marked anisotropy of these sources because of the low-energy radiation. The average emission averaged over 4π geometry and weighted for inverse square law may be as low as 94% of that for a point source (Nath *et al.*, 1993). Generally, when computer programs are used to calculate the dose distribution from an array of sources it is assumed that they are point sources because it is usually not possible to determine their orientation. However, a correction should be made to their activity to correct for anisotropy. Guidance on the modelling of the correction factor has been given by AAPM TG43 (Nath *et al.* 1995).

The use of iodine-125 for permanent implants can be compared with that of gold-198, since similar sites have been implanted. Although source and dose distributions are similar, the dose time–volume considerations are very different. From the typical gold grain implant using the Manchester system, 65–70 Gy would be given, typically with an initial dose rate of about 0.7 Gy h^{-1}. For iodine-125, the dose is typically 160 Gy MPD. Typical initial dose rates are 0.05–0.1 Gy h^{-1}, and the dose rate after 120 days is still 0.01–0.02 Gy h^{-1}. These low dose rates combined with the low energy of the radiation make the study of relative biological effectiveness (RBE) for iodine-125 permanent implants a difficult subject and complicate any comparison with gold-198 implants. Radiobiological considerations have also led to the use of palladium-103 rather than iodine-125 for permanent implants (Ling 1992). Because of its shorter half-life, Pd-103 delivers a higher initial dose rate than I-125 and this is more effective in the treatment of rapidly growing tumours. A nomogram for the calculation of the number of Pd-103 seeds and their spacing, similar to that for I-125, has been given by Anderson *et al.* (1993). An MPD of 115 Gy has been found to correspond to 150 Gy for I-125. The total seed strength for this prescription (in mCi) is given by $3.2 (d_a)^{2.56}$.

Some work has been done using higher activity iodine-125 seeds for temporary implants. Clarke *et al.* (1988) used ribbons of seeds with a total source strength with a mean of 500 μGy h^{-1} as a replacement for Ir-192, mainly for treatments of the breast.

6.6.5 The use of seeds to treat the prostate

The use of seeds to treat the prostate is described briefly. In most centres using seeds for carcinoma of the prostate, transperineal implantation with template guidance has supplanted open-laporotomy technique. A very high level of quality assurance is now applied to this technique to ensure optimum and accurate planning of treatment. A pre-implant volume study is performed with transrectal ultrasound to determine target volume and seed placement. The isodose plan is then performed and optimized, and source strength adjusted as necessary. The typical activity is 0.35 mCi for iodine-125 or 1.4 mCi for palladium-103. The prescription, based on

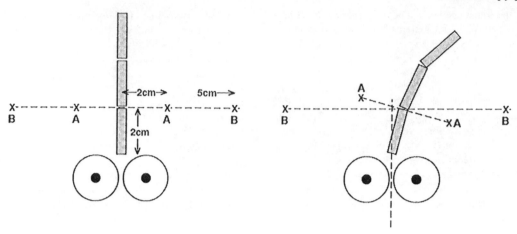

Figure 12.7 Source arrangement for treatment of the uterine cervix (Manchester system). Ideal geometry is shown on the left. The positions of points A and B for non-ideal geometry are shown on the right.

the AAPM TG43 dosimetry system (Nath *et al.* 1995), is normally 144 Gy minimum peripheral dose (MPD) for iodine-125 and about 110 Gy MPD for palladium-103.

The seeds are inserted transperineally in special 18-gauge, 21-cm needles using ultrasound and fluoroscopy to check the position of the needles and seeds as the operation progresses. In the post-planning stage, radiographs are taken and the special computer-planning system identifies each seed. Several hundred seeds could be located in this way but typically the implant will use about 100 seeds. The implant is reconstructed in 3-D and the isodose distribution can then be calculated.

6.7 Gynaecological intracavitary therapy

The early development of intracavitary therapy for gynaecological tumours was largely concerned with the design of applicator systems in parallel with the developments in dosimetry. A number of systems have been developed, most notably in Stockholm, Paris, Houston, and Manchester. Generally, all systems involve the use of a central line source in the uterus with two sources in the vaginal fornices within shaped applicators. In the Manchester system, the vaginal sources are contained within ovoids and held apart by a spacer.

These treatments involve relatively high doses, usually 74 Gy, given in two fractions each over a 1–3-day period separated by 1 week. Because of the high doses, accurate source positioning is essential to avoid damage to the critical tissues, which include the rectum and the bladder. For this reason, many of the developments have been concerned with applicator design (e.g. to include local shielding), patterns of loading, and methods of providing packing between the sources, and critical structures.

6.7.1 Manchester system

Early techniques for treating the uterine cervix involved the insertion of a specified quantity of radium into the uterus and vagina for a number of hours to give a combined milligram hours depending on the volume treated. The Manchester system attempted to deal more scientifically with the dosimetry by defining points at which to calculate the dose and giving a number of combinations of source strengths in the uterine tube and the vaginal ovoids to produce a similar isodose shape for different treatment volumes. It was considered that the tissue tolerance in the para-cervical triangles was the limiting factor for this treatment. This led to the designation of point A, at which the target dose is specified. Point A is defined to be 2 cm along the axis of the central tube (from the lower end) and 2 cm from it laterally. There are two interpretations of 'laterally' when the uterine tube is tilted in the AP view. The definition given by Meredith (1967) has point A rotating with the uterine tube (Figure 12.7), whereas other workers have interpreted laterally as meaning anatomically lateral. A further position, point B, is defined to be 5 cm from the mid-line at the same level as point A (Figure 12.7).

In many instances, the dose to point B is boosted by external beam irradiation. This is provided by coaxially opposed fields arranged to irradiate the whole pelvis, but with central shielding to protect the area that received the highest dose from the insertion. Commonly, a wedged central block is used to try to match the dose inhomogeneity from the brachytherapy treatment.

In the Manchester system, the uterine source consists of rubber tube containing one to three standard G-type sources, although sometimes a rigid tube has been used. Originally, these were radium sources, but now they are

Table 12.11 Source loadings and dose rates to point A for treatment of the uterine cervix using caesium-137 G-tubes (Manchester system)

Applicator	Loading 'units'	Dose rate at point A(mGy h^{-1})	
Intra-uterine			
Long	4 + 4 + 6	344	
Medium	4 + 6	342	
Short	8	273	
Ovoids		*Plus washer*	*Plus spacer*
Large	9 or (2 + 4 + 4)	189	183
Medium	8	190	188
Small	7 or (2 + 2 + 4)	190	189

The source strengths are defined in terms of 'units' that are normally 2.5 mg radium equivalent, which is equal to 18 μGy h^{-1}. The ovoids may be separated by a washer or spacer. For large and small ovoids the nominal loading can be achieved using three sources, as shown.

generally caesium-137. The sources are arranged with the source at the applicator tip having 50% more activity than each of the others. The recommended loadings of these sources are shown in Table 12.11, where the source strength is given in 'units' that were originally equal to 2.5 mg radium; this is equivalent to a nominal reference AKR of 18 μGy h^{-1}. The ovoids have three sizes and are loaded, as shown in Table 12.11. It is a recommendation in the Manchester system that the dose rate at point A should be taken from standard tables, which assume ideal geometry, i.e. with the uterine tube not tilted in the anterior–posterior view. The dose rates at point A for standard loadings are shown in the table. For long and medium uterine tubes, the total dose rate at point A is approximately 0.53 Gy h^{-1}, and for a standard prescription of 74 Gy the total treatment time is 140 or 70 h for each insertion.

Some radiotherapists prefer not to use the standard tables, but instead calculate point A dose for the actual source arrangement as described in Section 7.3.1. The dose rate at point B is generally 20–25% of the dose rate at A. This should not be derived from the ideal geometry, but should be calculated by reconstruction.

The loading of the sources in units of 2.5 mg radium equivalent cannot be achieved for the large and small ovoids with G-type tubes. One method of overcoming this is to use the next highest activity for the first insertion and a lower activity for the second, so as to achieve an average source strength as indicated in the table. Alternatively, the ovoids can be loaded with three sources with a total source strength approximately 10% greater than that recommended. The additional activity corrects approximately for the additional cross-filtration which occurs when bunches of sources are used.

Treatment of the body of the uterus can be undertaken using a similar technique but with proportionally more activity in the uterine tube than in the ovoids. This is typically 6–8 'units' (108–144 μGy h^{-1}) in each of the

ovoids and 16–32 'units' (288–576 μGy h^{-1}) in the uterine tube.

For treatment of the vagina, applicators were designed to contain a series of standard gynaecological tubes in a line within a Perspex cylinder. The strength of the tubes used could be changed according to the diameter of the applicator to give a similar dose rate at the surface.

The data given by Breitman (1974) can be used to calculate the dose rate at the surface of the vaginal applicator or at some distance from it. She gives dose rates for a range of transverse distances from standard sources and at a range of distances along the source axis, enabling a calculation of dose rate at any point when sources are arranged in line. The tables are for 1 mg radium equivalent caesium-137 sources. This can be scaled on the basis that 1 mg radium equivalent equals a reference AKR of 7.2 μGy h^{-1}.

6.7.2 Afterloading techniques for gynaecological insertions

The rationale for using afterloading systems was discussed in Section 5. At the present time, it is unusual not to use some form of afterloading. Manual systems have been used since the 1960s and are available commercially; one example is the system produced by Nycomed Amersham in which disposable applicators, which mimic the Manchester manual loading system, are supplied. These are inserted in theatre with the caesium subsequently being loaded after the patient returns to the ward. In this case, local shielding is required for the protection of nursing staff. Such systems are relatively inexpensive and are recommended if it is not possible to obtain a remote afterloading system for these treatments. However, from the radiation protection viewpoint, a remote system is preferred.

In addition to radiation protection, remote afterloading systems have the advantage of improved flexibility in source loading allowing dose distributions to be modified, for example, when the insertion geometry is not ideal. However, there may be a reluctance to make significant changes to standard dose distributions that have been established through many years of clinical experience.

One of the principal problems associated with remote systems is the radiobiology of higher dose rate treatments. Increased dose rates are almost invariably used, mainly because of the increased discomfort to the patient from the rigid applicators, which have to be attached to the afterloading machine. This has meant a reduction in treatment time from 3 days to, generally, 24 h or less. In addition, there may be a logistical problem in having expensive equipment tied up for 3 days at a time. Radiobiological problems are discussed in Section 8.

6.7.3 ICRU specification of dose in gynaecological cancer treatment

Although the Manchester system is inherently reliable for treatments given with the specified source arrangement, it is not easy to compare with other dosimetry systems. To enable dosimetry systems to be compared the ICRU published *Dose and volume specification for reporting intracavitary therapy in gynaecology* (ICRU 1985). This uses similar terminology to the ICRU report on external beam therapy (ICRU 1978) (see Chapter 7, Section 2), but with modified definitions, which are reproduced below.

Target volume

The target volume contains those tissues that are to be irradiated to a specified absorbed dose according to a specified time–dose pattern. For curative treatment, the target volume consists of the demonstrated tumour(s), if present, and any other tissue with presumed tumour.

Treatment volume

The treatment volume is defined as the volume enclosed by a relevant isodose surface selected by the radiotherapist and encompasses at least the target volume. In intracavitary therapy, it is not feasible to express the value of the isodose surface enclosing the treatment volume as a percentage of the dose at any point within the treatment volume. This is because of the steep dose gradient around the sources and the variation encountered in the techniques used. It is necessary to plan the treatment to include the target volume within the treatment volume.

Irradiated volume

The irradiated volume is that volume, larger than the treatment volume, which receives an absorbed dose considered to be significant in relation to tissue tolerance. The significant absorbed dose level can be expressed as a percentage (e.g. 50%) of the agreed dose level.

Reference volume

The reference volume is defined for the typical pear-shaped distribution produced by the Manchester system and is shown in Figure 12.8. It is the volume enclosed by the reference isodose surface and is defined by the three dimensions:

(1) the height d_h is the maximum dimension along the intra-uterine source and is measured in the oblique frontal plane containing the intra-uterine source;

(2) the width d_w is the maximum dimension perpendicular to the intra-uterine source and is measured in the same oblique frontal plane;

(3) the thickness d_t is the maximum dimension perpendicular to the intra-uterine source and is measured in the oblique sagittal plane containing the intra-uterine source.

The report also recommends that, to aid the study of combined intracavitary and external beam therapy, the absorbed dose at reference points related to bony structures, particularly the lymphatic trapezoid and the pelvic wall, should be reported as well as the dose to the

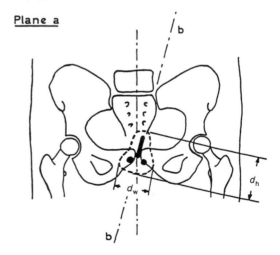

Figure 12.8 Dimensions of the reference volume for gynaecological treatment. Reproduced with permission from ICRU (1985).

bladder and rectum. A further recommendation is that the total reference air kerma of the sources should be stated. The total air kerma is the sum of the product of reference AKR and the time of insertion for each source.

The purpose of the ICRU recommendations is to provide standardized data for the comparison of different treatment regimes. When reporting clinical data it is stressed that, in addition to the parameters described above, a full description should be given of both the technique and the time–dose pattern employed.

6.8 Dosimetry for high dose-rate afterloading-treatment machines

The most common HDR source is iridium-192 with a nominal activity of 370 GBq (10 Ci). The older terminology for source strength is routinely adopted with HDR probably due to its simplicity. This source, which is used in both the MicroSelectron and GammaMed afterloading systems, is supplied by Mallinckrodt. They recommend an AKR constant of 110 μGy m^2 GBq^{-1} h^{-1} for their source pellet, corresponding to AKR equal to 4.07 cGy m^2 h^{-1}. This may be compared with the value in Table 12.1, 113 μGy m^2 GBq^{-1} h^{-1}.

The source is 3.5 mm long with a diameter of 0.6 mm. It is contained in a laser-welded stainless steel cable in the form of a pellet, 5.6 mm long, with a diameter of 1.1 mm. When not in use the source is kept in a shielded safe in the head of the unit.

In use, the source is stepped using regular spacing through a choice of applicators. Each applicator is attached to a specific outlet or channel. It is possible to program a patient specific arrangement of different times at each dwell position, and these to be specific to each channel. There are 18 available channels on a Micro-Selectron and 24 on the GammaMed machines. Channels dwell positions and times can be entered via a PC or by making use of a pre-programmed data card.

HDR brachytherapy has been successfully used for intracavitary and interstitial implants. Where its intended use is to replace an existing LDR technique, clinicians may wish to continue with the dosimetry technique they are acquainted with, whilst observing radiobiological changes at the new dose rate. The versatility of the units allows both Manchester and Paris dosimetry, by changing dwell points and/or dwell times in applicators, in some cases using identical applicator arrangements.

A purpose-built computerized-planning system is supplied with most makes of HDR afterloading unit. A library of existing applicator configurations may be included, or built up by the user to match local practice. When required, particular applicators can be selected, and information on the sections of the applicators and source-stepping distances being used can be fed in. A template of source dwell positions can then be automatically computed.

Commercial programs available today include dose optimization options. However, these should be used with caution, as few, if any, restraints or limits on dwell times are included. Careless use of optimization options may lead to unacceptably high doses at the applicator surface or non-target anatomical sites.

Programs calculate dose at a point by summing dose contributions from all dwell positions used. A full isodose distribution is produced, which can be viewed either in multiplanar orthogonal views, or in a more sophisticated 3-D representation. The calculation may be based on a nominal activity, e.g. 370 GBq/10 Ci source, or may take into account the source decay to a specified treatment date. In both cases, dose rate at a point will be calculated from this activity making use of the AKR factor or a Γ factor (see Section 3). Care is needed to ensure that the factor used by the computer in dose calculations is consistent with values used in measuring and defining source activity. It may not be possible to change this factor in the commercial program.

AAPM Task Group No. 43 (Nath *et al.* 1995) has recommended that future source strengths should be specified in terms of dose-rate constants in a water medium near the source, in order to overcome the problems of different exposure-rate and AKR-factor constants being used for the same radionuclide.

Both the Paris and Manchester systems are specific, both in the amount of radioactive material to be used for a given target volume and in the arrangement of sources. The clinician's prescription is then determined by the system itself. When computed isodoses are used for prescription, the rapid fall-off in dose around the source may mean that different clinicians prescribe to a different isodose level. Alternatively, the same isodose value may be chosen but it may have a different location due to the dwell position and time derived from the particular optimization program. It is, therefore, difficult to define a universally understood prescription method. The ICRU have proposed a list of parameters for prescribing a moving source prescription. These are listed in table 4.4 of ICRU Report 58 (ICRU 1997).

6.8.1 Optimization options available with commercial systems

Optimization in an HDR dose-calculation program is a process whereby individual dwell times are varied in order to achieve a best match of the resulting dose to that required at defined points. A mathematical function can be applied to describe the clinical situation. This function is maximized (or minimized) to provide a solution in terms of individual source dwell times. Correct and sufficient specification of dose points, as well as a very good mathematical match to the clinical situation, are prerequisites for a truly optimal solution. Where there are limited or no means of applying constraints regarding maximum doses to surrounding structures, solutions using commercial optimization programs may at best require some modification, and at worst prove inappropriate for clinical use.

Applicator dwell positions and reference point positions are stored in an orthogonal matrix. Dose reference points may be manually input, together with doses required at those points, or computer calculated to be at a specified distance from an applicator. In a geometrical approach adopted by one manufacturer, dwell positions themselves become the dose reference points requiring a specified dose throughout the implant. This approach works well, if dwell position spacing in the implant is uniform.

Whichever method of optimization is applied, it is the implanted or inserted positions in the applicators available to the HDR source that determine the choice of isodose distributions available. A bad implant can only be partially rectified by varying dwell times. Where applicators or catheters are non-uniformly distributed in the treatment volume, there may be comparatively large regions where no dwell position is possible. This can be countered partially by increasing the dwell time in the nearest neighbouring position. However, any increase in dose achieved in this way, will result in a proportional increase in dose – not only at the sites of these missing dwells or 'holes', but also close to the source dwell positions themselves. Whilst the time increase has a linear effect on dose, the distance effect follows the inverse square law. Compensating for missing available dwell positions may be restricted by limits to local dose around existing available dwell positions.

6.8.2 The Paris system and HDR dosimetry

Where there is a clinical requirement to apply the Paris system using HDR to match an existing LDR technique, catheters should be implanted in an identical arrangement to that already in use. Uniform activity along an iridium wire is stimulated using equal dwell times along a length similar to that used in a LDR implant. LDR dosimetry provides the linear source activity needed, and the treatment time for a required dose. Dwell times for a 370 GBq iridium-192 source can be calculated from these by dividing the total activity-time evenly between the dwell positions.

The Paris system produces a less homogeneous isodose distribution than either Manchester or optimized dose distributions. It may cause more irradiation of healthy tissue. However, a modified approach to the Paris system has been described by Van der Laarse and Prins (1994a). The length of the catheters is kept 0.5 cm inside that of the target area and reference isodose. Optimization points are defined between catheters along their whole lengths. The reference dose is taken as 85% of the

mean of these points doses. The concept is similar to a Paris system reference isodose equal to 85% of basal dose.

6.8.3 The Manchester system and HDR dosimetry

The Manchester interstitial dosimetry system provides dose homogeneity over a prescribed plane or volume to within ±10% of the specified dose. It can be applied to an HDR system with no further need for optimization. It does, however, refer to a prescribed dose 10% higher than the minimum expected in the target region. Therefore, for a dose prescribed to a minimum, 'Manchester' doses must be increased accordingly.

The Paterson–Parker tables in Table 12.5 can be used to determine the total dwell time for the implant by applying a conversation factor 0.0885. This converts reference air kerma per gray to dwell time (in seconds) per gray for a nominal 370 GBq source. It assumes that AKR is equal to 40.7 mGy m^2 h^{-1}. For example, for a 20 cm^2 area, the total dwell time required to deliver 10 Gy at 0.5 cm using a 370 GBq source would be $(286 \times 0.0885 \times 10) = 253$ s. The total dwell time is apportioned between the periphery and centre according to Manchester rules. Individual dwell times are obtained by spatially distributing these times uniformly over the peripheral and central dwell positions, as appropriate.

The implementation of HDR using Manchester dosimetry can be considered with reference to Figure 12.9. An orthogonal arrangement of catheters is used for the treatment of an area (including clinical margins) of L cm by W cm. The catheters have a separation of 1 cm and it is assumed that there is a single or a double plane with a separation of 1 cm. The source is used in dwell positions at 1 cm spacing. The ratio, P, of total dwell time in the periphery of the implant to the

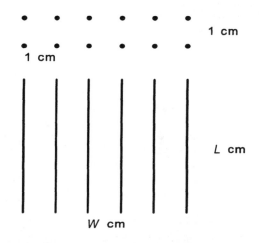

Figure 12.9 Orthogonal template for HDR catheters.

central dwell time is determined from the area using the data in Table 12.4. The time at each dwell position in the periphery and centre (T_p, T_c) to deliver a dose of D Gy is determined as follows:

Total number of peripheral dwells (i.e. at each position in the outermost catheters and at the ends of the central catheter) = $2n(L + W)$.

Total number of central dwells = $n(L - 1)(W - 1)$.

Therefore, $P = \dfrac{2n(L + W)T_p}{n(L - 1)(W - 1)T_c}$.

Total dwell time per Gy is determined for the area of the implant from the source strength–time product, A, from Table 12.5.

Total dwell time per Gy for a 370 GBq Ir-192 source = $0.0885 \times A$ s.

The total dwell time to deliver the prescribed dose can then be equated to the total dwell times in the periphery and in the centre of the implant:

$$0.0885\, A\, D = 2n(L + W)T_p + n(L - 1)(W - 1)T_c.$$

$$\text{Therefore, } T_p = \frac{0.0885A\, D}{2n(L + W)(1 + 1/P)}$$

$$\text{and } T_c = \frac{0.0885A\, D}{n(L - 1)(W - 1)(1 + P)}.$$

If the space between dwell positions is less than 1 cm (i.e. less than the needle separation), then the total dwell time required along each needle can be calculated and distributed evenly over the stopping positions, provided that the stopping positions, for central needles at their ends (peripheral stopping times) are kept the same.

For volume implants using the Manchester system, i.e. implants on more than two planes, reference should be made to Meredith (1967). The volume of the implant should be calculated, and times based on the modified Paterson–Parker tables in Table 12.5 (see Section 6.2.3) with the same conversion factor to dwell time or a 370 GBq Ir-192 source, i.e. 0.0885. The total time should then be divided between the planes and the distribution rules from Meredith (1967) applied to each plane. The time per plane should be distributed in proportion to the area of each plane, with external plane areas being weighted by a factor of 1.5.

Clinical example

Three-plane implant of the breast to treat a volume 6 cm wide by 6 cm long and 2 cm thick. The template for the implant has an orthogonal grid with seven 6-cm long wires at a 1-cm spacing. Calculation of dwell times assumes a Ir-192 source with an activity of 370 MBq. A time correction is required for the true activity at the time of treatment, although this may be done automatically by the afterloading machine.

Volume of implant = $6 \times 6 \times 2$ cm^3 = 72 cm^3.
From Table 12.5, source strength required = 458 μGy Gy^{-1}.
The total dwell time for 1 Gy is, therefore, $0.0885 \times 458 = 40.5$ s.
Since the area for each plane is the same, the Manchester system requires the time for each external plane to be weighted by a factor of 1.5 relative to the central plane, i.e. 37.5% of the total time.
The total dwell time for each external plane = $0.375 \times 40.5 = 15.2$ s Gy^{-1} and for the central plane = $0.25 \times 40.5 = 10.1$ s Gy^{-1}.
For an area of 36 cm^2, the ratio of dwell times in the periphery and in the central position of each plane, $P = 1$ (Table 12.4). Therefore, the number of peripheral and central dwell positions is: $2(6 + 6) = 24$ and $(6 - 1)(6 - 1) = 25$, respectively, in each plane.
Therefore, for the external planes, dwell times are given by:
$T_{p,e} = 15.2/(24 \times 2) = 0.317$ s Gy^{-1} in the periphery
and
$T_{c,e} = 15.2/(25 \times 2) = 0.304$ s Gy^{-1} in the central region.
In the central plane, the times are two-thirds of this, i.e. $T_{p,c} = 0.211$ s Gy^{-1} and $T_{c,c} = 0.203$ s Gy^{-1} for the peripheral and central positions, respectively.

Should 5-mm steps be used for the same catheter grid, there would then be 13 dwell positions in each catheter. The dwell times at the ends of the catheter would be the same to provide the same total dwell time at the end positions. For the 11 intermediate positions, the dwell times would be weighted by a factor of 5:11, i.e. 0.455.

The Manchester system can be used to determine an optimum distribution of sources before catheter insertion and of dwell times before prescription, i.e. it can be the starting point for planning. It is standard practice to use computer calculations to determine dose distributions for the reconstructed implant using the planned dwell times. Modifications to these can then be made if dose inhomogeneities are seen and if the total dose to the tumour volume differs from the prescription. In the example above, it was found that the tumour volume in the central plane was covered by the 85% isodose rather than the 90% as intended. The external catheter times in the central plane were, therefore, increased to match those in the external planes. Figure 12.10a shows the calculated dose distribution through the centre of the implant. The 90% isodose is that prescribed, 100% corresponds to the Manchester dose, and 110% shows the maximum predicted using Manchester dosimetry. Times rounded up to the nearest 0.1 s and increases to the central external catheter times resulted in an overall

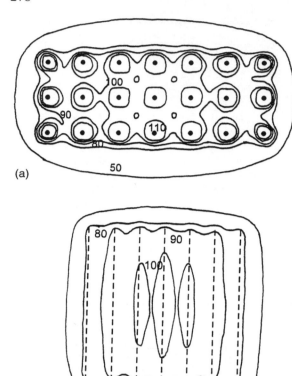

(a)

(b)

Figure 12.10 Isodose distributions for a 6 × 6 × 2 cm³ implant based on Manchester dosimetry rules to give 1000 cGy Manchester dose: (a) through the central plane; and (b) in the minimum dose plane between the catheters.

treatment time of 42.2 s Gy⁻¹, 104% of that predicted by the original Manchester calculation. Figure 12.10b shows the distribution in the minimum dose plane between the catheters.

6.8.4 Clinical prescriptions in HDR brachytherapy

Gynaecological insertions

In the UK, point A remains a standard prescription point in full gynaecological insertions. Dwell time weighting can be matched to the AKR contributions of standard LDR insertions. Where vaginal applicators are used, prescription is usually to a point, half-way along the prescribed length, 0.5 cm from the surface of the applicator.

Bronchial and oesophageal insertions

Bronchial and oesophageal insertions are usually single-line sources, which pass through the tumour site. A common prescription point is mid-way along the length of treatment at 1.0 cm from the applicator.

Interstitial insertions

Current prescription practice in interstitial brachytherapy, e.g. breast or prostate treatments, is predominantly to the minimum isodose covering the treatment volume, where a treatment volume is defined. Frequently, the final volume is determined at surgery and catheters are inserted to cover this volume. With breast insertions, it is recommended that dwell positions are kept 0.5 cm within the skin surface. Full skin dose, if required, is still possible by judicial weighting of dwell times in the source positions closest to the surface.

Moulds

Prescriptions for mould treatments are usually to the skin surface, 5 mm or more below an applicator bearing material. Materials used are approximately tissue-equivalent. Where treatment is required to some depth, it is possible to decrease the dose gradient using a greater thickness of material. If appropriate, the thickness of the mould can be locally varied, to restrict the dose to sensitive structures close to the treatment area.

6.8.5 Dose–volume histograms and choice of treatment plan

There are three types of dose–volume histogram (DVH), which may be used to analyse dose distributions in brachytherapy:

(1) cumulative dose–volume histogram;

(2) differential dose–volume histogram;

(3) natural volume–dose histogram.

In contrast to external beam irradiation, most computer-planning systems do not determine site-specific DVHs for brachytherapy, although several groups are working on this.

Cumulative dose–volume histograms

A cumulative DVH relates the total volume of tissue receiving a minimum specified dose from an implant as a function of dose. Provided a specified isodose is seen to narrowly cover the treatment volume, it can be considered as representative of the volume. Figure 12.11 is the DVH for the three-plane implant in Section 6.8.3. The rectangular area within the 90% box represents the prescribed implant dose. Higher dose values represent overdose, which may be welcome inside but unwelcome outside the treatment volume. For good dose homogeneity, this section of the curve should be as steep as possible. The dose to normal tissue volumes outside the required treatment volume is represented by the first section of the curve. For minimum dose to healthy tissue, this section of the curve should be shallow. Figure 12.12 shows how optimization may not always offer the best treatment option. Cumulative

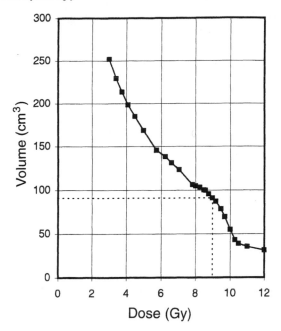

Figure 12.11 Cumulative DVH for the Manchester 10 Gy three-plane plan (see Figure 12.10). The planned treatment volume was 72 cm³.

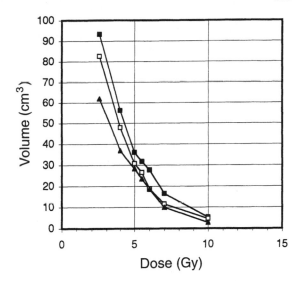

Figure 12.12 Cumulative DVHs for three different plans: (▲) Manchester dose: 5.5 Gy, minimum 5 Gy; (□) an optimized dose distribution to give 5.5 Gy to reference points along the mid-plane, and to enclose the treatment site within the 5 Gy isodose; (■) Paris dosimetry 5 Gy to 85% basal dose.

DVHs for three different dosimetry approaches to a two-plane breast implant have been plotted on the same graph. It can be seen that the optimized plan gives higher doses to normal tissue than the Manchester distribution.

Differential dose–volume histogram

A differential DVH relates the volume in a patient receiving a specific dose, to that dose. Where all source dwell positions are inside the treatment volume, and a reference isodose narrowly envelops this volume, it can be assumed that all doses higher than the reference dose are within the treatment volume. It is possible, therefore, to obtain some form of dose uniformity index from this information. Where the reference isodose includes healthy tissues, or organs at risk, and where it is not possible to have separate DVHs for the volume and specified sites, this uniformity index on its own may be misleading. It is necessary to consider the full 3-D isodose distribution before the selection of a plan can be made.

Future developments incorporating anatomical information from multiple CT slices in organ-specific differentials DVHs, may prove decisive in selecting a specific plan, e.g. in prostate implants, where rectal dose may be critical.

Natural volume–dose histogram

The natural volume–dose histogram introduced by Anderson (1986) is a mathematical method of suppres-

sing the over-riding inverse square law effect from the DVH curve, whilst preserving proportionality between volume and the area under the curve.

The differential DVH for an iridium-192 point source coincides practically with that of an ideal point source, and is given by:

$$\frac{dV}{dD} = -2\pi S^{3/2} D^{-5/2}. \tag{22}$$

For a function $u(D)$ defined as:

$$u(D) = -D^{3/2} + \text{constant} \tag{23}$$

it can be shown that:

$$\frac{dV}{du} = -\frac{4}{3}\pi S^{3/2}. \tag{24}$$

For a single-point source, the natural VDH is a flat curve.

Natural VDHs have been used to generate a series of dose-homogeneity indices (van 't Riet *et al.* 1993; van der Laarse and Prins 1994b). It must be remembered, however, that these relate to the dose distribution as a whole, and give no indication of whether the dose is in the right or wrong place.

6.8.6 Current and future developments in HDR planning

A full understanding of optimization programs and their clinical meaning is required to use these options correctly. The Manchester system, with its inherent optimization based on dose homogeneity and its long clinical history, can be used as an aid in HDR dosimetry, either in its own right or as a comparison to the plan produced by computerized optimization. Requirements for high- or low-dose regions in an even dose distribution can then be achieved by varying individual dwell times.

As computing systems develop, and planning and optimization algorithms become more sophisticated, the independent use of computerized-treatment planning in HDR brachytherapy will become a safer option. Some optimization programs now include restrictions on the variability of dwell times. Future developments will allow for more maximum and minimum variations in dose at specific points.

The introduction of multiple-slice CT and other diagnostic imaging data into the planning process, will allow more precise definition of target volumes and dose-limiting structures. The development of organ-site-specific differential DVHs, will aid in selection of a particular planning option. The full potential of HDR stepping source treatment as a fully planned method of radiotherapy, comparable with external beam, is still being developed. This process is only possible due to the versatility of the treatment units.

7. Practical aspects of absorbed dose calculation

Dosimetry systems are used to specify the distribution of sources in the volume to be treated in order to give the required dose or dose rate. Because of the practical difficulties of implantation, the sources are rarely positioned as prescribed. Therefore, it is usually necessary to make a retrospective calculation of dose rate from the implant in order to determine the overall treatment time.

The degree of sophistication of dose calculation will vary from centre to centre. In recognition of the highly heterogeneous nature of the dose distributions from these treatments, some therapists may consider it sufficient to calculate the area of the implanted sources. From this, and using Paterson–Parker tables, the total treatment time can be determined. This is the traditional approach, which requires the minimum calculation. Similarly, a measurement may be made of the average separation of implanted iridium wires that can be used for the calculation of basal dose rate. Alternatively, the therapist may require a full calculation of absorbed dose on a three-dimensional matrix in order to produce the isodose surfaces surrounding the implant. From the dose matrix it may be possible to derive the average dose in specified planes or the average basal dose rate according to the Paris system. Full dose calculation may be the most complete description of the implant, but the results can

be difficult to interpret and use for the specification of total treatment time.

7.1 Source-reconstruction methods

However the calculation is made, it is necessary to determine the geometry of the implanted sources. This is invariably done using an X-ray technique. In the simplest case in which the area of the implanted sources is to be derived, the easiest method is to take a single radiograph in a direction that is perpendicular to the plane of the implant. Direct measurement from the film and the application of an appropriate magnification factor will yield the area. This technique depends on the radiographs being taken at the correct angle, which may not be possible for certain implants, so that it is now more common to use computer programs to reconstruct the position of the implanted sources. The reconstructed implant can be viewed from any direction, enabling a more accurate calculation of area to be made. Reconstruction of the position of the sources also allows a complete calculation of dose distributions, and facilities for this are included in most treatment-planning systems.

Reconstruction of the position of sources requires the use of two radiographs. They must be taken at two different angles or through two different centres. The normal techniques are to take orthogonal views or to use two views at the same angle but with shifted centres. The orthogonal technique is the most common.

7.1.1 Orthogonal technique

Two orthogonal films are used to determine the co-ordinates of points within the patient relative to an origin, which is taken as the point at which the central axes of the beams intersect. Figure 12.13 shows a point P with co-ordinates x, y, z relative to the origin.

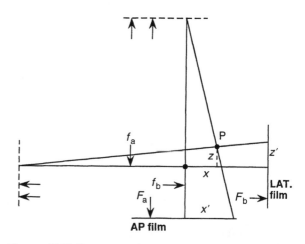

Figure 12.13 Reconstruction of the implant geometry from orthogonal radiographs.

Commonly, the two views are taken through anterior–posterior and lateral portals, but alternative arrangements can be used. In Figure 12.13, the distances from the focus to the origin are f_a, f_b with focus–film distances of F_a and F_b. The displacements of P from the origin measured on the two films are x' and z'. From simple geometry the x and z co-ordinates of P are given by:

$$x = x' \frac{f_a - Z}{F_a} \tag{25}$$

$$z = z' \frac{f_b - x}{F_b}. \tag{26}$$

Solving these equations yields:

$$x = x' \frac{f_a F_b - z' f_b}{F_a F_b - x' z'} \tag{27}$$

$$z = z' \frac{f_b F_a - x' f_a}{F_a F_b - x' z'}. \tag{28}$$

The displacement y from the original perpendicular to the x, z plane can be calculated from either film to give:

$$y = y'(a) \frac{f_a F_b - z' f_b}{F_a F_b - x' z'} \tag{29}$$

or

$$y = y'(b) \frac{f_b F_a - x' f_a}{F_a F_b - x' z'}. \tag{30}$$

in which $y'(a)$ and $y'(b)$ are the measured displacements in the A and B projections, respectively. The two equations should yield the same value of y.

The displacements measured on the film are generally much less than distances to the focus, so that approximate equations can be written:

$$x = \frac{x'}{M_a} \tag{31}$$

$$z = \frac{z'}{M_b} \tag{32}$$

$$y = \frac{y'(a)}{M_a} \quad \text{or} \quad y = \frac{y'(b)}{M_b} \tag{33, 34}$$

in which M_a and M_b are the magnification factors of the two films at the origin and are given by:

$$M_a = F_a/f_a \quad \text{and} \quad M_b = F_b/f_b. \tag{35, 36}$$

These approximations are sufficiently accurate provided that each point is displaced from the origin by distances that are only a few per cent of the distance from the focus to the origin. For larger arrangements of sources, the full equations should be used.

In principle, any X-ray set can be used to take the orthogonal views. Because of the radiation protection problems associated with the transport of patients containing high-activity sources, in the past some centres have preferred to use a mobile X-ray unit in the theatre or ward. Films taken in this way required the use of markers, such as rings, to enable the magnification factors to be calculated, and this compromised the accuracy of calculation. Most implants now involve some form of afterloading, so that the radiation protection problems no longer apply and the method of choice is to use the treatment simulator. This has a number of advantages.

1. The simulator is mechanically stable and can be set up accurately to the required angles.

2. The angles of the radiographs can be chosen to give the clearest view of the sources without obstructive anatomical features. In principle, these need not be orthogonal, but this would lead to a reduction in the accuracy of reconstruction.

3. The distance from the focus to the origin is the source–axis distance and is known accurately.

4. The distance from the focus to the image intensifier face is displayed; from this it is simple to calculate the focus–film distance.

5. The centre of the beam which marks the origin can be displayed using an appropriate graticule. Alternatively, it can be determined from the field wires.

Various jigs can be made to provide similar information with a diagnostic X-ray set, but there is a basic disadvantage arising from the lack of mechanical precision when compared with the simulator.

7.1.2 Shift technique

In this technique, two exposures are made from the same direction but with two separated beam centres (Figure 12.14). The shift technique can be used with a single film, but two films are usually preferred and are known as stereo-shift films. Typically, the centres of the two views are separated by 20 cm or more. The advantage of the method is that both films can be taken through the anterior–posterior portal to give a much clearer view of the sources than can be obtained on the lateral view required when orthogonal films are used. This is particularly true for small seeds. In addition, it can be easier with multiple-seed implants to match the individual sources in the two films.

Figure 12.13 represents the view taken through one point P in the implant when the X-ray source has been shifted a distance S along the y-axis. The height z of the point above the film can be calculated from its displacement y_1 and y_2 from a reference point O on the films. The reference point is a fixed marker with a known height z_0 above the film. The marker can conveniently be

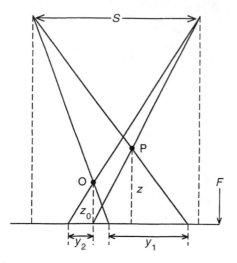

Figure 12.14 Reconstruction of the implant geometry from shift radiographs.

placed on the top of the examination couch. Then z is given by:

$$z = F \frac{(F - z_0)(y_1 - y_2) + S z_0}{(F - z_0)(y_1 - y_2) + SF} \qquad (37)$$

where F is the focus–film distance.

The height above the film can be used to calculate the magnification factor at P, and thus the x and y displacements from the axis of either film can be calculated provided that the axis is marked. It can be shown that the magnification factor M_p at P is given by:

$$M_P = \frac{(F - z_0)(y_1 - y_2) + SF}{S(F - z_0)}. \qquad (38)$$

It may be more convenient to take the stereo films with the fixed marker O positioned so that it is mid-way between the two beam axes, in which case the y co-ordinate of P with respect to O is calculated from the average displacement of P measured on the two films:

$$y = \frac{S(y_1 + y_2)/2}{(y_1 + y_2) - SF/(F - z_0)}. \qquad (39)$$

The x co-ordinate can be calculated from either film.

7.1.3 CT localization

A well-calibrated CT scanner can provide an accurate three-dimensional reconstruction of the implant and has the advantage of showing the anatomy. This permits the calculation of doses to normal tissues. However, a large number of thin slices are needed to avoid partial volume effects and to give sufficient precision. In addition, there

are few centres with the resources to use CT scanners for this purpose other than for special studies.

7.1.4 Stereotactic localization

Most systems for stereotactic brain implants and surgery have been built around the Brown–Roberts–Weels (BRW) system, which uses a frame pinned to the skull. A number of authors, e.g. Lutz *et al.* (1988), have adapted this system by incorporating a fiducial-marker box attached to the frame. A pair of orthogonal films allows the position of sources (or the marked tumour site) to be located accurately with respect to the BRW co-ordinate system.

7.2 Errors

The high dose gradient around implanted sources means that even small errors in calculation of position will result in large errors in dose rate calculation. For example, a 2 mm error in the separation between two 4 cm long sources, which are 10 mm apart, would result in an error in dose-rate at a point mid-way between the sources of approximately 20%. Thus it is vital to reduce these errors as much as possible.

Errors occur when reconstructing source positions from film using either the orthogonal or the stereo-shift method. When a simulator has been used for the films, the errors due to geometry should be small, provided that the geometric data have been recorded accurately. The two major sources of error are the precision of measurement of the radiographic data and patient movement. The position of each source can be measured directly from the film but, more commonly, there is direct input to the planning computer using a digitizer. Following reconstruction, the calculation of needle length, for example, should be used as a check against the true length of the needle. Patient movement between films is a particular problem for treatments of the breast with iridium wire implants. The two films should be taken under shallow breathing.

If the approximate equations with a single magnification factor are used, errors are introduced that increase with the distance of the focus from the origin. If the focus to origin distance is 100 cm, this error will be approximately 1% per centimetre displacement. The calculation of magnification factor from a ring or similar device is limited by the precision to which measurements can be made from the film. The accuracy to which films from a diagnostic set can be used depends on the accuracy of the geometric set-up.

In general, orthogonal films are superior to stereo-shift in terms of accuracy but, if seeds are used, stereo-shift is essential in order to identify individual seeds, in which case errors can be reduced by using a focus–film distance greater than 100 cm and shifting at least 60 cm.

7.3 Clinical applications

7.3.1 Gynaecological insertions

As in all brachytherapy applications, the calculation detail required by the therapist varies widely for different treatment protocols. In some centres, treatment time is based on standard source loadings and strengths; in others a full calculation is made for each patient based on the reconstruction of the source positions. Reconstruction of the sources is relatively simple because their position is standardized. The most accurate reconstruction makes use of orthogonal radiographs. Care is needed to ensure that the right and left ovoid sources are correctly identified in the lateral view. Care is also needed when determining the position of the ends of caesium tubes; because of their relatively large diameter, tubes that are fore-shortened in a particular view appear longer than they actually are. The point input to represent the end of the tube should be displaced from the end seen on the radiograph by a distance that depends on the tube radius.

Contrast medium in the bladder or rectum will show up these sensitive sites, but a rectal marker consisting of metal spheres in a catheter is more accurate for this accessible site. In the early use of remote afterloading, some centres used CT to study the position of the applicators in detail (Wilkinson *et al.* 1983). This allowed alterations to be made to the dose distribution – usually to reduce rectal or bladder doses – by changes to the machine program to alter active pellet positions, the total number of active pellets used, or the treatment time in one or more channels.

Dedicated brachytherapy treatment-planning programs that can produce isodose curves for the individual source loading of the applicators are available from the manufacturers of remote afterloading systems. The dwell time for the sources in each applicator can then be determined to give the desired dose to a given isodose level or to point A. The dwell times or the source loading can be altered following insertion to optimize the treatment, particularly in terms of reducing dose to the rectum or bladder as described above.

It is also possible to make rectal dose measurements using an appropriate detector, such as a solid state diode or a sealed ionization chamber (to avoid changes in sensitivity due to temperature). It is important with this type of measurement that it is accurate and representative of the dose rate to the rectum; accuracy can be ensured by careful calibration of the detector and regular checks of its sensitivity. Measurements should be made at several positions so as to avoid the single-measurement problem, which may produce an erroneously high or low value. There are special multiple-detector systems that allow this to be done so that the spatial distance between measuring points is very accurate. These measurements are best made in theatre so that the sources can be

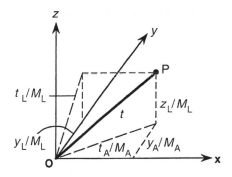

Figure 12.15 Calculation of magnification factor from orthogonal views of a needle implant.

repacked if unacceptably high dose rates are recorded. For afterloading systems, the measurement can be made with special low-activity sources and the result can be scaled up to the source strength to be used for treatment. Measurement and calculation should always be compared and an attempt made to reconcile the two results if there is a significant difference between them.

7.3.2 Needle implants

When active sources are implanted in theatre, it is often undesirable to move the patient to the simulator for localization films. Radiographs then need to be taken in theatre or on the ward. In this situation, the magnification factor for each film has to be determined. The standard method of obtaining magnification factors is to use a magnification ring of known dimensions placed as close as possible to the same height above the film as the implant. However, with needles it is possible, and very often preferable, to use one or more of the needles to determine the magnification.

In Figure 12.15 the needle is represented by the line OP. Its length is equal to t, with projected lengths in the anterior–posterior and lateral films given by t_A and t_L respectively. On each film, axes must be drawn about the point O to represent the anterior–posterior (z-axis) or lateral (x-axis) direction of the X-ray beams, as well as the common orthogonal y-axis. On the lateral film, the projected height of point P above the y-axis is given by z_L. If M_A and M_L are the magnification factors for the anterior–posterior and lateral films, respectively, then:

$$\left(\frac{t_A}{M_A}\right)^2 + \left(\frac{z_L}{M_L}\right)^2 = t^2. \tag{40}$$

The ratio R of the magnification factors can be determined from the ratio of the projected heights y_A and y_L of point P along the y-axes of the two radiographs:

$$R = \frac{y_A}{y_L} = \frac{M_A}{M_L}. \tag{41}$$

Therefore:

$$M_A = \left[\frac{t_A^2 + (z_L R)^2}{t^2}\right]^{1/2}. \tag{42}$$

Similarly, by measurement of the x displacement x_A of point P on the anterior–posterior film, it can be shown that:

$$M_L = \left[\frac{t_L^2 + (x_A R)^2}{t^2}\right]^{1/2}. \tag{43}$$

The equations are sufficiently accurate provided that the length of the needle is less than about 5% of the focus–film distance. Care is needed to ensure that the films are orthogonal and that they are positioned in a plane perpendicular to the axis of the beam.

If an orthogonal film pair is taken accurately, with the optimum view through the array of sources, it is possible to reconstruct the positions of the sources. This can usually be done using the digitizer of a treatment-planning computer. The operator locates an origin on each of the films and identifies each needle on both films. The task of identifying several needles can be facilitated by observing details such as the following:

(1) the orientation of the eyelet (if the eyelet can be seen clearly on one film it should show as solid on the orthogonal film);

(2) the relative heights of the needles on both films.

Once the reconstruction is complete some computer programs can display the implant from any angle required; however, it may be useful for the clinician to visualize the implant in three-dimensional space by constructing a model from the geometric co-ordinates.

7.3.3 Iridium-192 wire

Iridium-192 wire presents some special problems in source-preparation 'handling' and obtaining the information from radiographs in order to calculate doses accurately.

When the outer plastic tubing is implanted, the loading end is chosen, depending on accessibility. Nylon balls and lead discs are fitted to both ends of the tubing to hold it in place. The lead disc at the non-loading end may be fully crimped, but the one at the loading end is only partially crimped to allow the easy passage of the sheathed iridium wire.

The length of plastic tubing below the skin must be determined. This is achieved by a direct measurement of the length of a dummy source loaded into the tube with the position of the open end of the tube marked on it. If the non-loading end is fully crimped, the length below the skin is this length less the diameters of the nylon spacers and the length of the plastic tube emerging from the spacer at the loading end. The therapist specifies the position between the skin entry points at which the live iridium wire is to be positioned. This enables a calculation to be made of the length of inactive wire to be added to the active wire.

For the calculation of dose, radiographs must be taken as discussed previously. These are best taken on the simulator before the live sources are loaded. To show the position of the tubes, marker wires made of high atomic number material must be used. Copper is usually sufficient, but it may be difficult to distinguish thin copper wires when the image of the wire is superimposed on the edge of a rib, as may occur for breast treatments. For this reason, platinum wires may be preferred. The dummy wires themselves are encapsulated within a thin tube, and it is convenient if they are made up of alternate segments of wire and blank spaces, each of which is generally 10 mm long. This provides a second method of determining length by counting the number of segments between the lead discs. For multiple-plane implants, it may be more convenient to use dummy wires with segments of different lengths (e.g. 5, 10, and 15 mm) in each plane so that the sources can be more readily identified.

Reconstruction from the orthogonal radiographs, as discussed previously, requires input to the computer of matched points in the two views. This can be achieved by matching marker segments on the two films and assuming that the wire is straight between these points. Some computer systems do not need matched points for input other than fixed-end positions, which may be the lead discs. These systems interpolate the co-ordinates of the wires between the two views. Whatever system is used, the total length of wire between the end-points should be calculated and compared with the value that was measured directly. Any discrepancy greater than about 5% should be investigated to see whether a reconstruction error has been made.

Strictly, the Paris system requires the calculation of basal dose rate on the central transverse plane of the implant. However, because the wires are unlikely to be straight and parallel, it is better to calculate in two other planes and to average the basal dose rate for these three planes. The reference dose rate can then be calculated. The additional planes should be 10 mm either side of the centre, or 15 mm if the wires are longer than 100 mm. Planning systems generally divide the source into several equal segments. One approach, described by Mayles *et al.* (1985), is to treat these as point sources 10 mm apart.

8.   Radiobiological models

Doses in radiotherapy have mainly been derived empirically through the careful recording of clinical experience. The main end-points considered are tumour regression and recurrence, and normal tissue morbidity. Changes to treatment regimes have been guided by the application of radiobiological models, but these are based to a large extent on clinical data.

There are a number of problem areas in the consideration of doses for brachytherapy. The first concerns the aspects of dose inhomogeneity in the treatment volume. This is dealt with through the careful application of standard dosimetry systems as discussed in Section 6. The second concerns the difficulty in relating brachytherapy experience to that gained from external beam irradiation. In the latter case, treatments are normally given at dose rates between about 0.5 and 2 Gy min^{-1} in 15–35 fractions over a time period of 3–7 weeks. This is very different from standard, LDR brachytherapy regimes in which the dose rate is approximately 0.5 Gy h^{-1}, generally no more than two fractions are given, and treatment does not extend over a period much longer than 2 weeks. These treatment schedules cannot be equated easily. The third problem arises when trying to relate the experience of LDR brachytherapy to MDR and HDR. This has become particularly important with the introduction of remote-afterloading systems. This section is concerned with the radiobiological models that have been developed in order to deal with these problems.

The effects of dose rate on clinical outcome have long been understood. In the early days of the Manchester system, Paterson recommended the use of a correction to the treatment time for the standard implant, 7000 R (about 65 Gy) in 7 days. If the calculated time differed by more than 1 day from this, then 8 h were to be added for every additional 24 h, and conversely the time was to be shortened by 8 h per 24 h if the time was calculated to be 6 days or less.

One of the early models for equating the effects of different fractionation schemes for external beam therapy was the time–dose–fraction (TDF) model. It was adapted for continuous irradiation by Orton (1974). One of the problems in using the TDF model is that it does not differentiate between late and acutely responding tissues, which can lead to major errors in its application. For this reason, it is no longer recommended for use unless the changes in treatment schedule are relatively minor. It will not be described here.

A useful summary of this subject is given in Steel (1993).

8.1 Linear–quadratic model

The model that is now most widely accepted for tackling these problems is the linear–quadratic (LQ) model. The application of this model in brachytherapy is described by Dale (1985).

Cell survival s can be described in terms of two components, which have a linear and a quadratic dependence on dose D:

$$s = \exp -(\alpha D + \beta D^2) \tag{44}$$

in which α and β are constants and are characteristic of the tissues irradiated. The biological effect E of the irradiation is determined from the survival and is defined as:

$$
\begin{aligned}
E &= -\log s \\
&= \alpha D + \beta D^2
\end{aligned} \tag{45}
$$

or

$$\frac{E}{\alpha} = D\left(1 + \frac{D}{\alpha/\beta}\right). \tag{46}$$

The parameter E/α is sometimes referred to as the biologically effective dose (BED) or alternatively as the extrapolated response dose (ERD). This can be seen to be the product of dose and a function of dose described as the relative effectiveness (RE):

$$\mathrm{RE} = 1 + \frac{D}{\alpha/\beta}. \tag{47}$$

For fractionated therapy, in which n fractions of dose d are given separated by a time interval of at least 6 h, equation (46) can be modified to give:

$$(\mathrm{ERD})_n = nd\left(1 + \frac{d}{\alpha/\beta}\right) \tag{48}$$

and

$$(\mathrm{RE})_n = \left(1 + \frac{d}{\alpha/\beta}\right) \tag{49}$$

where the subscript n indicates that ERD and RE are for fractionated therapy. These equations can be used for external beam therapy and for HDR brachytherapy.

For continuous irradiation, such as that associated with LDR and MDR treatments, account must be taken of the repair of sublethal damage occurring during the time period of treatment. In this case the equation for RE is:

$$(\mathrm{RE})_T = 1 + \frac{KR}{\alpha/\beta} \tag{50}$$

where the subscript T indicates continuous irradiation over a time T, R (in Gy h^{-1}) is the dose rate, and K is given by:

$$K = \frac{2}{\mu}\left[1 - \frac{1 - \exp(-\mu T)}{\mu T}\right] \tag{51}$$

in which μ is the time constant for sublethal repair which is generally taken to be equal to 0.46 h^{-1} corresponding to a repair half-life of 1.5 h. It should be noted that in this equation the time T is the summed irradiation time of all the treatment fractions and not the time of each fraction. In this case ERD is given by:

$$(ERD)_T = RT(RE)_T. \tag{52}$$

It can be shown that, for small values of T, K becomes approximately equal to T so that equations (49) and (50) become identical, with d equal to RT.

Equation (51) is the exact method for the derivation of K. However, in practical cases, in which the irradiation time is generally greater than 10 h, an approximate relationship can be used:

$$K = \frac{2}{\mu}\left(\alpha - \frac{1}{\mu T}\right). \tag{53}$$

For times in excess of 100 h, corresponding to LDR, this can be further simplified to:

$$K = 2/\mu. \tag{54}$$

In order to match two irradiation schedules in terms of their radiobiological effectiveness, it is necessary to equate their ERDs. It should be emphasized that this comparison is only strictly correct if the overall treatment time, i.e. the time from the start of the first fraction to completion of the last fraction, is matched. This is because the LQ model as described here does not include any modelling for cellular repopulation.

Application of the equations generally requires a knowledge of the ratio α/β. It has been shown that, for a wide range of acutely responding tissues, α/β is approximately 10 Gy and this value has been widely adopted. It is believed that tumour response may best be described in this way, and so this value is also used for tumour effects. For gynaecological treatments in particular, the dose delivered is chiefly limited by late radiation effects. For these it has been shown that α/β lies in the range 2–4 Gy for most late-responding tissues.

Some examples will be given to illustrate the use of these equations in practice. In the examples in this text, a value of α/β of 3 Gy will be assumed for late responding tissues.

Example 1

This example is a special case in which the value of α/β cancels and complete radiobiological equivalence is achieved. This is for a comparison between HDR fractionated therapy and LDR treatment with a total time greater than 100 h for which equation (54) applies. It is assumed, in this example, that the total dose is the same, i.e. $nd = RT$. For radiobiological equivalence, the RE for the two schedules should be equated and use of equations (49) and (46) leads to:

$$KR = d$$

so that

$$n = \mu T/2 \approx T/4.$$

This simple equality leads to the conclusion that perfect matching to LDR therapy requires at least 25 treatment fractions to be given, which is clearly an impossibility.

Example 2

In this example, a conventional LDR treatment of the uterine cervix is to be matched to a MDR regime. For LDR treatment, the dose to point A is 0.53 Gy h^{-1}, the total dose is 75 Gy given in two fractions, and the total treatment time is 142 h. The MDR dose rate is 1.5 Gy h^{-1}.

For early effects ($\alpha/\beta = 10$) for LDR:

$$K = 2/0.46 = 4.35 \quad \text{(equation (54))}$$
$$ERD = 75(1 + 4.35 \times 0.53/10)$$
$$= 92.3 \quad \text{(equation (50) and (52))}.$$

For MDR and by re-arranging equations (50), (52), and (53):

$$T = \frac{\left[ERD(\alpha/\beta)\mu^2 + 2R^2\right]}{R\mu[\mu(\alpha/\beta) + 2R]}.$$

Therefore:

$$T = 38.1 \text{ h}$$
$$D = 38.1 \times 1.5 = 57.2 \text{ Gy}.$$

For late effects ($\alpha/\beta = 3$):

$$ERD = 132.6$$
$$T = 29.3 \text{ h}$$
$$D = 44.0 \text{ Gy}.$$

In this example, the LQ model indicates that the total dose for the MDR treatment should be reduced by 24% to give similar effects as LDR in the tumour and by 41% to match the late effects. Since late effects are the limiting factor in these treatments, the implication of these calculations is that MDR therapy is less effective than LDR.

Example 3

In this example, the LDR treatment in the previous case will be compared with an HDR schedule using six fractions over the same time period.

For early effects ($\alpha/\beta = 10$) it has been shown that, for LDR:

$$ERD = 92.3.$$

Therefore:

$$92.3 = 6d(1 + d/10) \quad \text{(equation (51))}$$
$$d = 8.4 \text{ Gy}$$
$$nd = 50.4 \text{ Gy}.$$

For late effects ($\alpha/\beta = 3$) and LDR:

$$ERD = 132.6.$$

Therefore:

$$132.6 = 6d(1 + d/3)$$
$$d = 6.8 \text{ Gy}$$
$$nd = 40.8 \text{ Gy}.$$

As in the previous example, a greater total dose reduction is required to match the late effects (46%) than to match the early effects (33%).

8.2 Clinical applications

The examples given in the previous section demonstrate the dilemma in going from LDR to MDR or HDR therapy, which is that it is predicted that there would be a greater degree of normal tissue damage to give the same level of tumour killing.

However, the equations should be used with great caution. One aspect that was not discussed above is the assumption that the dose at point A is the critical dose for both tumour and critical normal tissue. It may be necessary to make further calculations for other structures, e.g. the rectum and the bladder, based on the dose rates received from the two therapy regimes. If the doses at these structure at different relative to point A, then different conclusions may be drawn (Dale 1990).

Ultimately, the safest guide to optimum treatment schedules with these higher dose rates is the clinical experience gained with them. For the analysis of such clinical data it should be remembered that when remote afterloading is used instead of conventional LDR therapy, changes may have been made in applicator design and dose distributions, as well as in dose rate. Therefore, care should be taken in interpreting results that may not be affected only by dose rate.

The preceding discussion has implied that MDR and HDR treatments are radiobiologically inferior to those at LDR. However, it should be recognized that the benefits of afterloading systems, which use higher dose rates, extend beyond that of reducing radiation dose to staff. With afterloading there is the opportunity of positioning the applicators with greater care and ensuring that the packing between the sources and sensitive structures is adequate. There is the potential for optimization of the dose distribution after each insertion by altering the source-loading pattern. In addition, for HDR therapy, because treatment times are of the order of a few minutes, the applicators and packing are much more likely to remain in place than is the case for more protracted treatments.

9. References

American Association of Physicists in Medicine (1987). *Recommendations of task group no. 32: specification of brachytherapy source strength*. AAPM Report no. 21. American Institute of Physics, New York.

American Association of Physicists in Medicine (1997). Review on I-125 sealed source dosimetry implementation. *AAPM Newsletter*, March/April 1997. AAPM, Maryland.

Anderson, L.L. (1976). Spacing nomograph for interstitial implant of ^{125}I seeds. *Med. Phys.*, **3**, 48–51.

Anderson, L.L. (1986). A 'natural' volume–dose histogram for brachytherapy. *Med. Phys.*, **13**, 898–903.

Anderson, L.L., Kuan. H.M., and Ding, I.-Y. (1981). In *Modern interstitial and intracavitary radiation cancer management* (ed. F. George), pp. 9–15. Masson, New York.

Anderson, L.L., Moni, J.V., and Harrison, L.B. (1993). A nomograph for permanent implants of palladium-103 seeds. *Int. J. Radiat. Onc. Biol. Phys.*, **23**, 81–7.

Berger, M.J. (1968). Energy deposition in water by photons from point isotropic sources (MIRD pamphlet no. 2). *J. Nucl. Med.*, **9** (Supplement 1), 15–25.

Breitman, K.E. (1974). Dose–rate tables for clinical ^{137}Cs sources sheathed in platinum. *Br. J. Radiol.*, **47**, 657–64.

British Institute of Radiology (1993). *Recommendations for brachytherapy dosimetry*. Report of a Joint Working Party of the BIR and the IPSM. B.I.R. London

Casebow, M.P. (1984) Dosimetry tables for standard iridium-192 wire planar implants. *Br. J. Radiol.*, **57**, 515–8.

Casebow, M.P. (1985). 'Paris' technique implant dosimetry tables for 0.3 and 0.6 mm diameter ^{192}Ir wire. *Br. J. Radiol.*, **58**, 549–53.

Clarke, D.H., Edmundson, G.K., Martinez, R.C., Matter, R.C., and Warmelink, C. (1988). The utilization of I-125 seeds as a substitute for Ir-192 seeds in temporary interstitial implants: an overview and a description of the Willow Beaumount hospital technique. *Int. J. Radiat. Onc. Biol. Phys.*, **15**, 1027–33.

Dale, R.G. (1985). The application of the linear–quadratic, dose-effect equation to fractionated and protracted radiotherapy. *Br. J. Radiol.*, **58**, 515–28.

Dale, R.G. (1990). The use of small fraction numbers in high dose-rate gynaecological afterloading: some radiobiological considerations. *Br. J. Radiol.*, **63**, 290–4.

Dutreix, A., Marinello, G., and Wambersie, A. (1982). *Dosimétrie en curiethérapie*. Masson, Paris.

Gibb, R. and Massey, J.B. (1980). Radium dosage: SI units and the Manchester system. *Br. J. Radiol.*, **53**, 1100–1.

Hall, E.J., Oliver, R., and Shepstone, B.J. (1966). Routine dosimetry with tantalum-182 and iridium-192 wires. *Acta Radio. Ther.*, **4**, 155–60.

International Commission on Radiation Units and Measurements(1978). *Dose specification and reporting of external beam therapy with photons and electrons*. ICRU Report 29. ICRU, Bethesda.

International Commission on Radiation Units and Measurements (1985). *Dose and volume specification for reporting intracavitary therapy in gynaecology*. ICRU Report 38. ICRU, Bethesda.

International Commission on Radiation Units and Measurement (1997). *Dose and volume specification for reporting interstitial therapy*. ICRU Report 58. ICRU, Bethesda.

International Organization for Standardization (1990a). *Sealed radioactive sources classification* Draft ISO Technical Report 2919. ISO, Geneva.

International Organization for Standardization (1990b). *Sealed radioactive sources – leak test methods* ISO Technical Report 4862. ISO, Geneva.

Jones, C.H. and Bidmead, M.A. (1989). Calibration of the MicroSelectron HDR system. In *Brachytherapy 2* (ed. R.F. Mould), pp. 75–87. Nucletron International, Leersum.

Kornelsen, R.O. and Young, M.E.J. (1981). Brachytherapy build-up factors. *Br. J. Radiol.*, **54**, 136.

Krishnaswany, V. (1979). Dose tables for ^{125}I seed implants. *Radiology*, **132**, 727–30.

Kubo, H.D., Glasgow, G.P., Pethel, T.D., Thomadsen, B.R., and Williamson, J.F. (1998). Report of the AAPM radiation therapy committee task group no. 59: High dose-rate brachytherapy treatment delivery. *Med. Phys.*, **22**, 375–403.

Ling, C.C. (1992). Permanent implants using Au-198, Pd-103 and I-125: radiobiological considerations based on the linear–quadratic model. *Int. J. Radiat. Oncol. Biol. Phys.*, **23**, 81–7.

Löffler, E. (1989). Source calibration of iridium-192 wires: part of a quality assurance program. In *Brachytherapy 2* (ed. R.F. Mould), pp. 70–4. Nucletron International, Leersum.

Lutz, W., Winston, K.R., and Maleki, N. (1988). A system for stereotactic radiosurgery with a linear accelerator. *Int. J. Radiat. Oncol. Biol. Phys.*, **14**, 373–81.

Marinello, G., Valero, M., Leung, S., and Pierquin, B. (1985). Comparative dosimetry between iridium wires and seed ribbons. *Int. J. Radiat. Oncol. Biol. Phys.*, **11**, 1733–9.

Massey, J.B., Pointon, R.S., and Wilkinson, J.M. (1985). The Manchester system and the BCRU recommendations for brachytherapy source specification. *Br. J. Radiol.*, **58**, 911–3.

Mayles, W.P.M., Mayles, H.M.O., and Turner, P.C.R. (1985). Physical aspects of interstitial therapy using flexible iridium-192 wire. *Br. J. Radiol.*, **58**, 529–35.

Meisberger, L.L., Keller, R.J., and Shalek, R.J. (1968). The effective attenuation in water of the gamma rays of ^{198}Au, ^{192}Ir, ^{137}Cs, ^{226}Ra, ^{60}Co. *Radiology*, **90**, 953–7.

Meredith, W.J. (ed.) (1967). *Radium dosage – the Manchester system*, 2nd edn. Livingstone, Edinburgh.

Nath, R., Meigooni, A.S., Muench, P., and Melillo, A. (1993). Anisotropy functions for ^{103}Pd, ^{125}I, and ^{192}Ir interstitial brachytherapy sources. *Med. Phys.*, **20**, 1465–73.

Nath, R., Anderson, L.L., Luxton, G., Weaver, K.A., Williamson, J.F., and Meigooni, A.S. (1995). Dosimetry of interstitial brachytherapy sources: recommendations of the AAPM radiation therapy committee task group no. 43. *Med. Phys.*, **22**, 209–34.

National Radiological Protection Board (1988). *Guidance notes for the protection of persons against ionising radiations arising from medical and dental use.* HMSO, London.

Orton, C.G. (1974). Time–dose factors (TDFs) in brachytherapy. *Br. J. Radiol.*, **47**, 603–7.

Pierquin, B., Dutreix, A., Paine, C.H., Chassagne, D., Marinello, G., and Ash, D. (1978). The Paris system in interstitial radiation therapy. *Acta Radiol. Oncol.*, **17**, 33–48.

Rao, G.U.V., Kan, P.T., and Howells, R. (1981). Interstitial volume implants with I-125 seeds. *Int. J. Radiat. Oncol. Biol. Phys.*, **7**, 431–8.

Sakelliou, L., Sakellariou, K, Sarigiannis, K., Angelopoulos, A., Perris, A., and Zarris, G. (1992). Dose rate distributions around ^{60}Co, ^{137}Cs, ^{198}Au, ^{192}Ir, ^{241}Am, ^{125}I (models 6702 and 6711) brachytherapy sources and the nuclide ^{99}Tc^{m}. *Phys. Med. Biol.*, **37**, 1859–72.

Sayeg, J.A. and Gregory, R.C. (1991). A new method for characterizing beta-ray ophthalmic applicator sources. *Med. Phys.*, **18**, 453–61.

Shalek, R.J., and Stovall, M. (1969). Dosimetry in implant therapy. In *Radiation dosimetry*, Vol. III (ed. F.H. Attix and E. Tochlin), pp. 743–807. Academic Press, New York.

Steel, G.G. (1993). The dose rate effect: brachytherapy. In *Basic clinical radiobiology* (ed. G.G. Steel). Edward Arnold, London. pp 120–9.

Trott, N.G. (ed.) (1987). Radionuclides in brachytherapy: radium and after. *Br. J. Radiol.*, Supplement No. 21. BIR, London.

van der Laarse, R. and Prins, T.P.E. (1994a). The stepping source dosimetry system as an extension of the Paris system. In *Brachytherapy from radium to optimization* (ed. R.F. Mould, J.J. Battermann, A.A. Martinez, and B.L. Speiser), pp. 319–30. Nucletron, Veenendaal

van der Laarse, R. and Prins, T.P.E. (1994b). Comparing the stepping source dosimetry system and the Paris system using volume–dose histograms of breast implants. In *Brachytherapy from radium to optimization* (ed. R.F. Mould, J.J. Batterman, A.A. Martinez, and B.L. Speiser), pp. 352–72. Nucletron, Veenendaal

van 't Riet, A., te Loo, H.J., Mak, A.C.A., Veen, R.E., Ypma, A.F.G.V.M., Bos, J. *et al.* (1993). Evaluation of brachytherapy implants using the 'natural' volume–dose histogram. *Radiother. Oncol.*, **26**, 82–4.

Walsh, A.D., Dixon-Brown, A., and Stedeford, J.B.H. (1983). Calculation of dose distributions for iridium-192 implants. *Acta Radiol. Oncol.*, **22**, 331–6.

Wilkinson, J., Moore, C.J., Notley, H.M., and Hunter, R.D. (1983). The use of Selectron afterloading equipment to simulate and extend the Manchester system for intracavitary therapy of the cervix uteri. *Br. J. Radiol.*, **56**, 409–14.

10. Additional reading

Godden, T.J. (1988). *Physical aspects of brachytherapy*. Adam Hilger, Bristol.

Interstitial Collaborative Working Group (1990) *Interstitial brachytherapy: physical, biological and clinical considerations.* Raven Press, New York.

Williamson, J.F. (1995), Berlin pp 247–302. In *Radiation Therapy Physics* (ed. A. Smith). Spring–Verlag. Recent developments in basic brachytherapy physics.

Chapter 13

Unsealed-source therapy

M.A. Flower and S.J. Chittenden

1. Introduction

The use of unsealed sources of radioactivity for therapy is a small but growing branch of nuclear medicine and a unique form of radiotherapy. Techniques used in the diagnostic applications of nuclear medicine have already been described in a companion volume in this series (Sharp *et al.* 1998). Only those aspects that are specific to therapy applications of unsealed sources will be considered here.

As with brachytherapy (see Chapter 12), the radiation dose is delivered internally. However, whereas brachytherapy involves the use of solid sources implanted into tissues or inserted into body cavities, unsealed-source therapy involves the administration of radioactive material usually in a liquid form (as solution or colloid) using various methods of administration: ingestion; infusion into the vascular or lymphatic system; and injection into a body cavity or directly into a tumour.

Alternative names are often used for unsealed-source therapy. Systemic-radionuclide therapy is a common term, implying that the whole body is irradiated, but the treatment relies on the preferential uptake and prolonged retention of the agent by the tumour, resulting in a higher tumour to normal tissue dose ratio. Targeted-radionuclide therapy using unsealed sources (or 'magic bullets') implies that the labelled compound is highly selective, if the administration is systemic, or refers to a more direct route to the tumour (e.g. direct injection into a body cavity or cyst). Unsealed-source therapy has been used for over 50 years but new applications are continually being investigated. It can, in certain cases, deliver larger internal radiation doses more selectively to target tissue than external-beam radiotherapy. Another advantage is its ease of use, since it is usually a non-invasive procedure with relatively few side-effects.

Sections 2 and 3 deal with the choice of radionuclide and the dosimetry techniques used in biologically-targeted radionuclide therapy. General practical aspects including radiation protection are covered in Sections 4

and 5. Specific practical procedures relating to some of the clinical applications listed in Table 13.1 are described in Section 6. Finally, brief outlines of some of the new approaches in this field are described in Section 6.7.3.

2. Choice of radionuclide

2.1 Physical considerations

There are three basic considerations in choosing a radionuclide for unsealed source therapy:

(1) physical properties of the radionuclide (i.e. type and energy of emissions, and physical half-life);

(2) chemical properties required for localization and retention in the tumour (Murray and Ell 1998, p. 1041);

(3) methods of production (Leach *et al.* 1996, pp. 1905–14).

The types of radionuclide decay that are of greatest potential use in unsealed-source therapy are those that involve the emission of beta particles, Auger electrons, and alpha particles. ^{131}I and ^{32}P have been the most commonly used radionuclides, but their physical properties are not necessarily ideal. Other radionuclides, together with new pharmaceuticals, are being considered (Leach *et al.* 1996, pp. 1905–14).

2.1.1 Beta emitters

There is a wide choice of beta-emitting radionuclides for unsealed-source therapy and hence a flexibility in the choice of beta range in tissue. Table 13.2 lists the physical properties of beta emitters, with half-lives greater than 2 days, which either have been used or are of potential use in radionuclide therapy. The radionuclides are listed in order of increasing beta energy and only the most abundant beta and gamma radiations are included. The average energy of an emitted beta particle

Table 13.1 Examples of clinical applications of radionuclide therapy

Radionuclide	Pharmaceutical	Application
^{32}P	NaH_2PO_4	Polycythaemia vera, essential thrombocythaemia
^{32}P	$CrPO_4$	Intracavitary
^{89}Sr	$SrCl_2$	Relief of bone pain
^{90}Y ^{198}Au	Colloid	Radiation synovectomy
^{90}Y	Microspheres	Hepatic tumours
^{90}Y	Silicate colloid	Intracavitary
$^{90}Y/^{131}I$	Antibodies	Various tumours
^{114m}In	Lymphocytes	Lymphoma
^{131}I	NaI	Thyrotoxicosis, goitre, differentiated thyroid carcinoma
^{131}I	mIBG	Neural crest tumours
^{131}I	Lipiodol	Hepatic tumours
^{153}Sm	EDTMP	Relief of bone pain
^{153}Sm	PHYP	Intracavitary
^{165}Dy	FHMA	Radiation synovectomy
^{169}Er	Citrate colloid	Radiation synovectomy
^{186}Re	Sn-HEDP	Relief of bone pain

mIBG = metaiodobenzylguanidine.
EDTMP = ethylene diamine tetramethylenephosphonate.
PHYP = particulate hydroxyapatite.
FHMA = ferric hydroxide macroaggregates.
HEDP = hydroxyethylidine diphosphonate.
Data from Hoefnagel (1991) and references in Section 6.

is approximately one-third of its maximum energy and the maximum range in soft tissue, in mm, is approximately equal to the maximum energy, in MeV, multiplied by 5 (Holmes *et al.* 1987, p. 166). Although pure beta emitters (e.g. ^{32}P) may be considered as ideal from the point of view of delivering a high local dose whilst sparing tissues at a distance, radionuclides that emit gamma rays in addition to beta particles (e.g. ^{131}I) have the advantage that external counting and imaging techniques can be applied more easily to assess the uptake and distribution of the therapy agent. However, the gamma rays increase the whole-body dose to the patient.

The range of the beta particles is important in relation to the size of tumour to be treated. The relationship between the specific ionization and the range of beta particles in soft tissue with respect to beta energy is shown in Figure 13.1. High-energy beta particles provide radiation cross-fire, which can offset the problem of heterogeneous uptake in large tumours. These long-range beta particles are also better suited to the treatment of large volumes. If the beta emitter is uniformly distributed throughout the source volume, the dose rate will be uniform throughout this volume except for a reduction close to the outer edge. For very small tumours (less than a few mm in diameter), a large fraction of the total dose from beta particles emitted within the tumour could be deposited in surrounding tissues (Figure 13.2). Hence,

for the treatment of micrometastases, short-range electrons and alpha emitters would be more appropriate.

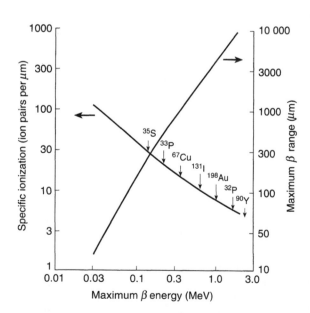

Figure 13.1 The relationships between the specific ionization and the range of beta rays in soft tissue with respect to the beta energy. Adapted from Spencer (1978).

Table 13.2 Physical properties of beta-emitting radionuclides for unsealed-source therapy

Radio nuclide	$T_{1/2}$ (Days)	$n_{i,np}$	$\bar{E}_{i,np}$ (MeV)	$n_{i,p}$	$\bar{E}_{i,p}$ (MeV)	Δ_{np} (g Gy MBq^{-1}h^{-1})	Δ_p (g Gy MBq^{-1}h^{-1})
Low-energy betas							
^{191}Os	15.4	1.00	0.038	0.26	0.129	0.078	0.046
^{35}S	87.4	1.00	0.049	–	–	0.028	–
^{33}P	25.4	1.00	0.077	–	–	0.044	–
^{45}Ca	163.0	1.00	0.077	–	–	0.044	–
^{199}Au	3.2	0.66	0.082	0.37	0.158	0.082	0.051
^{169}Er	9.3	0.55	0.101	–	–	0.060	–
^{67}Cu	2.6	0.57	0.121	0.49	0.185	0.089	0.066
^{47}Sc	3.4	0.68	0.143	0.68	0.159	0.093	0.062
^{177}Lu	6.7	0.79	0.149	0.11	0.208	0.085	0.020
^{161}Tb	6.9	0.67	0.154	0.22	0.025	0.113	0.020
Medium-energy betas							
^{131}I	8.0	0.89	0.192	0.81	0.364	0.109	0.219
^{153}Sm	2.0	0.43	0.229	0.28	0.103	0.156	0.035
^{143}Pr	13.6	1.00	0.314	–	–	0.181	–
^{198}Au	2.7	0.99	0.315	0.96	0.412	0.188	0.233
^{186}Re	3.8	0.73	0.362	0.09	0.137	0.198	0.012
^{111}Ag	7.5	0.93	0.363	0.07	0.342	0.204	0.015
^{143}Pm	2.2	0.97	0.363	0.03	0.286	0.210	0.006
High-energy betas							
^{89}Sr	50.5	1.00	0.583	–	–	0.336	–
^{32}P	14.3	1.00	0.695	–	–	0.400	–
^{114m}In	49.5	0.99[a]	0.777[a]	0.15	0.190	0.526	0.054
^{124}I	4.2	0.22	0.830	0.61[b]	0.603[b]	0.111	0.622
^{90}Y	2.7	1.00	0.935	–	–	0.539	–

n_i and $\bar{E}_i$ refer to the most abundant radiations (see Section 3.1 for definitions); Δ_{np} and Δ_p are the total equilibrium dose constants for non-penetrating and penetrating radiations, respectively.
[a] Emitted from daughter.
[b] ^{124}I decays via electron capture and positron emission. In addition to the photons listed, photons with $n_i = 0.451$, $E_i = 0.511$ are emitted following positron annihilation.
Data from ICRP (1983).

2.1.2 Auger-electron emitters

Radionuclides (e.g. ^{123}I, ^{125}I, ^{117}Sn) that decay by electron capture or internal conversion, emit low-energy characteristic X-rays and Auger electrons. Most of these electrons have very short range (<1 μm) and, therefore, are only of use in therapy if the source is attached, or very close, to the cell nucleus. The potential use of Auger-electron emitters specifically for radioimmunotherapy (RIT) has been discussed elsewhere (Humm 1986), and a recent review of targeted radiotherapy using Auger-electron emitters can be found in Leach *et al.* (1996, pp. 1973–92). Biological effects are critically dependent on the subcellular and subnuclear localization of Auger-electron emitters. Theoretical and experimental studies suggest that ^{123}I (with short half-life) is more effective than ^{125}I (with longer half-life). Potential methods of targeting include the use of analogues of DNA precursors (e.g. iodo-deoxyuridine) and of molecules that bind to DNA (e.g. growth factors or oligonucleotides). Unfortunately, heterogeneity of radionuclide uptake is a serious limitation on the success of targeted therapy with Auger-electron emitters. In order to facilitate targeting to tumours and to reduce toxicity in normal cells, direct injection of, for example, nucleosides labelled with Auger-electron emitters are being investigated (Kassis *et al.* 1996).

2.1.3 Alpha emitters

The advantages of alpha emitters (e.g. ^{211}At, ^{212}Bi) for radionuclide therapy are their short range (typically 50–90 μm, i.e. several cell diameters), high-linear energy transfer (LET) and hence increased biological effectiveness. A single alpha particle can deposit approximately 0.25 Gy in a 10 μm diameter cell nucleus (Humm 1986). This offers the possibility of combining cell-specific targeting with radiation of similar range. Preclinical studies with a variety of ^{212}Bi- and ^{211}At-labelled radiopharmaceuticals have produced exciting results

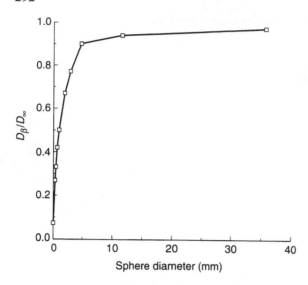

Figure 13.2 Graph of the ratio of the average beta dose D_β in a sphere to the dose D_∞ in an infinite volume containing the same radioactive concentration of ^{131}I, versus sphere diameter. Data taken from Malone (1975).

(Leach *et al.* 1996, pp. 1915–31). Several approaches have been explored, including labelled colloids, monoclonal antibodies, metabolic precursors, receptor-avid ligands, and other low molecular weight molecules. However, patient studies are not recommended until highly specific tumour targeting can be guaranteed. One way of achieving this would be by using routes of administration that confine the agent to the region of the tumour. Alternatively, alpha-emitting compounds could be used *in vitro*, e.g. to purge bone marrow and/or peripheral blood of tumour cells.

2.2 Radiobiological considerations

The radiobiology of unsealed-source therapy differs from that of external-beam radiotherapy owing to differences in dose distribution and dose rate (Leach *et al.* 1996, pp. 1871–84). At microscopic levels, the dose distribution is unlikely to be uniform, but this is not necessarily a disadvantage if it is caused by an increased uptake of the radiopharmaceutical in the target cells. In contrast to fractionated high dose-rate external-beam radiotherapy, unsealed sources deliver continuous irradiation at relatively lower dose rates. In addition, the dose rate varies during therapy, decreasing at a rate that depends on both the physical half-life of the radionuclide and the biological clearance of the compound.

From radiobiological considerations, continuous low dose-rate irradiation may be viewed as being a particularly effective type of radiotherapy, as it ensures that the differential sparing between tumour and normal tissues is maximized. A given dose has a reduced

biological effect if delivered at a low dose rate but the magnitude of this effect varies for different tissues: for early-responding tissues (bone marrow, epithelium) the effect is small; for late-responding tissues (vascular endothelium, nervous tissue, kidney) it can be large. Only at the later stages of therapy (low dose rate) will here be sparing of late-responding normal tissues.

The linear-quadratic (LQ) model for cell survival, applied originally to conventional radiotherapy (external beam and brachytherapy, see Chapter 12, Section 8), can also be applied to radionuclide therapy (Howell *et al.* 1998). The LQ model, when applied to unsealed source therapy has to be modified to allow for the period of accumulation of the radionuclide in the tissue of interest and to take into consideration the proliferation of normal and tumour tissues. These authors have shown that the modified LQ model can be helpful when choosing a radionuclide for a particular type of therapy. In particular, for a given therapeutic effect in a tumour, a longer-lived radionuclide can result in a lower detrimental effect on the bone marrow than a shorter-lived radionuclide. The optimal physical half-life is about 2–3 times the biological clearance half-time of the therapeutic compound in the tumour.

3. Dosimetry techniques

This section will show that it is impossible to achieve precise estimates of the magnitude and distribution of internal dose delivered from unsealed sources. As a result of the inherent large uncertainties, dosimetry calculations are often not performed for individual patients. However, with the advent of improved imaging and counting techniques, estimates of internal dose are becoming more commonplace. Even then, these are often retrospective dosimetry calculations performed using data acquired during therapy, rather than pretreatment planning.

The most widely used method of calculating absorbed dose for patients treated with unsealed sources has been developed by the Medical Internal Radiation Dose (MIRD) committee of the American Society of Nuclear Medicine (Loevinger *et al.* 1991). The aim of this committee was to develop a dosimetry system for diagnostic nuclear medicine, but the methods can equally well be used for unsealed-source therapy using beta emitters. However, for microdosimetry of small tumours or micrometastases, and when considering alpha or Auger-electron emitters, other computational methods have to be used (Leach *et al.* 1996, pp. 1941–1955). These methods require knowledge of the biodistribution of the radiopharmaceutical at the microscopic level, for which autoradiography plays an important role.

There are two useful software programs available for MIRD calculations. The first program is called MIR-

DOSE (Stabin 1996) and is available from Oak Ridge Institute for Science and Education (RIDIC 1997). The second, called MABDOSE (Johnson 1988), is aimed at dosimetry for radioimmunotherapy (Section 6.6) and allows the inclusion of a spherical tumour at any site in the body.

Although MIRD data are not expressed in SI radiation units, all data in this chapter are expressed in those SI-based units most commonly used for therapy applications. Hence, care must be taken when converting data derived from MIRD tables into SI units. The following is a useful conversion factor:

$$1 \text{ g rad } \mu\text{Ci}^{-1}\text{h}^{-1} = 0.27 \text{ g Gy MBq}^{-1}\text{h}^{-1}. \quad (1)$$

3.1 MIRD in theory

For the purposes of internal dose calculations, the body is considered as a set of source organs (i.e. those that have a significant uptake of the radiopharmaceutical) and a set of target organs (i.e. those that are being irradiated by the source organs). Target organs, as defined in MIRD, are any organs (or tissues) of interest for which the absorbed dose is to be estimated and, hence, can include normal tissues as well as tumours. Various configurations of source and target organs can be considered:

(1) target and source organs geometrically separated;

(2) target and source organs identical;

(3) source within target organ;

(4) source encompassing target organ.

For each pair of source and target organs, the following equation is used to calculate the absorbed $D_{t \leftarrow s}$ (in Gy) to a target organ from activity in a source organ:

$$D_{t \leftarrow s} = \frac{\tilde{A}_s}{m_t} \sum_i \Delta_i \phi_i \quad (2)$$

where $\tilde{A}_s$ is the cumulated activity in the source (in MBq h), m_t is the mass of the target organ (in g), Δ_i is the equilibrium absorbed dose constant for radiation of type i (i.e. the mean energy per nuclear disintegration) (in g Gy MBq^{-1} h^{-1}), and ϕ_i is the absorbed fraction (i.e. the fraction of the radiation of type i emitted from the source and absorbed by the target). The total dose to a single organ arising from radiation emitted by several source organs is simply the sum of the absorbed doses from all the source organs.

The cumulated activity $\tilde{A}_s$ is proportional to the total number of radioactive disintegrations that occur in the source organ, and depends on: the activity administered; the uptake of, retention by, and excretion from the organ; and the physical decay of the radionuclide. $\tilde{A}_s$ is equal to the time integral of the activity in the source organ:

Table 13.3 Nuclear data for the most abundant radiations emitted from ^{131}I

Radiation	n_i	E_i (MeV)	Δ_i (g Gy MBq^{-1}h^{-1})
Non-penetrating			
β_1	0.0200	0.0691	0.001
β_3	0.0664	0.0964	0.004
β_5	0.8980	0.1916	0.099
Penetrating			
γ_4	0.0578	0.2843	0.009
γ_9	0.8201	0.3644	0.172
γ_{12}	0.0653	0.6367	0.024
γ_{14}	0.0173	0.7228	0.007

Data from MIRD Pamphlet 10 (MIRD 1975a).

$$\tilde{A}_s = \int_0^\infty A_s(t)\mathrm{d}t \quad (3)$$

which is the area under the activity–time curve $A_s(t)$ for that organ.

It is helpful when considering both Δ_i and ϕ_i to separate the different emissions into non-penetrating radiation (beta particles and electrons) and penetrating radiation (X- and gamma rays). Δ_i (in g Gy MBq^{-1} h^{-1}) is given by:

$$\Delta_i = 0.576 n_i \overline{E}_i \quad (4)$$

where n_i is the mean number of the ith type of radiation emitted per disintegration, and $\overline{E}_i$ is the mean energy of the ith type radiation (in MeV). Δ_i is found from nuclear decay tables for each type of radiation emitted. MIRD tables (MIRD 1975a) list the values for most radionuclides used in nuclear medicine and, as an example, Table 13.3 lists the values of n_i, $\overline{E}_i$, and Δ_i for the most abundant radiations emitted from ^{131}I. The values of Δ_{np} and Δ_p (the total equilibrium dose constants for non-penetrating and penetrating radiations, respectively) listed in Table 13.2 are useful indicators of the gamma dose relative to the beta dose for each therapy radionuclide.

For non-penetrating radiation, ϕ_i is equal to: 0 when the target and source organs are geometrically separated; 1 when the target and source are the same organ; and 0.5 at a source–target interface. An example of the last case occurs when considering the absorbed dose to the wall of a body cavity containing radioactivity (e.g. to the bladder wall when the bladder contains radioactive urine).

For penetrating radiation, the fraction ϕ_i depends strongly on both the geometry of the source–target configuration and on the radiation energy. Values of ϕ_i derived from Monte Carlo calculations can be found in MIRD Pamphlet 5 (MIRD 1969) for various radionuclides and pairs of source and target organs.

Equation (2) can be simplified by the introduction of the mean dose per unit cumulated activity $S_{t \leftarrow s}$ (in Gy MBq^{-1} h^{-1}) defined by:

$$S_{t \leftarrow s} = \frac{1}{m_t} \sum_i \Delta_i \phi_i. \qquad (5)$$

Hence, the absorbed dose to a target organ from a single source organ is given by:

$$D_{t \leftarrow s} = \tilde{A}_s S_{t \leftarrow s}. \qquad (6)$$

Values of the mean dose per unit cumulated activity (known as S values) have been tabulated for a variety of radionuclides and for different source–target configurations in both standard man (MIRD 1975b) and children (NCRP 1983) and are now kept up to date on the Internet (RIDIC 1997).

The MIRD scheme for calculating the dose from internally administered radionuclides makes the assumption that the activity is uniformly distributed in the source organ. It also assumes that the shape, size, and position of the organs are as represented by the human phantom described in Pamphlet 5 (MIRD 1969). The MIRD scheme does not permit the determination of a maximum or minimum dose to each target organ considered, but simply provides the mean dose to the target volume. Evidence from micro-autoradiography and from miniature dosimeters suggests that the assumption of a uniform distribution of beta emitters and hence uniform irradiation of tissue is incorrect. There may be significant heterogeneity in the 10–100 μm range. For example, Sinclair *et al.* (1956) estimated that in the treatment of toxic diffuse and non-toxic nodular goitre with Na^{131}I, the maximum dose was typically 3 and 10 times the mean dose to the thyroid gland, respectively.

The limitations of the MIRD system specifically for RIT have been reviewed by Fisher (1994). Several groups are starting to produce 3-D dose distributions resulting from unsealed-source therapy in order to overcome some of these limitations. These dose distributions are derived from sequential registered SPECT images and either dose-point kernel convolution (e.g. Giap *et al.* 1995), which is only valid for homogeneous tissues, or patient-specific Monte Carlo techniques (e.g. Einhorn *et al.* 1996, pp. 367–72), which are more accurate but require longer computational times. Dose–volume histograms (see Chapter 9, Section 1.3.3) and tumour control probabilities can be derived from these 3-D dose distributions in the same way as for external-beam radiotherapy.

3.2 MIRD in practice

Apart from the limitations associated with the basic assumptions outlined above, the accuracy with which the internal dose can be estimated depends on the accuracy with which the parameters $\tilde{A}_s$ and $S_{t \leftarrow s}$ can be determined in practice.

3.2.1 Determination of cumulated activity, $\tilde{A}_s$

Sequential measurements of the activity $A_s(t)$ at various times t in each source organ of interest are required to determine $\tilde{A}_s$. Region of interest analysis on orthogonal views from a gamma camera is a common method used to assess organ uptake (Sharp *et al.* 1998, section 4.4.3). Counts in the patient images are compared with counts in the images of a phantom that simulates the patient geometry and contains a known amount of the appropriate radionuclide. Dead-time corrections may be necessary when the count rate is high during the first few days after a therapy administration. Alternatively, the count rates can be reduced (e.g. by the use of high-Z attenuation sheets or low-sensitivity collimators). Corrections are also needed for background activity in tissues surrounding the organ of interest and for variations in patient and source thickness.

None of the therapy radionuclides currently used is ideal for imaging with a gamma camera, as they are either pure beta emitters (e.g. ^{32}P) or the energies of the gamma rays emitted (e.g. from ^{131}I) are such that poor quality images are obtained (owing to penetration of and scattering in the collimator). Hence, alternatives to the gamma camera (e.g. stationary probe or whole-body scanner) may be preferred for quantitative measurements of organ uptake when dealing with therapy radionuclides. Other options are as follows:

(1) to perform a tracer study prior to therapy using a radioisotope more suited to gamma camera imaging (e.g. ^{123}I instead of ^{131}I, although the advantages offered by the lower energy photons (159 keV) are offset by the shorter half-life (13 h), which limits its use in the determination of $A_s(t)$ at $t > 72$ h);

(2) to use dual isotopes, i.e. a simultaneous injection of both imaging and therapy radionuclides (e.g. ^{51}Cr and ^{32}P (Ott *et al.* 1985) or ^{85}Sr and ^{89}Sr (Blake *et al.* 1986) for imaging and therapy, respectively);

(3) to image the bremsstrahlung radiation from beta emitters (Smith *et al.* 1988; Siegel *et al.* 1995).

Single-photon emission CT (SPECT) (Sharp *et al.* 1998, ch. 2; Rosenthal *et al.* 1995) may be used as an alternative to planar imaging (Figure 13.3). A calibration phantom is still needed, but the correction for activity in surrounding tissues is in general no longer required.

For a single organ or tumour, the activity–time curve is usually represented by a single exponential:

$$A_s(t) = A_0 \exp(-0.693t/T_e) \qquad (7)$$

where A_0 is the initial activity (in MBq) in the source organ (assuming rapid initial uptake), and T_e is the

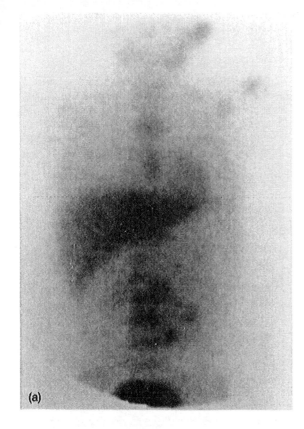

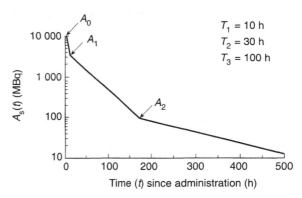

Figure 13.4 Typical three-phase activity–time curve for the whole body.

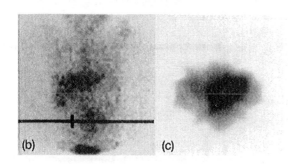

Figure 13.3 ^{123}I mIBG images at 24 h: (a) planar image (600 s anterior view); (b) planar image (20 s anterior view); (c) SPECT image at level shown in (b).

effective half-life (in hours) of the radiopharmaceutical in that organ, and is related to the physical and biological half-lives T_p and T_b by:

$$\frac{1}{T_e} = \frac{1}{T_p} + \frac{1}{T_b} \tag{8}$$

In this case, substituting equation (7) into equation (3):

$$\tilde{A}_s = 1.44 A_0 T_e. \tag{9}$$

When considering the whole body as the source organ, $\tilde{A}_s$ is determined from sequential measurements with a calibrated whole-body counter. Various detector geometries can be used (e.g. ceiling-mounted stationary detector, shielded scanning detector, or several fixed detectors in a shielded room). For pure beta emitters, the whole-body counter can be set up to detect the bremsstrahlung radiation. The activity–time curve for the whole body is usually represented by the sum of several exponential functions. $\tilde{A}_s$ can be determined by fitting straight lines to the log-linear activity–time curve (Figure 13.4) and using the equation:

$$\tilde{A}_s = 1.44\left[A_0 T_1 + \sum_{n=1}^{N-1} A_n(T_{n+1} - T_n)\right] \tag{10}$$

where A_n is the activity (in MBq) at the point of intersection between the nth and the $(n + 1)^{th}$ phases of excretion, T_n is the apparent effective half-life (in hours) of the nth phase of excretion, and N is the number of phases. For a three-phase activity–time curve, equation (10) simplifies to:

$$\tilde{A}_s = 1.44[(A_0 - A_1)T_1 + (A_1 - A_2)T_2 + A_2 T_3]. \tag{11}$$

The whole-body dose $D_{wb \leftarrow wb}$ due to activity in the whole body, is simple to obtain and useful as an indirect estimate of the gamma radiation dose to the blood and bone marrow, which could be dose-limiting organs. In addition to *in vivo* imaging and counting techniques, direct sampling of body fluids (e.g. blood and urine) may be used to determine their cumulated activity.

When the radionuclide is not uniformly distributed in the body, the basic MIRD equations need to be modified (Cloutier *et al.*, 1973) so that the dose to a target organ is not overestimated. Without these modifications, which require the whole body to be considered as the sum of the individual source organs plus the 'rest of body', the amount of radionuclide in a target organ would be included twice.

3.2.2 Determination of S values (and mass of target organ, m_t)

The mean dose per unit cumulated activity $S_{t \leftarrow s}$ is strongly dependent on the mass of the target organ. Hence, a small error in m_t may result in a large error in $S_{t \leftarrow s}$ and $D_{t \leftarrow s}$. In therapy applications involving children, appropriate S values can be obtained by interpolation from a plot of S values against m_t using data tabulated for standard children (NCRP 1983) and standard adults (MIRD 1975b).

Various methods can be used to assess organ mass. Palpation was used in the past but this was subjective and very inaccurate. Ultrasound, X-ray CT, and MRI all have excellent spatial resolution and can provide very precise measurements of the *anatomical* volume of an organ. However, the radiopharmaceutical may not be distributed throughout this entire volume and thus the mass of tissue within which the radionuclide is concentrated may be overestimated by these methods. Nuclear medicine imaging has relatively poor spatial resolution, but is the only means of assessing the *functional* volume (and hence mass) of tissue, which is the more relevant parameter for dosimetry calculations. It is important to quote whether an *anatomical* or *functional* mass has been used when reporting the results of dose calculations.

The accuracy with which the functional volume can be determined depends on the spatial resolution of the imaging system and on the radionuclide involved. As previously mentioned, therapy radionuclides have poor imaging characteristics. Taking ^{131}I as an example, the various ways of determining functional volume are, in order of increasing accuracy:

(1) planar imaging with ^{131}I (anterior, posterior and lateral views required);

(2) ^{131}I SPECT (Alaamer *et al.* 1994) (ideally using ultra-high resolution, high-energy collimators);

(3) ^{123}I SPECT tracer study prior to therapy (Gilland *et al.* 1994);

(4) ^{124}I positron emission tomography (PET) tracer study prior to therapy (Flower *et al.* 1994).

Provided the problem of production in sufficient quantities can be solved, ^{124}I is a potential therapy radionuclide since, as shown in Table 13.2, the values of Δ_{np} for ^{124}I and ^{131}I are virtually identical. As PET offers the most accurate means of assessing functional volume, other positron emitters are being considered for tracer studies prior to unsealed-source therapy (e.g. ^{64}Cu, ^{83}Sr, and ^{86}Y prior to ^{67}Cu, ^{89}Sr and, ^{90}Y therapy, respectively) (Leach *et al.* 1996, p. 1912)).

3.2.3 Determination of radioactive concentration, $A_s(t)/m_t$

Equation (2) has to be used when a tumour is considered as both the target and source organs, as S-values do not exist for this situation. The first term is the integral of the radioactive concentration, $A_s(t)/m_t$, in the tumour, and sequential quantitative tomographic imaging is the best method for estimating the radioactive concentration, as this avoids making errors on the separate assessment of $A_s(t)$ and m_t, which would be combined in quadrature.

3.2.4 Summary of minimization of errors

In contrast to external-beam therapy, for which dosimetry is very precise, the calculation of doses delivered during unsealed-source therapy is subject to large errors. In order to minimize these:

(1) check that the assumptions made in the MIRD schema are applicable;

(2) use the most accurate method available for determining m_t or $A_s(t)/m_t$;

(3) acquire as many data points over as long a time period as possible for the activity–time curve.

Radiation protection problems and count-rate limitations of the gamma camera make the early acquisition of data after therapy difficult. A combination of early measurements during a tracer study and late measurements following therapy administration is a reasonable compromise. However, the kinetics of the radiopharmaceutical may not be identical in the tracer and therapy studies, so extrapolation of data can also be subject to error.

3.2.5 Worked examples

In order to illustrate the methods outlined above, examples of typical dose calculations are outlined in Tables 13.4–13.6. Further examples of dose calculations, including dose to tumours and normal organs (e.g. blood and bladder), can be found elsewhere (Papanastassiou *et al.* 1995; Leach *et al. 1996, pp. 1933–1940, 1993–2008*).

3.3 Limiting organs

The dose that can be delivered to the tumour is limited by the maximum dose that can be tolerated by normal tissues. The dose-limiting organs for unsealed-source therapy depend on the route of administration and on the radiopharmaceutical. In systemic therapy, the dose-limiting organ is often the bone-marrow: if there is a risk of bone-marrow ablation, a bone-marrow harvest may be performed prior to therapy, for subsequent regrafting if necessary. For intrathecal administrations,

Table 13.4 Calculation of dose to thyroid remnant during ablation therapy with 3.7 GBq $Na^{131}I$

Data used

$$E_\gamma = 0.364 \text{ MeV only}$$
$$\bar{E}_\beta = 0.192 \text{ MeV only}$$
$$\Delta_\gamma = 0.172 \text{ g Gy MBq}^{-1}\text{h}^{-1}$$
$$\Delta_\beta = 0.099 \text{ g Gy MBq}^{-1}\text{h}^{-1}$$
$$\phi_\gamma = 0.026 \text{ (data extrapolated from MIRD (1969))}$$
$$\phi_\beta = 1$$
$$T_e = 193 \text{ h} \qquad (= T_p)$$
$$A_0 = 92.5 \text{ MBq} \qquad (=2.5\% \text{ uptake})$$
$$m_t = 8 \text{ g}$$

Using equations (2) and (9), the dose to the thyroid remnant from activity in the remnant is given by:

$$D_{\text{remnant} \leftarrow \text{remnant}} = \frac{1.44 \times 92.5 \times 193}{8} (0.172 \times 0.026 + 0.099) \text{ Gy}$$

$$= 3213 \, (0.0045 + 0.099) \text{ Gy}$$
$$= 330 \text{ Gy}$$

NB For simplicity, only the principal beta and gamma radiations (see *Table 13.3*) were considered in this example but the calculation illustrates that less than 5% of the dose is delivered by the penetrating radiation.

Table 13.5 Calculation of dose to whole body during ^{131}I mIBG therapy of a 5-year-old child with neuroblastoma

Data used

$$A_0 = 10\,000 \text{ MBq}$$
$$A_1 = 4000 \text{ MBq}$$
$$A_2 = 100 \text{ MBq}$$
$$T_1 = 10 \text{ h}$$
$$T_2 = 30 \text{ h}$$
$$T_3 = 100 \text{ h}$$
$$S_{\text{wb} \leftarrow \text{wb}} = 8.42 \times 10^{-6} \text{ Gy MBq}^{-1}\text{h}^{-1} \text{ (from NCRP (1983))}$$

Using equation (11), for a three-phase activity-time curve:

$$\tilde{A}_{\text{wb}} = 1.44 \, [(10\,000{-}4000) \times 10 + (4000{-}100) \times 30 + (100 \times 100)] \text{ MBq h}$$
$$= 2.7 \times 10^5 \text{ MBq h}$$

Using equation (6):

$$D_{\text{wb} \leftarrow \text{wb}} = 2.7 \times 10^5 \times 8.42 \times 10^{-6} \text{ Gy}$$
$$= 2.2 \text{ Gy}$$

NB In this example, the doses delivered during the three phases of excretion are in the ratio 32:63:5, showing that it is very important to obtain early measurements of whole-body retention (see Section 3.2.3).

the dose-limiting organ is the spinal cord. If there is high uptake in the liver, this could lead to radiation hepatitis and chronic veno-occlusive liver disease. The bladder is also at risk from radioactivity in the urine and patients should be hydrated and/or catheterized to reduce the dose to the bladder wall.

The dose-limiting organs for new agents are not necessarily known in advance and it is important that detailed dosimetry estimates and toxicity studies are performed for each new agent considered for unsealed source therapy.

4. General procedures

Having covered the theoretical aspects of radionuclide therapy, attention is now turned to the practical aspects, which are based on experience at the Royal Marsden

Table 13.6 Calculation of dose to peritoneal wall after intracavitary administration of 740 MBq ^{32}P chromic phosphate

Assumptions

^{32}P plates out onto surface of peritoneal cavity in a uniformly thin layer within 24 h
Surface area of peritoneum = 20 000 cm^2
Half-value depth in tissue = 0.08 cm (Taasan *et al.* 1985)
Tissue density = 1.0 g cm^{-3}
$T_e = T_p = 14.3$ days (i.e. no leakage from cavity)

Data used

$$
\begin{aligned}
m_t &= 20\ 000 \times 0.08 \text{ g} \\
&= 1600 \text{ g} \\
\Delta_\beta &= 0.4 \text{ g Gy MBq}^{-1}\text{h}^{-1} \\
\phi_\beta &= 0.5
\end{aligned}
$$

Using equation (9):

$$
\begin{aligned}
A_s &= 1.44 \times 740 \times 14.3 \times 24 \text{ MBq h} \\
&= 3.7 \times 10^{-5} \text{ MBq h}
\end{aligned}
$$

Using equation (2):

$$
\text{Dose to peritoneal wall} = \frac{3.7 \times 10^{-5}}{1600} \times 0.4 \times 0.5 \text{ Gy}
$$

$$
= 46 \text{ Gy}
$$

Hospital, Sutton. This section outlines the main procedures at each stage of unsealed-source therapy.

4.1 Consultation with the patient

Details of the treatment are described to the patient as soon as unsealed-source therapy is proposed, so that potential problems can be solved before the patient becomes radioactive. Information sheets or booklets are generally helpful to the patient at this stage. Details relevant to radiation protection may be easily obtained from the patient by completion of a questionnaire based on the checklist shown in Table 13.7. Female patients should not be pregnant or breast feeding at the time of radionuclide therapy and may need to avoid pregnancy for a given time afterwards.

4.2 Dosimetry and prescription of administered activity

The prescription of a nominal (empirical) activity is the current practice for most types of therapy. However, the administered activity may be tailored to the individual patient if dosimetry calculations (Section 3) are performed in advance (e.g. by using a small accurately measured quantity of the therapy radiopharmaceutical as a tracer). All dosimetry calculations are checked by a second suitably qualified person.

Table 13.7 Radiation-protection checklist when planning unsealed-source therapy

1. Patient name.
2. Radiopharmaceutical and activity.
3. Proposed date of administration.
4. Relevant details of any previous radionuclide therapy.
5. Patient's primary language. If not English, will an interpreter be necessary and/or available when treatment is given?
6. Where does the patient live? (e.g. house or nursing home).
7. Details of others at home, including ages of children.
8. Could children stay elsewhere for a few days if necessary?
9. Details of where the patient will stay after therapy, if not at home, and of others staying there.
10. Method of transport to home after therapy (e.g. taxi, public/private transport).
11. After therapy, will the patient have any contact with children or pregnant women? If so, what are the details?
12. Patient's occupation, if involving photography or other radiosensitive work.
13. Details of any factors likely to cause radiation protection problems during therapy (e.g. incontinence, poor mobility, blindness).
14. Other relevant details (e.g. check that patient is not pregnant nor breast feeding at time of therapy).

RADIONUCLIDE THERAPY

PRESCRIPTION AND REQUISITION

Full name of patient..... M r ... Samuel .. S.M.I.T.H ....

Hospital number.... 6.4.4.0.2.6 ..... Ward. Radio Iodine Therapy Unit

Please supply the following radioactive material

for use in.... R.T.U .... on. 2./.7./.91. at. 14:00

Isotope	Chemical form	Method of administration	Activity or radiation dose
^{131}I	m I BG	I/V	1·5Gy To Whole Body

Print name.... J. COURAGE ...... Signed... J. Courage
        (ARSAC holder/Deputy)

                          Date........ 14/6/91

CALCULATION OF ACTIVITY (if radiation dose specified by clinician)

Activity required... 5700 ... M Bq to give dose of .. 1·5 ....Gy

Calculated by .O. P. Theakston .... date. 11./.6./.91.

Checked by .... S. X. Wadworth .... date. 13./.6./.91.

ISSUE/DISPENSING

Sample number.. F.I. 86/1 ....

The required nominal activity of. 5700 MBq at. 1400 .on. 2./.7./.91.

was dispensed by. E.S.B. Fuller .... at. 13.30 .on. 2./.7./.91.

was checked by.. O.P. Theakston .... at 13:35 .on. 2./.7./.91.

ADMINISTRATION

Total activity administered. 5730 MBq at.. 14:15 .. on. 2./.7./.91.

Signed.. S. Neame .... Radiotherapist or delegated person

RADIATION CLEARANCE

Patient has residual activity of. 50 MBq at. 14:00 .on. 12./.7./.91.

Patient has radiation clearance for discharge after .. 14:00 .....

                          on. 12./.7./.91.

Yellow card to be issued *YES/NO

Signed.... S. X. Wadworth ....* Physicist/~~Nurse~~/~~Radiographer~~

* delete as appropriate

copies:- 1.Notes 2.Physics 3.Radiochemistry 4.Nuclear medicine 5.Clinic

Figure 13.5 Radionuclide therapy form.

4.3 Ordering and documentation

It is a legal requirement in the United Kingdom that a certificate is obtained from the Administration of Radioactive Substances Advisory Committee (ARSAC) to cover each type of radiopharmaceutical administration (Sharp *et al.* 1998, section 7.6.1) and that the order form for each radionuclide therapy is signed by the ARSAC licence holder (or his/her delegated deputy). An example of a suitable form, with sections completed at each stage of the therapy procedure, is shown in Figure 13.5. Additional documentation includes the consent form (signed by the patient), booking forms (e.g. for patient admission to hospital or dosimetry measurements during therapy), and dispensing sheets for the radiopharmaceutical.

4.4   Preparation for therapy

The patient may require special preparation for the therapy procedure, either in advance (e.g. by drugs or special diet), or on the day of administration (e.g. by hydration, cannulation, or sedation). The patient should have haematological and renal function tests prior to radionuclide therapy: poor renal function is generally a contra-indication for this type of treatment. Bone marrow harvest may be required in cases where myelosuppression is a possibility after therapy. Prior to administration, checks should be made that the patient's circumstances relative to radiation protection have not changed since the initial assessment. The patient's relatives may require information or training, particularly if they will be involved in nursing the patient. Preparation of the radiopharmaceutical (e.g. defrosting) and the administration room (e.g. covering of areas likely to become contaminated) may be required.

4.5   Dispensing

UK regulations require radiopharmaceuticals to be dispensed only in premises registered by the Environment Agency and authorized to keep, use, and dispose of radioactive substances in accordance with the Radioactive Substances Act (HMSO 1993). The dispensed activity must be measured (e.g. in a calibrated 'well-type' ionization chamber) and should be within 10% of the prescribed activity. Sample volume, density, homogeneity, positioning, and container may affect the response of a well chamber, particularly in the measurement of pure beta emitters. Correction for saturation effects may be necessary for assay of therapy activities. Therefore, the instrument should be calibrated and subject to regular quality control tests for the full range of situations and radionuclides encountered (Parkin *et al.* 1992; Sharp *et al.* 1998, section 5.5). All dispensed therapy activities should be checked by a second person. A small sample of the material may be taken for quality control tests (e.g. radiochemical purity or sterility) (Sharp *et al.* 1998, section 6.4).

4.6   Administration

It is current practice at our centre for the ARSAC licence holder (or delegated deputy) to carry out the clinical direction (and possibly the physical direction) of therapy administrations. A radiographer, physicist, or other suitably qualified person should also be present and may physically direct the administration. Typical procedures used are described in Section 6. In order to calculate the exact activity administered to the patient, the residual radioactivity in the equipment used for dispensing and administration (e.g. vial, syringes, tubing) must be measured accurately.

4.7   Monitoring and scanning during therapy

4.7.1   Patient measurements

Regular scans and whole-body counts, if performed, should be carried out with identical geometry and as frequently as possible. The measurements may be required for radiation protection purposes (Section 5) and/or dosimetry (Section 3). In the latter case, to provide maximum information, scans should commence as soon as the activity in the patient allows. Tests (e.g. on blood and urine) may be required to monitor progress and/or toxicity.

4.7.2   Personnel and environmental monitoring

Monitoring of dose rate, and for contamination of staff, equipment, and environment, must be carried out at each stage of the therapy procedure. Further details of monitoring, decontamination procedures and waste disposal can be found in Section 5 and in Sharp *et al.* (1998, ch. 7).

4.8   Discharge of patient and follow-up

The patient should only be discharged when they have radiation clearance (Section 5.4.7) and are medically fit to leave. Appointments for further measurements or scans may be required. The results of these measurements are reviewed at follow-up appointments.

5.   Radiation protection

Radionuclide therapy is one of the most hazardous procedures involving the use of ionizing radiations that is performed in hospitals, due to potential contamination, as well as high exposure-rates. Hence the physicist, as qualified expert, has a very important role.

   This section aims to draw attention to aspects of radiation protection, which are of particular importance in unsealed-source therapy. It is not intended to be a general guide to radiation protection in nuclear medicine, since the subject is covered elsewhere (Sharp *et al.* 1998, ch. 7). It is written to comply with UK legislation (HMSO 1985; HSC 1985; HMSO 1988; NRPB 1988; HMSO 1993) but the general principles are applicable in all countries (Sharp *et al.* 1998, section 7.9.6; ICRP 1990). The ARSAC license holder is responsible for ensuring that all persons involved with radionuclide therapy comply with legislation. UK regulations require a physicist to liase with the license holder to ensure that radiopharmaceuticals are administered safely and in accordance with accepted therapeutic practice.

   Unsealed sources can give rise to radiation doses, not only by external exposure, but also by internal exposure from absorption, inhalation, or ingestion. It is essential to take stringent precautions to minimize both possibilities during radionuclide therapy. Local rules and written systems of work must be followed during the relevant stages of the therapy procedure and great care taken to ensure that radiation exposure is as low as reasonably practicable at all times (known as the ALARP principle).

5.1 Laboratory procedures

Radiation protection principles of minimizing exposure time, maximizing distance from the source, and using shielding must be followed. The following points are particularly important.

1. Work surfaces should be protected from contamination by covering (e.g. with plastic-backed absorbent paper or trays).

2. Syringes must be shielded whenever possible. Lead or tungsten shields are suitable for gamma-emitting radionuclides. High activities of energetic beta-particle emitters can produce significant bremsstrahlung doses. Therefore, syringes ideally should be shielded with a combination of Perspex and lead (Williams *et al.* 1995).

3. Large activities of high-energy gamma emitters, such as ^{131}I, require thick shielding. These heavy items require careful handling.

4. The use of automatic dispensing and administration systems is recommended (Williams *et al.* 1995).

5. Volatile iodine may be released from compounds containing iodine: these should be prepared in a unit with extraction facilities to provide operator protection.

6. In addition to controlled-area warning notices, an audible dose-rate alarm is useful for a therapy dispensing area.

7. It is useful to allocate shielded space in or near the radioisotope laboratory, where contaminated items (including those returned from the administration area) may be stored prior to disposal or re-use.

5.2 Movement of sources within the hospital

During transport from the dispensing laboratory to the administration room (ideally nearby), the therapy radiopharmaceutical must be well-shielded and packaged to avoid spills in the event of an accident. A sturdy trolley is useful or, in appropriate situations, the radiopharmaceutical may be carried by hand in a shielded box. Two persons should be present during any movement of therapy activities in case of accidents.

5.3 Monitoring

5.3.1 Therapy areas and equipment

Contamination and exposure-rate monitors (calibrated for each radionuclide, e.g. in terms of the annual limit of intake), must be readily available and used at all stages of the therapy procedure. They should be suitable for the radionuclide used (e.g. an end-window Geiger counter for contamination monitoring of beta emitters, and a side-window Geiger counter or scintillation detector for gamma emitters).

5.3.2 Personnel involved with the therapy

1. During preparation, dispensing and administration of a therapy radiopharmaceutical, it is advisable to monitor finger dose (e.g. by using small LiF thermoluminescent dosimeters).

2. To assess dose from external exposure, a personal dosimeter (e.g. a film badge) must be worn. If shielding is used and a high dose rate is expected, above the level of the shielding, it is advisable to wear two dosimeters (i.e. on shielded and unshielded parts of the body).

3. An integrating personal dosimeter with direct read-out and a dose-rate alarm, is useful at high dose rates.

4. Staff who are at risk of inhalation of volatile radionuclides (e.g. ^{131}I) are advised to monitor both their chest (immediately after exposure) and thyroid (at 24 h) with a calibrated NaI scintillation detector.

5. Staff involved with therapy procedures should have regular whole-body counts to assess low-level contamination.

5.4 Procedures and facilities on the ward

All involved staff must be fully trained in the principles of radiation protection relevant to the therapy. It is recommended that physics staff organize teaching sessions on a regular basis and before therapy procedures that are infrequently carried out.

5.4.1 Room design

A purpose-built unit is advantageous for in-patient therapy procedures using unsealed sources. Facilities in the unit at our centre include the following: a separate room with *en suite* bathroom and toilet for each patient; extra shielding in the walls and floor (under the bed) of each room; a whole-body counter (compensated Geiger–Müller tube) in the ceiling above each bed; and a utility room with washing and drying machines (designated for use with radioactive-contaminated linen) and a macerator for disposal of lightweight contaminated waste (e.g. disposable crockery, nappies, and tissues).

5.4.2 Precautions against external exposure

During therapy procedures with high-energy gamma-emitting radionuclides (e.g. ^{131}I), precautions are usually necessary (at least for the early part of therapy) to minimize dose to attending personnel from external radiation as outlined below.

Shielding

Mobile lead shields may be necessary (e.g. for staff working close to the patient, and/or at the door of the room to shield visitors). If the patient is catheterized, the catheter bag should be placed in a lead pot (with lid) to reduce exposure to staff, and to prevent errors in measurements of whole-body counts.

Distance

Access to the treatment room is restricted to trained personnel, who should work at the maximum practicable distance from the patient.

Time

Residual activity in the patient (derived from whole-body retention measurements) is used to recommend a maximum time for staff to spend each day, at a given distance from the patient. This is based on a daily proportion of the yearly maximum dose allowed for radiation workers.

5.4.3 Precautions against contamination

During radionuclide therapy, body fluids of the patient (e.g. urine, perspiration, vomit, saliva, blood) may be radioactive, with consequent risk of contamination. As an example, the precautions listed below are those taken at our centre to avoid contamination during the treatment of thyroid carcinoma with $Na^{131}I$ (see Section 6.1.1). During other types of therapy, if there is less risk of contamination, it may not be necessary to carry out all of these procedures.

1. Prior to administration of the radionuclide, plastic-backed absorbent paper is taped to the floor around the patient's toilet and on other surfaces where contamination is likely.

2. The patient is confined to their own suite for the duration of the therapy, unless required to leave (e.g. for scans).

3. Before leaving their room, the patient showers and changes into clean clothing: overshoes are put on when leaving the room and removed on return.

4. Patients are advised to wear disposable underwear and slippers, and to use tissues instead of hand-kerchiefs, and are provided with disposable crockery and cutlery.

5. Access to the patient's room is restricted to trained personnel who are required to wear plastic over-shoes, aprons and gloves. These are discarded in designated plastic bags on exit from the room and treated as radioactive waste.

6. All staff who enter the patient's room or handle potentially contaminated items, must monitor themselves for contamination immediately afterwards. If contaminated, staff should proceed as in Sharp *et al.* (1998, section 7.5.6).

7. No item is removed from the patient's room unless first checked for contamination by trained staff.

8. Sampling of body fluids is avoided, if possible, in the first few days of therapy, when these samples are likely to be most radioactive. Specimens should be monitored and, if necessary, instructions on handling given to the laboratory testing the sample.

5.4.4 Warning signs and cautionary notices

After administration, exposure-rate measurements must be made around the treatment room and/or therapy unit. If necessary, warning signs must then be displayed clearly to indicate the designation of the area (i.e. controlled or supervised). The nature and activity of the radionuclide used, the date and time of administration and any relevant instructions to attending staff (e.g. use of protective clothing and recommended maximum time close to the patient) must also be displayed. In-patients at our centre wear a wristband, indicating they are radio-active, at all times until discharge.

5.4.5 Decontamination of linen

Bed linen and clothing used in our therapy unit are changed frequently and put into plastic bags. Each item is monitored subsequently and, if contaminated, is washed twice in the designated washing machine, dried, and remonitored. Items still contaminated are placed in labelled plastic bags and stored in a designated locked room until the remaining activity is negligible.

5.4.6 Disposal of contaminated waste

Liquid waste and patient excreta from our therapy unit are discharged into the sewage system via the designated patient toilet (within the authorization of our centre to dispose of radioactive waste). The toilet is flushed at least twice after each use to dilute any radioactive content.

Macerable solid waste is collected regularly by trained staff and macerated immediately. Unmacerable waste is placed in plastic refuse bags or 'sharps' bins, which are monitored, labelled, and stored until the level of radioactivity is low enough to permit disposal in conformity to standard hospital practice. Further details on the disposal of radioactive waste can be found in Sharp *et al.* (1998, section 7.8).

Table 13.8 Guidelines for maximum activity (in MBq) of patient, when leaving hospital, in relation to radiation protection restrictions

Radionuclide	Return to radio sensitive work, contact with children (< 10 MBq MeV)	No restriction[a] (< 50 MBq MeV)	Travel by public transport (< 150 MBq MeV)	Travel by private transport (< 300 MBq MeV)
[131]I	30	150	400	800
[198]Au colloid	30	150	400	800
[90]Y	100[b]	500	1500	3000
[32]P	300	1500	4500	9000
[89]Sr[c]	300	1500	4500	9000

[a]Except for radiosensitive work and contact with children.
[b]Special case due to bremsstrahlung consideration.
[c]Recommendations at our centre based on similarity to [32]P.
Adapted from NRPB (1988), p. 57.

5.4.7 Discharge of patient

The main factors that determine whether a patient may be given radiation clearance for discharge are as follows: the radionuclide administered, the residual activity in the patient, the home circumstances, and method of patient's transport to home. Consideration must also be given to the state of health and nursing requirements of the patient. For example, a patient treated with a pure beta emitter will not present an external radiation hazard, but might give rise to contamination if incontinent. It may be advisable to delay the discharge of such a patient, and/or to provide them with special instructions (e.g. regarding handling of contaminated laundry).

If the product of the patient's residual activity and the total gamma-ray energy does not exceed 10 MBq MeV, then no further radiation protection precautions are necessary. At levels greater than this, a patient might be discharged, but may have to observe certain restrictions after leaving the hospital (Table 13.8). All patients discharged at a level above 50 MBq MeV should be given an instruction card detailing the type and duration of restrictions (Figure 13.6). The instruction card should be carried by the patient until the date when restrictions cease.

When discharging a patient to another institution (e.g. nursing home, hospital) details of residual activity and estimates of activity excreted in the urine must be supplied. This will enable records to be kept in accordance with the Radioactive Substances Act (HMSO 1993).

5.4.8 Decontamination of room

After discharge of an in-patient, the treatment room is monitored for contamination and, if necessary, decontaminated by cleaning with proprietary detergents such as Decon (Sharp *et al.* 1998, section 7.5.7). Moveable items that cannot be adequately decontaminated, may be stored until remaining activity is negligible.

5.4.9 In the event of death of a patient

If a patient should die soon after receiving unsealed-source therapy, the Radiation Protection Adviser should be notified immediately. Precautions may be required (e.g. for post-mortem and/or regarding disposal of the corpse by burial or cremation). Activity limits for these procedures for the most common therapy radionuclides are listed in Table 13.9.

5.5 Contingency plans

Most incidents involving unsealed sources in hospitals do not warrant emergency action, but can be dealt with by trained staff working in the area (Sharp *et al.* 1998, sections 7.5.5–7.5.7) using a 'spill kit' (container of items useful for decontamination of personnel and equipment). However, contingency plans must be drawn up to cover the possibility of serious incident (NRPB

Table 13.9 Maximum activities (in MBq) of radionuclides for disposal of corpses without special precautions

Radionuclide	Post-mortem or embalming	Burial	Cremation
[131]I	10[a]	400[b]	400[b]
[90]Y colloid	200[a]	2000[c]	70[d]
[198]Au colloid	400[b]	400[b]	100[d]
[32]P	100[a]	2000[c]	30[d]
[89]Sr	50[a]	2000[c]	20[d]

The values in the second, third, and fourth columns relate to the greatest risk to those persons involved in the procedures.
[a]Based on contamination hazard (HMSO 1985).
[b]Based on dose rate external to the body (HMSO 1985).
[c]Based on bremsstrahlung dose at 0.5 m.
[d]Based on contamination hazard (HMSO 1985) assuming that these radionuclides remain in the ash.
Adapted from NRPB (1988), p. 60.

Hospital name and address: **INSTRUCTION CARD FOR PATIENTS TREATED WITH RADIONUCLIDES.** Patient name: Address: Patient hospital record no.: Department/ward: 1	This card should be carried at all times until : Radionuclide: Activity : Administered on : In case of difficulty hospital telephone no.: 2
Please observe the following instructions after you leave the Hospital:- (1) Do not travel by public transport until: (2) Try to avoid long journeys by public transport (i.e. any in which you might have to spend more than one hour in any one vehicle) until: (3) Do not return to work until: (4) Do not visit places of entertainment until: 3	(5) Avoid non-essential contact with adults until: (6) Avoid non-essential contact with children until: (7) Other: Consultant: Signature of Doctor: 4

Figure 13.6 Four-page instruction card given to patients on leaving hospital after unsealed source therapy. Adapted from NRPB (1988), p. 59.

1988, p. 71). In such an event, the Radiation Protection Supervisor for the area and the Radiation Protection Adviser must be informed. Equipment for use in an emergency involving unsealed sources (e.g. respirators, barriers for restricting access, portable monitors, and a list of useful telephone numbers) must be available. The effectiveness of contingency plans should be tested in training exercises using low-activity sources.

6.   Specific therapy procedures

This section describes some clinical applications of unsealed-source therapy. Only specific variations from the general procedures in Sections 4 and 5 are covered, so the following subsections should not be consulted in isolation. Most of the methods described are those followed at our centre and may differ from regimes elsewhere.

6.1   Thyroid carcinoma and thyrotoxicosis treated with Na^{131}I

Radioiodine has been used for many years for the safe and effective treatment of differentiated carcinoma of the thyroid and thyrotoxicosis (Hoefnagel 1991; O'Doherty *et al*, 1993; Shapiro 1993; Lazarus 1995; Murray and Ell 1998, ch. 80). Iodide is trapped by the thyroid and incorporated into the hormones triiodothyronine (T3) and thyroxine (T4), this metabolic activity providing the selective uptake and retention required for effective systemic radionuclide therapy.

6.1.1   Treatment of differentiated carcinoma of the thyroid

Patients are referred for radioiodine treatment for differential thyroid carcinoma after partial or total thyroidectomy. These treatments are always performed on an in-patient basis. It is current practice at our centre to prescribe 3 GBq Na^{131}I to ablate the thyroid bed remnants. Further treatments using at least 5.5 GBq are given to treat metastases, which are unlikely to take up iodine if there is substantial normal thyroid tissue remaining. The whole-body dose is typically about 0.5 Gy per administration at these levels. Higher administered activities (up to 11.1 GBq) are under investigation in order to increase absorbed doses, particularly in bone metastases. A number of centres are also carrying out dosimetry measurements to enable the administered activity to be optimized for each individual patient (e.g. Samuel and Rajashekharrao 1994).

Thyroid hormone replacement tablets (triiodothyronine (T3) or thyroxine (T4) prescribed after thyroidectomy) must be stopped well before radioiodine therapy to maximize uptake and hence dose to the thyroid. T3 and T4 are stopped 10 and 21 days, respectively, before therapy. For 3 weeks before therapy, the patient should avoid iodine rich foods (e.g. fish) and medicines containing iodine. X-ray examinations using contrast medium (which contains iodine) should also be avoided during this period. Prior to therapy, blood samples (for full blood count, chemistry, and thyroid function tests) and a chest X-ray are taken. A low level of thyroid stimulating hormone (TSH) predicts a poor therapeutic outcome and the use of recombinant human TSH prior to therapy to enhance the uptake of radioiodine is under investigation.

At our centre, a typical dosimetry study for radionuclide therapy of thyroid carcinoma commences with the administration of either 185 MBq Na^{123}I or 100 MBq Na^{124}I. Approximately 24 h later, the patient has a tomographic scan from which the tumour volume is determined. Immediately afterwards, the administration procedure and radiation protection restrictions necessary during therapy are explained to the patient. This includes advice to drink plenty of fluids and void frequently (to reduce bladder dose), and to suck sharp-tasting sweets (to reduce dose to salivary glands). The patient is given a prophylactic anti-emetic before administration and anti-emetics during therapy, as required.

Na^{131}I in capsule form is used at our centre for this type of therapy unless the patient has difficulty in swallowing. Capsules give a lower dose to the oral mucosa and avoid the possibility of a high-activity spill during dispensing or administration procedures. The activity ordered from the supplier is the exact amount required at the time of administration (allowing for physical decay).

The capsule is tipped from its shielded container into a plastic medicine cup. As quickly as possible, the patient tips the capsule from the cup into their mouth and swallows it with lukewarm water. After administration, the patient is confined to the treatment suite, and

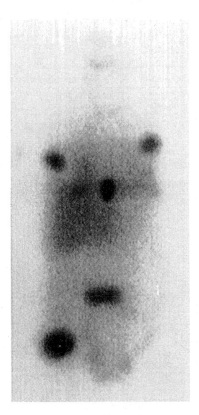

Figure 13.7 Whole-body Na^{131}I scan at 72 h (20-minute anterior view, acquired with scanning camera) showing metastases from differentiated thyroid carcinoma in bone and lung.

appropriate shielding and warning signs are put in place. The patient is advised to have a hot drink within 15 min of administration to help the capsule to dissolve.

Patient measurements are as follows: whole-body counts shortly after administration (i.e. before any excretion), then at least twice daily until discharge; scans at 24, 48, 72, and 144 h of areas required for dosimetry; whole body scan at 72 h (Figure 13.7); blood samples at 24, 48, 72, and 144 h for determination of protein-bound iodine (PBI) and dose to whole blood. The patient scans are compared with those of calibration phantoms to determine activity in the tumour(s). MIRD methodology (Section 3) is then used to calculate absorbed doses to the tumour(s), whole body and blood. Thyroid hormone replacement tablets are recommended immediately after the whole-body scan.

Most patients are discharged 3–5 days after administration. Six weeks later the patient returns for TSH and thyroglobulin (Tg) measurements. The whole-body scan and PBI results are used to determine whether further treatment is required. If these results are normal, a 400 MBq Na^{131}I whole-body scan and retention measurements may be performed 12 weeks post-discharge. These results, together with the Tg measurement, then determine whether additional treatment is required. Further therapies are carried out at a minimum interval of 3 months. Care should be taken with respect to the timing and activity of diagnostic administrations, as some centres have reported a 'stunning' effect, i.e. reduced uptake during $Na^{131}I$ therapy carried out within a few weeks of a diagnostic administration of $Na^{131}I$ of >100 MBq (Cavalieri 1996).

6.1.2 Treatment of thyrotoxicosis

The treatment policy for an overactive thyroid at many centres is to render the patient hypothyroid, preferably with a single dose of radioiodine, and to this end a wide range of administered activities have been used. The aim of our treatment, however, is to render the patient euthyroid, thus obviating the need for the patient to take thyroid hormone replacement tablets. In the past, our policy was to prescribe 75 MBq for Graves' disease and 400 MBq for toxic nodular goitre or thyrocardia. However, this often necessitated repeat treatments and/or rendered patients hypothyroid. With the availability of $Na^{124}I$ and PET scanning, it has been found that a single dose of 50–60 Gy to the functional thyroid volume has a high probability of rendering patients with Graves' disease euthyroid and the prescription has been changed to one of dose rather than activity (Flower *et al.* 1994). Preliminary follow-up data (Pratt *et al.* 1997) have shown that the percentage of patients rendered euthyroid at 12 months increased from 24% (after 75 MBq) to 53% (after 50 Gy to the functional thyroid).

The thyrotoxic dosimetry protocol at our centre first requires the patient to discontinue their carbimazole (or other anti-thyroid medication). Three days later the patient is given 15 MBq $Na^{124}I$ or 0.37 MBq $Na^{131}I$. Thyroid uptake measurements are carried out at 24, 48 or 72, and 144 or 168 h, to determine the effective half-life of iodine in the thyroid. The functional thyroid volume is determined by a PET scan at 24 h or indirectly by ultrasonography.

Equations (2) and (9) are used to determine the activity required to give the prescribed absorbed dose to the functional volume of the thyroid. This is usually less than 400 MBq of $Na^{131}I$ and therapy is performed on an out-patient basis. Occasionally, it may be necessary to admit the patient to hospital (e.g. if the patient has small children or requires specialized nursing). Patient preparation is similar to that for thyroid carcinoma (Section 6.1.1).

It is usual to administer the radioiodine orally, but in rare circumstances it may be given intravenously, in which case care must be taken to order $Na^{131}I$ suitable for injection. Liquid $Na^{131}I$ for oral administrations is dispensed from stock solution as necessary. The required activity is diluted with drinking water in a shielded

plastic container. The patient's dentures are removed before administration to prevent radioiodine collecting under them. The patient is given absorbent disposable towels to cough into should the need arise while swallowing the iodine. (This could prevent severe contamination over a large area.) The liquid is swallowed through a straw (to reduce the area of oral mucosa in contact with the radioiodine). The patient then swallows water used to rinse the plastic container and more water to rinse the mouth, before replacing dentures.

Most patients leave hospital immediately after administration, with appropriate instructions regarding radiation protection. Patient measurements consist of a scan (using a gamma camera with pinhole collimator) and thyroid uptake measurements, at 24 h after administration. (The scan is not essential if a PET scan was performed prior to therapy). Carbimazole is restarted 3 days after therapy. Thyroid function tests are carried out at regular intervals of 2–3 months initially, then at longer time intervals if no further therapy is required.

6.2 Treatment of neuroectodermal tumours with ^{131}I mIBG

There are several neuroectodermal tumours, such as neuroblastoma and phaeochromocytoma, for which treatment with mIBG (an analogue of norepinephrine) may be indicated (Hoefnagel 1991; Wafelman *et al.* 1994; Gaze and Wheldon 1996; Leach *et al.* 1996, pp. 1933–1940; Murray and Ell 1998, ch. 82). Neuroblastoma is a malignant tumour that occurs most frequently in young children. Therapy of this tumour with ^{131}I mIBG poses particular radiation protection problems due to the age of the patients. Treatment of adult neuroectodermal tumours is performed in a similar manner, but generally involves fewer radiation protection problems. All ^{131}I mIBG treatments are performed on an in-patient basis.

There are several techniques under development aimed at improving radiolabelled mIBG therapy. These are mainly concerned with the optimum scheduling of mIBG therapy and chemotherapy. Other approaches include multi-modality treatment, and the uses of hyperbaric oxygen and carrier-free mIBG to enhance the therapeutic (i.e. tumour to normal tissue) ratio (Gaze *et al.* 1995; Schwab and Pearson 1995, pp. 576–612; Gaze and Wheldon 1996).

It is current practice at our centre for the administered activity to be determined by pretherapy dosimetry with ^{123}I mIBG SPECT (Section 3), carried out no more than a few weeks prior to therapy. The patient must avoid drugs known to interfere with mIBG uptake for 10 days before the tracer is given. Thyroid blockade (e.g. via oral administration of Lugol's iodine 0.2 ml for a child; 0.3 ml for an adult, taken three times daily, or potassium iodide capsules 250–500 mg m^{-2} per day) is given for

2 days prior to the tracer and for 3 days afterwards. (It should be noted that Lugol's iodine tastes unpleasant and is best diluted in a palatable drink.)

Approximately 370 MBq ^{123}I mIBG is administered (183 MBq if the patient weighs less than 10 kg). Whole-body retention is measured using a NaI counter at administration and every few hours for at least 72 h SPECT scans for tumour dosimetry are taken at approximately 4, 24, 30, 48, 54, and 72 h. Tumour and/or normal organ activities are found by comparison with SPECT scans of calibration phantoms. MIRD methodology (Section 3) is then used to calculated absorbed doses to the whole body, tumour(s) and any normal organs of interest. From these results the activity to be administered for therapy is chosen.

Administered activities of ^{131}I mIBG for therapy are between 3 and 30 GBq and whole-body doses are generally between 1 and 2 Gy. When treating children, parents or relatives may be involved in nursing the patient during therapy (ICRP 1990, p. 34) so that the child does not feel so isolated. Prior to therapy, radiation protection restrictions and other details (e.g. the use of protective clothing and radiation monitors) are explained to the parents (and the child if old enough to understand). Sedation of a young child for the initial days of the treatment must be considered, especially if they would not otherwise cooperate with the necessary restrictions. Drugs that interfere with mIBG uptake must be avoided for at least 10 days prior to therapy. Thyroid blockade (as for the tracer) is started 48 h prior to therapy and continued for at least 2 weeks post-therapy. The exact length of time will depend on the activity retained by the patient.

Among the assessments carried out prior to therapy are: full blood counts; haemoglobin concentration; bone marrow trephine and aspirates; urine catecholamines and chest X-ray. Patients are sedated (if necessary) and catheterized (if incontinent of urine) before administration. Anti-emetics are prescribed for several days at the start of therapy. An intravenous infusion (IVI) of saline is used to hydrate the patient to 3 l m^{-2} per day for at least the first 24 h of therapy. Hydration commences before administration so that tubing connections in the administration system can be checked for leakage.

Therapy activities of ^{131}I mIBG are currently available in liquid or frozen form. In the latter case, administration must take place within 2 h of defrosting otherwise the radiochemical purity may be reduced. The required activity is drawn into a suitable syringe and the needle replaced with a short length of saline-primed, plastic tubing. The syringe is placed in a shielded pump on a reinforced trolley. (There are several automatic systems for dispensing and administration, which are currently under development, aimed at reducing radiation dose to personnel involved with these procedures.)

The mIBG is administered through a Hickman line or cannula, with saline from the IVI and mIBG flowing into the patient together (Figure 13.8a). The duration of infusion depends on whether or not the ^{131}I mIBG was frozen. If so, the infusion should take place over 30–60 min as soon as possible after defrosting: more rapid infusion may result in hypotensive or hypertensive crisis so appropriate drugs must be readily available. If the mIBG was not frozen, longer infusion times are possible as the radiochemical purity remains stable for up to 24 h. The patient's pulse and blood pressure must be monitored frequently (e.g. every 5 min for 2 h during and after administration, and at longer time intervals thereafter). On completion of administration, the saline IVI is used to flush out the syringe and tubing before the pump is disconnected.

Patient measurements are as follows: whole-body counts immediately after administration then typically every few hours until discharge, then at the same time points as the scans. Scans for dosimetry are carried out regularly (e.g. on days 3, 6, 8, and 10, and weekly thereafter for up to 1 month). Follow-up measurements include tests of urinary catecholamines, full blood counts, bone marrow biopsy, thyroid function tests, and scans using ^{123}I mIBG and ^{99m}Tc MDP. Therapy may be repeated, but at the higher levels of whole-body dose the interval between treatments should be at least 6 weeks to ensure that the full extent of any myelosuppression from the previous therapy is known.

6.3 Radionuclide therapy in the relief of pain from skeletal metastases

There are several radiopharmaceuticals under investigation for the palliative management of patients suffering from pain due to skeletal metastases (particularly from prostatic or breast carcinoma) (Hoefnagel 1991; Porter and Chisholm 1993; Leach *et al.* 1996, pp. 2027–42; Murray and Ell 1998, ch. 83). These include ^{32}P orthophosphate, ^{89}Sr chloride, ^{186}Re HEDP, ^{153}Sm EDTMP, and ^{117m}Sn (4+) DTPA. ^{186}Re, ^{153}Sm, and ^{117m}Sn have the advantage of suitable gamma emissions for imaging. To date only ^{32}P and ^{89}Sr have been used extensively (Porter and Chisholm 1993): the others are currently undergoing clinical trials (Bayouth *et al.* 1994; de Klerk *et al.* 1996; Krishnamurthy *et al.* 1997). Various methods of enhancing therapeutic efficiency are under investigation, including the use of bisphosphonates to improve retention of radionuclide in the tumour, prior treatment with radioenhancing chemotherapy agents and combination with external-beam radiotherapy. However, myelotoxicity is the dose-limiting factor in this type of therapy, therefore, methods of reducing bone marrow damage are also of importance (Porter and Chisholm 1993, pp. 49–55; Leach *et al.* 1996, pp. 2027–2042).

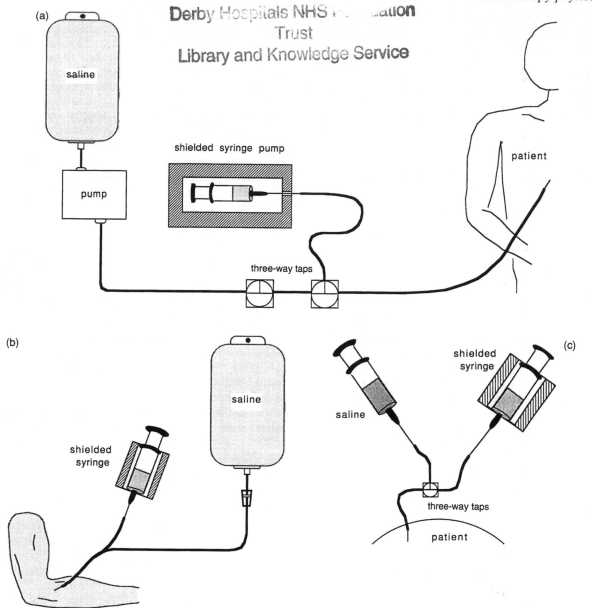

Figure 13.8 Schematic diagrams of equipment designed to minimize radioactive contamination and exposure typically used for the following administration procedures: (a) ^{131}I mIBG therapy; (b) ^{89}Sr therapy; (c) instillation into cyst or joint.

^{89}Sr chloride therapy at our centre is described below. Strontium is a calcium analogue and hence is taken up into bone. Studies have shown that uptake and retention of ^{89}Sr are much greater in metastatic bone lesions than normal bone (Blake *et al*. 1986). Treatment with ^{89}Sr is usually an out-patient procedure, unless the patient requires specialized nursing or is a contamination risk (only usually due to urinary incontinence). A fixed

activity of 150 MBq is currently prescribed at our centre. Any calcium supplements taken by the patient should be discontinued at least 2 weeks before administration. Low blood counts and/or significant bone marrow involvement are contra-indications for therapy with ^{89}Sr. Patients who are significantly incontinent of urine are catheterized before administration and for several days afterwards.

For administration of the ^{89}Sr chloride, a saline IVI is connected to a cannula inserted into a peripheral vein (Figure 13.8b). A low flow rate is set to check the system for leakage and the ^{89}Sr is then injected slowly into a small side branch of the tubing near the vein. After injection of the ^{89}Sr, the IVI is continued for a few minutes to flush the tubing, and is then used to flush the syringe. The syringe is removed and, after further flushing of the tubing, the IVI is disconnected.

In most cases, the patient leaves hospital immediately. Urinary excretion of ^{89}Sr is highest during the first 24 h after administration, and activity excreted after 1 week post-injection is normally less than 10% of the total excreted. Therefore, patients are advised to: take care with personal hygiene; flush the toilet twice after use; and wash urine-stained garments separately from other clothes for 1 week after administration. Some patients experience a brief increase in pain at about 48 h after treatment and should have adequate analgesia. A reduction in the patient's usual level of pain is not generally seen until 2–4 weeks after injection.

Full blood counts are measured regularly after therapy: maximum platelet depression usually occurs at about 6 weeks. If the patient has benefited from ^{89}Sr therapy but later relapses with pain at the initial or other sites, further treatments may be given (subject to adequate blood counts) at minimum intervals of 3 months. Follow-up ^{99m}Tc MDP bone scans may be carried out.

6.4 Treatment of polycythaemia vera with ^{32}P sodium phosphate

Polycythaemia vera (PV) is a proliferative disorder of the bone marrow resulting in increased production of red blood cells. PV may eventually lead to leukaemia and can cause thrombosis or haemorrhage due to increased blood viscosity. The disease may be treated by phlebotomy alone or phlebotomy supplemented by myelosuppression. Hydroxyurea and ^{32}P sodium phosphate have been used extensively as myelosuppressive agents: busulphan, recombinant anagrelide, and interferon-alpha are currently under evaluation (e.g. Vasserman 1976; Berk *et al.* 1986; Hoefnagel 1991; Parmentier and Gardet 1994; Bilgrami and Greenberg 1995; Berlin 1997; Murray and Ell 1998, ch. 81). ^{32}P is concentrated selectively by the mitotically active bone marrow cells and later incorporated into the calcium phosphate of adjacent bone, from which the marrow is irradiated further.

The procedure for treatment with ^{32}P sodium phosphate is outlined below. The Polycythaemia Vera Study Group (PVSG) recommend in initial activity of 85 MBq m^{-2} of body area with an upper limit of 185 MBq (Wasserman 1976). Oral administration requires a larger initial activity as only 70–80% of the activity is absorbed by the intestinal tract. Prior to therapy with ^{32}P, phlebotomy is carried out to reduce the haematocrit to about 45%. This increases blood flow to vital organs and reduces the risk of vascular accident. Therapy administration and discharge procedures are similar to those of ^{89}Sr chloride treatment (Section 6.3) and are performed on an out-patient basis. Full blood counts are required for follow-up every 2–3 months. If no significant response is obtained after 12 weeks, the treatment is repeated with the administered activity increased by 25%. If necessary, further increases of 25% may be carried out every 12 weeks to a maximum of 260 MBq in one treatment. However, the procedure at some centres is to administer a fixed activity at each treatment: in our case 185 MBq. After remission, retreatments should be restricted to 6-monthly intervals, and phlebotomy carried out as required. Long-term follow up by the PVSG has shown that patients treated with ^{32}P have an increased risk of developing leukaemia and other (non-haematological) malignancies. For this reason, the PVSG has recommended that treatment with ^{32}P is generally reserved for patients over the age of 70 (Berk *et al.* 1986).

6.5 Instillation of radiocolloids into body cavities and cysts

Radiocolloids are used to treat both benign and malignant disease by instillation into body cavities and cysts (Hoefnagel 1991; Murray and Ell 1998, ch. 85 and 95). There are three main applications of this type of therapy. First, radiation synovectomy, which is carried out for chronic synovitis mainly due to rheumatoid arthritis. If this condition is not treated it leads to pain and loss of movement of the joints (Smith *et al.* 1988; Deutsch *et al.* 1993; Edmonds *et al.* 1994; Siegel *et al.* 1994; Clunie *et al.* 1995; Murray and Ell 1998, ch. 95). The second area of application is in the reduction of fluid produced inside cystic brain lesions, which can cause severe pressure effects on surrounding normal tissue (Taasan *et al.* 1985; Pollock *et al.* 1995). The third application is the treatment of malignant effusions and micrometastases in the serous cavities (peritoneum, pericardium and pleura) e.g. from ovarian or lung carcinoma (Ott *et al.* 1985; Hoefnagel 1991; Vergote *et al.* 1993; Pattillo *et al.* 1995; Murray and Ell 1998, ch. 85). The following radiocolloids are among those that have been used: ^{32}P chromic phosphate (CrPO$_4$), ^{90}Y and ^{169}Er citrates, ^{90}Y silicate, ^{198}Au colloid, ^{165}Dy FHMA and ^{153}Sm PHYP.

Most of the colloidal particles are assumed to plate out on the cavity/cyst wall after administration and thus remain fixed on the surface requiring treatment. Therefore, the radionuclides used for therapy are chosen to match the beta range to the thickness of surface to be treated so that underlying tissues are spared. For example, in radiation synovectomy [169]Er colloid (mean beta range in tissue = 0.3 mm) is used mainly to treat joints in the fingers, whilst ^{90}Y colloid (mean beta range = 3.6 mm) is commonly used to treat knee joints.

There is usually a small amount of leakage of radiocolloid from the body cavity during treatment, which may concentrate in lymph nodes. This may be an advantage in malignant conditions, but is otherwise undesirable. There is generally less leakage when colloids with larger particles (e.g. FHMA with mean particle diameter 5 μm) are used. In the case of radiation synovectomy, many centres co-inject corticosteroids, which reduce inflammation and may help to retain the radiocolloid with the joint. The main problem encountered with this type of therapy, however, is uneven distribution of colloid (and hence absorbed dose) on the cavity surface. To a certain extent this may be predicted by tracer scans of a gamma-emitting colloid prior to therapy. (Pattillo *et al.* 1995). However the distribution has been found to vary substantially over several days in some cases (Vergote *et al.* 1993).

Dosimetry calculations require an estimate of the surface area to be treated from which the mass may be calculated. Dilution techniques and/or scanning may be used to assess volume and hence surface area of cavities (Taasan *et al.* 1985; Pattillo *et al.* 1995; Pollock *et al.* 1995). A cyst or serous cavity should be aspirated prior to injection of colloid to remove the bulk of fluid, since dilution decreases the delivered dose. However, enough fluid must be left (or added) to aid even distribution of the radiocolloid (Tulchinsky and Eggli 1994). Administered activities vary according to the radionuclide used and the surface area to be treated. Typically <100 MBq $Cr^{32}PO_4$ is used to give a dose of 100–400 Gy to the surface of a brain cyst, 185 MBq ^{90}Y silicate delivers a dose of approximately 100 Gy to the synovium of a knee joint and 400–4000 MBq $Cr^{32}PO_4$ is used to give approximately 30–300 Gy to the peritoneal surface.

Figure 13.8c shows a method of administration suitable for instillation of a colloid into a cyst or joint via a three-way tap. Saline, from a syringe connected to the other arm of the tap, is used to flush the radioactive syringe and tubing after administration. Flushing is essential, since colloids settle out quickly and a large proportion of the radioactivity could remain in an unflushed syringe; however, in the case of small cysts and joints the flushing volume should also be small. Leakage back up the needle track is rare, but dressings from the area should be monitored.

After administration, the patient should change position regularly to promote even distribution of the colloid, except in the case of synovectomy, where the joint is flexed and extended once or twice, then held still by a bandage or splint, for a time dependent on the half-life of the radionuclide used. This is necessary as

movement increases leakage from the joint. The uniformity of distribution of the therapy radionuclide can be assessed using scans of a tracer amount of a gamma-emitting colloid or by bremsstrahlung imaging/counting (Ott *et al.* 1985; Smith *et al.* 1988; Vergote *et al.* 1993; Siegel *et al.* 1994, 1995).

6.6   Treatment with radiolabelled antibodies

The development of labelled monoclonal antibodies (mAbs), which bind to tumour-associated antigens, has lead to the possibility of radioimmunotherapy (Humm 1986; Hoefnagel 1991; Bruland 1995; Einhorn *et al.* 1996; Wilder *et al.* 1996; Murray and Ell 1998, ch. 84). However, there are a number of difficulties with this type of therapy, which have limited its success to date. The main problems are outlined below, along with some of the suggested solutions that are currently under evaluation. Further details can be found in Reilly *et al.* (1995), Einhorn *et al.* (1996), Wilder *et al.* (1996), and Stoldt *et al.* (1997).

6.6.1   Problem 1

Tumour uptake of intravenously administered radio-labelled antibody is both low (typically <0.01% injected activity per gram) and heterogeneous.

Solutions

1. Intracavitary/intratumoural administration.

2. Prior to treatment increase tumour vascular permeability with vasoactive drugs or mAbs conjugated with vasoactive or proinflammatory agents.

3. Use hyperthermia, external radiation or recombinant interferon to increase uptake.

4. Use cocktails of different mAbs.

5. Use mAbs fragments which distribute more evenly through tumour nodules due to their low molecular weight.

6. Use a pretargeting technique (Stoldt *et al.* 1997) to improve tumour to normal tissue uptake and retention. Bifunctional antibodies have been used in pretargeting procedures. One method allows time for the bifunctional antibody to localize in the tumour and for excess antibody to clear from the blood/normal organs before a radiolabelled water-soluble hapten is administered. This small molecule binds to mAbs in the tumour and the excess is quickly excreted. Several pretargeting procedures are based on the avidin/biotin system. Avidin is a glycoprotein with very high affinity for biotin – a water solution vitamin. One three-step approach predoses with biotinylated mAbs, followed later by an avidin 'chase'. This increases the number of binding sites available in the tumour and removes

excess biotinylated mAbs from the circulation. The final step is the administration of radiolabelled biotin. Multi-step approaches require careful attention to the dosage and timing of each step to ensure success.

6.6.2 Problem 2

Uptake and retention of radiolabelled mAb in the blood and normal organs are too high.

Solutions

1. Use small molecular weight mAb fragments, which are cleared faster than intact mAb.

2. Pretargeting techniques as in solution (6) above and variations thereof, e.g. the saturation of circulating free antigen by preinfusion of cold antibody or the administration of a second antibody after the radiolabelled mAb to form an immune complex, which is cleared rapidly from the blood.

3. Use plasmaphoresis or extracorporeal immunoadsorption to remove excess mAbs from the blood.

4. Reinfuse bone marrow or peripheral stem cells following high dose radioimmunotherapy.

6.6.3 Problem 3

Metabolism of immunoconjugates resulting in loss of conjugate from the tumour and uptake of the radiolabel into normal organs.

Solutions

1. Increase tumour retention of the radiolabelled mAb by the use of more stable linkage chemistry.

2. Reduction of blood/normal tissue retention by the use of more metabolizable chemical linkages.

6.6.4 Problem 4

Immune response either to the murine mAb (HAMA response) or to the agent conjugated to the mAb (e.g. avidin). Apart from the risk of an allergic reaction by the patient, these responses result in faster elimination from the blood and hence lower tumour uptake of the radiolabelled antibody on subsequent administrations.

Solutions

1. Use antigen binding fragments: these are less immunogenic than intact mAbs.

2. Use chimeric (murine variable regions fused to human constant regions) mAbs or CDR grafted humanized mAbs (murine complementarity-determining regions grafted onto a human antibody framework) to reduce immunogenicity significantly. However, both of these have the disadvantage that they are eliminated more slowly from the blood than murine mAbs.

3. Treat patients with depressed immune response (e.g. as in B-cell malignancies).

The use of radiolabelled antibodies is not yet a standardized procedure except where large research studies are in progress. Owing to their biological nature, their efficacy and safety are unpredictable in the individual patient, and sterile procedures and medical supervision are particularly important. Since antigens are not tumour-specific, it is essential to use a monoclonal antibody that shows good immunoreactivity with the tumour (established by immuno-cytochemistry) and as little cross-reactivity with normal tissues as possible. A tracer-labelled study should be carried out to obtain a true evaluation of specificity *in vivo*, and the clearance time from normal tissues (DeNardo *et al.* 1996; Leach *et al.* 1996, pp. 2009–26). Examples of techniques for dosimetry measurements and calculations after radio-immunotherapy are given in Papanastassiou *et al.* (1993), Weber and Kassis (1993), Fisher (1994), Breitz *et al.* (1995), Papanastassiou *et al.* (1995), and Einhorn *et al.* (1996).

A regime that has been used with encouraging results to treat B-cell lymphoma (Kaminski *et al.* 1996) is performed with ^{131}I labelled anti-CD20 (a murine monoclonal antibody directed against the CD20 B-lymphocyte surface antigen expressed by B-cell lymphomas) and is described below. The patient must have normal hepatic and renal function, <25% lymphoma cells in the marrow and must have no history of allergy to foreign protein.

A tracer study is performed in which 685 mg of unlabelled anti-CD20 is infused over 60 min followed immediately by 15–20 mg of anti-CD20, labelled with 185 MBq ^{131}I infused over 30 min. Tumour and normal organ dosimetry are calculated from whole-body retention and gamma camera measurements taken for at least 5 days after infusion. Thyroid blockade for both the tracer and therapy administrations continues for at least 14 days after infusion.

At least 1 week after the tracer administration 685 mg unlabelled anti-CD20 is infused as before, followed by 15–20 mg anti-CD20 labelled with a therapeutic activity of ^{131}I. The exact activity depends on the whole-body dose required, which in this study was restricted to not more than 0.85 Gy (resulting in tumour doses of up to 26 Gy). Blood cell and platelet counts are determined weekly for at least 6 weeks following therapy. Hepatic enzyme, renal function, and electrolyte studies are performed at 2, 6, and 12 weeks after therapy, then every 3 months thereafter. Serum thyrotropin is measured every 3 months. Peripheral blood B and T cells are measured by flow cytology at study entry, 6, and 12 weeks after therapy, then every 3 months until the number of B cells is normal. Serum immunoglobulin is measured at the same time. Serum is tested for HAMA before each tracer and therapy administration then at 2, 6, and 12 weeks after therapy. Retreatment is carried out after 12 weeks, if remission has not been achieved.

6.7. Other types of radionuclide therapy

6.7.1 Intra-arterial infusion for treatment of hepatic malignancies

This type of therapy is based on the fact that hepatic tumours derive their blood supply almost entirely from the hepatic artery, whilst normal liver is supplied mainly by the portal venous system. Thus, administration of radiopharmaceutical into the hepatic artery can be used to deliver high doses to small liver tumours. Various radiopharmaceuticals have been investigated (Hoefnagel 1991; Kassis *et al.* 1996; Murray and Ell 1998, ch. 85) including ^{131}I Lipiodol and Ethiodol, which have now generally been replaced by ^{90}Y glass microspheres (Andrews *et al.* 1994; Ho *et al.* 1996).

The patient must have satisfactory haematologic, hepatic, renal, and pulmonary function prior to treatment. In addition to these tests, ^{99m}Tc colloidal, CT and, in some cases, ultrasonic scans of the liver are performed. Prior to radionuclide therapy, angiography is carried out to investigate the hepatic circulation. If the vascular flow is such that colloidal particles would not be confined to the liver, then appropriate hepatic arteries may be occluded (e.g. using stainless steel coils or Ivalon particles).

The positioning of the intra-arterial catheter (in the hepatic artery distal to the origin of the gastroduodenal artery) and the rate of infusion are crucial to the success of this therapy. After catheter placement, it is usual to perform a ^{99m}Tc-labelled MAA perfusion study. The degree of deposition of the radionuclide in the lungs and/ or gastro-intestinal (GI) tract due to arteriovenous shunting is assessed from gamma-camera scans. The lung dose may be the limiting factor in the determination of the activity to be given for therapy. It has been estimated that 30 and 50 Gy are the lung tolerances for single and multiple treatments, respectively (Ho *et al.* 1997). An additional limit of 70 Gy for the dose to non-tumourous, but cirrhotic, liver has been suggested by the same group. Significant radioactivity in the GI tract is a contra-indication for therapy. Some centres administer angiotensin II immediately before the diagnostic and therapy colloids. This agent constricts normal, but not abnormal, vasculature and thus enhances the flow of colloid into the tumour and away from normal tissues.

The administered activity is calculated according to the mass of the liver (volume determined from CT scans) and up to 5 GBq has been administered per treatment. It is essential to flush out syringes and tubing used in the administration procedure to avoid leaving large residual

activities in these items. Bremsstrahlung scans may be carried out after therapy. Although it is difficult to determine the distribution of radioactivity in the liver accurately, it is estimated that absorbed doses of up to 750 Gy have been given to hepatic tumours using this approach (Ho *et al.* 1997). Side-effects include fever, raised liver enzymes, and GI tract disturbance. Follow-up measurements include haematologic and liver function tests, and chest X-rays.

6.7.2 Direct instillation of radiopharmaceutical into solid tumours

The administration of radiopharmaceuticals directly into solid tumours (Order *et al.* 1994; Chittenden *et al.* 1995; Siegel *et al.* 1995; Kassie *et al.* 1996) has been carried out mainly with radiolabelled colloids or antibodies. The rationale behind this approach is that the therapy agent will be retained to a large extent within the tumour volume, thus improving the therapeutic ratio.

As an example, intralesional administration of ^{131}I-labelled anti-tenascin antibody has been used at our centre for the treatment of patients with relapsed high-grade glioma (Chittenden *et al.* 1995). Pretreatment assessments included full blood counts, liver enzyme, urea and electrolyte, thyroid function and serum HAMA tests, and CT/MRI scans. Patients were given thyroid blockade from 2 days before, to 7 days after, infusion. Administration was performed via one or two catheters placed under stereotactic guidance. Up to 600 MBq radiolabelled mAb was infused by syringe pump at a rate of 50–100 μl per hour. (Small volumes and slow rates of infusion are required to avoid leakage of the radio-labelled-mAb back along the catheter track.)

Whole-body gamma-camera scans were taken typically on days 1, 2, 3, 4, 6, 8, and 11 after therapy to assess activity distribution outside the tumour. ^{131}I SPECT scans of the brain were carried out at the same time points and compared to scans of calibration phantoms to assess tumour activity. Whole-body retention was measured twice daily during therapy. Blood samples were taken twice daily initially, then daily until the patient was discharged. Total urine collection was carried out for each patient: the collection interval was 6 h for the first few days of therapy, then every 12 h until the patient was discharged. The activity in blood and urine samples were determined by comparison with an ^{131}I standard in a gamma counter. Tumour and normal organ doses were calculated according to MIRD methodology (Section 3): whole-body doses were 0.2 Gy or less and tumour doses 7–95 Gy in this study. Follow-up measurements during and after therapy were as follows: haematologic, liver and renal functions were tested every other day until the patient was discharged, weekly for 6 weeks then monthly; thyroid function tests and CT/MRI scans were performed monthly and serum was checked for HAMA response at 4 and 7 weeks after treatment.

6.7.3 New approaches

It seems likely that the future success of targeted radiotherapy using unsealed sources will involve various combinations of therapeutic agents and treatment modalities, in addition to the more direct routes of administration mentioned above (Sections 2.1.2, 2.1.3, 6.5, 6.7.1, 6.7.2).

Examples of combinations are:

(1) cocktails of beta emitters with different ranges, to treat tumours of variable size (Leach *et al.* 1996, pp. 1911–2);

(2) cocktails of radionuclides with different half-lives, e.g. to produce both rapid response and prolonged symptom relief in palliation of bone pain (Leach *et al.* 1996, pp. 2027–42);

(3) cocktails of radionuclides with different types of emissions, i.e. beta emitters combined with Auger-electron emitters or alpha emitters (Leach *et al.* 1996, p. 1988);

(4) cocktails of different mAbs to improve targeting in radioimmunotherapy (Wilder *et al.* 1996).

The rationale behind the use of multiple-treatment modalities in relation to tumour size is illustrated in the following example. In neuroblastoma therapy, total body irradiation or chemotherapy could be used to control micrometastases and small tumours <1 mm in size, ^{131}I-mIBG could treat tumours with dimensions between 1 mm and 1 cm, while external-beam radiotherapy could be directed at easily-detected large tumour masses >1 cm (Gaze *et al.* 1995). The use of radiosensitizing agents to maximize damage to tumours and the use of agents to protect tissues such as the bone marrow during radionuclide therapy are also being explored.

7. References

Alaamer, A.S. Fleming, J.S., and Perring. S. (1994). Evaluation of the factors affecting the accuracy and precision of a technique for quantification of volume and activity in SPECT. *Nuc. Med. Commun*, **15**, 758–71.

Andrews, J.C., Walker, S.C., Ackerman, R.J., Cotton, L.A., Ensminger W.D., and Shapiro B. (1994). Hepatic radioembolization with yttrium-90 containing glass microspheres: preliminary results and clinical follow-up. *J. Nucl. Med*. **35**, 1637–44.

Bayouth, J.E., Macey, D.J., Kasi, L.P., and Fosella, F.V. (1994). Dosimetry and toxicity of Samarium-153-EDTMP administered for bone pain due to skeletal metastases. *J. Nucl. Med*., **35**, 63–9.

Berk, P.D., Goldberg, J.D., Donovan, P.B., Fruchtman S.M., Berlin N.I., and Wasserman L.R. (1986). Therapeutic recommendations in polycythemia vera based on polycythemia vera study group protocols. *Semin. Hematol*., **23**, 132–43.

Berlin, N.I. (ed.) (1997). Polycythemia vera. *Semin. Hemat*., **34** (1).

Bilgrami, S. and Greenberg, B.R. (1995). Polycythemia rubra vera. *Semin. Oncol*., **22**, 307–26.

Blake, G.M., Zivanovic, M.A., McEwan, A.J., and Ackery, D.M. (1986). Sr-89 therapy: strontium kinetics in disseminated carcinoma of the prostate. *Eur. J. Nucl. Med*., **12**, 447–54.

Breitz, H.B., Durham, J.S., Fisher, D.R., and Weiden, P.L. (1995). Radiation-absorbed dose estimates to normal organs following intraperitoneal ^{186}Re-labeled monoclonal antibody: methods and results. *Cancer Research*, Supplement, **55**, 5817s–22s.

Bruland, Ø.S. (1995). Cancer therapy with radiolabelled antibodies. An overview. *Acta Oncologica*, **34**, 1085–94.

Cavalieri, R.R. (1996). Nuclear imaging in the management of thyroid carcinoma. *Thyroid*, **6**, 485–92.

Chittenden, S., Thomas, R., Hall, A., Smith T., Flux G., Brada M. *et al.* (1995). Dosimetry of intralesional ^{131}I-monoclonal antibody (Mab) therapy in patients with recurrent high grade gliomas. In *Radioactive isotopes in clinical medicine and research. Advances in pharmacological sciences* (Bergman, H. and Sinzinger, H., ed.) pp. 29–34. Birkhäuser Verlag, Basel, Switzerland.

Cloutier, R.J., Watson, E.E., Rohrer, R.H., and Smith, E.M. (1973). Calculating the radiation dose to an organ. *J. Nucl. Med*., **14**, 53–5.

Clunie, G., Lui, D., Cullum, I., Edwards J.C.W., and Ell P. (1995). Samarium-153-particulate hydroxypatite radiation synovectomy: biodistribution data for chronic knee synovitis. *J. Nucl. Med*., **36**, 51–7.

de Klerk, J.M., van het Schip, A.D., Zonnenburg, B.A., Van Dijk A., Quirijnen J.M.S.P., Blijham G.H. *et al.* (1996). Phase 1 study of rhenium-186-HEDP in patients with bone metastases originating from breast cancer. *J. Nucl. Med*., **37**, 244–9.

DeNardo, D.A., DeNardo, G.L., Yuan, A. Shen S., DeNardo S.J., Macey D.J. *et al.* (1996). Prediction of radiation doses from therapy using tracer studies with iodine-131-labeled antibodies. *J. Nucl. Med*., **37**, 1970–5.

Deutsch, E., Brodack, J.W., and Deutsch, K.F. (1993). Radiation synovectomy revisited. *Eur. J. Nucl. Med*., **20**, 1113–27.

Edmonds, J., Smart, R., Laurent, R., Butler P., Brooks P., Hoschl R. *et al.* (1994). A comparative study of the safety and efficacy of dysprosium-165 hydroxide macro-aggregate and yttrium-90 silicate colloid in radiation synovectomy- a multicentre double blind clinical trial. *Br. J. Rheumatol*., **33**, 947–53.

Einhorn, J. *et al.* (ed.) (1996) Papers from 4th Scandinavian symposium on radiolabelled monoclonal antibodies in diagnosis and therapy of cancer. *Acta Oncologica*, **35**, (3).

Fisher, D.R. (1994). Radiation dosimetry for radioimmunotherapy. An overview of current capabilities and limitations. *Cancer Suppl*., **73** (3), 905–11.

Flower, M.A., Al-Saadi, A., Harmer, C.L., McCready V.R., and Ott R.J. (1994). Dose–response study on thyrotoxic patients undergoing positron emission tomography and radioiodine therapy. *Eur. J. Nucl. Med*., **21**, 531–6.

Gaze, M.N. and Wheldon, T.E. (1996). Radiolabelled mIBG in the treatment of neuroblastoma. *Eur. J. Cancer*, **32A**, 93–6.

Gaze, M.N., Wheldon, T.E., O'Donoghue, J.A., Hilditch T.E., McNee S.G., Simpson E. *et al.* (1995). Multi-modality megatherapy with [^{131}I]meta-iodobenzylguanidine, high dose melphalan and total body irradiation with bone marrow rescue: feasibility study of a new strategy for advanced neuroblastoma. *Eur. J. Cancer*, **31A**, 252–6.

Giap, H.B., Macey, D.J., Bayouth, J.E., and Boyer, A.L. (1995). Validation of a dose-point kernel convolution technique for internal dosimetry. *Phys. Med. Biol*., **40**, 365–81.

Gilland, D.R., Jaszczak, R.J., Turkington, T.G., Greer K.L., and Coleman R.E. (1994). Volume and activity quantitation with Iodine-123 SPECT. *J. Nucl. Med.*, **35**, 1707–13.

Health and Safety Commission (1985). *Approved code of practice: the protection of persons against ionising radiation arising from any work activity.* HMSO, London.

HMSO (1985). *Ionising Radiations Regulations 1985.* (SI 1985 No. 1333). HMSO, London.

HMSO (1988). *Ionising radiation (protection of persons under-going medical examination or treatment) regulations 1988.* (SI 1988 No. 778). HMSO, London.

HMSO (1993). *The Radioactive Substances Act.* HMSO, London.

Ho, S., Lau, W.Y., Leung, T.W.T., Chan M., Ngar Y.K., Johnson P.J. *et al.* (1996). Partition model for estimating radiation doses from yttrium-90 microspheres in treating hepatic tumours. *Eur. J. Nucl. Med.*, **23**, 947–52.

Ho, S., Lau, W.Y., Leung, T.W.T., Chan M., Johnson P.J., and Li A.K.C. (1997). Clinical evaluation of the partition model for estimating radiation does from yttrium-90 microspheres in the treatment of hepatic cancer. *Eur. J. Nucl. Med.*, **24**, 293–8.

Hoefnagel, C.A. (1991). Radionuclide therapy revisited. *Eur. J. Nucl. Med.*, **18**, 408–31.

Holmes, R.A., Volkert, W.A., and Logan, K.W. (ed.) (1987). Therapies in nuclear medicine. *Nucl. Med. Biol.*, **14** (3).

Howell, R.W., Goddu, S.M., and Rao, D.V. (1998). Proliferation and the advantage of longer-lived radionuclides in radioimmunotherapy. *Med. Phys.*, **25**, 37–42.

Humm, J.L. (1986). Dosimetric aspects of radiolabeled antibodies for tumor therapy. *J. Nucl. Med.*, **27**, 1490–7.

International Commission on Radiological Protection (1983). *Radionuclide transformations. Energy and intensity of emissions.* ICRP Publication 38. *Ann. ICRP*, **11–13**.

International Commission on Radiological Protection (1990). *Recommendations of the ICRP.* ICRP Publication 60. *Ann. ICRP*, **21**.

Johnson, T.K. (1988) MABDOS: a generalized program for internal radionuclide dosimetry, *Computer Methods Programs Biomed.*, **27**, 159–67.

Kaminski, M.S., Zasadny, K.R., Francis, I.R., Fenner M.C., Ross C.W., Milik A.W. *et al.* (1996). Iodine-131-Anti-B1 radioimmunotherapy for B-cell lymphoma. *J. Clin. Oncol.*, **14**, 1974–81.

Kassis, A.I., Adelstein, S.J., and Mariani, G. (1996). Radiolabelled nucleoside analogs in cancer diagnosis and therapy. *Quart. J. Nucl. Med.*, **40**, 301–19.

Krishnamurthy, G.T., Swailem, F.M., Srivastava, S.C., Atkins H.L., Simpson L.J., Walsh T.K. *et al.* (1997). Tin-117m(4+)DTPA: pharmacokinetics and imaging characteristics in patients with metastatic bone pain. *J. Nucl. Med.*, **38**, 230–7.

Lazarus, J.H. (1995). Guidelines for the use of radioiodine in the management of hyperthyroidism: a summary. *J. Roy. Coll. Phys. Lond.*, **29**, 464–9.

Leach, M.O. *et al.* (ed.) (1996). Targeted radionuclide therapy of cancer. *Phys. Med. Biol.*, **41** (10), 1871–2042.

Loevinger, R., Budinger, T.F., Watson, E.E. Beddoe A.H., Boyer A.L., Dance D.R., Evans D.H., Ferrari M. *et al.* (ed.) (1991). *MIRD primer for absorbed dose calculations.* Society of Nuclear Medicine, New York.

Malone, J.F. (1975). The radiation biology of the thyroid. *Curr. Top. Radiat. Res. Q.*, **10**, 263–368.

Medical Internal Radiation Dose committee (1969). *Absorbed fractions for photon dosimetry.* MIRD Pamphlet 5. Society of Nuclear Medicine, New York.

Medical Internal Radiation Dose committee (1975a). *Radionuclide decay schemes and nuclear parameters for use in radiation dose estimation.* MIRD Pamphlet 10. Society of Nuclear Medicine, New York.

Medical Internal Radiation Dose committee (1975b). *Absorbed dose per unit cumulated activity for selected radionuclides and organs.* MIRD Pamphlet 11. Society of Nuclear Medicine, New York.

Murray, I.P.C. and Ell, P.J. (ed.) (1998). *Nuclear medicine in clinical diagnosis and treatment*, Vol. 2 (2nd edn), Ch. 78–85 and 95. Churchill Livingstone, Edinburgh.

National Council on Radiation Protection and Measurements (1983). *Protection in nuclear medicine and ultrasound diagnostic procedures in children.* NCRP Report 73. NCRP, Washington, DC.

National Radiological Protection Board (1988). *Guidance notes for the protection of persons against ionising radiations arising from medical and dental use.* HMSO, London.

O'Doherty, M.J., Nunan, T.O., and Croft, D.N. (1993). Radionuclides and therapy of thyroid cancer. *Nucl. Med. Commun.*, **14**, 736–55.

Order, S.E., Siegel, J.A., Lustig, R.A., Principato R., Zeiger L.S., Johnson E. *et al.* (1994). Infusional brachytherapy in the treatment of non-resectable pancreatic cancer: a new radiation modality (preliminary report of the phase I study). *Antibody Immunoconjugates and Radiopharmaceuticals*, **7**, 11–27.

Ott, R.J., Flower, M.A., Jones, A., and McCready, V.R. (1985). The measurement of radiation doses from P32 chromic phosphate therapy of the peritoneum using SPECT. *Eur. J. Nucl. Med.* **11**, 305–8.

Papanastassiou, V., Pizer, B.L., Coakham, H.B., Bullimore J., Zananiri T., and Kemshead J.T. (1993). Treatment of recurrent and cystic malignant gliomas by a single intracavitary injection of ^{131}I monoclonal antibody: feasibility, pharmacokinetics and dosimetry. *Br. J. Cancer*, **67**, 144–51.

Papanastassiou, V., Pizer, B.L., Chandler, C.L., Zananiri T.F., Kemshead T., and Hopkins K.I. (1995). Pharmacokinetics and dose estimates following intrathecal administration of ^{131}I-monoclonal antibodies for the treatment of central nervous system malignancies. *Int. J. Radiat. Oncol. Biol. Pys.*, **31**, 541–52.

Parkin, A., Sephton, J.P., Aird, E.G.A., Hannan, J., Simpson A.E., and Woods M.J. (1992). Protocol for establishing and maintaining the calibration of medical radionuclide calibrators, and their quality control. In *Quality standards in nuclear medicine* (Hart, G.C. and Smith, A.H., (ed.), Ch. 5. (IPSM Report 65). IPSM, York.

Parmentier, C. and Gardet, P. (1994). The use of 32 phosphorus (^{32}P) in the treatment of polycythemia vera. *Nouv. Rev. Fr. Hematol.*, **36**, 189–92.

Pattillo, R.A., Collier, B.D., Abdel-Dayem, H., Ozker K., Wilson C., Ruckert A.C.F. *et al.* (1995) Phosphorus-32-chromic phosphate for ovarian cancer: I. Fractionated low-dose intraperitoneal treatments in conjunction with platinum analog chemotherapy. *J. Nucl. Med.*, **36**, 29–36.

Pollock, B.E., Lunsford, L.D., Kondziolka, D. *et al.* (1995). Phosphorus-32 intracavitary irradiation of cystic craniopharyngiomas: current technique and long-term results. *Int. J. Radiat. Oncol. Biol. Phys.*, **33**, 437–46.

Porter, A.T. and Chisholm, G.D. (ed.)(1993). Palliation of pain in bony metastases. *Semin. Oncol.*, **20** (No. 3, Supplement 2).

Pratt, B.E., Flower, M.A., McCready, V.R., Harmer C.L., and Ott R.J. (1997). Results of PET dosimetry in the treatment of thyrotoxicosis by ^{131}I. In *Radioactive isotopes in clinical medicine and research*, Vol. **XXII** (Bergman, H., Kroiss, A., and Sinzinger, H., ed.), pp. 313–8. Birkhäuser Verlag, Basel, Switzerland.

Reilly, R.M., Sandhu, J., Alvarez-Diez, T.M., Gallinger S., Kirsh J., and Stern H. (1995). Problems of delivery of monoclonal antibodies. Pharmaceutical and pharmacokinetic solutions. *Clin. Pharmacokinet.*, **28**, 126–42.

RIDIC (1997). Compendium of *S*-values for radionuclides and phantoms employed in MIRDOSE. In *Radiation internal dose information centre (RIDIC)*. Oak Ridge Institute for Science and Education. [http://www.orau.gov//edsd/ridic.htm]

Rosenthal, M.S., Cullom, J., Hawkins, W., Moore S.C., Tsui B.M.W., and Yester M. (1995). Quantitative SPECT imaging: a review and recommendations by the focus committee of the Society of Nuclear Medicine Computer and Instrumentation Council. *J. Nucl. Med.*, **36**, 1489–513.

Samuel, A.M. and Rajashekharrao, B. (1994). Radioiodine therapy for well-differentiated thyroid cancer: a quantitative dosimetric evaluation for remnant thyroid ablation after surgery. *J. Nucl. Med.*, **35**, 1944–50.

Schwab, M. and Pearson, A.D.J. (ed.) (1995). Genetics, cellular biology and clinical management of human neuroblastoma. *Eur. J. Cancer*, **31A** (No. 4, special issue).

Shapiro, B. (1993). Optimization of radioiodine therapy of thyrotoxicosis: what have we learned after 50 years? *J. Nucl. Med.*, **34**, 1638–41.

Sharp, P.F., Gemmell, H.G., and Smith, F.W. (ed.) (1998). *Practical nuclear medicine* (2nd edn). Oxford University Press, Oxford.

Siegel, H.J., Luck, J.V., Siegel, M.E., Quines C., and Anderson E. (1994). Hemarthrosis and sinovitis associated with hemophilia: clinical use of P-32 chromic phosphate synoviorthesis for treatment. *Radiology*, **190**, 257–61.

Siegel, J.A., Zeiger, L.S., Order, S.E. and Wallner P.E. (1995). Quantitative bremsstrahlung single-photon emission computed tomographic imaging: use for volume, activity, and absorbed dose calculations. *Int. J. Radiat. Oncol. Biol. Phys.*, **31**, 953–8.

Sinclair, W.K., Abbatt, J.D., Farran, H.E.A., Harriss E.B., and Lamerton L.F. (1956). A quantitative autoradiographic study of radioiodine distribution and dosage in human thyroid glands. *Brit. J. Radiol.*, **39**, 36–41.

Smith, T., Crawley, J.C.W., Shawe, D.J., and Gumpel, J.M. (1988). SPECT using bremsstrahlung to quantify ^{90}Y uptake in Baker's cysts: its application in radiation synovectomy of the knee. *Eur. J. Nucl. Med.*, **14**, 498–503.

Spencer, R.P. (ed.) (1978). *Therapy in nuclear medicine*. Grune and Stratton, New York.

Stabin, M.G. (1996). MIRDOSE: Personal computer software for internal dose assessment in nuclear medicine. *J. Nucl. Med.*, **37**, 538–46.

Stoldt, H.S., Aftab, F., Chinol, M., Paganelli G., Luca F., Testori A. et al. (1997). Pretargeting strategies for radio-immunoguided tumour localisation and therapy. *Eur. J. Cancer*, **33**, 186–92.

Taasan, V., Shapiro, B., Taren, J.A. Beierwaltes W.H., McKeever P., Wahl R.L. et al. (1985). Phosphorus-32 therapy of cystic grade IV astrocytomas: technique and preliminary application. *J. Nucl. Med.* **26**, 1335–8.

Tulchinsky, M. and Eggli, D.F. (1994). Intraperitoneal distribution imaging prior to chromic phosphate (P-32) therapy in ovarian cancer patients. *Clin. Nucl. Med.*, **19**, 43–8.

Vergote, I.B., Winderen, M., De Vos, L.N. and Trope C.G. (1993). Intraperitoneal radioactive phosphorus therapy in ovarian carcinoma. Analysis of 313 patients treated primarily or at second-look laparotomy. *Cancer*, **71**, 2250–60.

Wafelman, A.R., Hoefnagel, C.A., Maes, R.A., and Beijnen, J.H. (1994). Radioiodinated metaiodobenzylguanidine: a review of its biodistribution and pharmacokinetics, drug interactions, cytotoxicity and dosimetry. *Eur. J. Nucl. Med.*, **21**, 545–59.

Wasserman, L.R. (1976). The treatment of polycythemia vera. *Semin. Hematol.*, **13**, 57–78.

Weber, D.A. and Kassis, A.I. (ed.) (1993). Radiolabeled antibody tumor dosimetry. *Med. Phys.*, **20**, (No. 2, Part 2, special Supplement).

Wilder, R.B., DeNardo, G.L., and DeNardo, S.J. (1996). Radio-immunotherapy: recent results and future directions. *J. Clin. Oncol.*, **14**, 1383–400.

Williams, L.E., Ettinger, L.M., Cofresi, E., Raubitschek A.A., and Wong Y.C. (1995). A shielded, automated injector for energetic beta-emitting radionuclides. *J. Nucl. Med. Technol.*, **23**, 29–32.

8. Recommended reading

Some of the references and review papers (Holmes *et al.* 1987; Hoefnagel 1991; Deutsch *et al.* 1993; O'Doherty *et al.* 1993; Porter and Chisholm 1993; Shapiro 1993; Weber and Kassis 1993; Fisher 1994; Bruland 1995; Schwab and Pearson 1995; Einhorn *et al.* 1996; Gaze and Wheldon 1996; Leach *et al.* 1996; Wilder *et al.* 1996; Berlin 1997; Murray and Ell 1998, chapters 78–84 and 95; Sharp *et al.* 1998) are particularly useful and recommended for further extended reading.

Chapter 14

Quality assurance in radiotherapy physics

A.L. McKenzie, T.M. Kehoe, and D.I. Thwaites

1. Introduction

Traditionally in radiotherapy, the term '*quality assurance*' has been applied to programmes for checking the performance of radiotherapy equipment and for measuring, against agreed criteria, the characteristics and parameters of the output from the equipment, such as radiation beams, images or treatment plans. These programmes are intended to give assurance that, ultimately, radiation dose will be delivered to target volumes with specified accuracy. It is possible to produce such programmes for all of the equipment and techniques described in this book, but, taking a wider view, it becomes clear that, while these programmes are *requirements* for quality, they are not sufficient in themselves to give the desired *assurance*.

Strictly, these requirements for quality should be called *quality control* programmes, and should be supported by an infrastructure of requirements at deeper levels, with the most fundamental levels being the strategic planning of the service to be provided and the overall management of the physics department and oncology centre.

As an illustration, consider the weekly monitor unit calibration of a linear accelerator (i.e. the measurement of dose delivered per monitor unit to a water phantom in standard geometry). In order for the physics department to be able to assure the director of oncology that the linear accelerator will be correctly calibrated every week, a system of requirements must be put in place to ensure that:

1. the ionization chambers used for the weekly calibrations have current calibration factors, the forms or charts that are available for determining the linear accelerator calibration are also current, in that they contain the current calibration factors for any ionization chambers that may be used, and that any obsolete forms or charts have been removed;

2. the physics department's set of protocols ('work instructions') for calibrating linear accelerators is up-to-date and consistent with national standards and codes of practice, and has replaced any obsolete set of work instructions;

3. physics staff have been trained to use the department's current set of work instructions for calibrating linear accelerators;

4. physics staff are available to perform the linear accelerator calibration (including contingency arrangements for unexpected absence) on the agreed weekly basis;

5. physics staff are aware of their own responsibilities with regard to the calibrations, and understand the responsibilities of others in the management structure;

6. the physics department negotiates resources for maintaining an adequate level of staffing and for procuring and maintaining dosimetry equipment and any other facilities that may be necessary to support the weekly calibration;

7. the physics department regularly reviews its strategy for providing service, including a dosimetry service, in collaboration with the director of the radiotherapy department.

Notice that the earlier quality requirements in this list are more directly concerned with the desired measure of quality (in this case, regular, accurate calibration of a linear accelerator), whereas the later requirements are more concerned with the structure and management of the physics department and the provision of a physics service. While the importance of all of the requirements in this particular case is clear, it is only in the last decade that the significance of the management-oriented requirements has been formally recognized in radiotherapy by incorporating them into quality assurance systems.

In the UK, the trigger for this was an error in the calibration of a new cobalt-60 source in a treatment unit. The error resulted in the overdosing of 207 radiotherapy patients before the miscalibration was detected by a national audit (Thwaites *et al.* 1992). As a result, the UK government Department of Health commissioned a working party to report on quality assurance in radiotherapy, and the working party recommended that quality assurance should be formalized along the lines of international quality standard ISO 9002:1987 (ISO 1987), which was, itself, based largely on the earlier British quality standard BS 5750 (BSI 1979). The current British, European and international versions of this quality system, namely BS EN ISO 9002:1994, EN ISO 9002 and ISO 9002:1994 are all identical (ISO 1994b). Another standard, called ISO 9001 (ISO 1994a), is identical to ISO 9002 except that the scope extends to design of the service or product. In referring to either ISO 9001 or ISO 9002, sometimes the generic title 'ISO 9000' is used.

The decision to adopt ISO 9002 as the basis for radiotherapy quality systems was pivotal. Instead of accepting the limited approach of requiring that radiotherapy quality control procedures be formalized, the working party recognized the management issues raised by the miscalibration (McKenzie 1996) and opted for ISO 9002 as a comprehensive system that included management issues within its scope.

In 1991, two centres in the UK were chosen by the Department of Health as pilot sites for interpreting the rather general language of ISO 9002 into practical radiotherapy terms (Bristol Oncology Centre and the Christie Hospital, Manchester). All other centres were then required to develop their own systems, using the Bristol and Manchester systems as models, if they so wished. In the Netherlands, the government has required that quality systems be set up in radiotherapy based on ISO 9001 (Leer *et al.* 1995). The European Society for Therapeutic Radiology and Oncology (ESTRO) has developed a system that incorporates the requirements of ISO 9001 (Thwaites *et al.* 1995).

These quality systems are meant to apply to the clinical and nursing, as well as the physics, aspects of radiotherapy, and whether the physics quality system is formally part of an integrated system or whether it is distinct for managerial reasons depends on the local management structure, but, in the latter case, clearly there must be a seamless interface between the physics quality system and that of the radiotherapy centre.

1.1 Other approaches to quality assurance

Other approaches to quality assurance have been published, e.g. American Association of Physicists in Medicine (1994) and World Health Organization (1988), and it is important to understand the differences between such systems and systems in which the requirements of ISO 9000 are given prominence. In the AAPM and WHO documents, for example, the emphasis is on programmes for quality control. Where quality management is discussed in these documents, it is done so without the formalism of ISO 9000, and in less forbidding terms. However, the point about ISO 9000 is that it is essentially a checklist of good management practices without any one of which any quality system will be incomplete and may fail. A good quality system should, therefore, at least contain all the elements of ISO 9000. Better systems will go further – while still containing ISO 9000 as an essential component – by requiring the incorporation of the highest quality standards and the pursuit of continuous quality improvement.

Because of its essential role in good quality assurance, it is helpful to know the basis of ISO 9000, despite its superficially unattractive construction. The following discussion of ISO 9000 should make it possible to build upon its management infrastructure, so that the quality control programmes of the American Association of Physicists in Medicine (AAPM 1994), the World Health Organization (WHO 1988), and the Institute of Physics and Engineering in Medicine (IPEM 1999) may be incorporated as necessary.

2. Contents of a quality assurance system for radiotherapy physics

The ISO 9001 standard lists 20 requirements for a quality system, labelled 4.1–4.20. Some physics departments would not include design of their service (requirement 4.4) or servicing their products (requirement 4.19) within their scope. Failure to meet any of the other requirements, however, will result in an inadequate physics service.

The requirements of ISO 9001 are listed in a fairly haphazard way, and the internal structure of the system may be appreciated more readily by dividing it into three inter-dependent components:

1. Control of the activities in radiotherapy physics.

2. Management of the radiotherapy physics service.

3. Control of the quality system itself.

These are considered in detail below, with the relevant requirements of ISO 9002 indicated in parentheses. Since requirements 4.4 and 4.19 refer to design and servicing, which may be omitted from the system, only 18 requirements are listed. It must be borne in mind that these form the minimum set required for a working quality system, and that other measures should be considered, such as the need continually to seek out and incorporate the highest standards against which to measure the physics service. In the 2000 revision of ISO 9000, the numbering of the requirements is changed, but the division into three principal components still applies.

2.1 Control of the activities in radiotherapy physics

This is the most familiar aspect of quality assurance. It covers all of the activities in radiotherapy physics that affect, directly or indirectly, the accuracy of radiation treatment in the radiotherapy department. However, it goes beyond the traditional focus, which is limited to work such as treatment planning and quality control of equipment performance, and instead, encompasses activities that must be carried out to support such work.

1. Purchasing radiotherapy physics equipment, such as ionization chambers and treatment planning computers. (4.6)

2. Care of equipment supplied by the radiotherapy department, such as linear accelerators during calibration and patients' notes during treatment planning. (4.7)

3. Control of the work in radiotherapy physics, which ultimately affects the accuracy of radiotherapy treatment, such as treatment planning and quality control of radiotherapy equipment. This will involve producing work instructions and action levels. (4.9)

4. Independent checking, at appropriate stages, of work that ultimately affects the accuracy of radiotherapy treatment. This will include checking treatment plans and calibrations of linear accelerators, with signatures to confirm the checks. (4.10)

5. Checking and calibrating equipment used for radiotherapy physics work, such as computer treatment-planning systems and ionization chambers. (4.11)

6. Marking equipment clearly with the status of checks and calibrations by indicating the date of tests and the next due date. (4.12)

7. Handling and storing work output, such as treatment plans and records of calibrations. (4.15)

8. Maintaining the traceability of work, such as the beam data used in patients' treatment plans or the brachytherapy sources used to treat individual patients. (4.8)

2.2 Management of the radiotherapy physics service

9. Assessing the resources needed for maintaining a quality service. Formally identifying the responsibilities of staff in the radiotherapy physics department, including appointing a quality management representative with specific responsibility for the quality system and who will produce a policy for quality in the department. Holding regular meetings called 'management review meetings' at which the performance of the quality system is reviewed, future needs of the service, including training requirements, are identified, and the wider impact of developments in radiotherapy physics and oncology is discussed. (4.1)

10. Meeting regularly with the director of the radiotherapy department so that the details of the service provided by the radiotherapy physics department are clear and agreed. This may include agreeing to priorities or negotiating more resources as the requirements of the director change. (4.3)

11. Implementing training needs identified by management review and documenting such training. (4.18)

2.3 Control of the quality system

At the management review meeting, evidence of the future needs and the recent performance of the quality system is considered, and the quality system is modified as a result. The feedback nature of this process is illustrated in Figure 14.1. The components of the process are:

12. The quality system. The quality management representative is responsible for producing and maintaining the documentation of the quality system, including descriptions of the work processes and planning for future changes to the system as requirements of the service develop. (4.2)

13. Document control. The quality management representative must control documents by ensuring that they are appropriately checked before being issued. A master list will ensure that copies of up-to-date documents are available as required and that obsolete documents are removed promptly, archiving them, if necessary, for legal reasons. (4.5)

14. Internal quality audit. Staff within the radiotherapy physics department should carry out independent audits to check the quality system and to see that procedures are being followed correctly. Reports of non-conformities detected by the audit will be used to initiate corrective and preventive action and will be included in the quality records analysed at management review meetings. (4.17)

15. Non-conformities in the service. These may be inadvertent or deliberate. Examples of the former include mistakes, incidents, delays, supplier problems, and problems with the system itself, all of which may be detected within the radiotherapy physics department or highlighted by complaints from the radiotherapy department. An example of a deliberate non-conformity would be using an ionization chamber beyond its due date of recali-

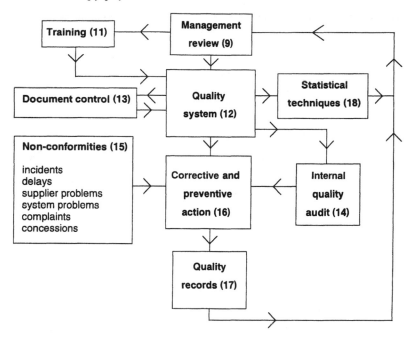

Figure 14.1 Control of the quality system. The feedback nature of the processes that control the quality system itself is shown. Numbers in brackets refer to the system requirements as described in the text.

bration because a standard intercomparison chamber was temporarily unavailable when other evidence, such as ^{90}Sr checks, validated the calibration factor in use. In this case, the deliberate deviation from the procedure would be formally sanctioned by a concession form. Concessions forms and reports of all non-conformities are used in initiating corrective and preventive action, and are included in the quality records analysed at management review meetings. (4.13)

16. Corrective and preventive action. Each concession form and non-conformity report is used:

    (1) to analyse the cause of the problem to which it refers;
    (2) to put it right; and
    (3) to take steps to avoid a recurrence of the problem.

    Procedures in the quality system may have to be amended as a result. (4.14)

17. Quality records. The quality management representative will maintain quality records showing the performance of the quality system. These records will include reports of mistakes, incidents, delays, supplier problems, non-conformities detected by audit, and problems with the system itself, and will be considered at the management review meeting. (4.16)

18. Statistical techniques. The possibility of using statistical techniques to assess the performance of the service should be considered. A simple example might be to categorize the different type of treatment plans produced and to find the time taken to produce plans in each category. The results of the analysis will be reported to the management review. (4.20)

3. Quality audit

Quality audit is a systematic independent review of a quality assurance programme or a quality system. It can be used to test both the implementation, or operation, of the system and the effectiveness, or performance, of the system. Thus, both procedural and practical audit are involved. Either can be applied at any level of the radiotherapy process. Quality audit of any type must be against predetermined standards, linked to those that the quality system, or part, is aiming to achieve and it should require action if these standards are not met. Thus, quality audit should be regular and form part of a quality cycle or loop.

Independence in the context of quality audit means that the methods of review must be independent of the procedures and processes under consideration, i.e. using evaluation techniques and equipment, where necessary, that are external to the system under test. Total independence implies external personnel. Alternatively, if audit is internal to the institution, independence ideally means personnel who are not responsible for the performance of the product or process under review. Internal quality audit of a quality management system has been discussed above (Section 2.3) as a necessary part of the control of a quality system. Section 6 discusses external audit for the purposes of accreditation of a quality management system.

Practical audit can take many forms, depending on the part of the radiotherapy process under test, but essentially it requires peer professionals to undertake the audit. This professional audit can be multidisciplinary or single discipline, again depending on the area of radiotherapy audited and the scope of the audit. In particular, it encompasses clinical and medical audit of practice and of outcome. Internal practical audit can be applied to a wide range of the technical stages and processes of radiotherapy in a given department. One particular example, which can be considered as an internal audit of the quality of treatment delivery and all prior contributing processes, is the systematic use of *in vivo* dosimetry and portal imaging to verify treatment to within prestated tolerances. Practical audit schemes carried out by an external organization (external practical audit) are discussed in Section 7.

4. Structure of the quality system

The purpose of a quality system is to provide management control over the activities that affect the quality of service delivered. No system is static, every system is complex. Using these as a starting point will aid the design and operation of a successful system.

When implementing a quality system, it is a common mistake to focus on the documentation of current best practice while placing less emphasis on the people working both with and within it. ISO 9000 is a documented system but it should be recognized that the system is essentially a framework upon which to hang policies and to define service specifications and other performance criteria. People are the key to delivering both a quality service and the operation of a control system designed to assure the effectiveness of that service (see Figure 14.2).

A well-designed system will have taken into account the *people* aspects, resulting in a balance between incurred bureaucracy and effectiveness consistent with the aims of the service.

4.1 The policy statement

The policy statement is a very important part of the system: it is the goal against which current performance

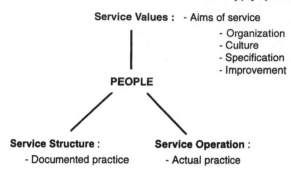

Figure 14.2 The complete quality system.

is regularly assessed. The aims of the system need to be defined by management and clearly understood by all. The policy statement is often used to define and communicate this, although it should be noted that a written policy is not a requirement of ISO 9000.

4.2 Quality system documentation

The structure of typical documentation is shown in Figure 14.3. The quality policy manual (level 1) is mandatory and acts as a route-map for auditing, a sales brochure for external consumption, and a statement of commitment to service quality for internal consumption. It contains the policy statement and outlines the scope of the activities covered within the system and how these activities are organized and controlled (through statements of responsibilities). ISO 9001:1994 has 138 'shall's scattered amongst 20 defined clauses, and all of these must be addressed by the quality system. Even if a clause is not implemented within a system, this must be stated explicitly in the manual. The clauses specify the methods by which management control of the assurance of a quality service can be demonstrated.

Management must, therefore, design the system to be specific for its own needs. By necessity, each system must be unique and must reflect the needs of the service,

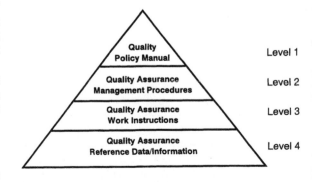

Figure 14.3 Typical documentation structure.

the environment within which the service is delivered, the staff charged with delivering it, and the organizational structure governing it.

The activities stated in the level 1 manual refer to the details documented in the remaining levels 2–4:

1. Level 2 contains procedures.
2. Level 3 documents are workplace instructions.

Convention has it that level 4 contains reference data or other information, and sometimes level 4 is combined with level 3. ISO 9000 does not specify requirements for this documentation and in practice levels 2–4 take many formats. For reference, advice can be sought from the International Standards Organization document ISO 10013 *Guidelines for developing quality manuals* (ISO 1995).

4.3 Level 2 quality assurance management procedures

The management requirements for controlling an activity are stated in a level 2 procedure. The term 'procedure' should be thought of as a shorthand way of writing '*quality assurance management procedure*'. This document normally has a standard layout with, typically, the following headings as a minimum: aim or objective, scope, responsibilities, associated documentation, and method. The method outlines important parts of the task, describing, ideally, chronological details of *what* must be done, *by whom, when, to what tolerances,* and, *what happens when tolerances are exceeded.*

4.4 Level 3 quality assurance work instructions

Any details of the tasks are deferred to level 3. These workplace or work instructions are typically referenced from a parent procedure and expand on the outline in that procedure by describing *how to carry out the required task.* The detail must be sufficient only to enable that task to be undertaken safely, and to the necessary quality standard by personnel approved to perform that task. In other words, a certain amount of experience and expertise is not only acceptable but desirable *but this must be defined within the documentation.*

4.5 Design of system documentation

The system is not designed to be a substitute for training of appropriately qualified staff but is a statement of good management and current practice, and hence acts as a reminder to competent staff with a temporary memory loss! This is a very important concept: the people in the system should already know how to perform their tasks, and they will only need to use the documentation at times of uncertainty. All documentation should, therefore, be brief, unambiguous, clearly laid out, and readily accessible.

The system designer must give careful thought to the location of each document. Will they be stored electronically or in hard copy? If the latter, then how many copies? How will they be bound? Will procedures be kept separate from level 3 documents? How will document control be accomplished?

For auditing purposes, every procedure must be audited at a defined frequency depending on its criticality, i.e. its impact on service quality. Only a selection of level 3 instructions are audited with the procedures. Hence, to reduce the quantity of work required during audit, it is preferable to minimize the number of procedures. Documentation may also be reduced by absorbing work instructions into procedures where that is possible, keeping in mind the circumstances under which they will be used.

Clearly there are competing demands regarding the number of procedures and other documentation present. There is no unique model for this. Management must make a decision based on local needs, remembering that the system is dynamic, and that it can and should be altered as and when necessary.

5. Practical implementation

5.1 Local development

Whilst there are many possible approaches to the detailed layout and content of a quality system, the basic underlying elements are essentially similar, as discussed in the previous sections. However, it cannot be overemphasized that the quality system and quality manual to be used in a given department must be designed in-house. Local development provides major benefits, not least those of 'ownership' of the system by the personnel in the department. Thus, initial planning and development of a quality system can draw on the experience and guidance offered by other centres' work, or by national or international guidelines e.g. those from ESTRO (Leer et al 1998), but the final structure and documentation must be tailored to specific local needs, methods, and organization, and must be drawn up by the local personnel involved in the work. The following sections provide a basic framework and sequence for beginning the implementation of a quality system. For completeness some previous points may be briefly repeated.

5.2 Setting up a quality-management structure

1. First, it is vital that the departmental management is committed to the achievement of quality, in part because the introduction and implementation of a

comprehensive quality system will require resources.

2. The quality management representative (QMR) should be appointed to be responsible for co-ordinating the process. An existing member of staff with a commitment to quality and an understanding of the issues is required.

3. A quality assurance committee (QAC) may be set up. The size and composition depend on the size of the department and the scope of the system. All relevant groups should be represented. At this stage the QAC can aid and support the QMR. In particular, they can communicate the aims and progress of the quality activities to the staff from the very beginning, to ensure that each member of staff understands, supports, and feels part of, any changes. In addition, they can act as channels for comment and criticism from staff back into the system as it develops.

5.3 Defining the scope of the quality system

1. The scope of the quality system must be decided and defined, using national and international guidelines as one starting point for discussion and using the aims and objectives of the department as another. These will help to form the basis of the department's quality policy.

2. For each part of the system, quality standards need to be defined and adopted. In many areas, these may be relatively easy to formulate, as there are many sets of recommendations relating to specific measurable endpoints (e.g. accuracy and precision of the dosimetric and geometric delivery of treatment). These frequently give rise to standards at other contributing points, which are necessary to achieve this (e.g. the specification, acceptance, and on-going quality control tolerances for equipment or pro-cesses) and many of these may already be in use in the department. However, other areas of a compre-hensive quality system may not have readily available standards and these will have to be developed to suit local requirements.

3. One way to approach the development of standards, where none are available, is to measure current performance, ask if this is acceptable, and set an initial standard, which can be realistically met. The aim is then gradually to improve, as appropriate, thereby using the system continually to improve quality.

4. If the system for physics is an independent one reflecting the management structure, there must be detailed discussion with the rest of the radiotherapy centre's quality team to ensure that the overall system is seamless, integrated, and comprehensive.

5.4 Deciding the tasks and the time scale

An inventory of the existing quality structure and procedures can be constructed.

1. This includes general areas, such as:
   (a) a description of the management structure of the department, defining existing relationships, roles and responsibilities of individuals and groups;
   (b) a description of the department's assets and consumables, and the ways in which they are purchased, managed, controlled, and replaced for optimum use and quality;
   (c) a description of the department's policies on staff qualifications, training and continuing professional development, to ensure that roles and responsibilities continue to be properly held and developed.

2. The department's operational processes can then be listed. All areas of work defined to be within the scope of the quality system can be split into appropriately sized elements. Existing written or unwritten procedures, etc., can be listed for each. Gaps can then be identified and prioritized. This begins to quantify practical tasks and to link them to the outline scope and policy. It involves as many staff as possible in the process from the outset. In addition, it builds in the existing local culture and methods, where appropriate.

3. From this inventory, the scale of the initial task can be assessed and a realistic time scale can be drawn up.

5.5 Preparing and implementing quality-system documentation

1. The various levels of documentation for each area of work should be prepared by the staff working in those areas. Many of these may already exist and it will simply be a case of putting them into a uniform format. Others may exist in unwritten form and they will need to be formalized. Others will not exist at all and these will need to be developed. In each case, the layout and content should comply with the locally agreed structure for quality system documentation (Sections 4.3–4.5).

2. Documents, when accepted, should be dated and issued in accordance with the document control system (Section 2.3 (13)).

3. Staff will require training in any new approach to work brought about by the implementation of the quality-system requirements.

4. There should be ample opportunity in the initial testing phase of any new procedures, to comment on and modify the system, if necessary. The endpoint should be a system that assures the quality standards

adopted by the department, but which is flexible enough to allow improvements in service. It should not stifle innovation, but rather should assist the safe and structured introduction of change. It is not an end in itself, but rather should serve the needs of the department. Therefore, it should be dynamic and open in operation. Any unnecessary bureaucracy identified at this, or later, stages should be removed.

5.6 Controlling the quality system

1. The QMR should develop the mechanisms for control of the quality system (Section 2.3) in parallel with the rest of the development phase, so that these are being put into place at the same time as the rest of the system is implemented.

2. Depending on the composition of the QAC, it may act as the management review group. Alternatively the management review group may consist of the QAC and additional members from the department's management team.

3. On-going internal audit and management review should be operated in a way that ensures that problems are identified quickly and are dealt with efficiently, and that improvements are introduced smoothly and speedily. It is important to foster a climate of openness in the department to ensure that problems (or potential problems) are reported freely and that the reasons for change are understood and can be questioned.

5.7 External audit

The department needs to decide whether to take part in external audit. As discussed in Section 3, this can be one or both of two types. External system audit linked to an accreditation process is one way to demonstrate compliance openly and outwardly with the requirements of a quality system structure. External practical audit is a means to demonstrate the achievement of specific quality standards. These are discussed in the next two sections.

6. Accreditation of the quality system

6.1 The role of certification

The role of certification may be understood by considering the positions of both a supplier of a service and a buyer who wishes to purchase the service.

Before purchase, the buyer investigates the service specification and its value for money. A series of 'important questions' are asked, which need appropriate answers before there can be assurance that the service is likely to meet requirements. Alternatively, the service may be so expensive or critical that the buyer wants the assurances to form part of a contract.

The supplier of the service is happy not only to give those assurances, but is comfortable with the idea of them forming part of a contractual obligation. However, it is frustrating to continually expend resources in agreeing to the same type of questions from successive customers. So, as part of the service specification all the common questions are collected together and the responses to them are independently assured by a respected third party. Potential buyers may or may not be satisfied with this independent assessment. However, every buyer is likely to have a number of supplementary questions specific to their own needs and, naturally, the supplier will accommodate these also.

The ISO 9000 model is analogous to the 'important questions' and is applied in exactly the same way as described above. Certificated systems have 'passed' an *assessment* against the international standard for the appropriate model. Organizations have been *certificated* by a suitably qualified independent body. The buyer knows the body is qualified because it is *accredited* by an appropriate national authority.

6.2 The certification process

1. Desk-top audit (sometimes called documentation assessment): typically, the level 1 quality policy manual is 'tested' for compliance with the requirements of the stated quality assurance model, i.e. ISO 9001 or ISO 9002 standard.

2. System audit: a check that a documented quality system is being complied with in practice.

The first system audit is the initial assessment when certification is achieved (or deferred until remedial work has been done). All clauses in the standard are checked by sampling a range of procedures across the breadth of the departments covered by the scope of the system. This is equivalent to passing a driving test, i.e. the system is 'safe' to be certificated.

Subsequent system audits are called surveillance visits. These are typically bi-annual and involve an in-depth check of operational against documented performance for all clauses and all involved departments over a period of 2–3 years. Emphasis also shifts from assessment against minimum requirements, to improvements aimed at making the system more effective.

6.3 Potential benefits of certification

A lot of the potential benefits are achieved prior to accredited certification. So why become certificated? There may be no choice if it is a contractual requirement. However, if there is a choice, the following advantages may be considered:

1. Certification proves the system does indeed meet the requirements of the standard.

2. The certificate is tangible 'reward' for a considerable resource investment.

3. It acts as a driver encouraging continual commitment to the system.

4. The display of a certification body symbol can be used as a marketing tool.

5. Effectiveness of the quality system must be demonstrable. It is difficult to see how this can be achieved without the rigour of independent assessment.

6. In order to maintain the certificate, the organization embarks on a process of continual improvement of the quality of service in partnership with the certificating body. This is, perhaps, the most important point.

6.4 Beyond certification

Some improvements in service provision arise from internal maintenance of the system but this is not the whole picture. The ISO 9001 or 9002 standard is designed only as a model for quality assurance management to be applied at the purchaser-supplier interface. Through documentation it provides a framework by which management can control the work practices of people. It does not provide mechanisms to encourage management to develop people policies, such as motivation, education, and development, teamwork, etc. Yet the purpose of the framework is to help people to deliver a quality service see (Figure 14.2). The standard is described in ISO 9000–1:1994 (ISO 1994c) clause 6 as 'the stakeholder-motivated approach'. Concentrating on people issues, as well as service specifications, performance criteria for all processes that directly or indirectly affect the quality of service to patients, and improvements in all these processes is termed 'the management-motivated approach'. The latter is more overtly incorporated into the 2000 revision of ISO 9000, but was already outlined in the ISO 9004 series of standards (ISO 1991, 1993, 1994d). Clause 6 concludes with:

The quality system implemented in this management-motivated approach will normally be more comprehensive and fruitful than the model used for demonstrating the adequacy of the quality system.

Without certification, it is unlikely that a quality-assurance management-control system will mature into a comprehensive quality-management system.

7. External practical audit

7.1 Dosimetry intercomparisons

External practical audit could be of any area of the radiotherapy process. However, most have been external

dosimetry intercomparisons. Various types have been carried out in association with the organization of clinical trials (e.g. CHART (Aird *et al.* 1995); EORTC (Johansson *et al.* 1986, 1987); RPC (Hanson *et al.* 1994)). Some of these have been set up specifically as audits of the dosimetry of patients entered into the trial (and so are quality-control programmes, as seen from the perspective of the trial) and some have encompassed a relatively wide range of parameters. However, they have been limited to centres participating in such trials. In addition, there have been a number of national or regional dosimetry intercomparisons, in which doses have been measured in all individual departments in that geographical area, by means of external independent equipment and techniques. The methods and results of many of these have been reviewed (Thwaites and Williams 1994; Thwaites 1994). Most audits have been at the level of beam calibration (e.g. Wittkamper *et al.* 1987; Thwaites *et al.* 1992; Nisbet and Thwaites 1997), whilst a smaller number have tested multi-beam planned situations in geometric, semi-anatomic or anatomic phantoms (e.g. Wittkamper *et al.* 1987; Thwaites *et al.* 1992). The typical aim of an intercomparison has been to establish the currently achieved accuracy and precision of radiotherapy dosimetry in a given country or region, and not to provide an audit as such. However, they have, by default, provided an audit of the dosimetry of the centres involved, and they have provided a basis and a methodology for subsequent regular dosimetry audit.

7.2 Routine dosimetric audit

More recently, there has been a growing emphasis on developing systems for routine external dosimetric audit available to all centres on a regular basis. These have been initially implemented at the level of external checking of dosimetry and equipment performance, partly because it is relatively straightforward to implement systematic checks in these areas, quality standards being well defined, and partly because it is important, as a first step, to ensure that the quality of the 'dosimetric infrastructure' in each institution is being achieved, because of the potential for lack of quality at these stages to affect the treatment of significant numbers of patients. Some of the characteristics of a dosimetric quality audit are:

(1) potentially of wider scope than a typical intercomparison;

(2) audit tolerances predefined;

(3) feedback from the auditors to each centre is mandatory, with points for action identified;

(4) a response is required from the centre, where appropriate;

(5) some degree of procedural audit of the processes being tested should be included;

(6) audit should be repeated regularly at an appropriate frequency.

The two main approaches are to use mailed TLD dosimetry systems, or to use ionization chamber systems and site visits. No one system is best for all circumstances. The resources available influence the choice of audit structure and method, and, therefore, the scope and precision of the system. Flexibility is necessary to allow different levels of practical audit to be applied to suit the local situation. Structures should be designed that enable simpler levels to be tested first, but allow for development to more complex levels as appropriate, and where there is adequate local support.

7.3 Mailed dosimeter audit systems

The long-established IAEA/WHO mailed TLD system for Co-60 calibration testing has been extended to megavoltage X-ray beam calibration testing (Svennsson *et al.* 1994), and a system for electron beams has been piloted. The EORTC and ESTRO systems have adopted a similar approach (Hanson and Johansson 1991; Dutreix *et al.* 1993). At the same time, the IAEA, RPC, and European systems have jointly developed more complex mailable phantoms, for possible use in testing other single-beam characteristics and for simple multi-beam planned irradiations (Hanson 1994, Bridier et al 1999). These mailed systems are based on a developing network of local, national, or regional link centres, which act as the communication link between co-ordinating and dosimeter read-out centres and the individual institutions.

7.4 Audit systems based on on-site visits

Other countries and regions have developed audits based on site visits, which allow greater flexibility of approach, both in what can be tested and in the associated procedural audit. These systems are more appropriate for centres that prefer, and can support, detailed audit of a more complex nature and are within acceptably close distances for site visits to be manageable and cost-effective. Finland, for example, has a central national centre with a statutory duty to carry out dosimetric audit, without which radiotherapy centres cannot be licensed. The US has a national centre (RPC), providing mailed TLD and site visits, but with no regulatory requirement that centres participate.

In the UK, *interdepartmental audit* has grown out of the national photon dosimetry intercomparison, which was organized on a basic network structure. The use of networks provides a flexible framework into which various types and levels of audit can be fitted to suit local or national needs and conditions (Thwaites 1996). The UK network comprises seven regional groups, each of which carries out some form of interdepartmental audit, whereby centres are audited by peer professionals from other centres within the group. A steering group, set up by the national professional body (currently the IPEM) co-ordinates the system, issues some basic recommendations and guidelines, and ensures occasional cross-linking of the groups. In addition, it is important that there are some points of linkage to other international audit networks.

Part of the UK recommendations include a minimum audit content, comprising annual visits and checking beam calibration on at least one megavoltage photon beam and testing a three-field planned treatment in a geometric phantom similar to that used in the original national dosimetry intercomparison. In practice, most of the groups have developed their systems to include more than the minimum recommendation (Bonnett *et al.* 1994; Thwaites 1996), some including methods employing semi-anatomic phantoms to test more complex treatment planning and delivery, and to move nearer to audit of full clinical dosimetry, i.e. nearer to the level of patient-treatment delivery.

As an example, the 'Scottish+' group carries out annual audits, but with a hierarchy of tests of different levels of the radiotherapy dosimetry chain over a roughly 5-year cycle. At the first level, tests are made of basic geometric and mechanical performance of treatment equipment, of chamber and beam calibration, of beam quality and other single-field parameters, and procedural audit is carried out on procedures, tolerances, frequencies, and records of basic dosimetry and equipment quality control in the centre. Allied to this, a geometric phantom is used to audit the basic practical planning methods and data with the simple three-field planned irradiations, and procedural audit is carried out on planning methods and quality control. Subsequent levels utilize a semi-anatomic phantom designed to simulate a number of treatment situations, and to test more realistic planned irradiations that incorporate previous levels into the tests. At the same time as each of these visits there is flexibility to audit other areas, such as electron beam calibration, kV beam dosimetry, brachytherapy dosimetry, etc..

7.5 Participation in external practical-audit systems

External practical audit is an effective means of identifying discrepancies if they are present, albeit only at the necessarily limited levels that can be tested. Meeting the audit criteria provides confidence to local personnel that their quality assurance procedures are achieving those defined quality standards and that their performance is consistent with others in the field. Therefore, participation is strongly recommended by a number of sets of national and international radiotherapy quality assurance guidelines.

The type of external practical audit system available to any given department will depend on their location. All departments in the world potentially have access to one or other of the mailed systems, within their capability to cope with demand. Currently, these can only provide routine audits of beam output on a regular basis. However, they are evolving. In a growing number of countries, centres have access to audit systems utilizing site visits. Although these are more expensive, they are more flexible and wide-ranging, and have the potential to evolve more easily to test more complex situations, whilst still incorporating basic audit as appropriate. There is a role for both types, depending on local circumstances, requirements, and resources. In some circumstances a combination may be appropriate, where the more detailed audit may be used at less frequent intervals (possibly to include use after the introduction of some new piece of equipment or process) and the cheaper audit may be used in intervening periods.

Whilst this discussion has concentrated on dosimetric audit, it may be noted that the principles can be readily applied to other areas of radiotherapy, including those involving multidisciplinary interaction and the development of external practical audit into these areas may be useful.

References

Aird, E.G.A., Williams, C., Mott, G.T.M., Dische, S., and Saunders, M.I. (1995). Quality assurance in the CHART clinical trial. *Radioth. Oncol.*, **36**, 235–45.

American Association of Physicists in Medicine (1994). Comprehensive QA for radiation oncology. Report of AAPM Radiation Therapy Committee Task Group 40. *Med. Phys.*, **21**, 581–618.

Bonnett, D.E., Mills, J.A., Aukett, R., and Martin-Smith, P. (1994). The development of an inter-departmental audit as part of a physics quality assurance programme for external beam therapy. *Br. J. Radiol.*, **67**, 275–82.

Bridier, A., Nystrom, H., Ferreira, I., Gomola, I. and Huyskens, D. (1999) A comparative description of three multipurpose phantoms for external audits of photon beams in radiotherapy *Radioth Oncol.* (in press)

British Standards Institution (1979). *BS 5750: Part 2: 1979.* BSI, London.

Dutreix, A., van der Scheuren, E., Derremaux, S., and Chavaudra, J. (1993). Preliminary results of a quality assurance network for radiotherapy centres in Europe. *Radioth. Oncol.*, **29**, 97–101.

Hanson, W. (1994). Simple geometric phantom to be used in the IAEA network. In *Radiation dose in radiotherapy from prescription to delivery*, pp. 311–16. IAEA, Vienna.

Hanson, U. and Johansson, K-A. (1991). Quality audit of radiotherapy with EORTC mailed in-water TL-dosimetry. *Radioth. Oncol.*, **20**, 191–96.

Hanson, W., Stovall, M., and Kennedy, P. (1994). Review of dose intercomparison at a reference point. In *Radiation dose from prescription to delivery*, pp. 121–30. IAEA, Vienna.

Institute of Physics and Engineering in Medicine (1999). *Physical aspects of quality control in radiotherapy.* IPEM Report 81. IPEM, York.

International Organization for Standardization (1987). *ISO 9002–1987 Quality systems – model for quality assurance in production and installation.* ISO, Geneva.

International Organization for Standardization (1991). *ISO 9004–2: 1991 Quality management and quality system elements – Part 2: Guidelines for services.* ISO, Geneva.

International Organization for Standardization (1993). *ISO 9004–4: 1993 Quality management and quality system elements – Part 4: Guidelines for quality improvement.* ISO, Geneva.

International Organization for Standardization (1994a). *ISO 9001: 1994 Quality systems – model for quality assurance in design, development, production, installation and servicing.* ISO, Geneva.

International Organization for Standardization (1994b). *ISO 9002: 1994 Quality systems – model for quality assurance in production, installation and servicing.* ISO, Geneva.

International Organization for Standardization (1994c). *ISO 9000–1: 1994 Quality management and quality assurance standards – Part 1: Guidelines for selection and use.* ISO, Geneva.

International Organization for Standardization (1994d). *ISO 9004–1: 1994 Quality management and quality system elements – Part 1: Guidelines.* ISO, Geneva.

International Organization for Standardization (1995). *ISO 10013: 1995 Guidelines for developing quality manuals.* ISO, Geneva.

Johansson, K-A., Horiot, J.C., Van Dam, J., Depinoy, D., Sentenac, I., and Sernbo, G. (1986). Quality assurance control in the EORTC co-operative group of radiotherapy. 2. Dosimetric intercomparison. *Radioth. Oncol.*, **7**, 269–79.

Johansson, K-A., Horiot, J.C., and van der Scheuren, E. (1987). Quality assurance control in the EORTC co-operative group. 3. Intercomparison in an anatomical phantom. *Radioth. Oncol.*, **9**, 289–98.

Leer, J.W.H., Corver, R, Kraus, J.J.A.M., v.d. Togt, J.Ch. and Buruma O.J.S. (1995). A quality assurance system based on ISO standards: experience in a radiotherapy department. *Radioth. Oncol.*, **35**, 75–81.

Leer, J.W., McKenzie, A., Scalliet, P., and Thwaites, D.I. (1998) *Practical guidelines for the implementation of a quality system in radiotherapy.* ESTRO Physics for Clinical Radiotherapy Booklet No. 4. ESTRO Brussels.

McKenzie, A.L. (1996). Would the two most serious radiotherapy accidents in the UK have occurred under ISO 9000? In *Radiation incidents* (ed. K. Faulkner and R.M. Harrison), pp. 40–44 BIR, London.

Nisbet, A. and Thwaites, D.I. (1997). A dosimetric intercomparison of electron beams in UK radiotherapy centres. *Phys. Med. Biol.*, **42**, 2393–409.

Svensson, H., Zsdánsky, K., and Nette, P. (1994). Dissemination, transfer and intercomparison in radiotherapy dosimetry: the IAEA concept. In *Measurement assurance in dosimetry*, pp. 165–75. IAEA, Vienna.

Thwaites, D.I. (1994). Uncertainties at the end point of the basic dosimetry chain. In *Measurement assurance in dosimetry*, pp. 239–56. IAEA, Vienna.

Thwaites, D.I. (1996). External audits in radiotherapy dosimetry. In *Radiation incidents* (ed. K. Faulkner and R.M. Harrison), pp. 21–28 BIR, London.

Thwaites, D.I. and Williams, J.R. (1994). Radiotherapy dosimetry intercomparisons. In *Radiation dose in radiotherapy from prescription to delivery*, pp. 131–42. IAEA, Vienna.

Thwaites, D.I., Williams, J.R., Aird, E.G., Klevenhagen, S.C., and Williams, P.C. (1992). A dosimetric intercomparison of mega-voltage photon beams in UK radiotherapy centres. *Phys. Med. Biol.*, **37**, 445–61.

Thwaites, D., Scalliet P., Leer J.W., and Overgaard, J. (1995). Quality assurance in radiotherapy. European Society for Therapeutic Radiology and Oncology advisory report to the Commission of the European Union for the 'Europe Against Cancer Programme'. *Radioth. Oncol.*, **35**, 61–73.

Wittkamper, F.W., Mijnheer, B.M., and van Kleffens, H.J. (1987). Dose intercomparison at the radiotherapy centres in The Netherlands. 1. Photon beams under reference conditions and for prostatic cancer treatment. *Radioth. Oncol.* **9**, 33–44.

World Health Organization (1988). *Quality assurance in radiotherapy*. WHO, Geneva.

Index